The **ART** and **SCIENCE** of
FACELIFT SURGERY

The ART and SCIENCE of FACELIFT SURGERY

SECOND EDITION

JOE NIAMTU, III, DMD

DIPLOMAT, AMERICAN BOARD OF FACIAL COSMETIC SURGERY

DIPLOMAT, AMERICAN ASSOCIATION OF ORAL & MAXILLOFACIAL SURGEONS

MEDICAL DIRECTOR

NIAMTU COSMETIC FACIAL SURGERY

RICHMOND, VIRGINIA

ELSEVIER

Elsevier
1600 John F. Kennedy Blvd.
Ste 1800
Philadelphia, PA 19103-2899

THE ART AND SCIENCE OF FACELIFT SURGERY, SECOND EDITION ISBN: 978-0-443-12136-4

Previous edition copyrighted 2019.

Senior Content Strategist: Lauren Boyle
Content Development Specialist: Meredith Madeira
Publishing Services Manager: Shereen Jameel
Senior Project Manager: Manikandan Chandrasekaran
Senior Designer: Miles Hitchen

Printed in the United States of America

Last digit is the print number: 9 8 7 6 5 4 3 2 1

Dedication

This book is dedicated to my late brother James Niamtu a special education teacher who loved teaching and my later father Joseph Niamtu, Jr, a World War II veteran who passed away at 97 years old.

Contributors

Jonathan Cook, MD
Plastic Surgeon
Private Practice
Sanctuary Plastic Surgery
Boca Raton, Florida

Barry DiBernardo, MD
Adjunct Clinical Professor
Department of Plastic Surgery
University of Pittsburgh
Pittsburgh, Pennsylvania

Kian Karimi, MD, FACS
Facial Plastic Surgeon
Dr. Kian Karimi Nasal and Facial Plastic Surgery
Los Angeles, California

Amit Kochhar, MD
Director
Facial Nerve Disorders
Pacific Head and Neck Surgery
Pacific Neuroscience Institute
Santa Monica, California

Gregory P. Mueller, MD, FACS
Plastic Surgeon
Private Practice Plastic Surgery
University of Nebraska, College of Medicine
University of Nebraska–Lincoln
Beverly Hills, California

Abdul Nassimizadeh, MD, MBChB, BMedSci, FRCS (ORL-HNS)
Clinical Entrepreneur Fellow
Ear, Nose, and Throat
University Hospital Birmingham
Birmingham, United Kingdom

Laxmeesh Mike Nayak, MD
Facial Plastic Surgeon
Private Practice
Nayak Plastic Surgery
St. Louis, Missouri

Joe Niamtu, III, DMD
Diplomat, American Board of Facial Cosmetic Surgery
Diplomat, American Association of Oral & Maxillofacial Surgeons
Medical Director
Niamtu Cosmetic Facial Surgery
Richmond, Virginia

Michael Oca, BS
Medical Student
School of Medicine
University of California
San Diego, California

Abraham Pathak, MD
Plastic Surgeon
Department of Plastic Surgery
Kh Plastic Surgery
New York City, New York

Malcolm D. Paul, MD
Clinical Professor
Department of Plastic Surgery
University of California
Irvine, California

Jason N. Pozner, MD
Adjunct Clinical Faculty
Plastic Surgery
Cleveland Clinic Florida
Weston, Florida

Voluntary Associate Professor
Department of Surgery
University of Miami Miller School of Medicine
Miami, Florida

Robert James Troell, MD, FACS
President
Beauty by Design

Adjunct Professor, Surgery
School of Osteopathic Medicine, Touro University Nevada
Las Vegas, Nevada

PREFACE

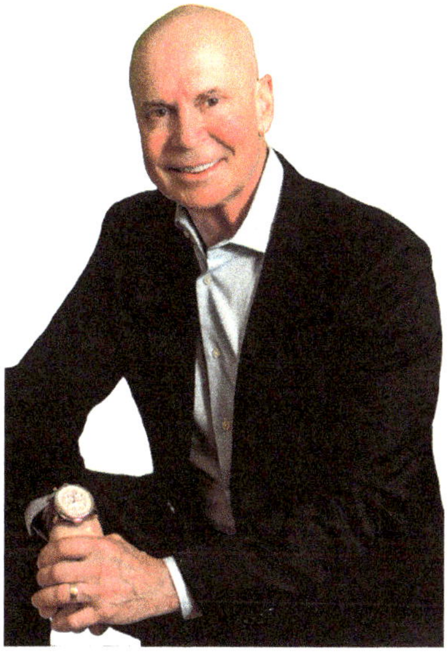

I have a long-standing author/publisher relationship with Elsevier Incorporated, which is the largest medical publisher in the world. It has been an honor to author my comprehensive textbook *Cosmetic Facial Surgery*. I was also privileged to be asked to author a second edition of this textbook. In this day of multimedia and electronic learning, being asked for a second edition is indeed an honor.

The purpose of this book is to provide an overview of facelift and neck lift surgery in a manner to serve as an educational tool for beginners and experts. Appealing to a broad audience requires both basic and advanced instruction. In my early days of cosmetic surgery, I held on to every word of my textbooks, and a good foundation is paramount to patient safety and predictable outcomes. I hope this text provides other surgeons with a similar experience.

I have worked hard to truly make this a "new" edition. I have added new contributors, new procedures, hundreds of new pictures and diagrams, and all new videos that accompany this book. I wrote the previous edition as a sole author but included some talented surgeons in this edition to increase the breadth of the material.

A phrase that will echo throughout this book is "patient safety and predictable outcomes." These concepts are truly the crux of cosmetic surgery. This text does not espouse to be the last word or represent singular techniques for facelift surgery. It does, however, provide a balanced view of time-tested techniques utilized by the author, contributors, and surgeons around the world.

It has truly been an honor to write the previous edition of this book and have it translated into multiple languages including Spanish and Chinese. I hope this edition reaches even more surgeons around the world.

Thank you for putting your time into reading the book; authoring it has truly been a labor of love.

JOE NIAMTU, III, DMD

Acknowledgments

Textbook acknowledgments usually are retrograde by recognizing people who have shaped the author's education and life, and I have done this in previous editions.

In this second edition of the text, I am doing an antegrade acknowledgment by recognizing individuals who came after my education.

I therefore am acknowledging the thousands of young surgeons all over the world that I have directly or indirectly trained over the past 4 decades. Their quest for knowledge, their curiosity of cosmetic surgery, and their youthful enthusiasm served as "educational caffeine" for me. Their energy gave me the energy to become and stay immersed in this profession far beyond the average surgeon. This meant that cosmetic surgery became a lifestyle, not a job. It has been rare for any conversation, day, or weekend in my life not to have something to do with cosmetic facial surgery.

It took many after-work hours to write this book, make videos, and teach courses, but it has been a labor of love. The best thing any student can do to honor their teacher is to pass the knowledge on to the next generation.

I am so lucky to have had this opportunity to educate and learn.

Always be a teacher, always be a student, and always be curious.

JOE NIAMTU, III, DMD

Contents

VIDEO CONTENTS

CHAPTER 1

What Is a Facelift? History and Semantics

Joe Niamtu, III

Chapter Outline

A "facelift" is not a new operation and has been surprisingly similar to the procedure performed over a century ago (Fig. 1.1).

Charles Conrad Miller was born in 1881 and died in 1951. He is regarded as a "featural surgeon" and one of the first surgeons to perform elective aging face surgery. In a 1907 cosmetic surgery article, he wrote the following which still resonates today:

> *This class of work is a special field, worthy of the closest study of the ablest of our profession, for he who operates or treats those cases has the future happiness and Peace of Mind of the patients at stake.*
>
> *Operations for improving the appearance cannot be botched. The operator must be skillful and fully capable in this field more than any other. It is my earnest desire to encourage men throughout the country to give this subject careful attention, before it promises to be, for many years, a most profitable and satisfactory specialty.*
>
> *The criminal carelessness of advertisers is unbelievable to those who have not seen the results of their utter disregard for patients. Many patients have consulted me who have been mutilated by advertisers, and I have yet to find one, who before submitting to the advertiser for treatment, had not consulted a regular physician in good standing. These ethical physicians, while ridiculing the desires of patients, could not conceal the fact that they were totally ignorant of this special subject.*
>
> *If a physician wishes to retain the respect of his patients for his opinion, he must at least be acquainted with the subject so as to be able to discuss it intelligently with those who bring the subject to his attention, otherwise we cannot blame patients for disregarding advice given.*
>
> *(Miller 1907, 286)*

The crux of the Miller's article is that no surgeon should operate outside of the scope of their training and knowledge. I say often in this text, surgeons should crawl before they walk, walk before they run, and run before they fly. Cosmetic facial surgery is an exciting specialty and one should never put patients at risk with one's undertrained exuberance.

New articles in the scientific literature have grown exponentially over the past 75 years (Fig. 1.2). The earliest facelift procedures consisted of a short skin flap only, which over the years progressed to extended skin flaps that included pre- and postauricular incisions. Generally, these procedures only addressed skin excess, and the longevity was much shorter than today's contemporary lifts. Platysmaplasty was another procedure introduced to improve the result. The next biggest advance came when surgeons began recognizing and addressing the superficial musculoaponeurotic system (SMAS) layer, which led to numerous techniques to tighten the SMAS. Today's facelifts are a combination of all of these techniques and can include SMAS plication, SMASectomy, deep plane SMAS, and subperiosteal dissections. Liposuction and liposculpture were improvements, and finally, "additive" facelift procedures to augment facial anatomy such as fat transfer and facial implants continued to make facelift surgery more natural. There are many other techniques that fell in and out of favor during the past 50 years and are beyond the scope of this chapter. Today's contemporary facelifts will be discussed in depth in the remainder of this text.

Twenty five years ago the answer to "What is a facelift?" used to be a simple, but now due to social media and inaccurate marketing, many things are called a "facelift." This is unfortunate and confusing to the consumer. Various types of providers perform procedures with skin tightening devices, threads, fat, fillers, platelet-rich plasma, or neurotoxins and refer to them as a facelift, a blatant misuse of the term. I am not sure there is a singular answer to the question, and it depends on who you ask. I think most surgeons would agree that a "facelift" is a procedure that uses pre- and postauricular incisions and a submental incision with some type of submentoplasty (platysmaplasty) performed through the submental incision. Pre- and postauricular flaps are undermined in the subcutaneous plane to various

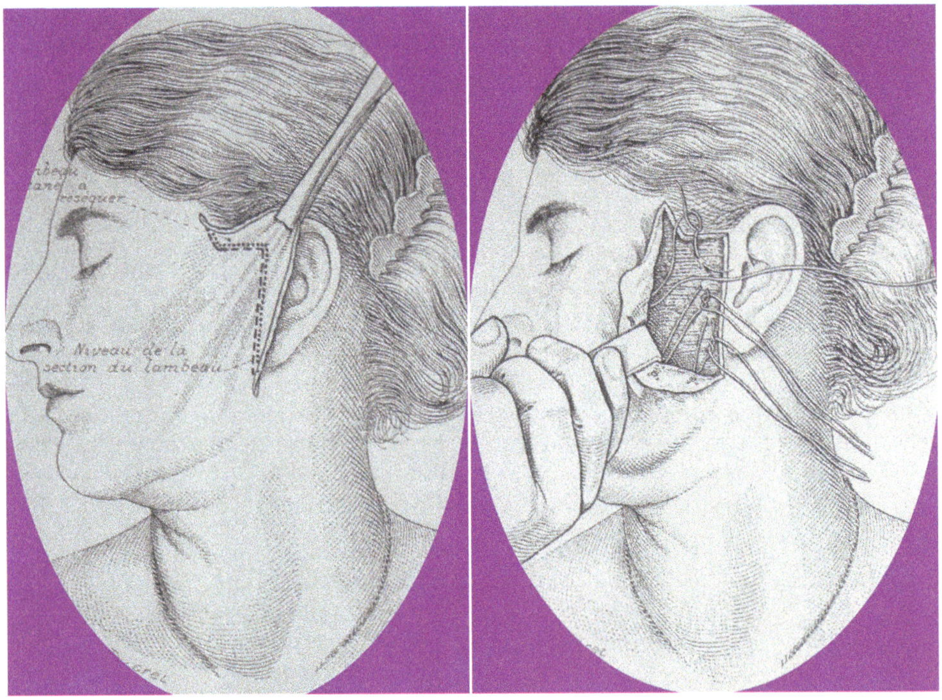

Fig. 1.1. This illustration from a 1924 textbook is dramatically similar to today's contemporary procedures. *(From Niamtu J. Cosmetic Facial Surgery, 2nd ed. Philadelphia, PA: Elsevier; 2018:35, Fig. 3.3.)*

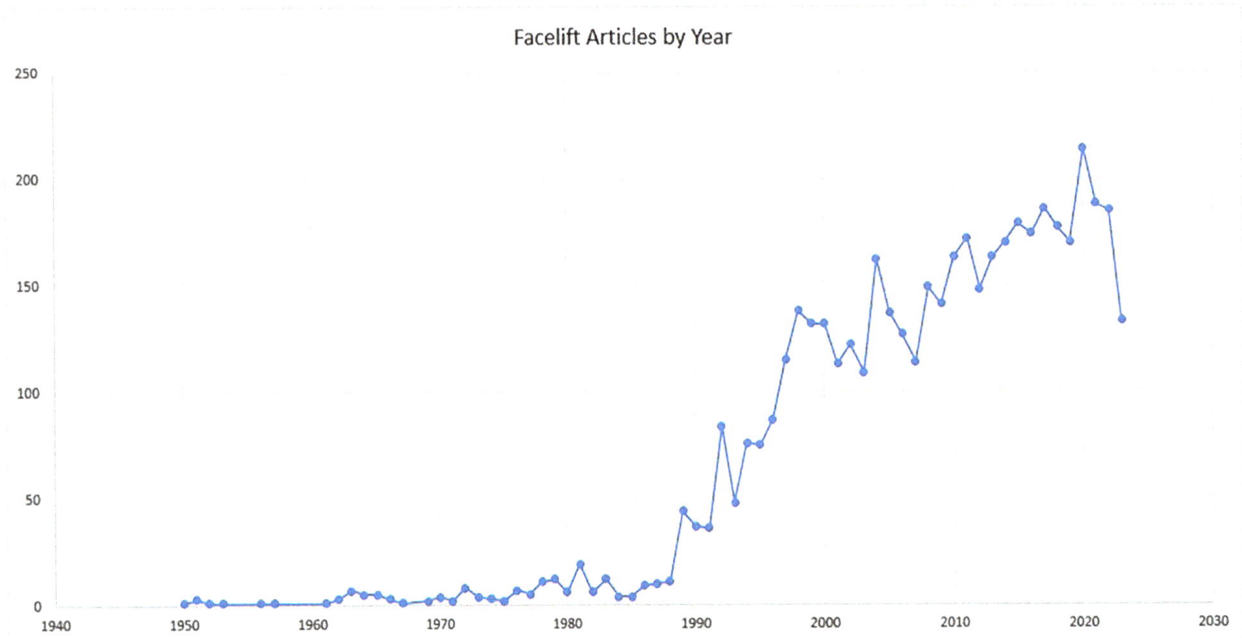

Fig. 1.2. The exponential abundance of scientific articles on "facelift" have increased over the past 70 plus years. *(Data from PubMed. www.pubmed.com. Last accessed September 2023.)*

distances, and some type of SMAS (superficial musculoaponeurotic system) tightening is performed. With the previous description, many subtypes of skin, fat, and SMAS treatment can be performed. Finally, concomitant ancillary procedures may be performed that include brow and forehead lift, blepharoplasty, facial implants or fat transfer, rhinoplasty, and skin resurfacing. Some surgeons omit the submentoplasty; some surgeons omit the posterior incision. The more that is omitted, the less the result and longevity of the procedure.

Many patients are still confused with the term "full facelift." This also means different things to different surgeons, but to me, it is a throwback from the days when the previously described facelift included a coronal browlift, hence addressing the "full face." In my experience this approach has fallen out of favor for more conservative techniques with less complications. The term "full facelift" is also misleading because it would imply that there also exists a "half facelift."

Some surgeons consider a facelift and a neck lift two separate procedures and reflect that in their fee. Once again, I personally consider a facelift to include a neck lift in the same procedure.

Other types of facelifts also include "short scar" or "weekend" facelifts, that generally only use a preauricular (or a very minimal postauricular incision) with or without submentoplasty.

Then, as mentioned earlier, there are numerous minimal incision lifts that do very little for aging and should not be categorized as a facelift.

Social media has done much to muddy the waters. Although accurate publicity is a good thing, much information on social media is misleading, marketing oriented, or totally false. Also, through social media, various surgeons promote their technique as "the only way" to perform a procedure. Deep plane facelift technique is a good example. It is frequently touted as a new breakthrough technique. Although it is a well accepted and usually effective means of performing a facelift, it is not new but rather 40 years old and certainly not the only way. Many patients are led to believe that no other facelift technique is acceptable! This is just a singular example of social media bias.

Call it what you want, just make sure you are accurately describing the actual procedure and being honest with the patient. Once again, safe surgery with predictable outcomes is paramount.

For the remainder of this text (unless otherwise specified), the term "facelift" will describe:

- Pre- and postauricular incisions and submental incisions
- Skin undermining
- SMAS and platysma techniques

These procedures primarily address the lower face and neck. I personally think "comprehensive facelift and neck lift" is also accurate nomenclature.

What Does a Facelift Do?

This is a very important question and requires a very accurate answer for patients. As mentioned earlier, social media has made things worse with unfounded techniques and overpromise. What a facelift will do and what a facelift won't do has to be accurately understood by the surgeon and patient.

A facelift primarily addresses the lower face, jowls, and neck. It does nothing for the upper face and minimally influences the midface (Fig. 1.3).

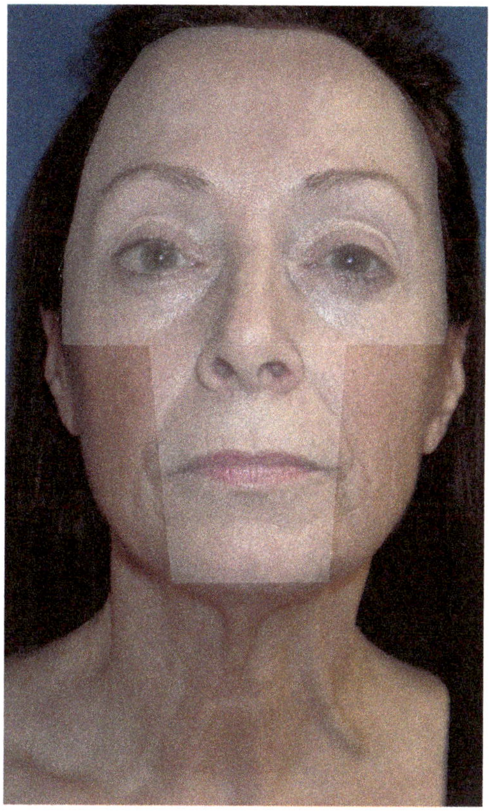

Fig. 1.3. This image shows the areas typically *not addressed* by most common facelift techniques. Cheeks and nasolabial folds may be improved but the more superior and medial the anatomy is, the less it is affected by a facelift. The central oval of the face has no improvement from facelift and neck lift.

As stated previously, a facelift is most effective on the lower face, especially the jowls and neck skin (Fig. 1.4). And these are the areas that patients will point out as bothering them at consultation.

To the reader: please note that the before and after images in this book will always constitute the before image on the left-hand side and the after image on the right-hand side.

As lower facial aging progresses, the jawline becomes squared off (Fig. 1.5, *left*). A facelift will restore the youthful taper of the aging face (Fig. 1.5, *right*).

Patients will frequently show the surgeon what changes they anticipate by pulling their skin back with their hands. Depending on the positioning of their hands this may be accurate or inaccurate (Fig. 1.6).

A facelift is not an operation for wrinkles. It may improve some facial rhytids by stretching the skin but will have no effect on the central face (Fig. 1.7). Laser skin resurfacing (or similar procedures) performed before, during, or after a facelift are required to truly address wrinkling (Fig. 1.8).

A facelift is also not an operation to treat obesity. Although it may improve face and neck features from skin tightening and liposuction, patients with high body mass index may be poor candidates for facelift surgery (Fig. 1.9). This is true from a surgical result standpoint, and these patients also frequently have more comorbidities and potential anesthesia complications. Some surgeons will not operate on patients with body mass indexes higher than 32. Again, what to expect and what not to expect from a procedure is absolutely imperative and must be discussed in the preoperative period. An unhappy patient returning after surgery thinking that they would have a slim face and neck is something to be avoided. Asking a patient to lose weight before surgery is no different than asking them

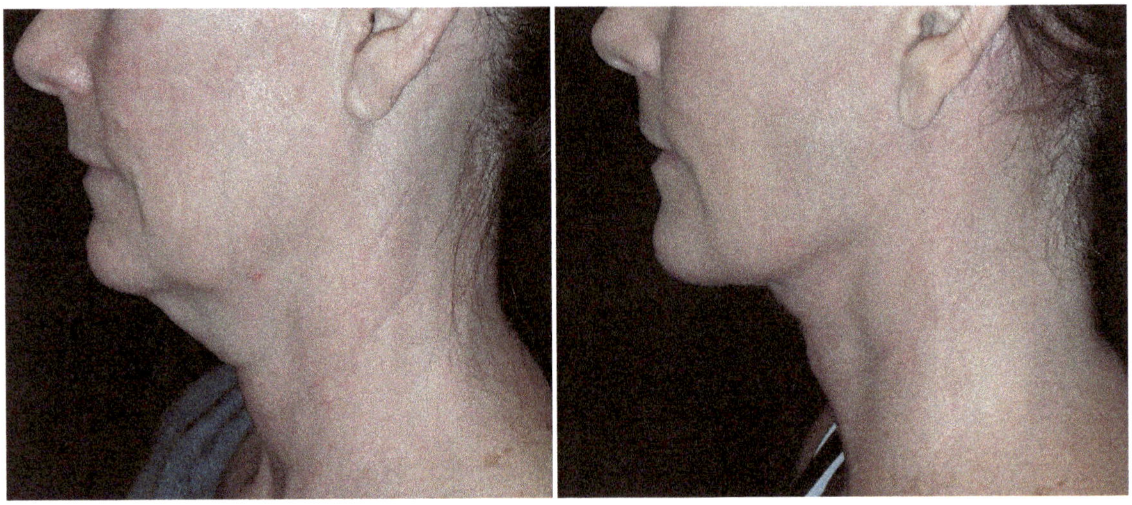

Fig. 1.4. A facelift has its most dramatic effects on the lower face and neck by improving jowls and excess neck skin. *Left* image is before and the *right* image is after the procedure.

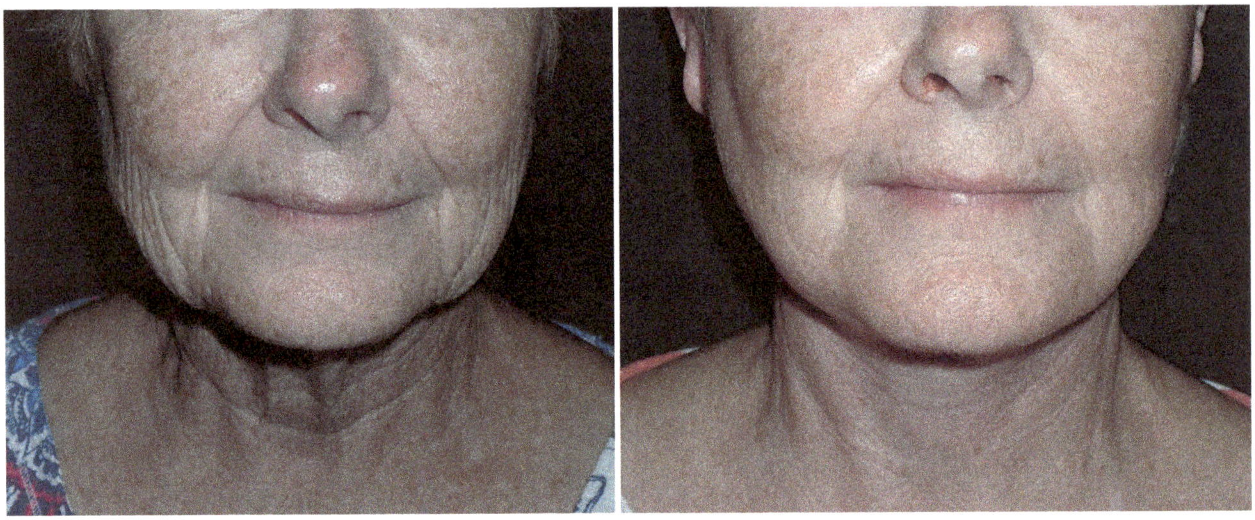

Fig. 1.5. The aging face become ptotic with a squared jawline (*left*). A well-done facelift will restore the youthful taper of the chin and mandible (*right*).

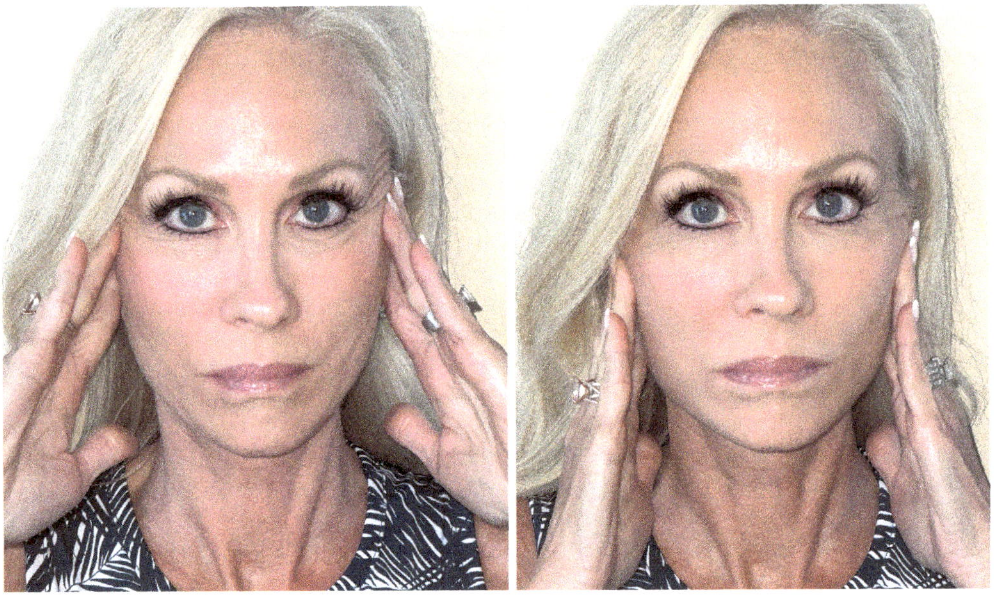

Fig. 1.6. Patients frequently present asking for "just this little tuck." The left image shows a position with unnatural vectors and distorts the mid and upper face anatomy. Placing the hands lower and elevating the lower face in a superolateral direction is a more accurate representation of an actual result.

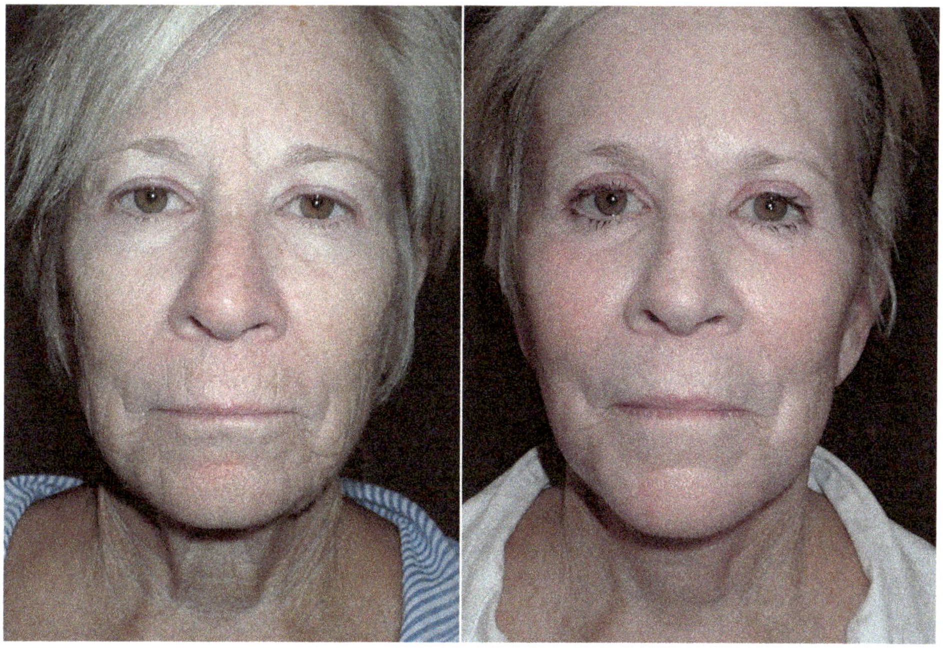

Fig. 1.7. This patient is shown before (*left*) and after facelift and neck lift (*right*) with concomitant perioral laser resurfacing. The lower face and neck are improved but most of the patient's wrinkles are only minimally improved from skin stretching.

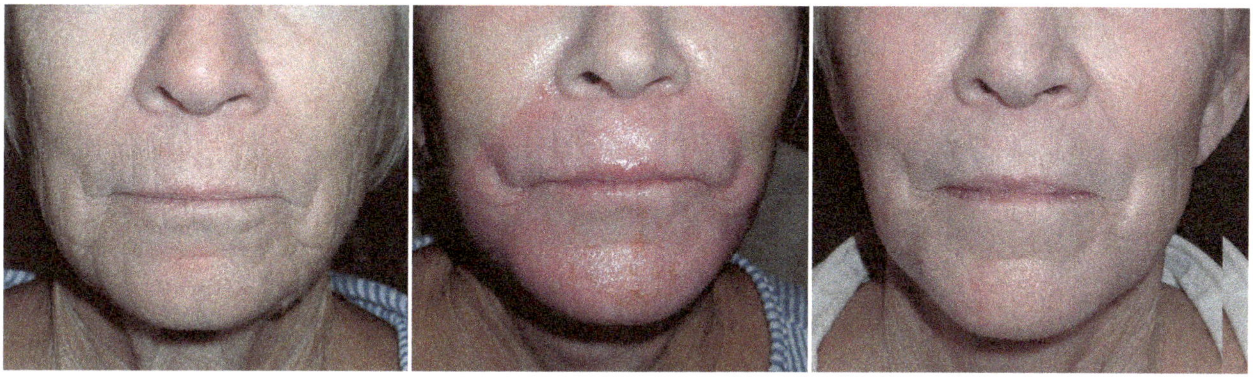

Fig. 1.8. The patient is shown here before facelift with simultaneous perioral CO_2 laser skin (*left*) resurfacing, 1 week after the facelift with perioral laser resurfacing (*center*), and 3 months after facelift and neck lift with concomitant CO_2 laser resurfacing (*right*). It is important that patients understand that a facelift in and of itself is not a treatment for wrinkles. Although it may improve some facial rhytids merely by stretching the skin, significant skin wrinkling will require other resurfacing procedures.

to quit smoking or control their blood pressure. This must be discussed in a medical manner, and most patients usually understand this necessity without being offended. Never sugarcoat a result.

As will be discussed later in chapters of this book dealing with patient evaluation, it is important that the patient understand the limitations of a facelift. This includes the requirement for simultaneous procedures to improve regions of the face and neck that will not be addressed solely by the facelift procedure. When a patient returns to the office after a facelift only and complains that their brow position hasn't changed, it is indicative of the surgeon failing to explain the true effects of the procedure to a patient. This is why the consent process is so important, and should describe not only what the procedure will do but what the procedure won't do (Fig. 1.10).

I started out this chapter by attempting to define what a facelift is. As you have seen, it is not a simple answer, and many factors enter into what defines an accurate answer. The most important thing is, regardless of what one calls the procedure, that the patient understands what to expect and what not to expect. Semantics are far less important than expectations.

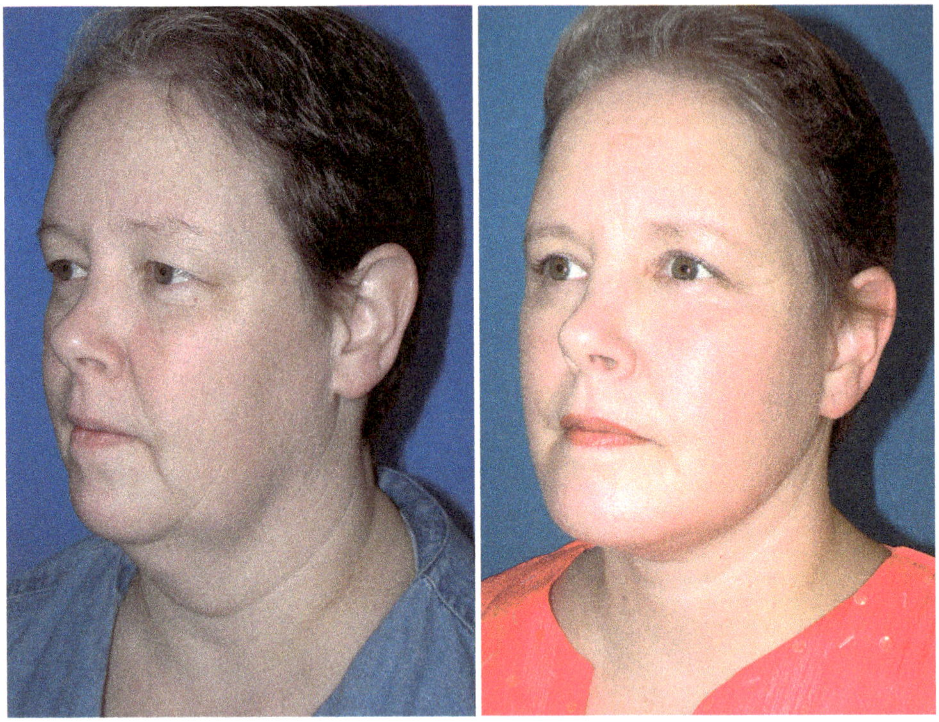

Fig. 1.9. This patient with a high body mass index is shown before (*left*) and after surgery (*right*) consisting of facelift, neck lift, chin implant, and blepharoplasty. This type of result is, in my experience, is as good as it can get, and most patients may have a lesser result.

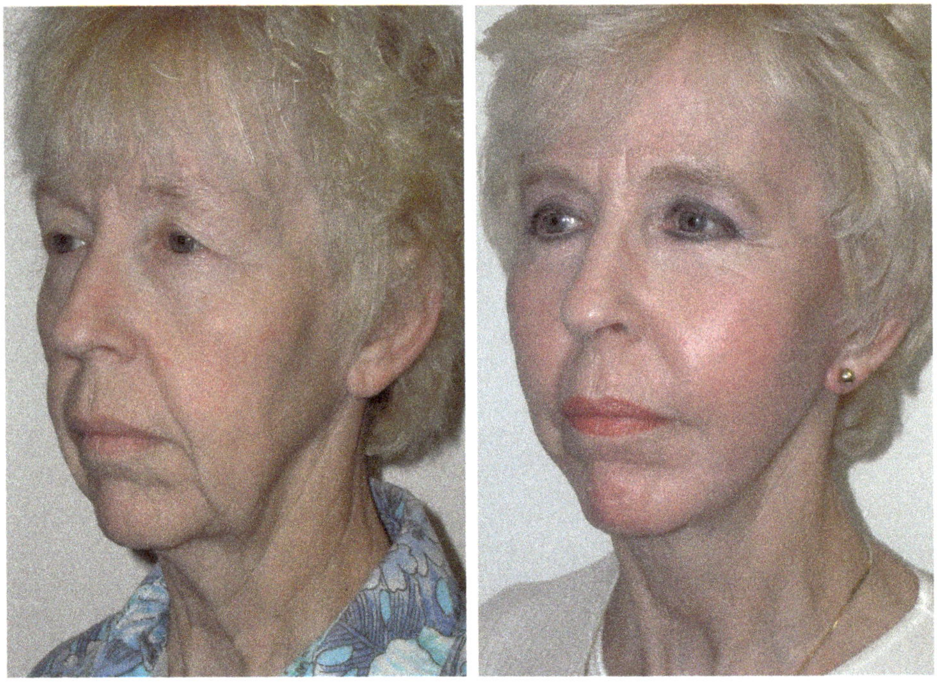

Fig. 1.10. It is important for patients to understand what a facelift will do and what it won't do, and the frequent necessity for multiple procedures that may occur before, during, or after the facelift. Multiple procedures are frequently required to address other areas of the face and neck that may not be improved with the facelift by itself. This patient is shown before (*left*) and after (*right*) a neck lift, upper and lower blepharoplasty chin implants, cheek implants, and full-face CO_2 laser resurfacing. All of these procedures were performed in the same surgical session.

Further Reading

Miller CC. Outstanding alae nasi. *Am J Derm Genitorurin Dis.* 1907;11:286.

CHAPTER 2

The Facial Aging

Joe Niamtu, III, Abraham Pathak

Chapter Outline

Some of the basics of facial aging are discussed in this chapter. This chapter will focus more on skin, midface, and lower facial aging. It is important that the reader also note that specific anatomic aging changes are also discussed in individual chapters within this text. It is important for all surgeons to understand and conceptualize that facial aging is a three-dimensional process and occurs in all hard and soft tissues, and as some people say, "We age from the inside out."

A youthful face consists of tight, full, and well-defined balanced features that we associate with vigor, beauty, and self-confidence. Young faces have smooth areas of transition throughout the facial thirds. The aging face, on the other hand, progresses to a ptotic, droopy, wrinkled state with loss of definition. These changes can be falsely perceived as tired, sick, or angry expressions. The aging face can have very distinct transition zones between facial thirds, such as sagging lids, bulging lower lid fat, ptotic cheeks, and the loss of smooth contour of the chin and mandibular border. Facial aging is three-dimensional and occurs with all hard and soft tissues.

Aging is a physiologic process of the body in response to the passage of time. Since the beginning of time, people have sought treatments to retard or reverse aging. Aging is a complex process that involves all of the hard and soft tissues of the body on a subcellular level.

Despite being a universal process, a complete knowledge of facial aging continues to elude us. Numerous theories and anatomical observations continually evolve our understanding of the morphological aging process.

Contemporary aging theory includes observation of sex-independent spatial changes, narrowing of the eyelid aperture, retrusion of the nasal alae into the cheek together with the thinning of the upper lip unit accentuating the nasolabial crease, and the gradual definition of the jowl fat pad over time (Fig. 2.1). Changes occur along the surface planes of the face but at right angles, underlining the multidimensional processes of facial aging.

It is paramount that all surgeons, and all patients for that matter, have an understanding of facial aging, which is the crux of cosmetic diagnosis and surgery.

As most cosmetic facial surgery patients are female, the nuances of metabolic aging influences are significant. Menopause produces decreased estrogen levels with elevated androgen levels, which contribute to epidermal and dermal changes. The decrease in basal metabolic rates (in men and women) facilitates weight gain and fat distribution in unwanted places such as thighs, abdomen, hip, buttocks, face, and neck. Add the effects of childbearing to the skin and muscle, and it is easy to understand the aging process in females. Subcutaneous fat also decreases, which affects the support of the skin. The face and neck are rich in glandular structures, which are less frequently discussed in volume loss but are probably moderate contributors. Skeletal muscles can undergo 50% atrophy with aging, and osteoporosis plays a key role in bone resorption, as the majority of women in their fifth decade are osteoporotic. Osteoporotic changes also occur in males and in both sexes contribute to facial skeletal and dental resorption. As the facial skeleton shrinks, even more soft tissue support is lost. Bone in the aging face is more prone to resorption in specific areas such as the orbital rims, maxilla and piriform region, and anterior

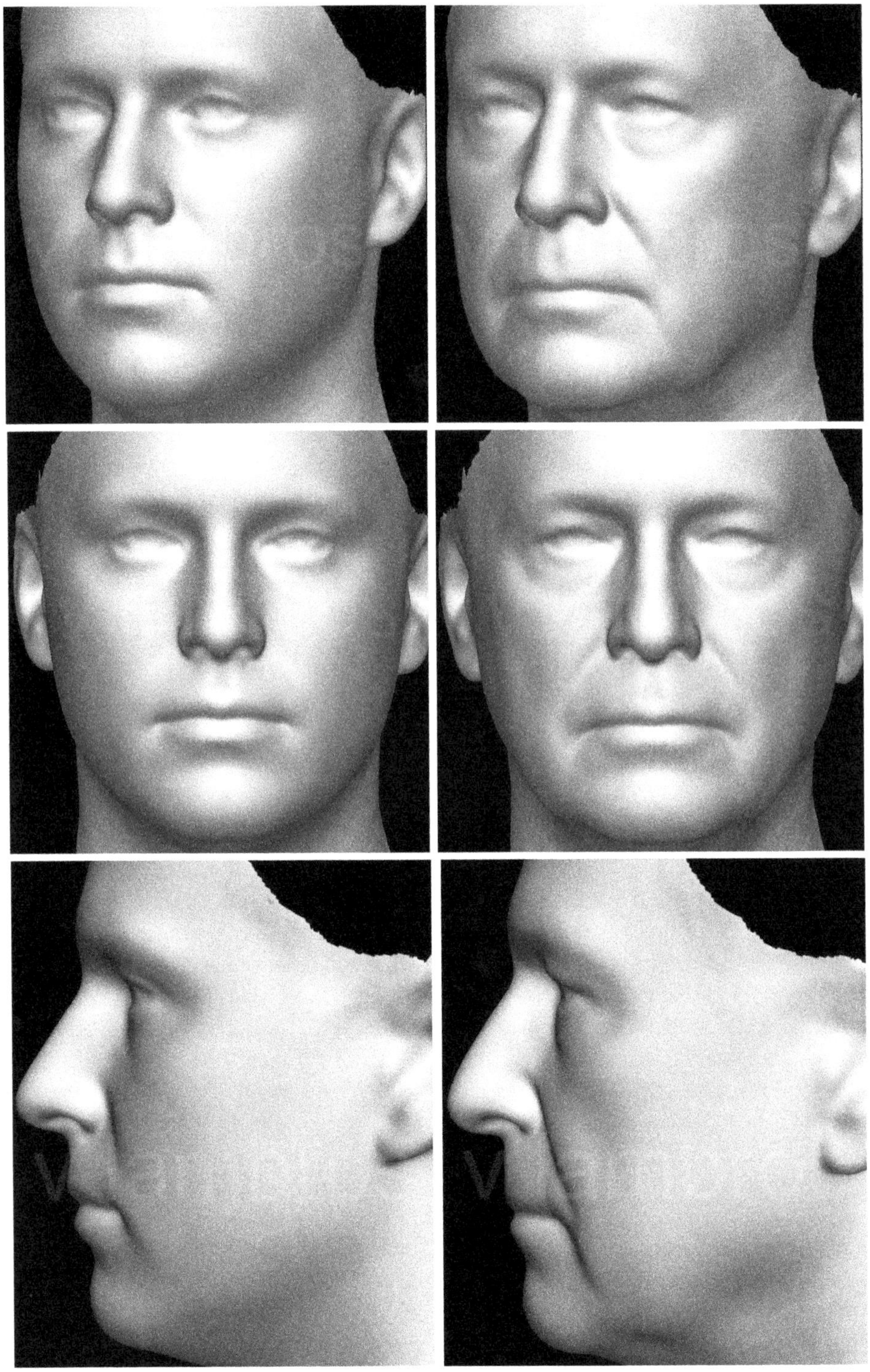

Fig. 2.1. Comparative image transitions of the average young and old male face showing the spatial changes of narrowing of the eyelid aperture, retrusion of nasal alae into the cheek with a thinning upper lip unit accentuating the nasolabial crease, and demarcation of the jowl fat pad. *(Courtsey Dr. Val Lambros.)*

mandibular and prejowl regions (Fig. 2.2). In addition to this, ligamentous attachments from bone to soft tissue tether the overlying soft tissue and contribute to hollowing when bone loss drags down the soft tissue anatomy.

One unique factor to facial aging is that in most cultures, the face is exposed. Clothes can masquerade somatic aging, but the face, neck, and hands give it all away.

As with all other theories or processes, surgeons and anatomists argue about what exactly happens during aging. Although most surgeons agree that atrophy, ligamentous laxity, and ptosis are causative factors, others argue against this. It is universally agreed, however, that aging is a gradual process of structural weakening, and its clinical effects begin in the third decade and progress throughout an individual's lifetime. Aging can be described as a process of deflation similar to the transition from grape to raisin.

Babies and toddlers have full rounded faces with full convex contours. This is, in part, from the small skeleton supporting the

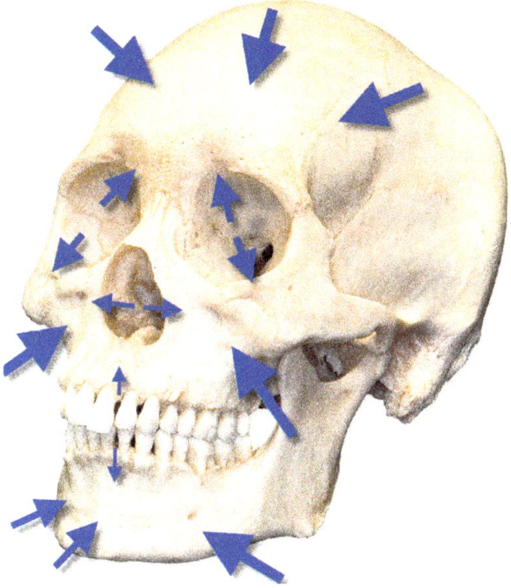

Fig. 2.2. Osseous resorption accounts for many aging changes. The *arrows* show common regions of bony atrophy, which cause loss of support for overlying soft tissue anatomy.

generous fat compartments in infancy. Adolescence includes rapid but disharmonious growth of bone, cartilage, muscle, and fat, which produces a sometimes-awkward appearance in the preteen years. Through the teen years, puberty produces secondary sexual characteristics including rapid growth phases, which produce hereditary but predictable and distinguishable facial changes. Middle age brings the onset of aging changes that progress until death (see later discussion). The cycle of aging is such that infants have large orbits and smaller maxillae, which make their midfacial characteristics resemble an aged person. As the midfacial skeleton grows, the infant takes on the midface of youth. Continued aging produces widening of the orbits with simultaneous maxillary and piriform resorption, which makes the aged person resemble an infant. Truly the cycle of life. Although some parts of the facial skeleton resorb with age, some areas such as the mandible enlarge, underlining the multifactorial and dynamic changes that contribute to the aging facial skeleton.

The youthful face is tapered like an upside-down egg, due to the distinct volume and tight tissue retention (Fig. 2.3, *top*). The aging face is more of a reverse taper, similar to a right-side-up

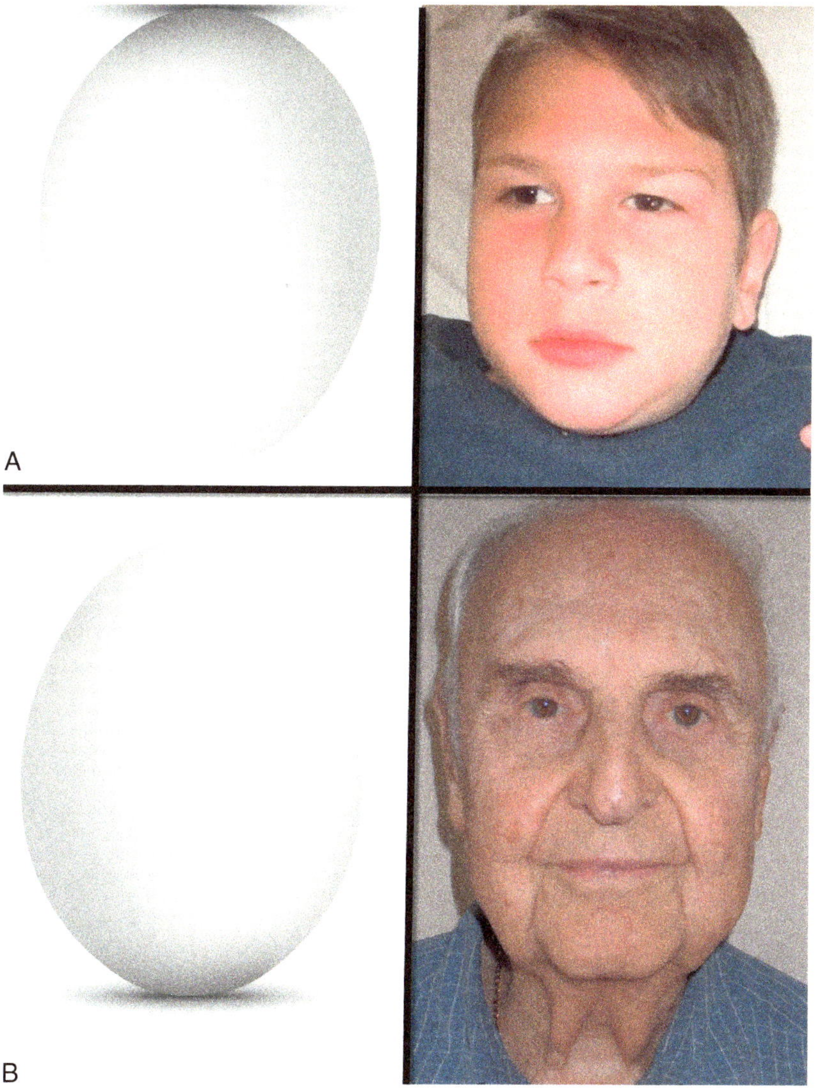

Fig. 2.3. The *upper* images show a young youthful face, which is tapered toward the jawline similar to an upside-down egg. The *lower* image shows an 80-year-old patient with a squared-off lower face similar to a right-side-up egg.

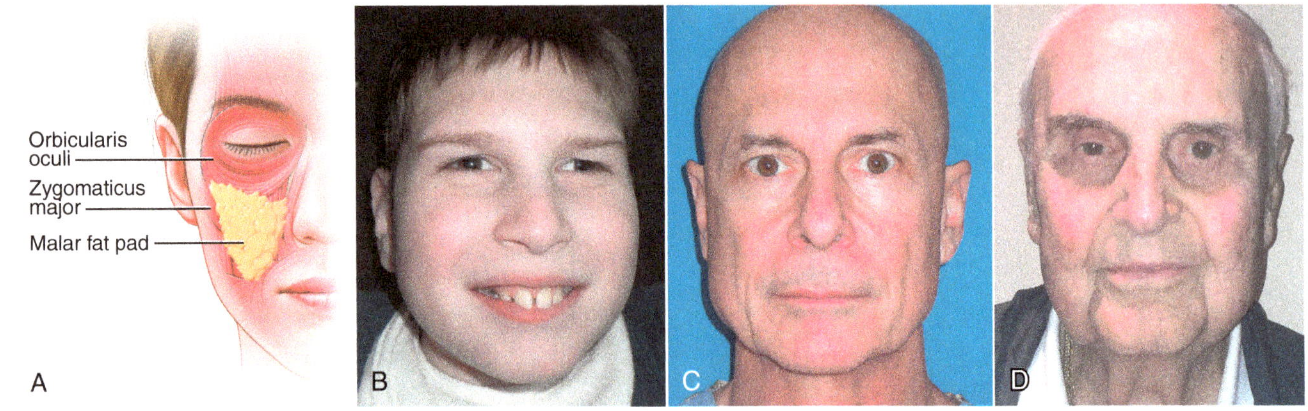

Fig. 2.4. The malar fat pad, youthful skeleton and undamaged skin complete the youthful midface. Descent of the malar fat pad, skeletal changes and aging and sun damaged skin contribute to the loss of the youthful, volumized. Ptotic changes also occur in the lower face and neck. Figure A shows relevant anatomy of the youthful midface. Figure B shows the author's 8 year old son, Figure C shows the author at 56 years of age and his father at 83 years of age. This family tree illustrates facial aging over three generations.

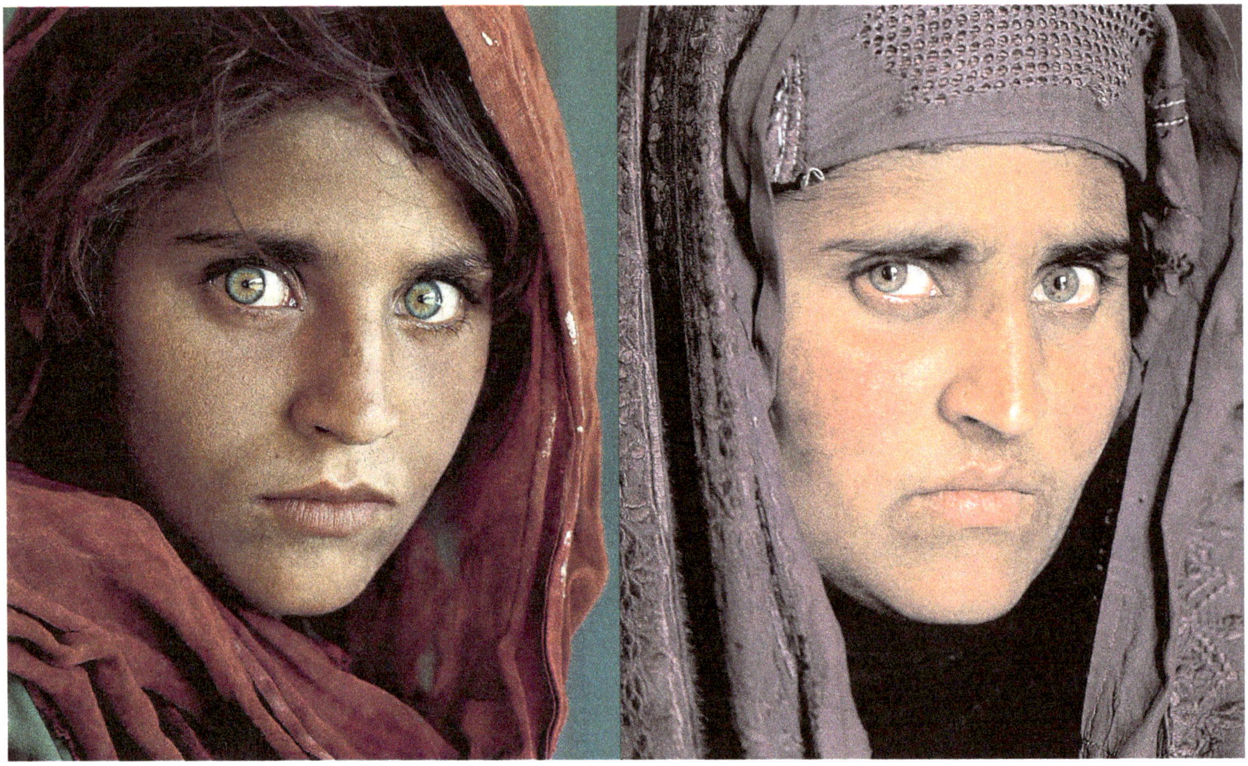

Fig. 2.5. This young patient shows classic beauty in her youthful features. These do not necessarily carry over in adulthood.

egg, due to the descent of volume and fat compartment changes (Fig. 2.3, *bottom*). Fig. 2.4 shows aging changes in three generations of the same family.

Aging changes are not only from volume loss and support changes but also due to intrinsic and extrinsic factors (Box 2.1).

Beauty does not necessarily transcend aging. Individuals deemed pretty or beautiful in their youth may not seem so in adulthood (Fig. 2.5).

Box 2.1. Comprehensive aging factors

Intrinsic aging factors	Extrinsic aging factors
Cellular senescence	Ultraviolet radiation
Decreased proliferative capacity	Environmental factors (ozone, etc.)
Decreased cellular DNA repair capacity	Tobacco use
Chromosomal abnormalities	Ethanol abuse
Hormone reductions	Gravitational effects
Gene mutation	Elasticity changes
Hard, soft, and dental structure loss	Emotional stress

Skin

It is interesting that biologic aging can sometimes exceed chronologic aging, and we all know 45-year-olds who look

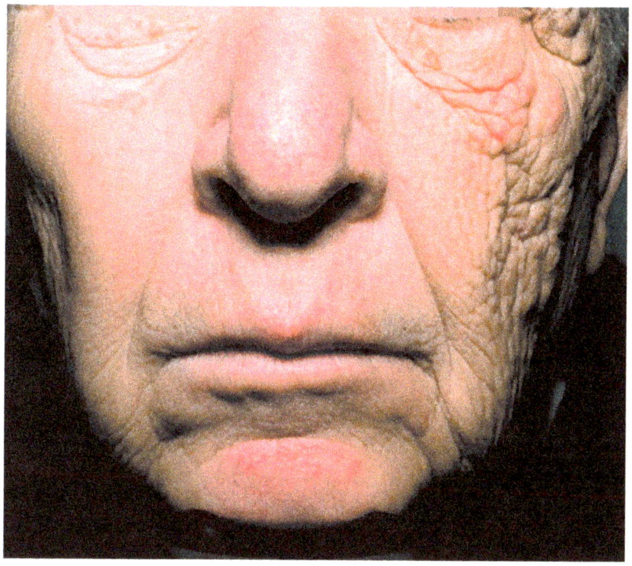

Fig. 2.6. This image shows unilateral advance skin actinic damage on a career truck driver whose left side faced the window.

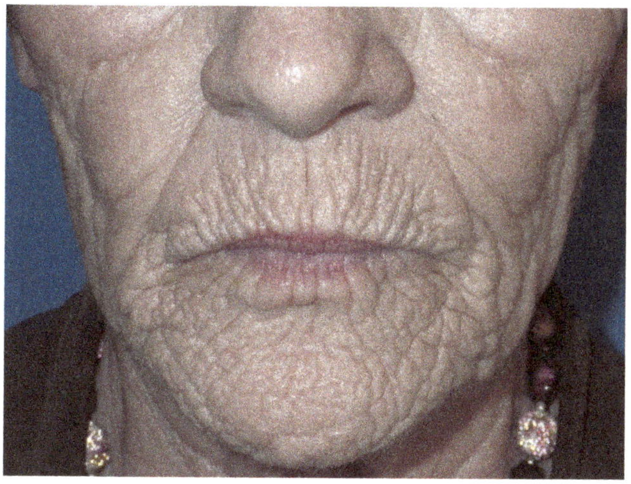

Fig. 2.7. This image shows a 65-year-old female with advanced skin aging, likely from sun damage and genetic predisposition.

60 or the inverse. Fig. 2.6 left shows a career truck driver with obvious accelerated actinic damage on the driver's side that is exposed to more sun and wind, and Fig. 2.7 shows a 65-year-old female with both hereditary and acquired aging (intrinsic and extrinsic).

The skin serves as the canvas of the face, revealing the deflation and atrophic changes of the various underlying components. Like the exposed hands, it rarely gets respite from the ravaging effects of the environment. Extrinsic factors—such as sun exposure, stress, and smoking—can accelerate the effects of aging.

Contributing to exogenous skin aging is the decrease in skin functions that occur with age. These include decreases in cell replacement, injury response, barrier function, sensory perception, immune and vascular responsiveness, thermoregulation, sweat production, sebum production, and vitamin D production. As normal regulatory pathways become dysfunctional with age, both the rejuvenation and healing processes of the skin are impaired. Recent studies have pointed to the dysfunction of the hypoxia-inducible factor (HIF)-1α regulatory pathway as a primary contributor to the decline of both processes. The dermis is thicker on areas of the face that are less mobile (e.g., forehead and nose) and thinner on areas of the face with increased movement (e.g., lower eyelids).

Genetic contributions to skin aging result in numerous biochemical, histologic, and physiologic changes. These changes include a reduction of vascularity, increased dermal/epidermal thickness, collagen changes, proteoglycan and dermal cellularity, and loss of elastic fibers.

Cumulative photodamage can be seen in almost every patient by comparing the sun-exposed and sun-protected areas of skin. The most obvious clinical cutaneous aging changes include markedly increased skin roughness, mottled hyperpigmentation, loss of elasticity, wrinkling, and sallowness.

Photoaging causes functional and anatomic modifications in the exposed regions. Ultraviolet B (UVB) radiation produces direct damage on the DNA of skin cells and also modulates the activity of cytokines and adhesion molecules. Ultraviolet A (UVA) radiation initiates the formation of reactive oxygen species (ROS), which also damages nuclear and mitochondrial DNA and activates matrix metalloproteinases (MMPs).

Histologically, the effects of skin photoaging include epidermal thickening, keratinocyte atypia, loss of polarity, and increased melanogenesis (Box 2.2 and Fig. 2.8). A fragmented and disorganized dermal fibrillar network is present and forms amorphous groups. Collagenous changes occur in the appearance of fragmented collagen fibrils, senescent fibroblasts, loss of function of glycosaminoglycans, and alterations in the cutaneous microvasculature.

Contributing to exogenous skin aging is the decrease in skin functions that occur with age. These include decreases in cell replacement, injury response, barrier function, sensory perception, immune and vascular responsiveness, thermoregulation, sweat production, sebum production, and vitamin D production. The dermis is thicker on areas of the face that are less mobile (e.g., forehead and nose) and thinner on areas of the face with increased movement (e.g., lower eyelids).

Lifestyle and hereditary factors are significant contributors to the aging equation. Some aging factors are controllable, and others are not. Studies of monozygotic twins have revealed that aging is affected greatly by environmental and lifestyle factors, as measured by physical appearance. The factors that exert the greatest influence seem to be substance or alcohol abuse, sun exposure, and emotional distress.

Box 2.2. **Pathologic changes of photodamaged skin**

- Thickened, more basket-woven stratum corneum
- Thinner, more atrophic epidermis
- Epidermal atypia
- Irregular melanin dispersion in the epidermis
- Decreased glycosaminoglycans in the dermis
- Abnormal-appearing elastic fibers in the dermis

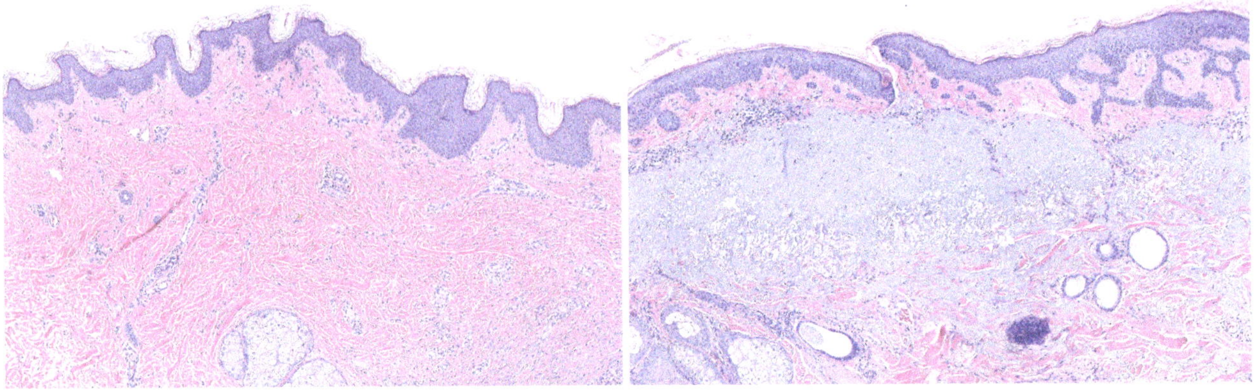

Fig. 2.8. The *left* image shows a hematoxylin and eosin stain of healthy skin showing normal stratum corneum, normal epidermal thickness, no atypical epidermal cells, normal rete ridges, and healthy collagen bundles. The *right* image shows the same stain of photodamaged skin showing thinning of the epidermis, flattening of the rete ridges, and solar elastosis in the dermis. *(Courtesy Dr. Jonhan Ho, Assistant Professor, University of Pittsburgh Medical Center.)*

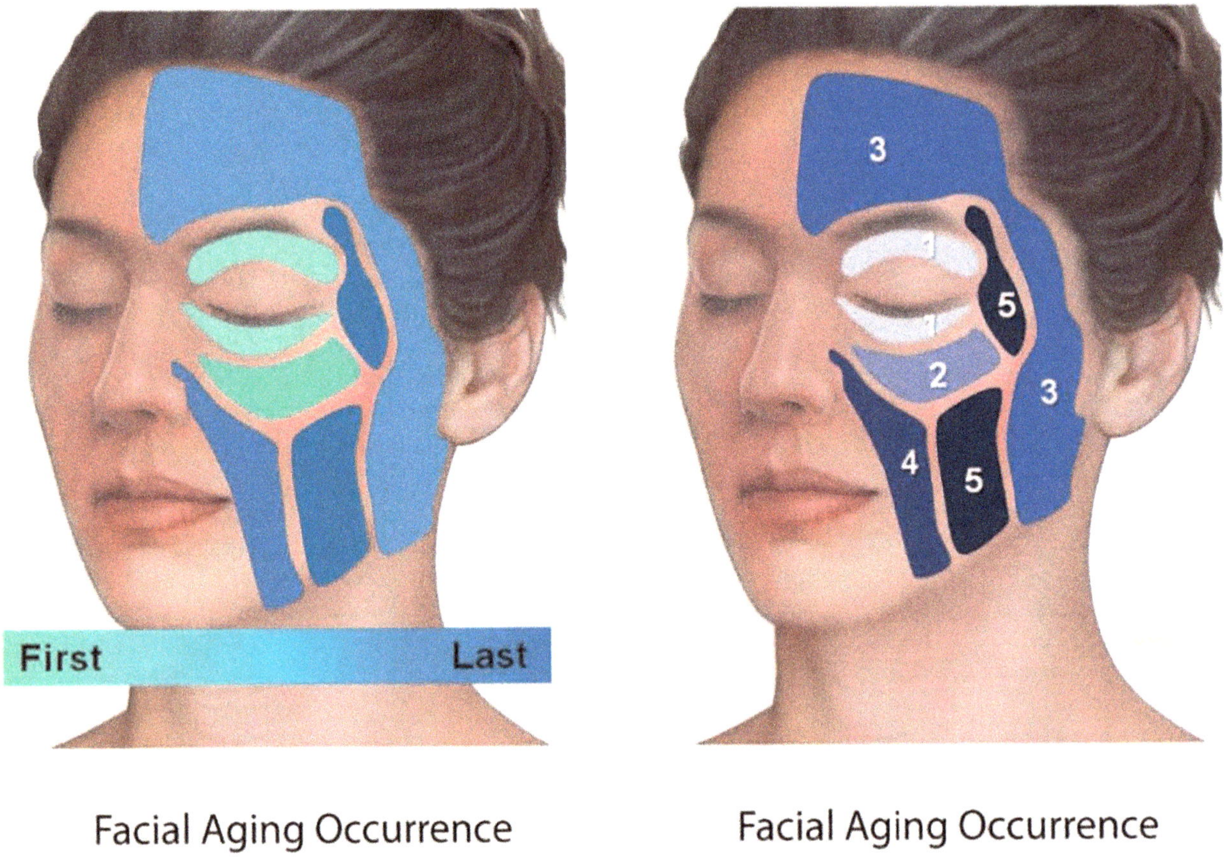

Fig. 2.9. Commonly observed sequence of facial fat compartment deflation in facial aging. *(Courtsey Dr. Rod Rohrich and PRS-Global Open forum.)*

The Relationship of Facial Fat in Aging

Once thought to be a continuous structure anatomically, the subcutaneous fat of the face has been revealed by Rohrich and Pessa to be highly compartmentalized with vascularized fibrous septal boundaries separating individual facial fat compartments (Figs. 2.9 and 2.10).

The nasolabial fat and jowl fat are separate distinct compartments. The periorbital fat is divided into superior, inferior, and lateral compartments. The malar fat is divided into the medial, the middle, and a larger lateral temporal-cheek fat spanning the height of the face from the cervical subcutaneous fat to the lateral-most compartment of the forehead. The forehead similarly has three compartments with the central, middle, and lateral temporal-cheek fat. Some compartments such as the periorbital and malar fat pads tend to deflate earlier in middle age, and others deflate later in life. In the youthful face the transition between these subcutaneous compartments is smooth, whereas variable deflation among compartments in the aging face render distinguishable abrupt contour changes. This volumetric understanding of facial aging continues to elicit

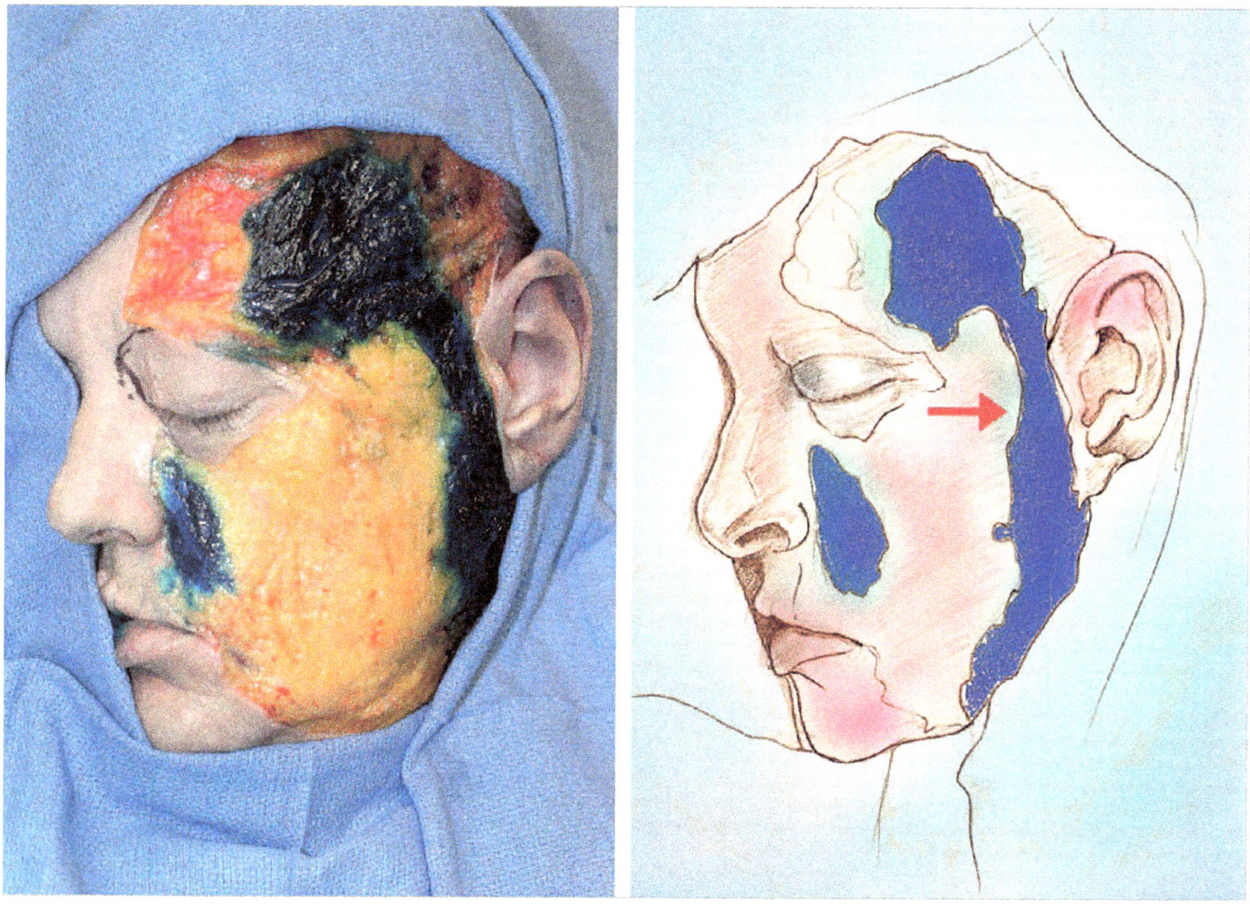

Fig. 2.10. Rohrich and Pessa injected methylene blue dye into cadaveric specimens, allowing dye diffusion to delineate the natural septal boundaries of the facial fat compartments. The unique broad expanse of the lateral temporal cheek compartment was highlighted in this manner (*arrow*). *(Reproduced from Rohrich RJ, Pessa JE. The fat compartments of the face: anatomy and clinical implications for cosmetic surgery. Plast Reconstr Surg. 2007, 119:2219–2227).*

interest and influence the techniques employed in facial rejuvenation today.

Midface and Lower Facial Aging

The cheeks are the foundation of the midface and basically are composed of the superficial and deep malar fat pads. In youth, the malar fat pads are full and in a superior and somewhat lateral position. With aging, the fat undergoes atrophy, and the malar fat pad becomes ptotic with underlying osseous resorption.

In youth the skin is held taut over the bone by several types of retaining ligaments. The taxonomy of these connective tissue structures varies. Anatomists describe "osteocutaneous" ligaments that represent fibrous bands with osseous (periosteal) origins and dermal insertions. The zygomatic and mandibular retaining ligaments are representative of "true" osteocutaneous retaining ligaments. The masseteric ligaments attach from muscle to dermis.

An additional support system is formed by the coalescence of the superficial and deep fasciae and referred to as *septae* and *adhesions*. These "soft tissue to soft tissue" retaining structures occur in the temple and lateral orbit. These various vascularized fascial networks partition the fat compartments and lend support against gravitational forces (Fig. 2.11).

It is of note that, clinically, the zygomatic and mandibular ligaments must be transected to truly free up the subcutaneous plane

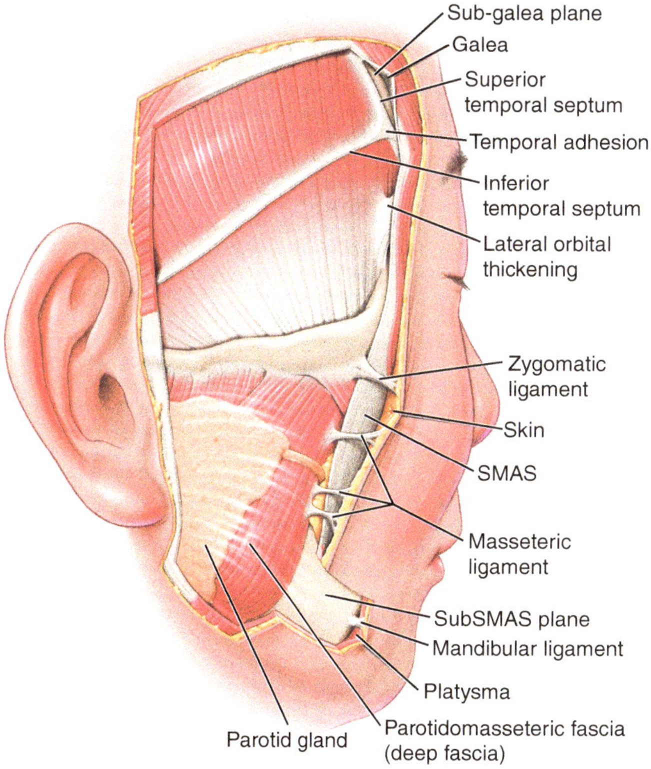

Fig. 2.11. The true ligaments and other connective tissue connections that stabilize the soft tissues of the face. *SMAS*, Superficial musculoaponeurotic system.

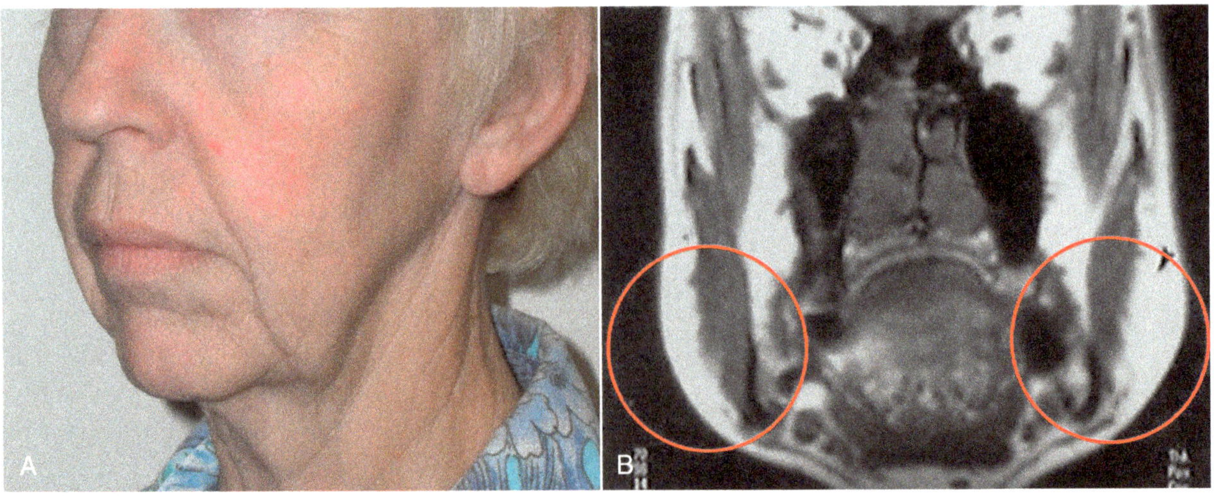

Fig. 2.12. The jowls consist of ptotic superficial musculoaponeurotic system, muscle, fat, and skin (*left*). This MRI scan (*right*) shows the ptotic fat and ptotic soft tissue accumulations that constitute the jowls.

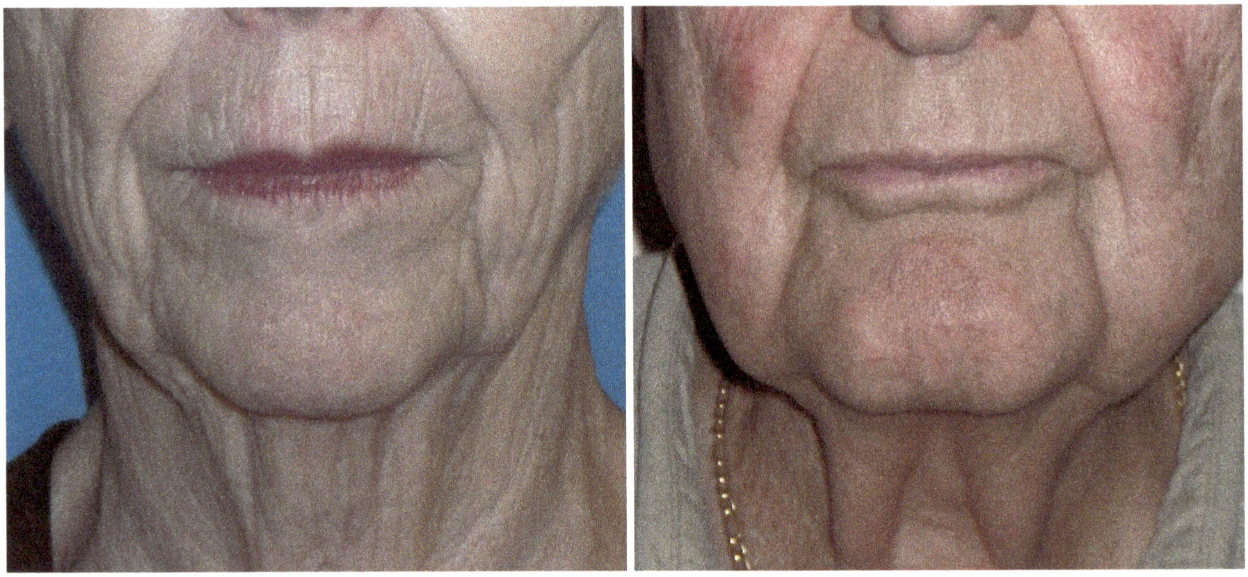

Fig. 2.13. These images illustrate perioral changes including nasolabial folds, melomental folds, chin ptosis, and jowling.

from the deeper planes during facelift surgery. The zygomatic ligaments, also referred to as *McGregor's patch*, represent a resistant region of dissection in the cheek, with its unsympathetic vascularity earning it the appellation as the "bloody gulch" among surgeons.

Weakening of all of the aforementioned ligaments also contributes to tissue descent, including the malar fat pads and buccal fat pads. In essence, the cheeks promote the jowls (Fig. 2.12). These volumetric and gravitational midface changes, coupled with photodamage, loss of tooth structure, and skeletal changes, all contribute to the drawn, gaunt, or hollow midface.

Jowls

As described, a series of ligaments keep the facial tissues taut in youth, and the laxity associated with aging allows cheek and jowl ptosis. In youth, a tight well-defined mandibular border is present. With aging, the combination of ligamentous laxity from the masseteric cutaneous and mandibular ligaments, superficial musculoaponeurotic system (SMAS) and soft tissue ptosis, photodamage, midface descent, and weight gain obscures the mandibular definition. Jowling is a result of ptotic fat compartment, as well as the buccal fat, descent, and the overlying skin changes. Superior and inferior jowl fat compartment position change is seen in patients with ptotic jowls, suggesting a shift of volume inferiorly. Dehiscence of the mandibular septum allows fat to flow across the mandibular border into the submandibular fat compartment. In addition, dermal muscular attachments are weak in the cheek, mandibular angle, and neck, which also contribute to cheek, jowl, and neck aging. Buccal fat is separate from jowl fat. Jowl fat is separate from the submandibular fat by a "septum" of connective tissue adherent to the mandibular body. Jowling is treated with SMAS facelift, liposuction, and skin resurfacing procedures. Figs. 2.13 and 2.14 show the ptotic deep tissues that constitute jowling.

In addition to jowling, the descent and/or herniation of the buccal fat pads can add to lower facial fullness, ptosis, and aging (Figs. 2.15–2.17).

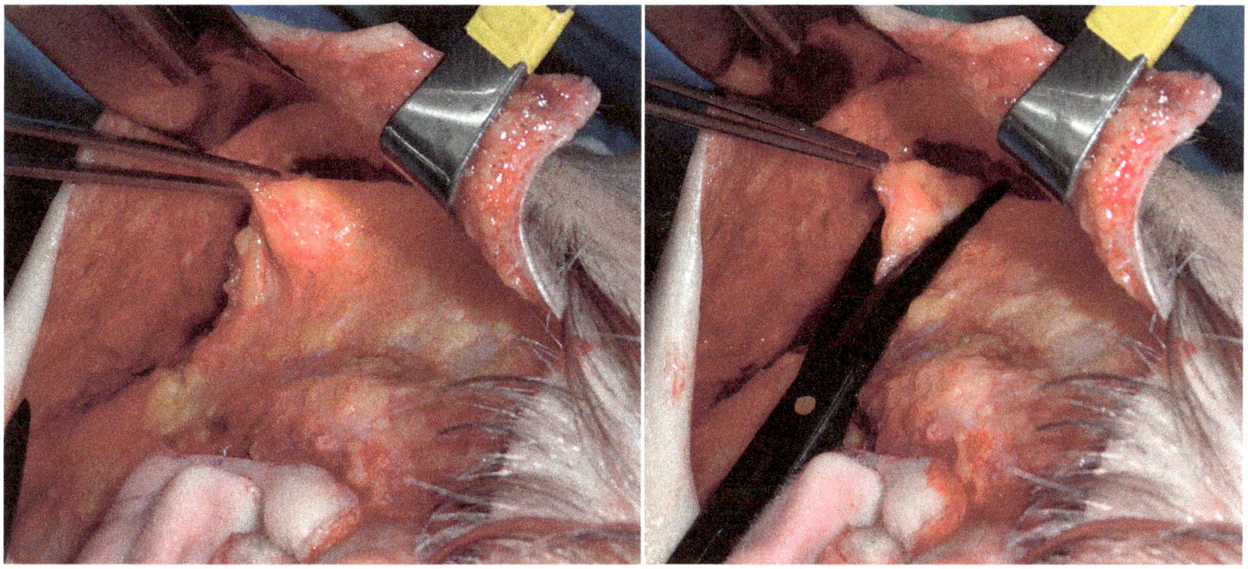

Fig. 2.14. The *left* image shows a forceps elevating the ptotic superficial musculoaponeurotic system and related soft tissue during facelift surgery that constitutes the jowl, and the *right* image shows jowl reduction.

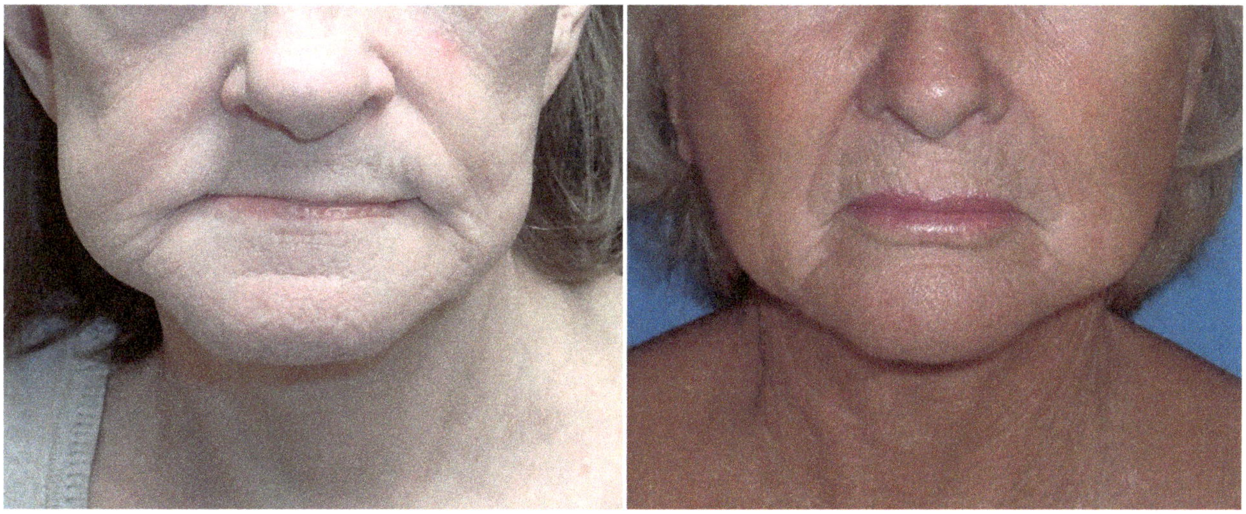

Fig. 2.15. These two patients exhibit typical lower facial aging changes that are amplified by buccal fat accumulations that can result in fullness and ptotic appearance.

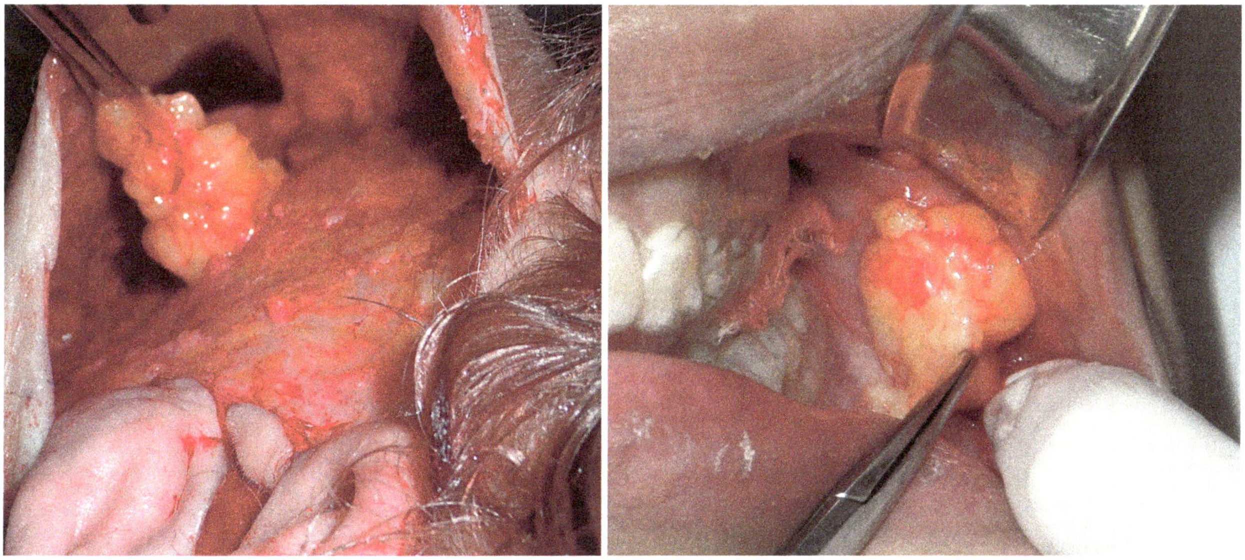

Fig. 2.16. Lower facial rejuvenation frequently includes buccal fat pad reduction. The *left* image shows the buccal fat being reduced during facelift, and the *right* image show an intraoral approach for reducing the buccal fat pad.

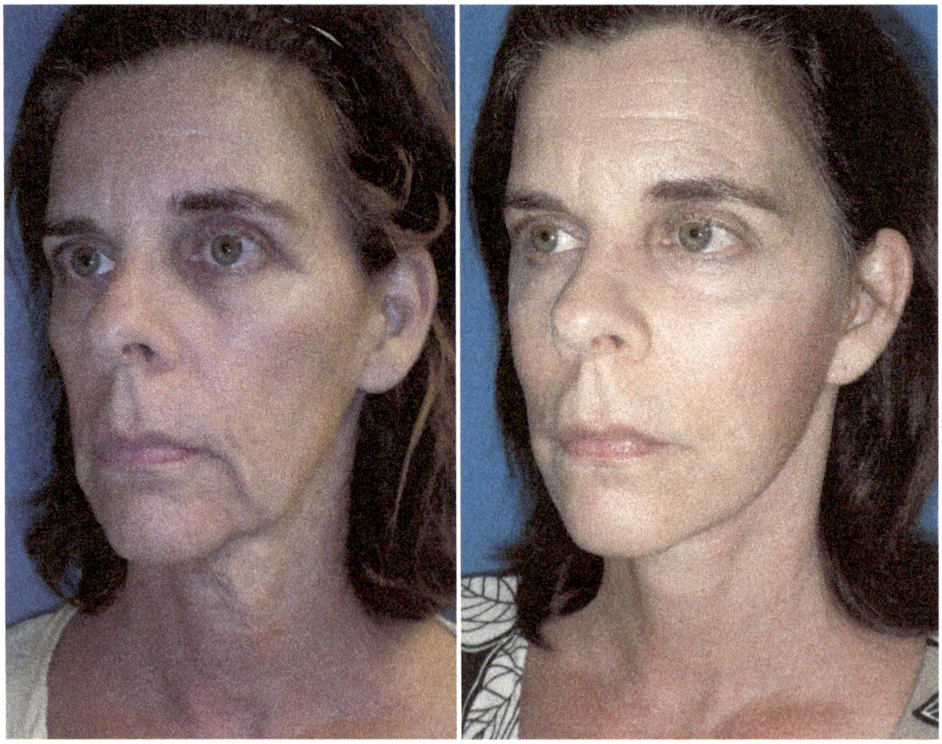

Fig. 2.17. Jowling is one of the primary reasons that patients seek facelift and neck lift surgery. The *left* image shows the patient with heavy jowling, and the *right* image shows the same patient after facelift and neck lift.

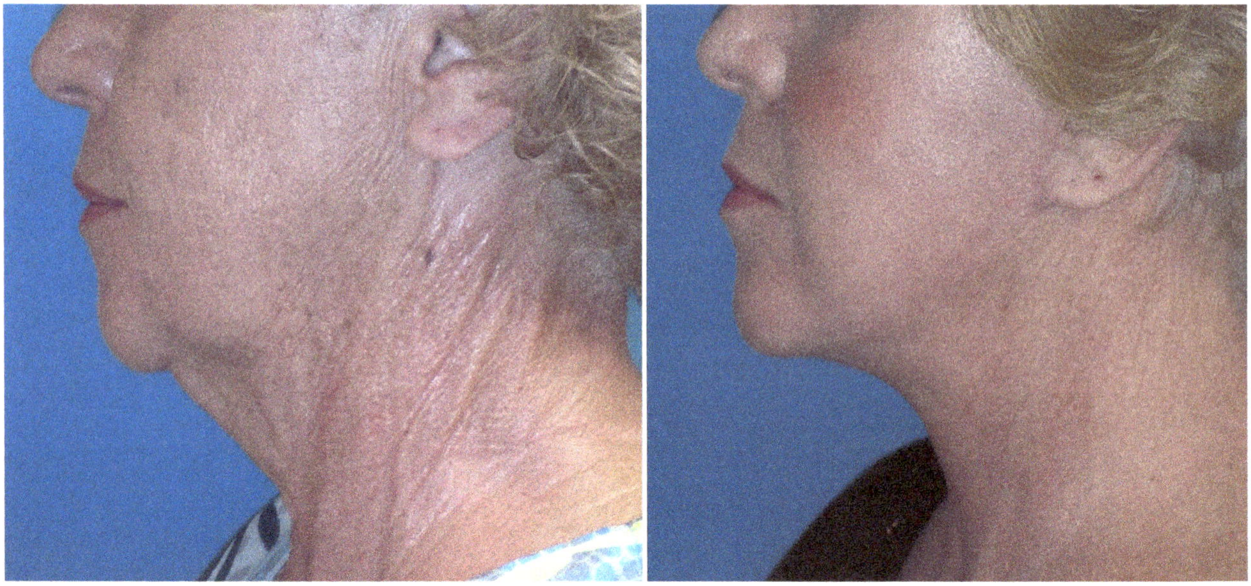

Fig. 2.18. The *left* image shows a patient 72-year-old female with soft tissue chin ptosis. The *right* image shows the same patient after facelift and neck lift with simultaneous chin implant.

Chin and Submental Region

The chin and submental area undergo significant aging changes. The submental region is well defined in most young people, and numerous changes occur throughout life. Generalized fat deposition with changes in the hyoid structure and muscular support can affect youthful submental sling. This produces a loss of definition of the cervicomental angle, fat deposition, and loss of chin definition with generalized fullness of the submental region. Because of skin changes, fat atrophy, muscle atrophy, dental changes, and contributing submental anatomy, the chin can become quite ptotic, especially in females. Generalized weight gain with aging also decreases the definition of the chin. A "witch's chin" is a term describing chin ptosis with soft tissue excess in females (Fig. 2.18). Loss of tone of the mentalis dermal insertions also contributes to chin aging. Chin aging is treated with chin implants, lifting procedures, injectable fillers, and submentoplasty.

Neck

"I hate my neck" are words that cosmetic facial surgeons hear on a daily basis. There is no more demoralizing feature to aging patients than excess and floppy neck skin and fat deposition (Fig. 2.19).

Platysmal banding begins in the late fourth decade and results in two separate cord-like structures from the mandibular border extending down the neck (Fig. 2.20).

The appearance of platysmal bands and neck fat is associated with dehiscence of fascia and atrophy of the platysma. Generalized weight gain and fat deposition can obscure the definition of the jaw. The aging neck skin and thin platysma muscle often appear to represent a single unit, although they are separate layers. Sagging skin is also a strong contributor to the aging neck, and this laxity is evident during a facelift procedure (Fig. 2.21) Ptotic submandibular glands also contribute to the aging neck and may present as fullness in the lateral submandibular region.

Treatment options in the neck are very limited and other than rhytidectomy (sometimes isolated platysmaplasty and submentoplasty), very few rejuvenation options exist. Newer technologies such as the suture suspension procedure and skin tightening with energy are evolving but cannot compete with traditional rhytidectomy for the improvement of excess neck skin. Fig. 2.22 summarizes many of the soft tissue cervicofacial aging changes, Table 2.1 lists aging changes by decade, and Figs. 2.23 and 2.24 illustrate aging throughout life span.

The Facial Aging Process From the "Inside Out"

Arthur Swift, MD,[1] Steven Liew, MD,[2] Susan Weinkle, MD,[3] Julie K Garcia, PhD,[4] and Michael B Silberberg, MD, MBA[5]

Gender Differences: Do Females and Males Age the Same?

In a 2019 three-dimensional study, Windhager et al., quantified some interesting facial aging data. Despite variation in lifestyle and environment, the first signs of human facial aging show between the ages of 20 and 30 years. It is a cumulative process of changes in the skin, soft tissue, and skeleton of the face. As quantifications of facial aging in living humans are still scarce, the authors in this study set out to study age-related changes in three-dimensional facial shapes using geometric morphometrics (Figs. 2.25–2.27). They collected surface scans of 88 human faces (aged 26–90 years from Croatian patients). Based on a geometric morphometric analysis of 585 measurement points (landmarks and semi-landmarks), they modeled sex-specific trajectories of average facial aging. Their results showed age-related facial shape change was similar in both sexes until around age 50, at which time the female aging trajectory turned sharply.

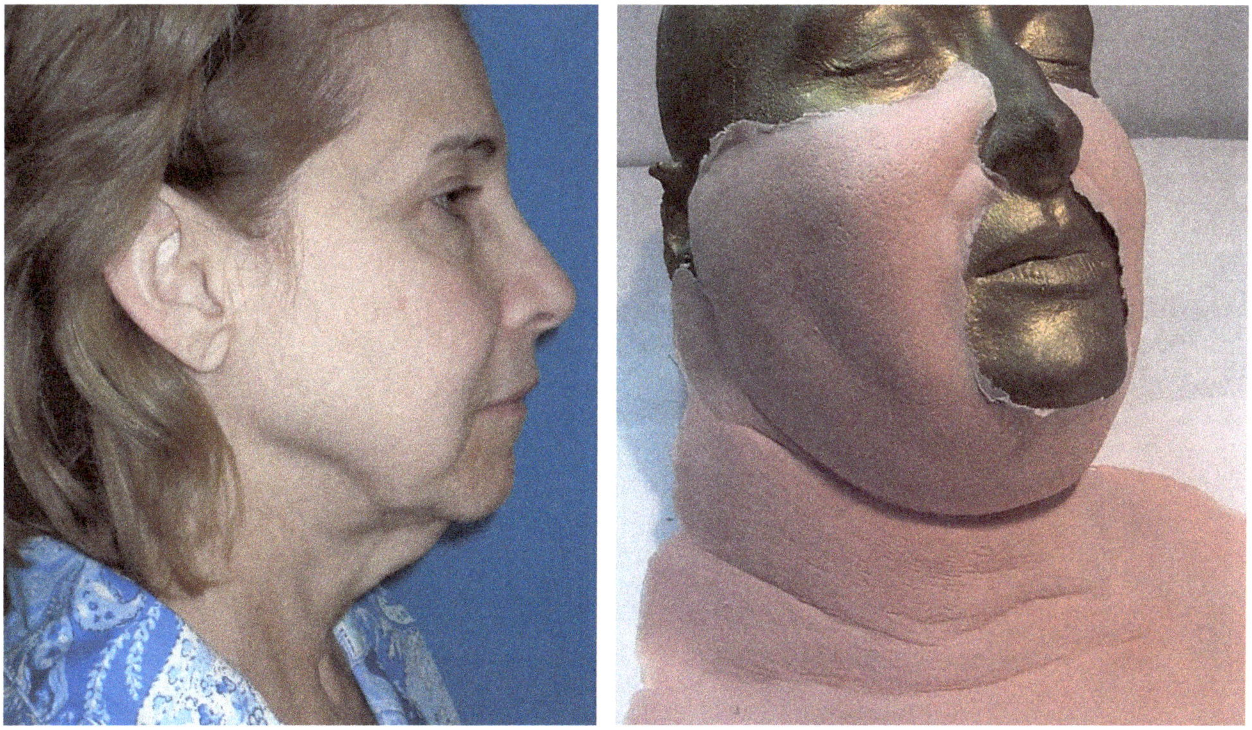

Fig. 2.19. The *left* image shows neck skin excess, and the *right* image shows a Hollywood "fat suit," which is how actors are made to look older with fat deposition and skin excess.

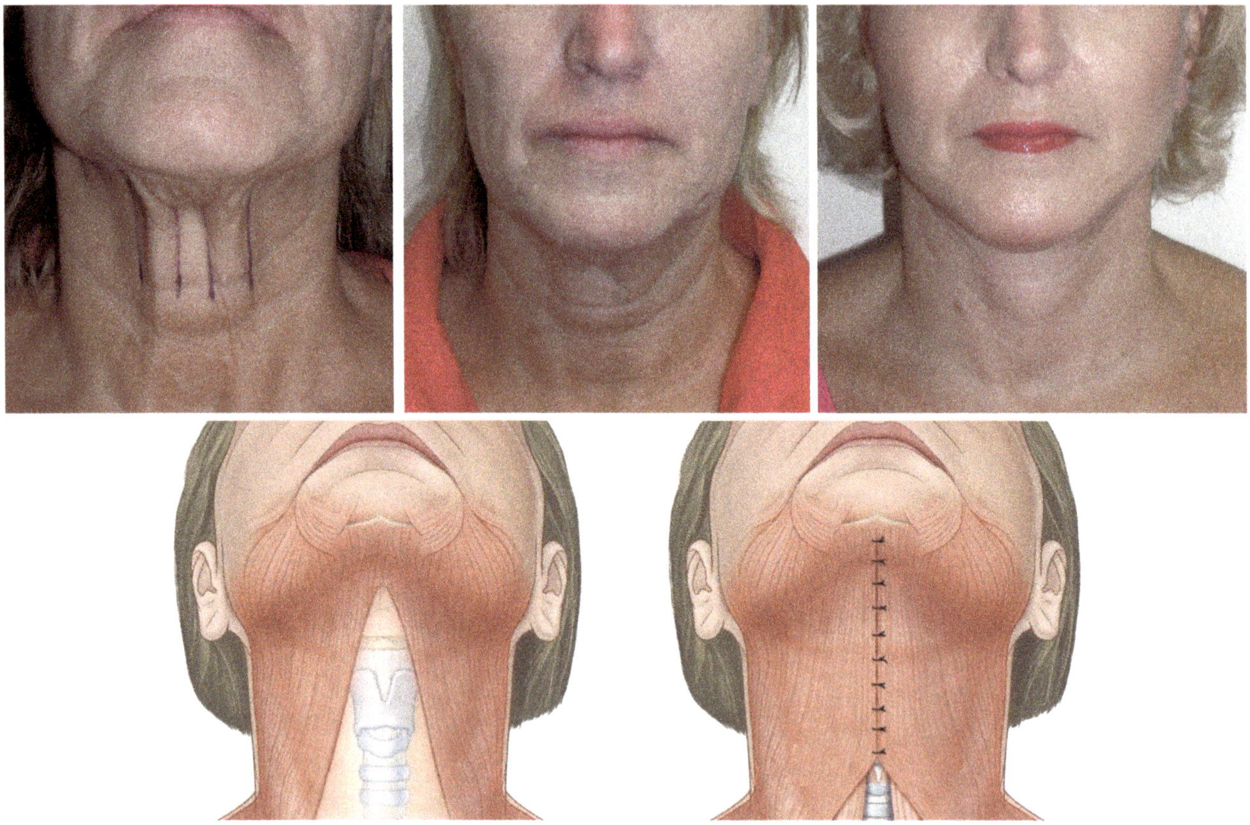

Fig. 2.20. The *upper left* image shows typical platysmal banding in the aging neck. The *upper middle* images shows banding before face and neck lift, and the *upper right* images show corrected platysmal banding after surgery. The *bottom left* image shows a representation of dehisced platysmal bands, and the *bottom right* image shows a graphic representation of sutured platysmal bands.

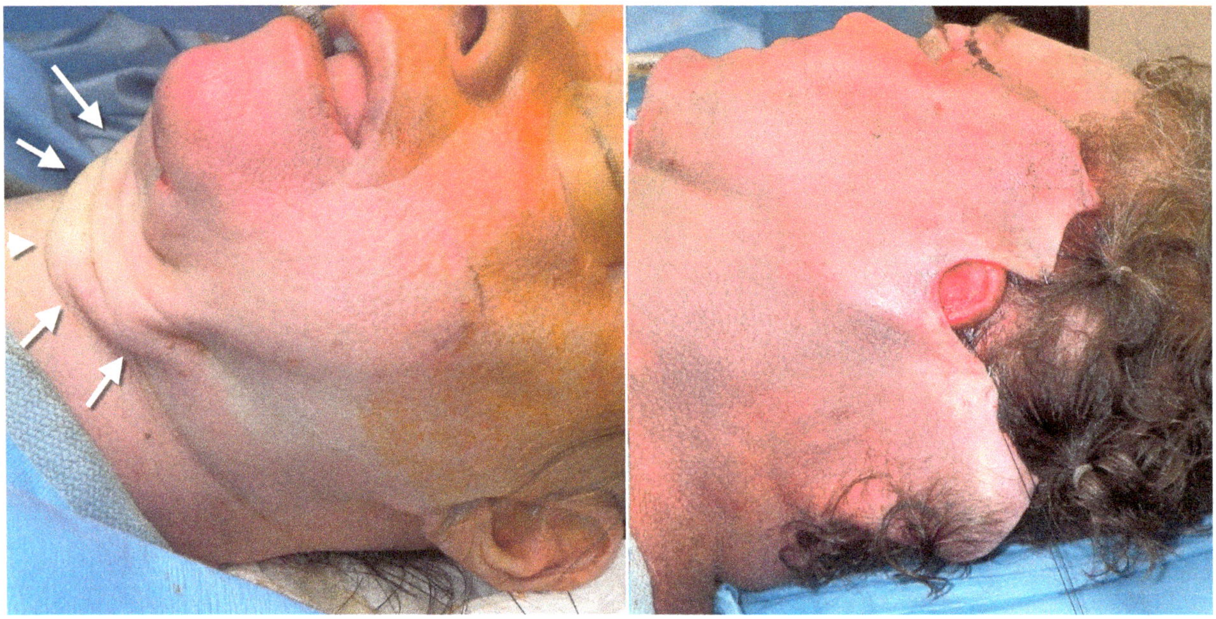

Fig. 2.21. The *left* image shows a patient immediately after platysmaplasty. The *right* image shows excess skin that is mobilized in this procedure and translates into significant skin excess that is removed during the facelift procedure to rejuvenate the lower face and neck.

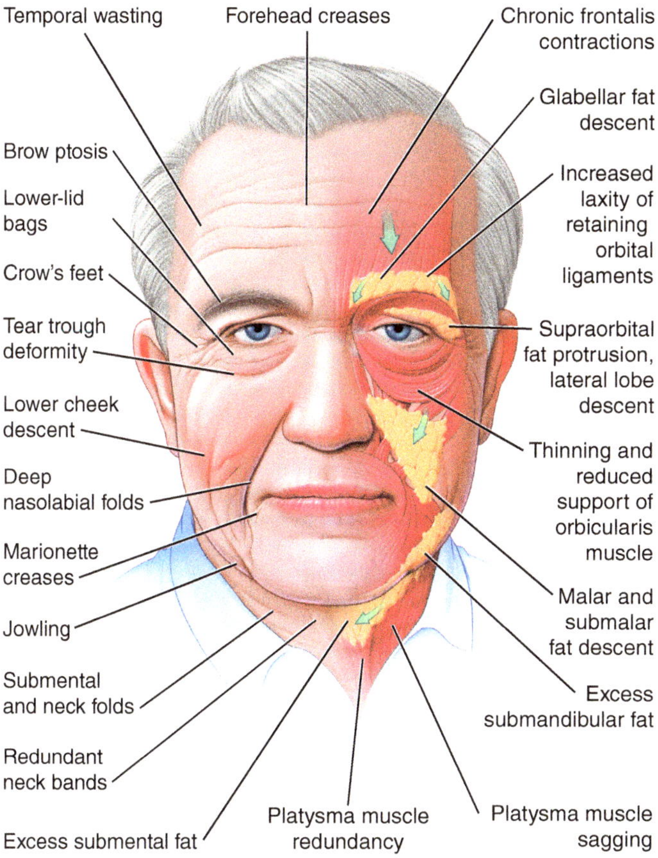

Fig. 2.22. Most of the aging changes discussed in this chapter are categorized in this drawing.

The overall magnitude of facial shape change (aging rate) was higher in women than men, especially in early postmenopausal females. Aging was generally associated with a flatter face, sagging soft tissue ("broken" jawline), deeper nasolabial folds, smaller visible areas of the eyes, thinner lips, and longer nose and ears. In postmenopausal women, facial aging was best predicted by the years since their last menstruation and

Age (yr)	Changes
30s or earlier	Forehead and glabellar lines appear
	Eyebrows may begin to descend
	Upper eyelid skin increases, and eyes appear smaller
	Fine lines around the lower eyelids and crow's feet emerge
	Tear trough lines and infraorbital fat become more prominent
	Midface aging begins
	Nasolabial folds form
	Lip thinning begins
	Alterations in skin texture and pigmentation appear
40s	Forehead, glabellar, and crow's feet lines deepen
	Eyebrows may continue to descend
	Upper eyelid skin increases in laxity and descends
	Tear trough elongates and the inferior orbital rim becomes visible
	Midface loses projection, hollows, and appears to descend
	Nasolabial folds deepen
	Lips thin and perioral lines develop
	Oral commissures and marionette lines become noticeable
	Chin begins to rotate/elongate
	Jawline loses definition
50s	Dynamic glabellar and forehead lines deepen and remain noticeable in repose
	Upper eyelid drooping increases
	Tear trough and lower eyelid scleral show worsens
	Nose begins to droop

From Swift A, Liew S, Weinkle S, Garcia JK, Silberberg MB. The facial aging process from the "inside out." Aesthet Surg J. 2021;41:1107–1119.

Table 2.1. Major manifestations of aging by decade of life.

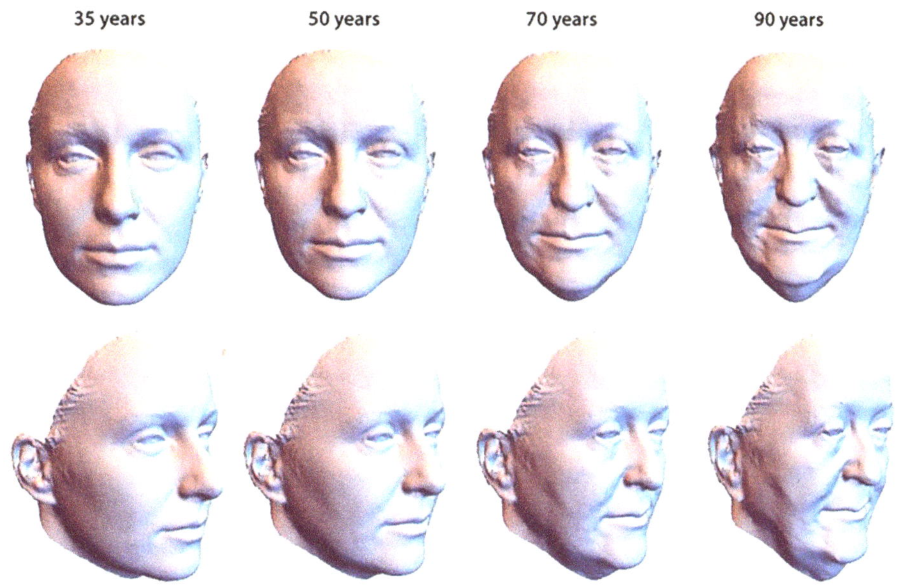

Fig. 2.23. This image shows a representation of female aging at 35 years of age, 50 years of age, 70 years of age, and 90 years of age. *(From Windhager S, Mitteroecker P, Rupić I, Lauc T, Polašek O, Schaefer K. Facial aging trajectories: a common shape pattern in male and female faces is disrupted after menopause. Am J Phys Anthropol. 2019;169:678–688.)*

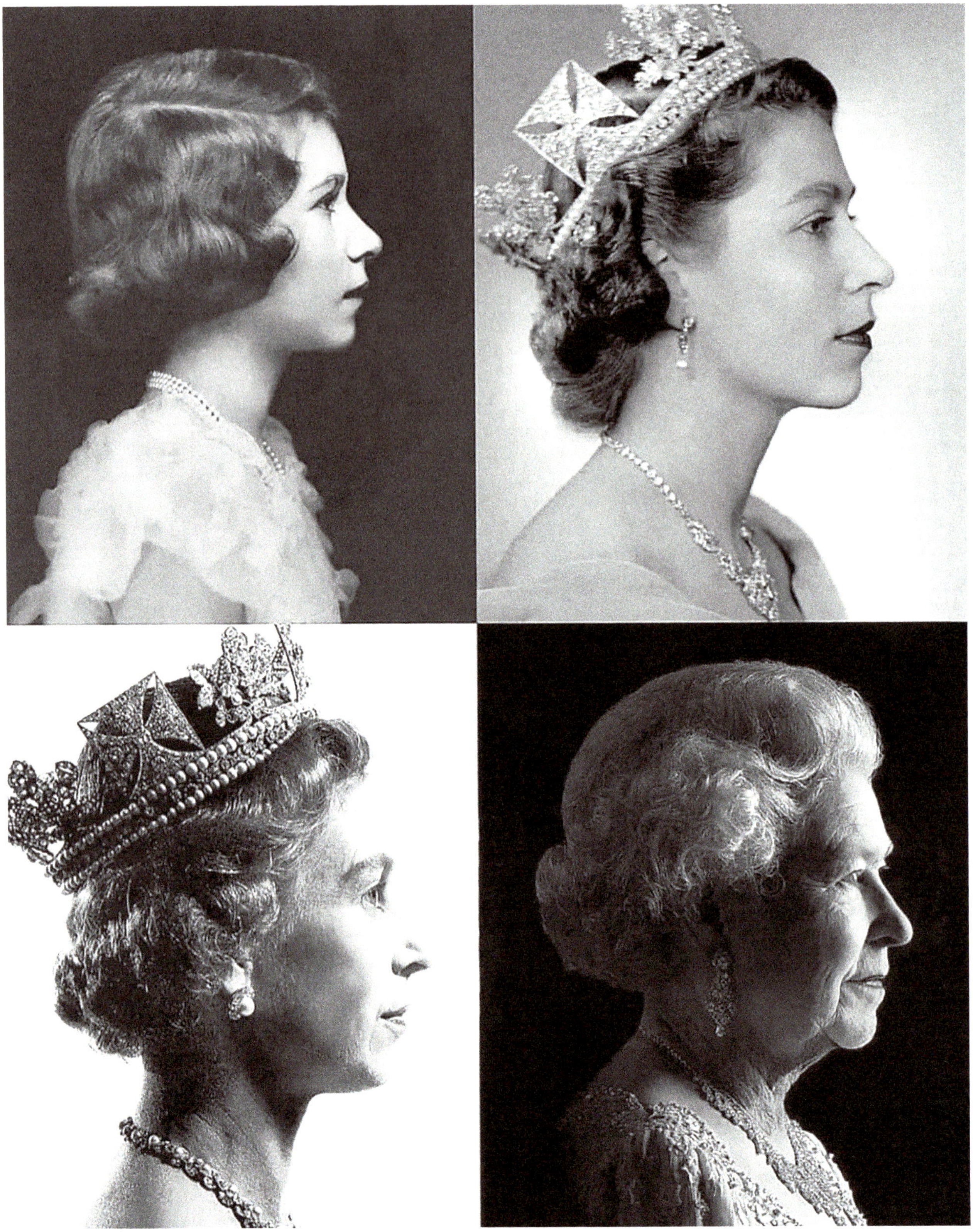

Fig. 2.24. Aging is inevitable and transcends money, power, and privilege. This image shows the graceful aging of the former Queen Elizabeth II.

was mainly attributable to bone resorption in the mandible. The authors surmised that "with high spatial and temporal resolution, we were able to extract a shared facial aging pattern in women and men, and its divergence after menopause. This fully quantitative three-dimensional analysis of human facial aging may not only find applications in forensic and ancient human facial reconstructions, but shall include lifestyle and endocrinological measures, and also reach out to studies of social perception." As technology increases, facial aging will become more understood and quantified.

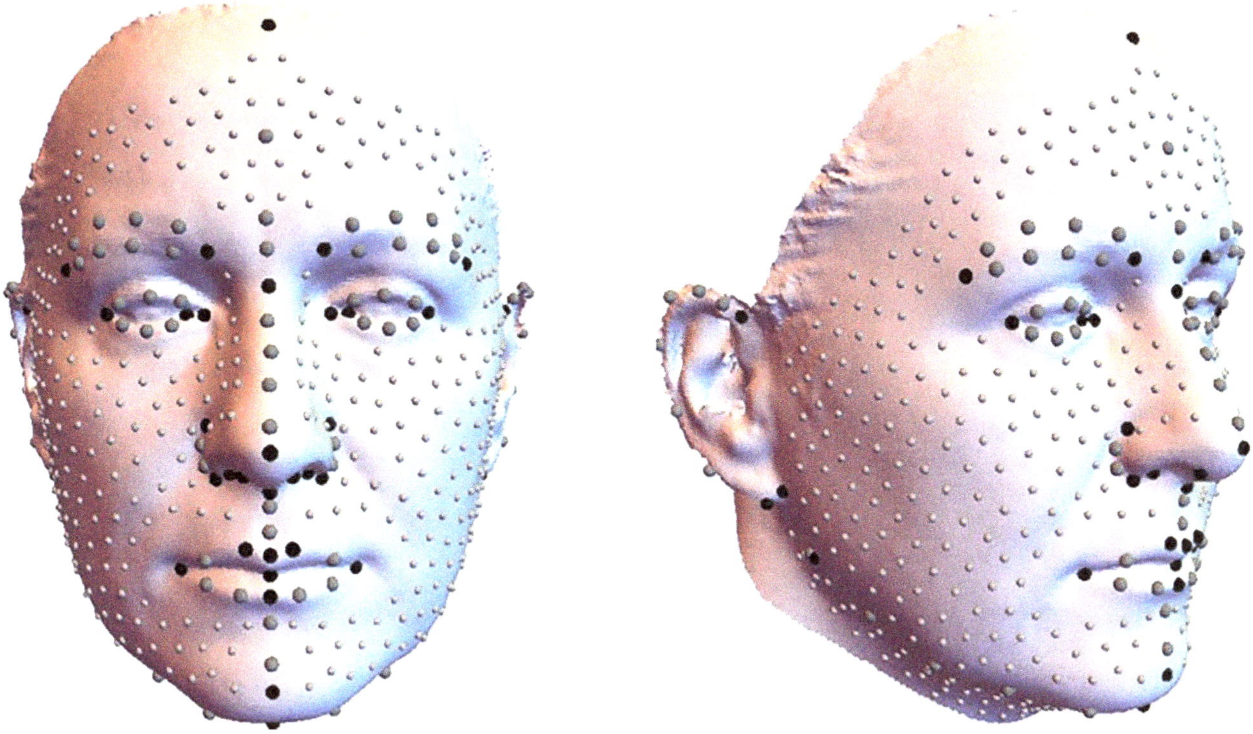

Fig. 2.25. Landmark scheme. Facial surface (sample average) with the 40 fixed landmarks (*black spheres*), 64 curve semi-landmarks (*large gray spheres*), and 481 surface semi-landmarks (*small gray spheres*) used in the analysis. *(Courtesy Sonja Windhager.)*

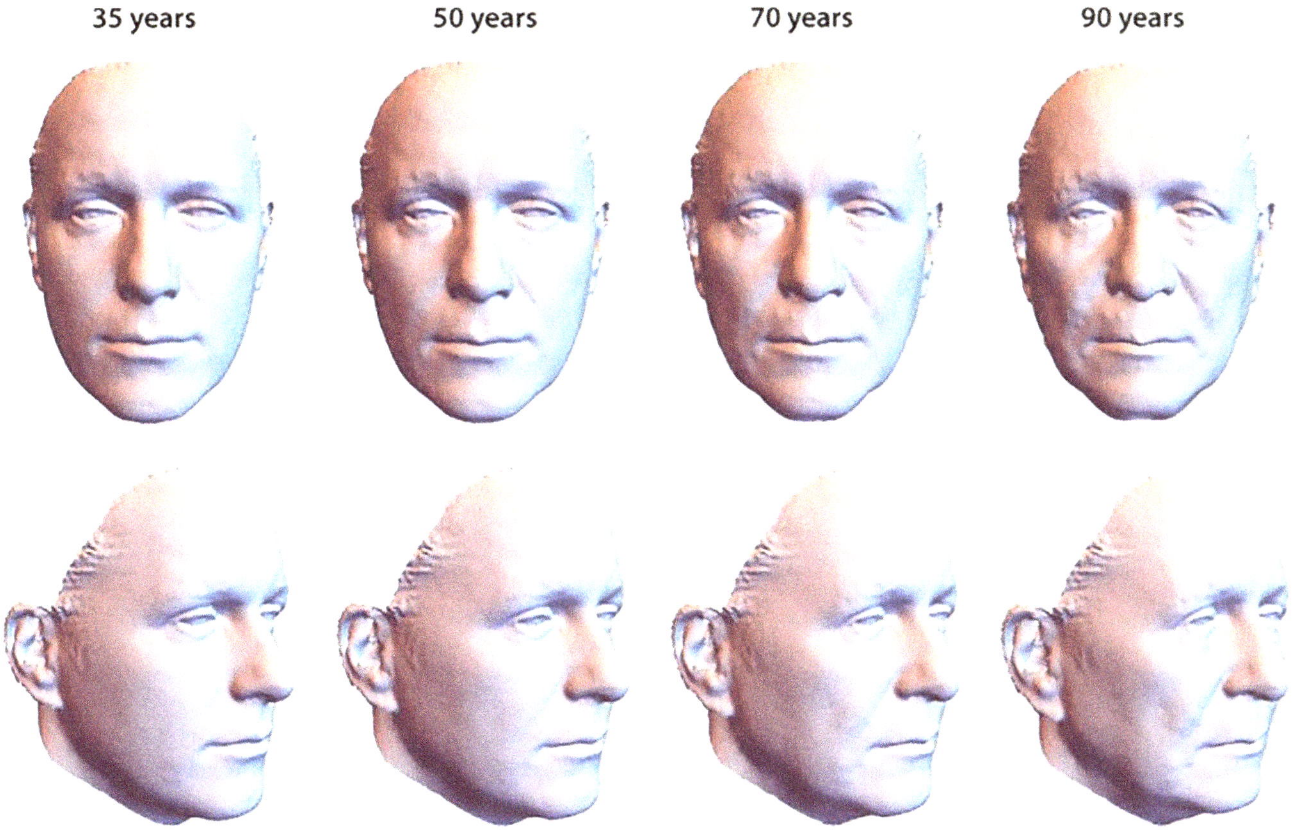

Fig. 2.26. Visualization of male facial aging derived from a linear regression of shape on age ($P < .001$, $n = 32$). The predicted 90-year-old face extrapolates the actual age range sampled. With increasing age, the face flattened, jowls formed, nasal tips dropped, eyelids drooped, and lips thinned. *(Courtesy Sonja Windhager.)*

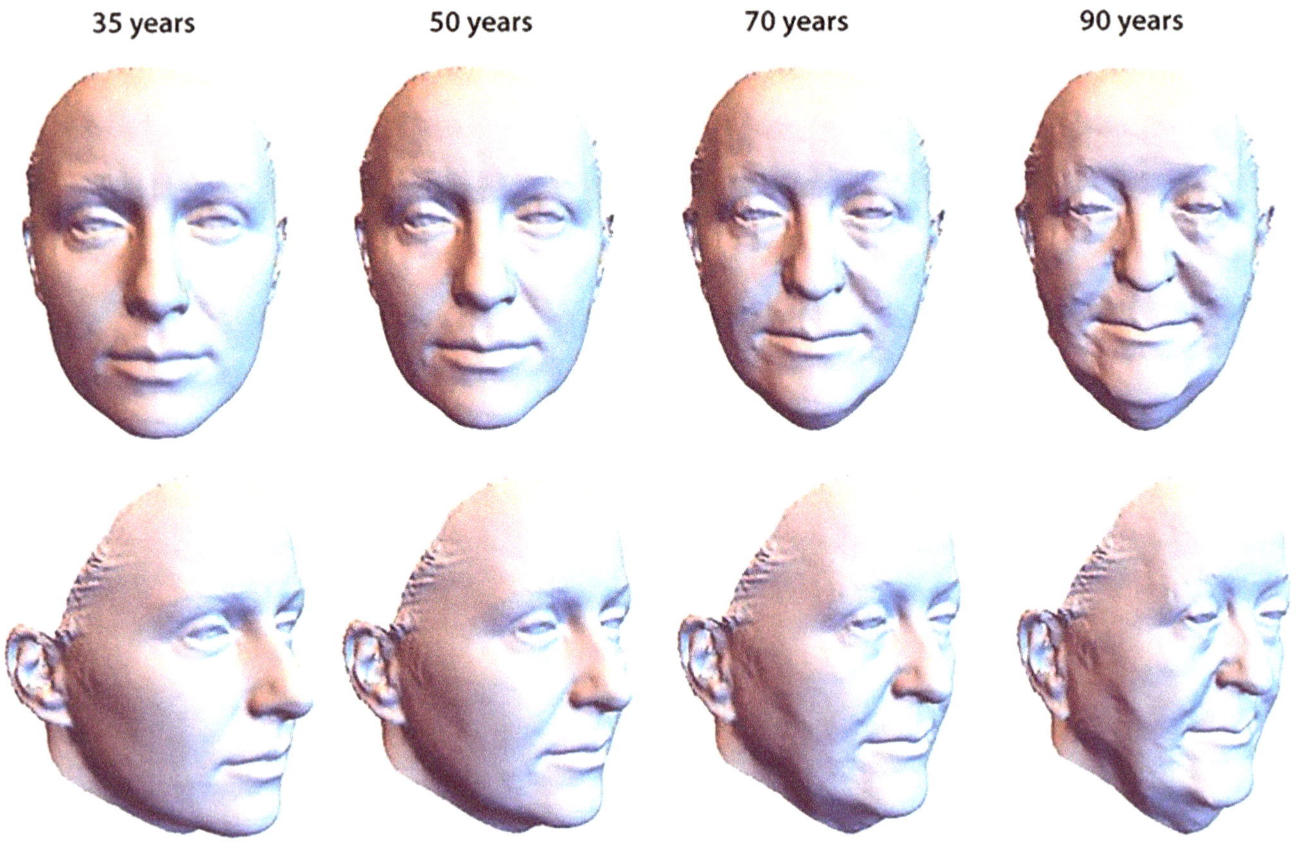

Fig. 2.27. Visualization of female facial aging in women younger than 55 years was derived from a linear regression of face shape on women aged ≤54 years ($P < .0001$, $n = 23$). Broadly, the predicted 70-year and 90-year faces are extrapolations of premenopausal aging to depict the shape changes more legibly. Aging in younger female faces resembled the male pattern, yet at about twice its pace. *(Courtesy Sonja Windhager.)*

Further Reading

Antel DE. How environmental and lifestyle choices influence the aging process. *Ann Plast Surg.* 1999;43:585–588.

Barron-Hernandez YL, Tosti A. Bimatoprost for the treatment of eyelash, eyebrow and scalp alopecia. *Expert Opin Investig Drugs.* 2017;26:515–522.

Defatta RJ, Williams EF. Evolution of midface rejuvenation. *Arch Facial Plast Surg.* 2009;11:6–12.

El-Domyati M, Attia S, Saleh F, et al. Intrinsic aging vs. photoaging: a comparative histopathological, immunohistochemical, and ultrastructural study of skin. *Exp Dermatol.* 2002;11:398–405.

Faerber TH. Evaluation of the aging face. In: Niamtu J, ed. *Oral and Maxillofacial Surgery Clinics of North America: Cosmetic Facial Surgery.* Philadelphia, PA: Saunders; 2000:523–530.

Farkas LG, Posnick JC, Hreczko TM. Anthropometric growth study of the ear. *Cleft Palate Craniofac J.* 1992;29:324–329.

Ferrario VF, Sforza C, Ciusa V, et al. Morphometry of the normal human ear: a cross-sectional study from adolescence to mid-adulthood. *J Craniofac Genet Dev Biol.* 1999;19:226–233.

Guinot C, Malvy DJ, Ambroisine L, et al. Relative contribution of intrinsic vs extrinsic factors to skin aging as determined by a validated skin age score. *Arch Dermatol.* 2002;138:1454–1460.

Heathcote JA. Why do old men have big ears? *BMJ.* 1995;311:1668.

Hill 3rd RH, Czyz CN, Kandapalli S, et al. Evolving minimally invasive techniques for tear trough enhancement. *Ophthal Plast Reconstr Surg.* 2015;31:306–309.

Jenkins G. Molecular mechanisms of skin ageing. *Mech Ageing Dev.* 2002;123:801–810.

Klein AW, ed. *Tissue Augmentation in Clinical Practice.* New York, NY: Taylor & Francis; 2006:141–238.

Krutmann J, Grewe M. Involvement of cytokines, DNA damage, and reactive oxygen intermediates in ultraviolet radiation-induced modulation of intercellular adhesion molecule-1 expression. *J Invest Dermatol.* 1995;105:67S–70S.

Lambros VS. Facial aging: a 54-year, three-dimensional population study. *Plast Reconstr Surg.* 2020;145:921–928.

Lambros VS. Discussion: quantitative evaluation of volume augmentation in the tear trough with a hyaluronic acid-based filler: a three-dimensional analysis. *Plast Reconstr Surg.* 2010;125:1523–1524.

Liu TC, Chen YS. Aging and external ear resonance. *Audiology.* 2000;39:235–237.

Ma W, Wlaschek M, Tantcheva-Poor I, et al. Chronological ageing and photoageing of the fibroblasts and the dermal connective tissue. *Clin Exp Dermatol.* 2001;26:592–599.

Makrantonaki E, Zouboulis CC. William J. Cunliffe Scientific Awards. Characteristics and pathomechanisms of endogenously aged skin. *Dermatology.* 2007;214:352–360.

Mally P, Czyz CN, Wulc AE. The role of gravity in periorbital and midfacial aging. *Aesthet Surg J.* 2014;34:809–822.

Motosko CC, Khouri KS, Poudrier G, Sinno S, Hazen A. Evaluating platelet-rich therapy for facial aesthetics and alopecia: a critical review of literature. *Plast Reconstr Surg.* 2018;141:1115–1123.

Pessa JE, Slice DE, Hanz KR, et al. Aging and the shape of the mandible. *Plast Reconstr Surg.* 2008;121:196–200.

Pessa JE, Zadoo VP, Mutimer KL, et al. Relative maxillary retrusion as a natural consequence of aging: combining skeletal and soft tissue changes into an integrated model of midfacial aging. *Plast Reconstr Surg.* 1998;102:205–212.

Pessa JE, Zadoo VP, Yuan C, et al. Concertina effect and facial aging: nonlinear aspects of youthfulness and skeletal remodeling and why, perhaps, infants have jowls. *Plast Reconstr Surg.* 1999;103:635–644.

Pottier F, El-Shazly NZ, El-Shazly AE. Aging of orbicularis oculi: anatomophysiologic consideration in upper blepharoplasty. *Arch Facial Plast Surg.* 2008;10:346–349.

Reece EM, Pessa JE, Rorich RJ. The mandibular septum: anatomical observations of the jowls in aging—implications for facial rejuvenation. *Plast Reconstr Surg.* 2008;121:1414–1420.

Rohrich RJ, Pessa JE. The fat compartments of the face: anatomy and clinical implications for cosmetic surgery. *Plast Reconstr Surg.* 2007;119:2219–2227.

Rohrich RJ, Ghavami A, Mojallal A. The five-step lower blepharoplasty: blending the eyelid-cheek junction. *Plast Reconstr Surg.* 2011;128:775–783.

Rubin M. *Manual of Chemical Peels.* Philadelphia, PA: Lippincott-Raven; 1995.

Schiller JD. Lysis of the orbicularis retaining ligament and orbicularis oculi insertion: a powerful modality for lower eyelid and cheek rejuvenation. *Plast Reconstr Surg.* 2012;129:692e–700e.

Stevens HP, Willemsen JC, Durani P, et al. Triple-layer midface lifting: long-term follow-up of an effective approach to aesthetic surgery of the lower eyelid and the midface. *Aesthetic Plast Surg.* 2014;38:632–640.

Stuzin JM, Baker HL, Gordon TJ. The relationship of the superficial and deep facial fascias: relevance to rhytidectomy and aging. *Plast Reconstr Surg.* 1992;89:441–451.

Swift A, Liew S, Weinkle S, Garcia JK, Silberberg MB. The facial aging process from the "inside out." *Aesthet Surg J.* 2021;41:1107–1119.

Tan R, Osman V, Tan G. Ear size as a predictor of chronological age. *Arch Gerontol Geriatr.* 1997;25(2):187–191.

Wan D, Amirlak B, Rohrich RJ, et al. The clinical importance of the fat compartments in midfacial aging. *Plast Reconstr Surg Global Open.* 2013;1:92.

Wang XY, Bi ZG. UVB-irradiated human keratinocytes and interleukin-1alpha indirectly increase MAP kinase/AP-1 activation and MMP-1 production in UVA-irradiated dermal fibroblasts. *Chin Med J.* 2006;119:827–831.

Windhager S, Mitteroecker P, Rupić I, Lauc T, Polašek O, Schafer K. Facial aging trajectories: a common shape pattern in male and female faces is disrupted after menopause. *Am J Phys Anthropol.* 2019;169:678–688.

Wulf HC, Sandby-Moller J, Kobayasi T, et al. Skin aging and natural photoprotection. *Micron.* 2004;35:185–191.

Yahoo Answers. Do noses or ears grow larger as we age? Is this true? http://answers.yahoo.com/question/index?qid=20060919041955AAEyteP.

Yang C, Zhang P, Xing X. Tear trough and palpebromalar groove in young versus elderly adults: a sectional anatomy study. *Plast Reconstr Surg.* 2013;132:796–808.

Zufferey JA. The nasolabial fold: an attempt of synthesis. *Plast Reconstr Surg.* 1999;104:2318–2320.

CHAPTER 3

Facelift Anatomy

Joe Niamtu, III

Chapter Outline

I personally think that there exists a time when a young surgeon suddenly begins to subconsciously visualize anatomy in three dimensions subconsciously. By this I mean that when this surgeon is operating on the side of the face, they can "see" the facial nerve, parotid duct, facial artery and vein, parotid gland, and so on. Obviously, this applies to any surgeon anywhere on the body. This does not happen overnight, as younger surgeons tend to think in two dimensions. When a person truly understands anatomy, it becomes 3D.

Facial anatomic expertise is imperative to performing competent facelift surgery and avoiding complications. Facelift surgery and anatomy are inseparable, and great surgeons are great anatomists. An organized way to discuss facial anatomy is to consider the progressive layers encountered during the procedure from skin to bone (Figs. 3.1 and 3.2).

Layers of the face:

Layer 1: skin
Layer 2: subcutaneous
Layer 3: superficial fascia (musculoaponeurotic)
Layer 4: areolar plane
Layer 5: deep fascia

Layer 1: Skin

The first (outermost) layer concerned in facelift anatomy is the skin. Facial skin varies in thickness, being thinnest in the eyelids and thickest on the nasal tip and forehead. The dermal plexus of blood vessels nourishes the skin (and facelift flap) and must always be respected. The handling of lipocutaneous flaps in cosmetic facial surgery should be as gentle as other procedures in which flap vascularity is essential to its survival. During facelift dissection, several millimeters of fat is left adherent to the dermal undersurface to protect this area and enhance flap viability. Many surgeons recommend a flap 5 mm in thickness. A general rule is that there should be fat on both sides of the facelift flap.

Layer 2: Subcutaneous

The next layer is the subcutaneous layer. This is the layer that is between the dermis and superficial musculoaponeurotic system (SMAS). The subcutaneous layer is basically a safe layer in the face and can be undermined in the subcutaneous plane without damaging significant anatomic structures. This layer is of varying thickness depending upon the location and patient. The subcutaneous layer is plentiful in the cheeks and anterior neck but is extremely thin in the postauricular mastoid region. Very mobile structures, such as the lips and eyelids, have very little subcutaneous fat. Connective tissue fibers known as "retinacular cutis" originate at the periosteum and travel through the deep layers to terminate in the dermis. The subcutaneous layer becomes thickened over the malar region, where dissection can be tenuous. This tissue is attached to the malar periosteum by retaining ligaments that run from the underlying periosteum through the malar pad and insert into the dermis. This area is very tenacious and because of its fibrous nature provides resistance when dissecting; it is referred to as "McGregor's patch." Brisk bleeding is also frequently seen in the area due to accompanying vasculature. The thickest layer of subcutaneous fat underlies the nasolabial folds.

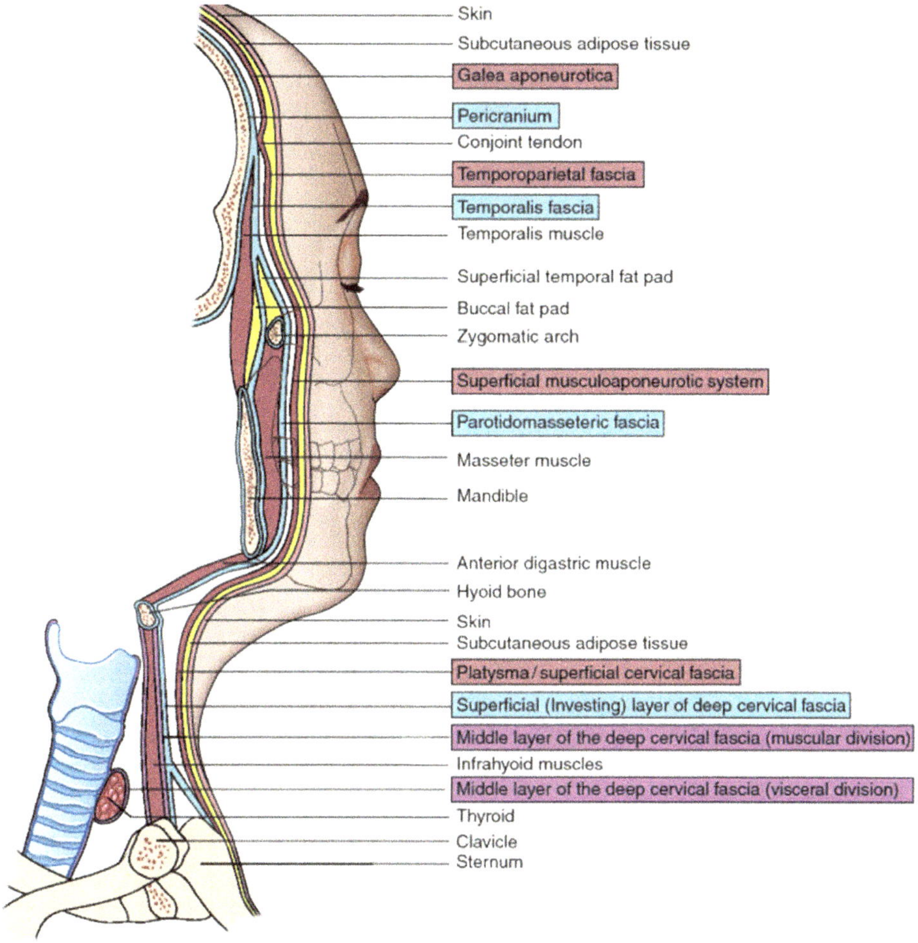

Fig. 3.1. Grouping the soft tissue layers of the face and neck. The brown color signifies the superficial layers, the purple color signifies the intermediate layers, and the blue color signifies the deep anatomic layers.

Layer 3: Superficial Fascia (Musculoaponeurotic)

The third layer is the superficial facial fascia (SMAS) layer. This layer separates the overlying subcutaneous fat from the underlying parotidomasseteric fascia and facial nerve branches and envelopes the facial mimetic muscles including orbicularis oculi, zygomatic major and minor, risorius and platysma. The SMAS does not invest the masticatory muscles, which are deeper.

The superficial fascia (Table 3.1 and Figs. 3.1 and 3.2) is formed from scalp to neck by:

- The galea aponeurotica (which splits to envelope the frontalis and occipitalis)
- The superficial temporal fascia (also called "temporoparietal fascia")
- The superficial facial fascia (SMAS) in the cheek region (which splits to envelope the midface mimetic muscles)
- The superficial cervical fascia (which splits to envelope the platysma).

The Superficial Musculoaponeurotic System

Understanding all of the aforementioned layers is essential to understanding and safely performing facelift surgery. Although each layer is complex in its own right, the SMAS is the most controversial layer, and its nomenclature is used correctly and incorrectly by surgeons and authors alike. The SMAS layer is a fibrofatty muscular layer in the cheek. It has been described by many leading authors and is said to be continuous with the galea in the scalp, the temporoparietal fascia in the temporal region, and the superior cervical fascia in the neck. This structure was initially described by Dr. Paul Tessier Fellows, Dr. Vladimir Mitz, and Dr. Martine Peyronie as muscular and fibrous tissue and termed the "superficial musculoaponeurotic system." They stated the SMAS exists in the parotid and cheek regions and invests the muscles of facial expression. In their original 1976 article, the authors state, "To us, the SMAS appears to be a fibromuscular network located between the facial muscles and the dermis, one which covers the facial motor nerves." They note that the SMAS separates two layers of fat in the face into superficial and deep layers. Their work also implied that the SMAS was continuous with the platysma.

Various authors contest Mitz and Peyronie's finite description of the SMAS and related layers, and some surgeons do not agree that there is any such thing as the SMAS at all. Reviewing the historic literature on the SMAS is, to say the least confusing and frequently contradictory.

I think most contemporary surgeons will agree the SMAS separates the subcutaneous fat from the underlying parotidomasseteric fascia. When a surgeon states that they pick up the SMAS,

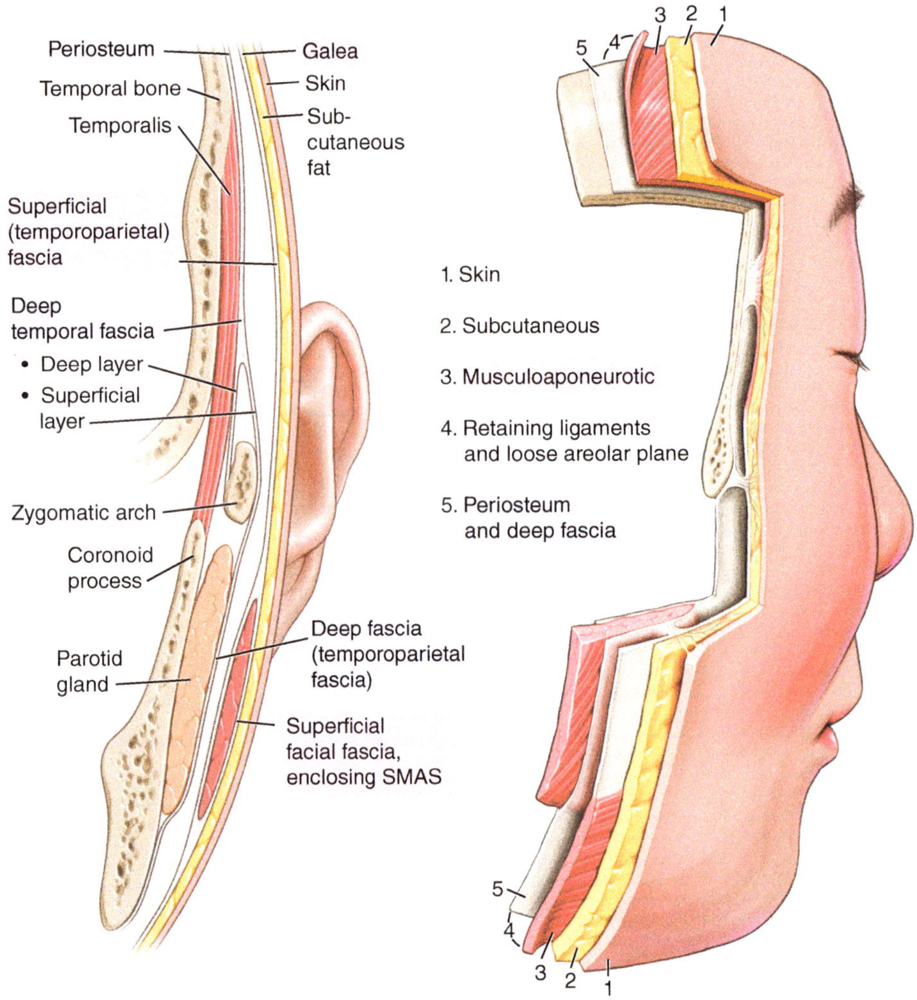

Fig. 3.2. Soft tissue anatomical layers of the face. Superficial layers are show in pink boxes and deep layers in the purple boxes.

Layer 3
Superficial Fascia (Musculoaponeurotic)

The galea aponeurotica
(which splits to envelope the frontalis and occipitalis)

The temporoparietal fascia
(also called superficial temporal fascia)

The superficial musculoaponeurotic system
(in the cheek region, also called the superficial facial fascia which splits to envelope the midface mimetic muscles)

The superficial cervical fascia
(which splits to envelope the platysma)

Table 3.1. The superficial fascial layers are listed from cephalad to caudad.

in reality they are picking up the subcutaneous adipose tissue and connective (aponeurotic) tissue above the parotidomasseteric fascia. This fibro-fatty-muscular tissue is what is frequently plicated, excised, imbricated, and otherwise managed in facelift surgery. Whether you agree or disagree with concepts about the embryology and histology, the remainder of this text will refer to the "SMAS" as the tissue between the dermis and parotidomasseteric fascia. The subcutaneous tissue and SMAS may be histologically and microscopically separate layers, but in actual surgery they are picked up, cut, pulled, and sewn as a single layer. Teleologically, this makes sense, as the physiologic function of the SMAS is to more effectively transfer mimetic muscle movement to the facial skin by septae that extend from the SMAS to the dermis. In theory, this would allow kinetic amplification, allowing the face to move more as a unit (as opposed to each individual muscle), thus making expression more efficient. When traction is placed on this layer, it moves all of the superficial layers of tissue, including the mimetic muscles, and basically repositions the deep ptotic facial tissues in the desired vector to reset the facial "mask" (Fig. 3.3).

All motor nerves providing movement of the facial muscles are deep to the SMAS plane (under the deep fascial layer).

Layer 4: Areolar Plane

This is a less defined layer that contains facial spaces, retaining ligaments, and the facial nerve branches.

Layer 5: Deep Fascia and Periosteum

This consists of the periosteum over bone and the deep fascia of the face and neck.

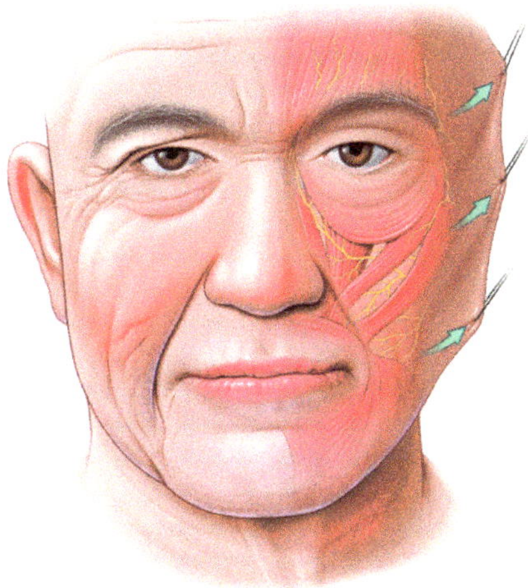

Fig. 3.3. Elevating the superficial musculoaponeurotic system (SMAS) allows resuspension of the ptotic deep tissues of the mid and lower face. Significant mobility and elevation occur at the neck and jawline. The midfacial tissues are more bound down and have less mobility. Virtually all techniques of contemporary rhytidectomy involve some form of SMAS management.

The deep layer of fascia is formed by:

- The periosteum in skull
- Temporalis fascia in the temple region (Over bony structures such as zygoma and cranium, this layer is indistinguishable from periosteum.)
- The parotidomasseteric fascia (deep facial fascia)
- The investing layer of the deep cervical fascia

Below these layers lie the muscles of mastication, the salivary glands, and principal neurovascular structures.

Staying superficial to the parotidomasseteric fascia (deep fascia) is a safe level of protection during facelift surgery, as the facial nerve branches lie inferior to this plane.

These fascial layer descriptions can be very confusing as they have multiple names and are frequently mischaracterized in various texts and diagrams. I believe the easiest way to understand them is to appreciate the two layers of fascia in the head and neck: superficial and deep. The first layer is the superficial fascia, which includes the galea, temporoparietal fascia, SMAS, and the superior cervical fascia (Table 3.1, Figs. 3.4 [*left*], 3.5, and 3.6). The second layer is the deep fascia which includes the periosteum of the skull, the temporalis fascia, the parotidomasseteric fascia, and the deep cervical fascia (Table 3.2, Figs. 3.1, 3.2, 3.4 [*right*], and 3.5–3.7).

The loose areolar plane lies between these two fascial layers, which accounts for the gliding mobility of the tissues in these areas.

Author's note:

What can become confusing is the deep temporal fascia. The outer temporalis fascia is intimate to the temporalis muscle and is often referred to as the "superficial layer of deep temporal fascia." This layer splits at the zygomatic arch and is separated by a fat pad as shown in Figs. 3.1 and 3.2. The lateral split of tissue is referred to as the "superficial layer of the deep temporal fascia" and the medial layer of the split is referred to as the "deep layer of the deep temporal fascia." Some surgeons mistakenly call the fascia on the cranial side of the temporalis muscle the "deep layer of deep temporalis fascia." This is not the case, and as stated in the previous sentence, the "deep layer of the deep temporalis fascia" occurs after the split on the arch. Many surgeons simplify this nomenclature by simply referring to these layers as "temporalis fascia."

Surgically speaking, this plane is "tiger territory"! Although this plane can be violated and navigated by experienced surgeons, many complications can be encountered by inadvertent entry by novice surgeons. Fig. 3.8 shows the facial nerve branches in relation to the face, and Fig. 3.9 shows the facial nerve branches crossing the masseter muscle under the masseteric fascia.

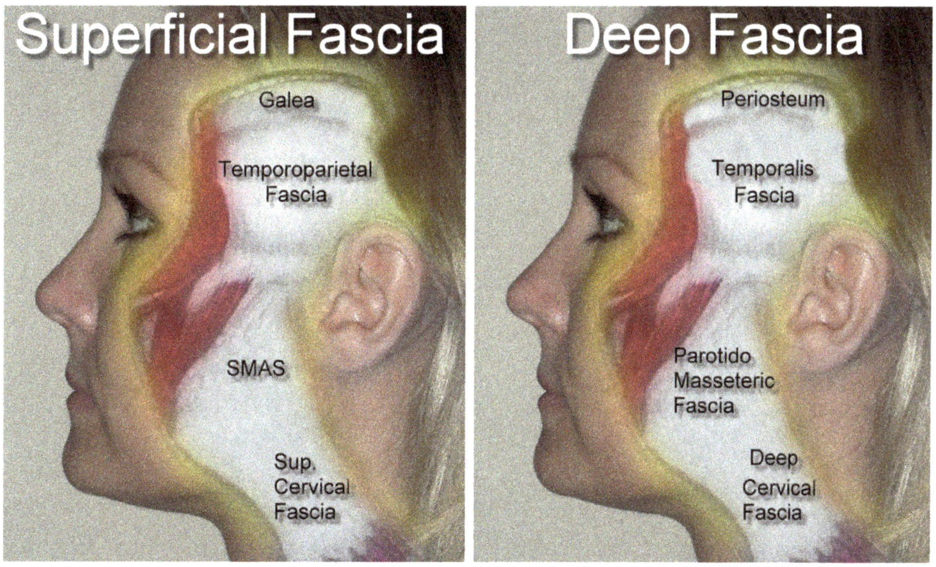

Fig. 3.4. This image is meant as the author's representation of a more complex and detailed true anatomic diagram. This simplification is used for explanation of the superficial fascia layers (*right*) and the deep fascial layers (*left*). *SMAS*, Superficial musculoaponeurotic system.

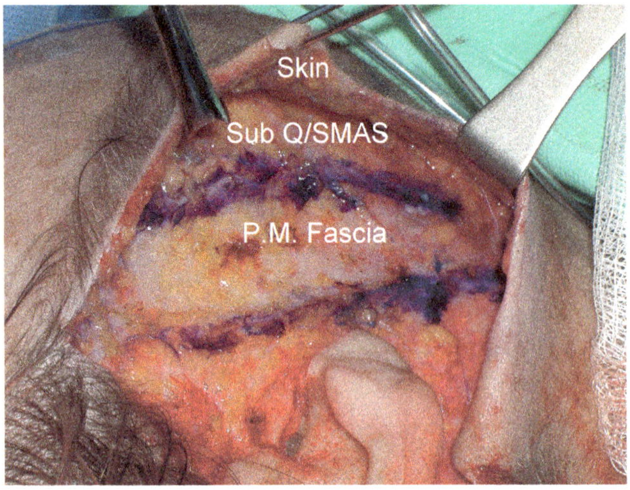

Fig. 3.5. A clinical image on a live patient shows the various layers encountered during faceilft surgery including the skin, subcutaneous fat and SMAS layer, and the parotidomasseteric fascia layer.

Layer 5 Deep Fascia
The periosteum in skull
The superficial layer of the deep temporal fascia in the temple region (over bony structures such as zygoma and cranium, this layer is indistinguishable from periosteum)
The parotidomasseteric fascia (deep facial fascia)
The investing layer of the deep cervical fascia

Table 3.2. The deep facial fascia layers are listed from cephalad to caudad.

The parotid gland is also very important in facelift surgery, as the facial nerve branches are deeper in the parotid gland until they emerge at the anterior border of the gland and cross the masseter muscle. Novice surgeons frequently limit their SMAS treatment to an area over the actual parotid gland. More experienced surgeons, or those performing deep plane dissections, can dissect more distally. Keeping any SMAS-tightening procedure over the confines of the parotid gland is the safest route for inexperienced surgeons. It is this sub-SMAS junction of parotid gland and masseter muscle that constitutes one of the major danger zones in facelift surgery. The parotidomasseteric fascia is very thin over this region, and the underlying facial nerve branches are vulnerable (Fig. 3.9). There is a sub-SMAS loose areolar tissue plane that extends from the anterior border of the parotid to the anterior border of the masseter. When performing deep plane (subSMAS) dissection, spreading instruments or the surgeon's finger can frequently be used to separate this loose areolar layer.

Another reason the facial nerves are protected in deep plane dissection is that most nerves innervate the mimetic muscles on their inferior surface (under the muscle). The only muscles of facial expression that have superficial (on top of the muscle) innervation are the deepest lying muscles—the levator anguli oris, the buccinator, and the mentalis—which are all innervated on their anterior surfaces (Fig. 3.10). These muscles are also the deepest of the facial mimetic muscles. Again, this level of dissection should be limited to experienced surgeons only, to prevent motor nerve damage. Staying over the parotid and above the parotid fascia is the safest anatomic area for novice facelift surgeons.

Several other structures are frequently encountered in facelift surgery and are particularly vulnerable to injury. The sternocleidomastoid muscle (SCM) is a significant landmark because the external jugular vein (Figs. 3.11 and 3.12, p. 31) and greater auricular nerve are intimate and traverse this muscle in the midlateral neck at a region known as Erb's point (also called McKinney's point) (Figs. 3.13 and 3.14, p. 31).

The greater auricular nerve originates from the cervical plexus, composed of branches of spinal nerves C2 and C3. It provides sensory innervation for the skin over parotid gland and mastoid process and both surfaces of the outer ear. The external jugular vein and greater auricular nerve lie deep in the SMAS and are protected as long as the dissection remains in the subcutaneous plane. The subcutaneous tissue becomes very thin in this part of the neck, and the dermis is sometimes intimate to the fascia of the sternocleidomastoid muscle, which can jeopardize the nerve and vein (Figs. 3.15 and 3.16, pp. 31–32). The greater auricular nerve is the most commonly injured nerve in facelift surgery.

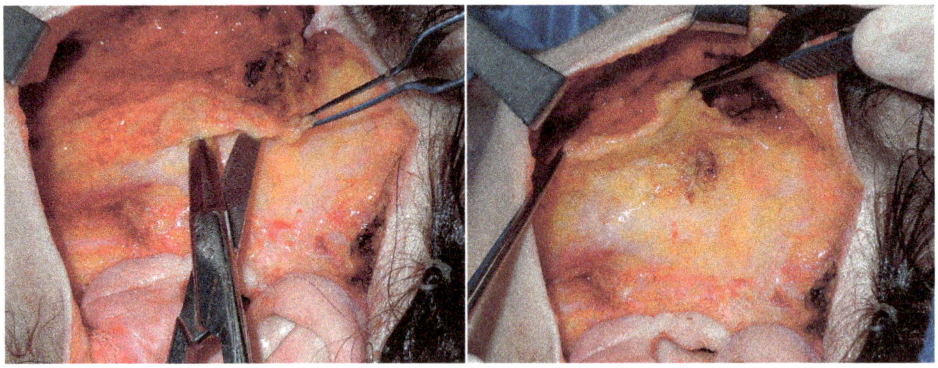

Fig. 3.6. This image shows the superficial musculoaponeurotic system being elevated above the parotidomasseteric fascia as performed in "deep plane" facelift.

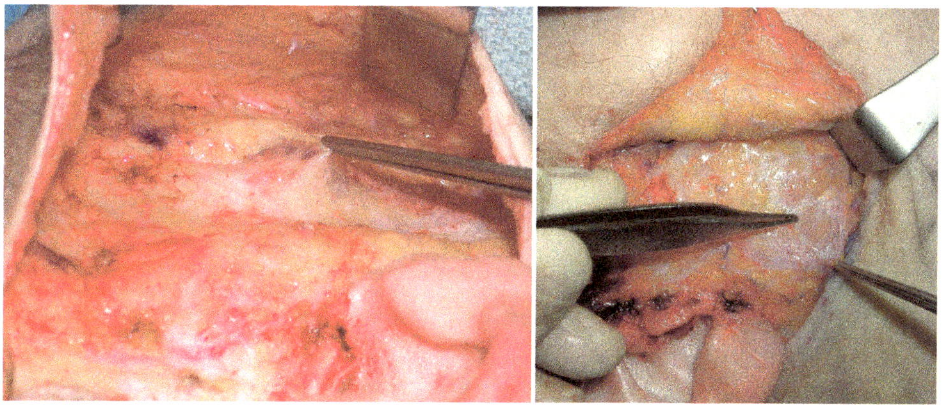

Fig. 3.7. The thin parotidomasseteric fascia (deep fascia) is elevated with forceps during a facelift procedure. The facial nerve branches and parotid duct lie inferior to this layer.

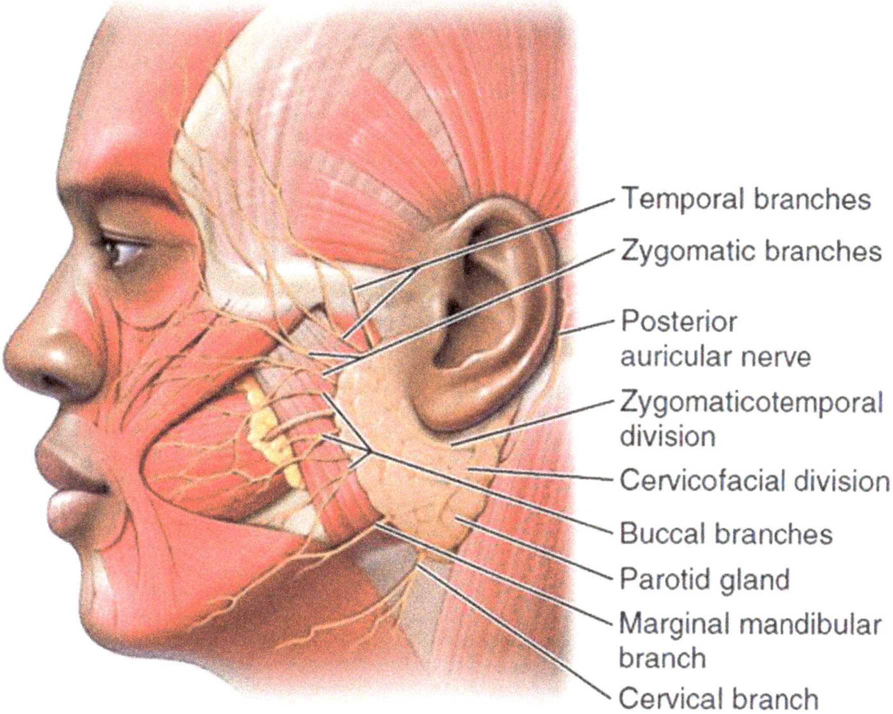

Fig. 3.8. The facial nerve branches are protected within the body of the parotid gland, but are vulnerable as they exit the gland.

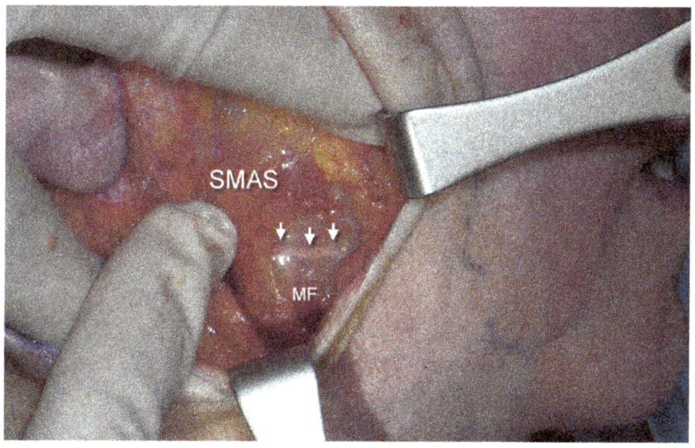

Fig. 3.9. This intraoperative facelift image shows the superficial musculoaponeurotic system (*SMAS*) layer and the underlying glistening masseteric fascia (*MF*), revealing a facial nerve branch (*arrows*) directly underneath. It is this region at the junction of the distal parotid and masseter where the facial nerve branches are particularly vulnerable.

Also of note is that the spinal accessory nerve (cranial nerve XI) exits the posterior border of the SCM also at the level of Erb's point (Fig. 3.16). Technically, Erb's point was classically described as a point where the cervical plexus exits from behind the posterior border of the sternocleidomastoid muscle. The four cutaneous nerves of the cervical plexus are the lesser occipital nerve, great auricular nerve, transverse cervical, and supraclavicular nerve. The scientific literature has many different descriptions of "Erb's" point, and many articles describe the spinal accessory and greater auricular nerve emerging from Erb's point; this description will be used in this text.

This nerve enters the posterior triangle to innervate the trapezius muscle and can be exposed between the posterior border of the SCM and the anterior border of the trapezius muscle. The platysma muscle stops at the midsternocleidomastoid muscle and only skin, a variable amount of fat, and fascia

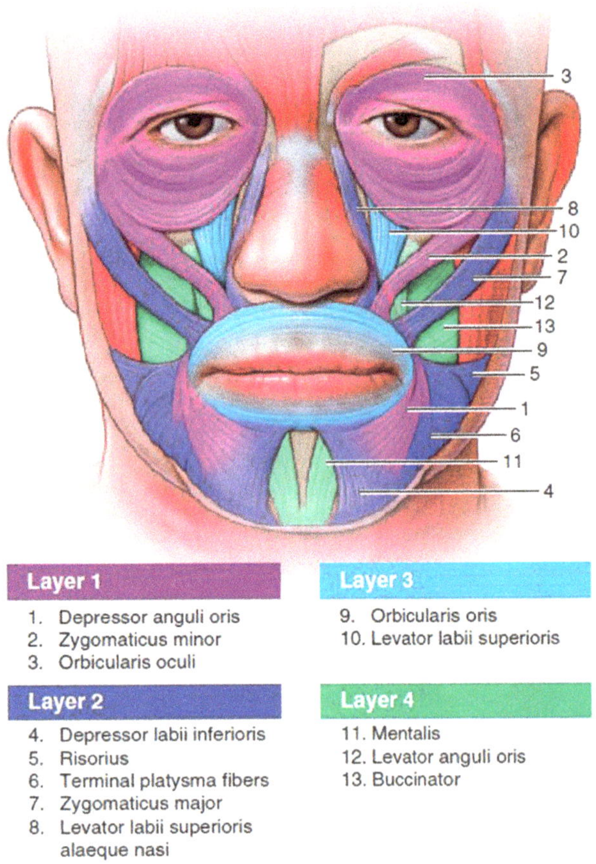

Fig. 3.10. The facial mimetic muscles are protected in deep playing facelift surgery because they are innervated from their inferior (under)surfaces The exception is the buccinator, levator labii superioris, and the mentalis muscles, which are the deepest lying muscles and are innervated on their outer surfaces.

overlie the spinal accessory nerve, making it prone to injury. Surgeons must remain extremely vigilant to avoid sensory and motor nerve damage in this region.

Much has been discussed about neuroanatomy during the facelift procedure; however, the face and neck are some of the most vascular portions on the body and blood supply, knowledge of vascular anatomy, and hemostasis are critical factors in cervical facial rhytidectomy (Fig. 3.17).

The facial artery in vein (branches of the external carotid and jugular veins respectively) provides profusion and return to the facial structures. The vascular pattern closely parallels the course of the facial nerves. Competent surgeons always have a subliminal picture of the underlying anatomy in all steps of an operation. Facelift surgery, like all surgical procedures that involves vascular eye flaps, relies on nourishment of the flap for viability (Fig. 3.18, p. 33). A decrease in blood flow can cause flap necrosis and significant scarring while hemorrhage can cause other complications including hematoma.

The deepest layer in the face is the periosteum and underlying bone. During a facelift, some surgeons perform subperiosteal dissection over the maxilla and mandible in an effort to mobilize the deepest tissue planes to better free the ptotic facial tissues as well as to allow this plane to scar down during healing in hopes of maintaining the lifted position. Cheek and chin implants are frequently performed in conjunction with facelift surgery, and this related subperiosteal dissection may provide additional deep tissue mobilization.

The youthful face is partially suspended by retaining ligaments that support the skin over the facial bones. These ligaments become lax with age and in part are responsible for the sagging of facial tissues. These connective tissue

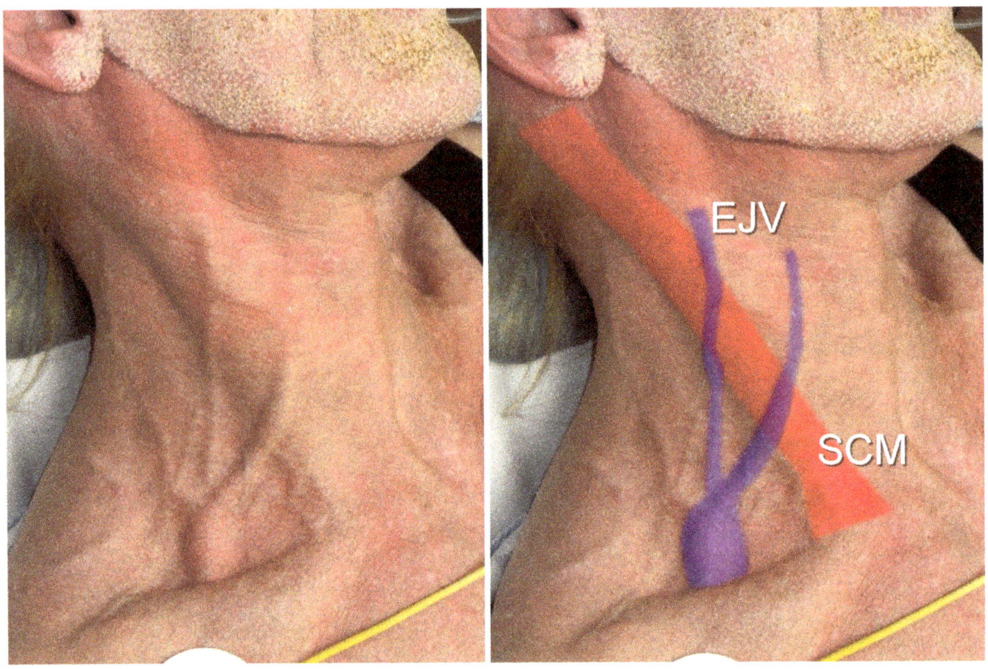

Fig. 3.11. The sternocleidomastoid muscle (*SCM*) is an important landmark in facelift and neck lift surgery for numerous reasons. The external jugular vein (*EJV*) with unusual branching is shown in this patient crossing the SCM.

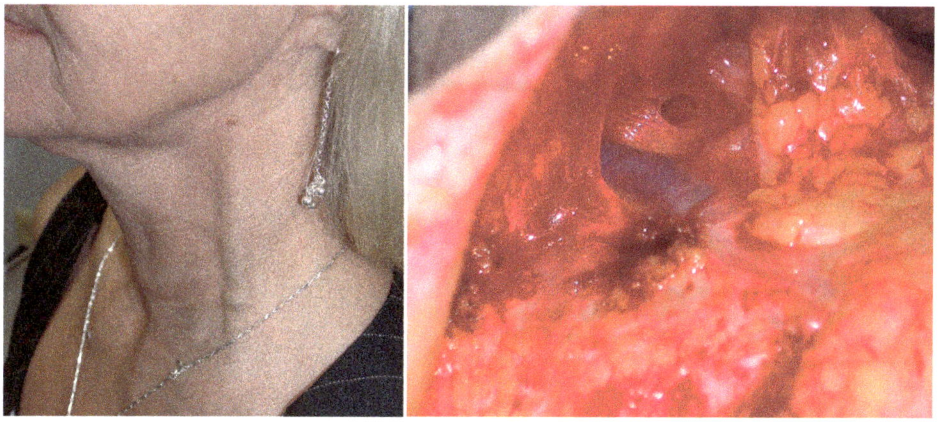

Fig. 3.12. The external jugular vein is shown in a patient preoperatively on the *left* and intraoperatively on the *right*.

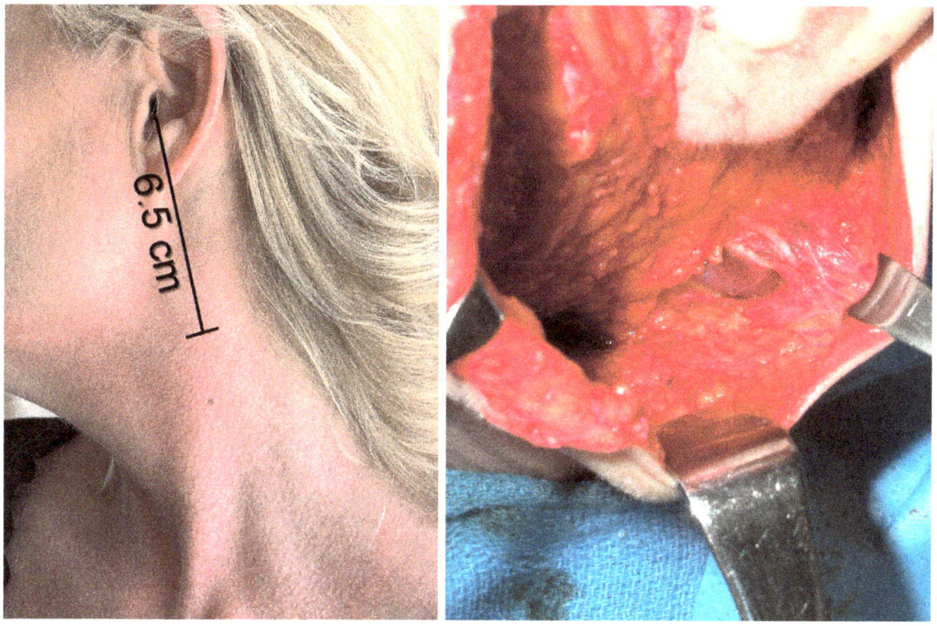

Fig. 3.13. The greater auricular nerve crosses the sternocleidomastoid muscle approximately 6.5 cm inferior from the external auditory canal (*left*) and is frequently anatomically associated with the external jugular vein as shown in the *right* image.

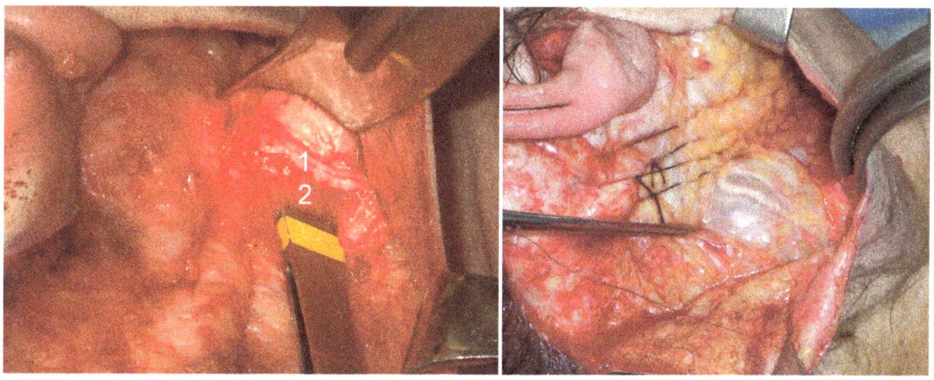

Fig. 3.14. The left image shows the greater auricular (1) in close approximation to the external jugular vein (2). The right image shows the greater auricular nerve lying under the thin fascial layer.

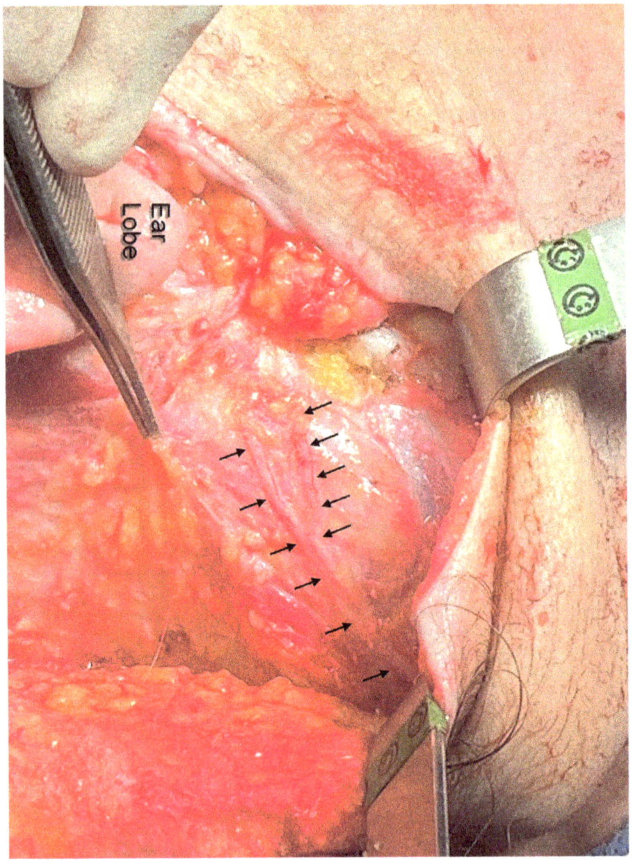

Fig. 3.15. The greater auricular nerve bifurcates to supply sensation to various regions pre- and postauricularly.

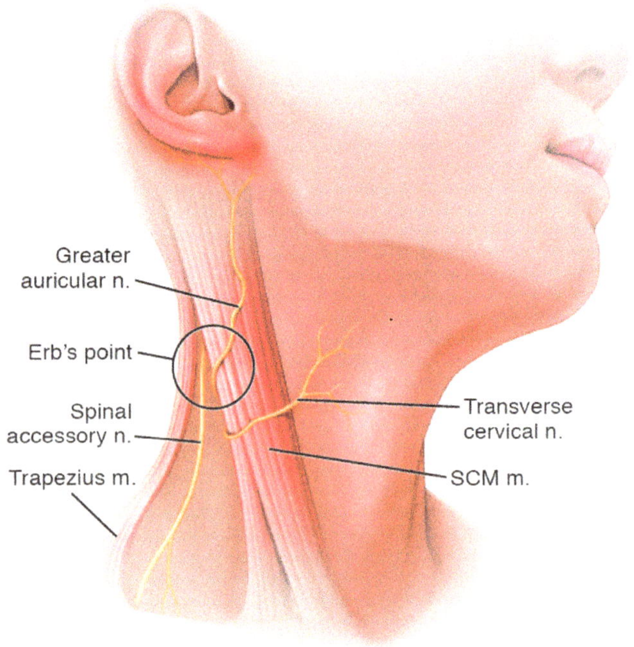

Fig. 3.16. The greater auricular (sensory nerve) and the spinal accessory nerve (motor nerve, cranial nerve XI) both exit the posterior portion of the sternocleidomastoid muscle (*SCM*). The greater auricular nerve crosses the belly of the SCM and is the most commonly injured sensory nerve in facelift surgery. The spinal accessory nerve has a significantly lower rate of injury but is well documented. *m.*, muscle; *n.*, nerve.

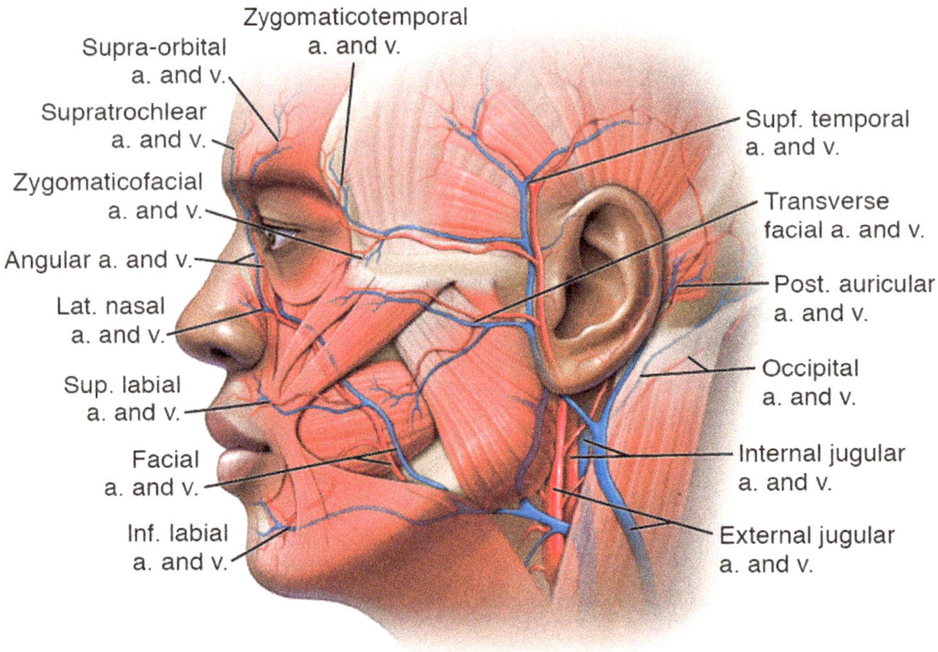

Fig. 3.17. The vascular supply to the face is illustrated. *a.*, artery; *v.*, vein.

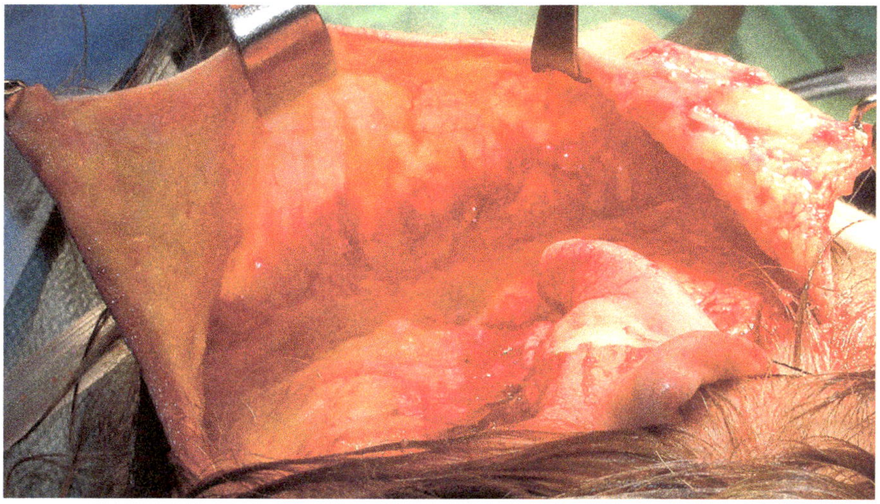

Fig. 3.18. The facelift flap (shown trans illuminated) is nourished by many delicate vessels form the dermal plexus, and any insult to the flap such as over traction, compression, excessive heat or cold can compromise its viability.

ligaments can course from bone to dermis (osteocutaneous ligaments) or from soft tissue to dermis (cutaneous ligaments). The exact name and location of these ligaments is described differently (and sometimes conflictingly) by various authors and texts. Regardless of the various names and anatomic descriptions, these ligaments can be appreciated by the surgeon when performing facelift dissection. The mandibular and zygomatic ligaments present noticeable adhesions that hamper tissue mobilization unless they are released. When the mandibular and or zygomatic ligaments are separated from the dermis, the previously bound tissue becomes noticeably mobile. Release of the masseteric and platysmal retaining ligaments is also performed in most facelift procedures. Fig. 3.19 shows a rendition of the approximate position of these retaining ligaments and Fig. 3.20 shows naturally occurring septae and adhesions that bind the superficial layers to the deeper layers. Retaining ligaments function similarly.

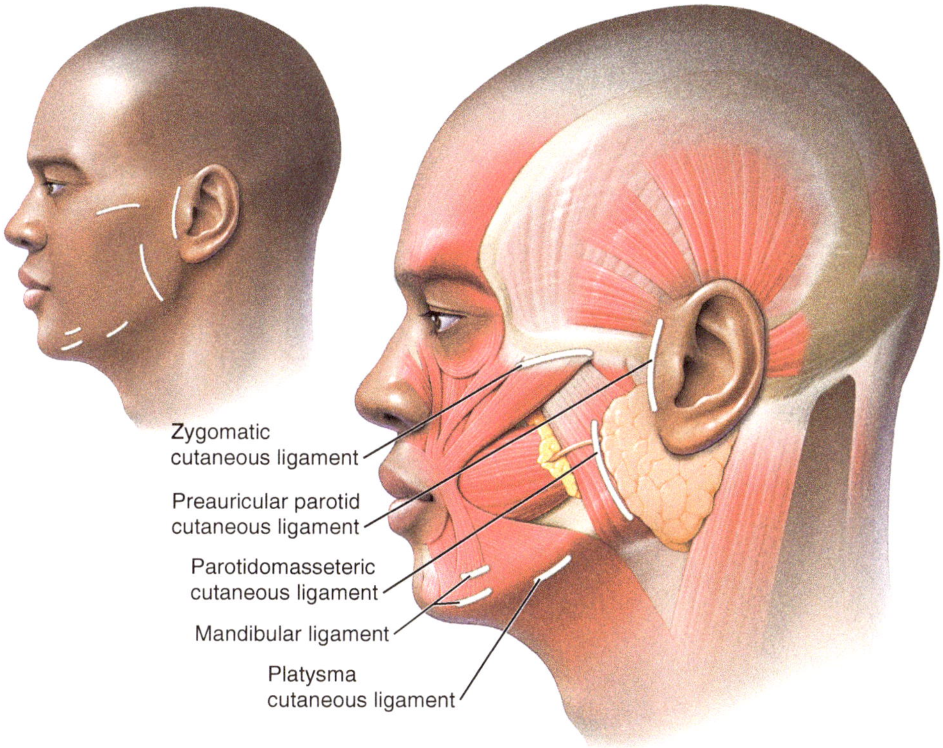

Fig. 3.19. Selected retaining ligaments are shown. These adhesions bind the dermis in numerous areas of the face and neck and require release during facelift dissection.

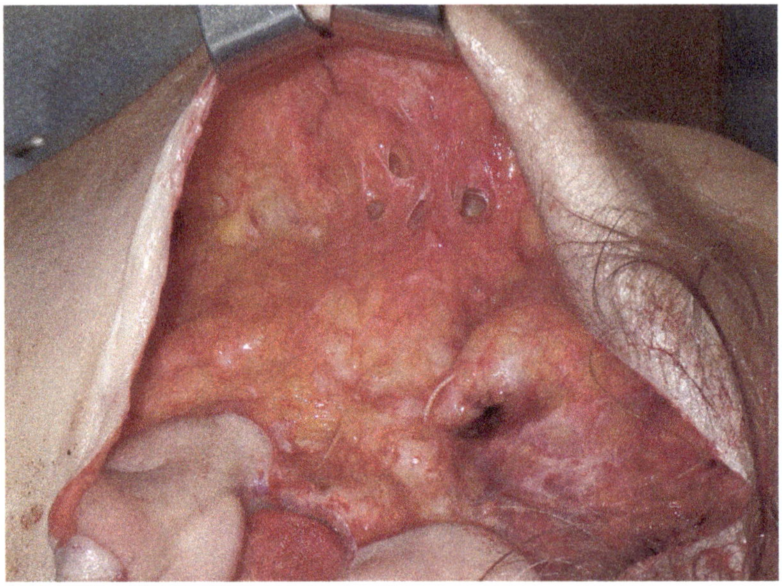

Fig. 3.20. This image shows fibrous septal adhesions in the zygomatic region of the cheek during facelift dissection. Although these structures do not represent the exact ligament per se, they do illustrate naturally occurring adhesions and the necessity of release for proper tissue mobilization.

Further Reading

Jacono AA. Face-lift surgical techniques. *Facial Plast Surg Clin North Am.* 2020 Aug;28(3):xv–xvi.

Kim SH, Choi BG, Chung KJ. Modified **deep-plane facelift** and lower midface lifting using **deep** fat compartment mobilization and zygomaticus major muscle plication. *Plast Reconstr Surg.* 2023 May 15.

Jacono AA, Bryant LM, Alemi AS. Optimal **facelift** vector and its relation to zygomaticus major orientation. *Aesthet Surg J.* 2020 Mar 23;40(4):351–356.

Hu S, Perkins SW. The extended superficial musculoaponeurotic system **deep plane facelift**. *Facial Plast Surg.* 2022 Dec;38(6):575–583.

Jacono AA, Alemi AS, Harmon JJ, Ahmedli N. The effect of a novel platysma hammock flap during extended **deep plane facelift** on the signs of aging in the neck. *Aesthet Surg J.* 2022 Aug 1;42(8):845–857.

CHAPTER 4

Evaluating and Understanding the Cosmetic Surgery Patient in the Preoperative Experience

Joe Niamtu, III

Chapter Outline

Physical Plant: Nonsurgical Spaces

If you perform cosmetic surgery, you have to have an office that is as nice as your biggest competitor. I say this because it is not uncommon for cosmetic surgery patients to seek multiple consultations. They are likely to see your competitors, and if their office grossly outshines yours, you are already at a disadvantage. Having said this, a poor surgeon with a great office will not succeed, but cleanliness and presentation are paramount. Always remember, these are elective patients seeking upper-class luxury surgery. They shop at high-end stores, stay at high-end hotels, and go on high-end vacations. They are used to being pampered and being in nice surroundings (Figs. 4.1 and 4.2). The cosmetic surgery office needs to be set up with this in mind. Having said this, many of my patients are middle class or blue collar, but they are spending outside of their means and expect the same environment as do wealthier patients. If you are just starting your journey, a typical medical space (Fig. 4.3) is not suitable for attracting cosmetic surgery patients in most markets. They simply expect more.

The cosmetic surgery office should be clean, pleasant, and in most practices decorated to accommodate females, since the majority of cosmetic patients are women. Consider your experience at a very high-class hotel and try to duplicate that in your business. You need to think Louis Vuitton and not Walmart. Obviously, this may be a challenge for the new surgeon out of training, but it should be a continual goal. "Concierge care" is a new buzzword, but most successful practices have known these secrets for a century. The entire goal is to get the patients' attention and for them to come and go with positive impressions. They have to realize that you are special and "do it different" and that means "better different." A patient greeter, providing drinks and snacks, assisting patients with paperwork, and having educational material available, underlines your commitment to patient service. Conveniences such as available computers or iPads and a wireless connection are contemporary amenities. If you figure out how to treat your patients special, you will be way ahead of the pack.

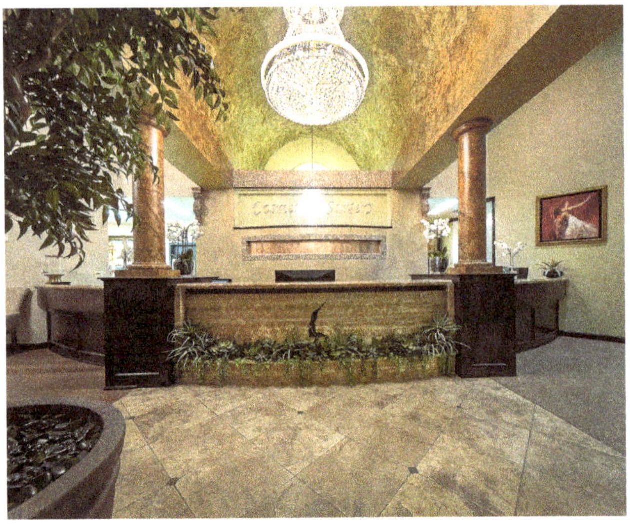

Fig. 4.1. Many cosmetic surgery offices have elegant interiors that cater to high-end patients. *(Courtesy Dr. Angelo Cuzalina.)*

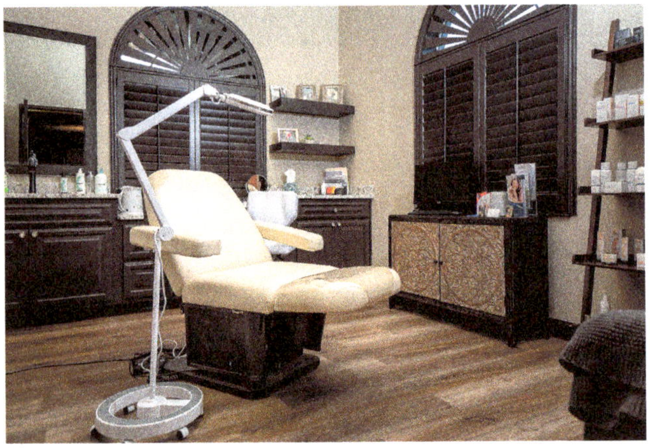

Fig. 4.2. Cosmetic surgery offices should be clean, bright, modern, and spa-like. A dingy medical space is not competition. *(Courtesy Dr. Pam Werschler.)*

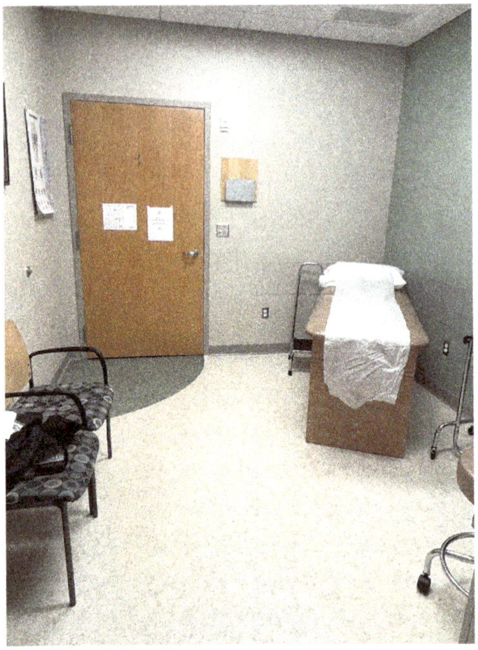

Fig. 4.3. An office similar to this may be commonplace in medicine, but not in cosmetic medicine.

Physical Plant: Surgical Spaces

Surgical spaces are discussed in Chapter 5.

Understanding the Cosmetic Surgery Patient and the Team Approach for the Office

The cosmetic surgery patient is truly a different animal than many of the patients we experience in residency or a specialty practice. The biggest difference is that these are elective patients seeking an upper-class luxury. When treating a patient for trauma or malignancy, they are grateful for your skills as they are emergent and may be lifesaving. Cosmetic surgery, on the other hand, is totally elective and expensive and never emergent. Nobody "needs" elective cosmetic surgery. Fortunately, the vast majority of these patients have positive outcomes and are happy with their treatment. Many cosmetic surgery patients may also have significant biopsychosocial implications that complicate normal interaction. Some of them have unrealistic expectations, some are body dysmorphic, and some are having surgery for the wrong reasons. In these cases, they may be unhappy with perfectly acceptable surgical results, and this is when things can become problematic. One of the best ways to become a great cosmetic surgeon is to choose the right patients and avoid the wrong ones. This is a skill that usually takes decades to master and will be addressed later in this chapter.

There is no more important aspect of the cosmetic surgery experience than the initial patient consult. As they say, you never get a second chance to make a first impression, and the first impression occurs when the patient phones the office to make an appointment. Unfortunately, this is where a lot of patients are lost. Having personable, friendly, energetic staff answering the phone can be one of your best referral sources. Many patients tell me they actually saw three or four other surgeons, but the professionalism and attitude of my staff persuaded them to come to my office.

A good staff, which I refer to as a team, is your most valuable asset. They can make your job fun and exciting or miserable and chaotic. Like any sport, assembling the perfect team takes much work and planning and can take years to get right (Fig. 4.4).

Many barriers between the initial phone call and the operating room can be eliminated by an astute front desk person. We refer to this position as a patient representative. A compassionate patient representative can alleviate many patient apprehensions and get the prospective patient into the office.

An exceptional patient service representative knows how to answer the telephone with a smile and make patients feel comfortable. The first question they ask is the caller's name, which they use frequently throughout the conversation, as everyone likes to hear their own name. A great front desk person can convert a question into a consult. If a patient calls to inquire how much you charge for a facelift, a poor employee with tell them the fee and the conversation is over. An exceptional employee will ask the patient their name. If the patient answers "Anne," the patient representative responds, "Thanks for calling, Anne. Dr. Niamtu has one of the busiest facelift practices on the East Coast and performs over 100 facelifts a year. He has developed his own specialized technique over the past 24 years focusing on patient safety with natural results. He has written numerous textbooks on the subject, gives lectures, and teaches other doctors internationally on his technique. We would love for you to come for a personal consultation. Can we set something up now?"

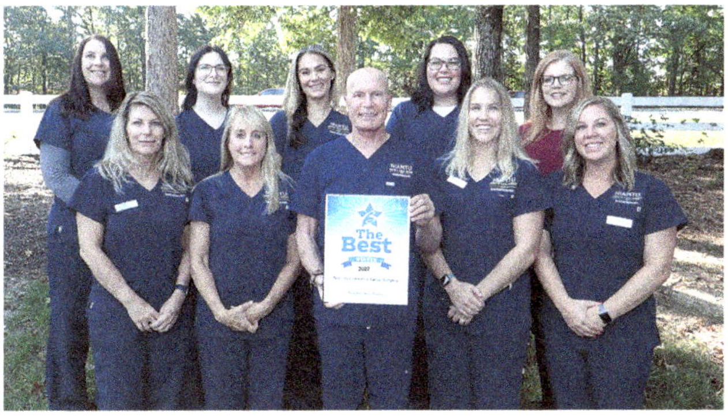

Fig. 4.4. A competent, energetic staff with unconditional focus on patient care can make your job so enjoyable that you never want to retire. This team has helped me win "Best Cosmetic Surgeon" in my city 29 times.

This great patient service representative has now converted a patient with a question into a patient with an appointment. Great patient service representatives are priceless and poor ones can run your business into the ground.

All of our patient representatives are familiar with all of our procedures and can discuss them accurately with prospective patients. All receptionists in our office spend time in the operating room observing procedures, and we also cross-train all our surgical assistants to answer the phones and make appointments. This cross-training allows all employees to appreciate the work of their peers and also means that they can fill in in a pinch.

Just like sports teams, the consistent branding is paramount and includes the use of logos, trademarks, pictures, and so on for all office and marketing materials. All of the printed materials, scrubs, signage, and so on should identify the presence of the team (Fig. 4.5).

The Art of the Consult

So much of what happens on the day of initial consultation can drive whether a patient signs up for surgery or decides to get more opinions. If they are impressed and treated in an incredible manner by an energetic, compassionate, and enjoyable staff, they are much more likely to return for surgery. Always remember that many patients, by default, will see numerous surgical practices for their problem. You have to show them love and make them want to come back. In short, you have to be better than the others.

From the time the patient drives into your parking lot, they must be impressed, and the doctor and team must make sure that everything is in order. Are you easy to find? Is the traffic negotiable? Is it easy to park? Are the grounds and building clean and classy? All of these small elements serve to add up to a final analysis and choice on the part of the patient.

When the patient walks in our door, they are greeted personally, and our staff signs them in and serves them snacks and/or drinks (almost everyone wants some) and makes small talk. If we are running behind, the patients are informed and kept up to date. It is a bad idea to make a new consult patient wait because it sends a very bad signal, so it is important to schedule new patients during predictable times where the office schedule does not run over. If you are running behind, you need something for the patient to do. Getting them from the reception room to a consult room breaks up the wait.

The patient should be escorted from the lobby to the consult room by the person who will be assisting the doctor at the

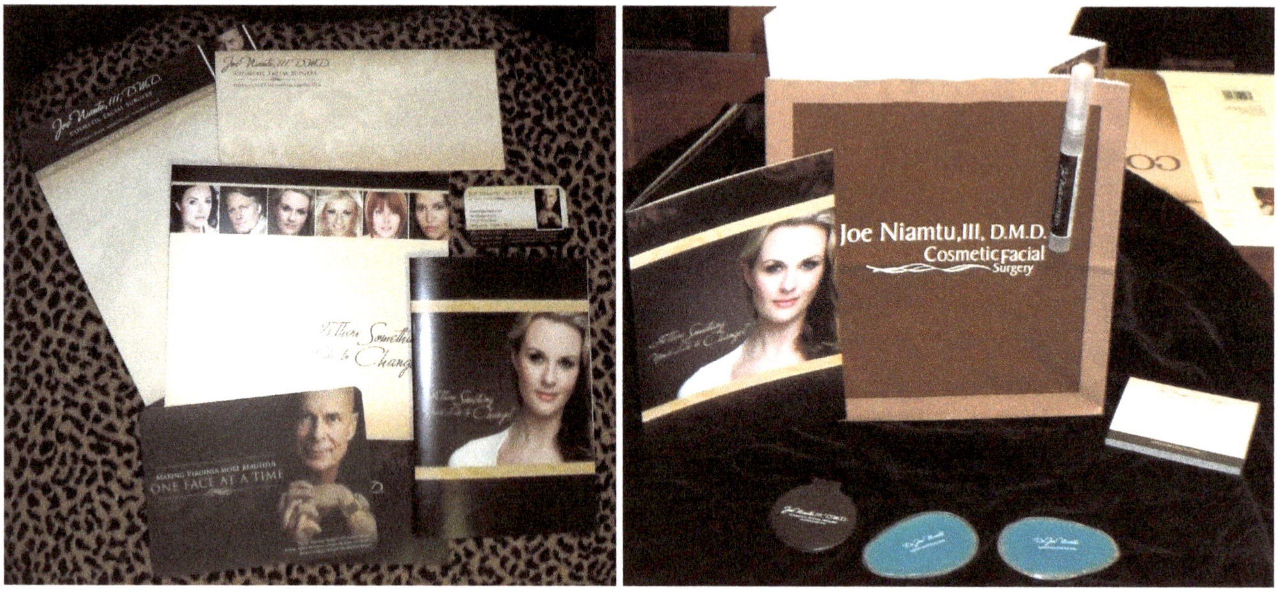

Fig. 4.5. Consistent branding is important in conveying the team concept.

consult. Furthermore, this person should accompany the same patient throughout their entire surgical experience, and this one-on-one bonding is extremely powerful at building relationships. The prospective patient should see smiles and positive energy from every single employee. Once in the consult room, they need something to do if there will be a wait. Having informational literature on hand or better yet, having them spend time on your website getting information about perspective procedures that will be discussed is a great occupier. Many surgeons have videos of them discussing procedures, and this is a great time to use them.

In my practice, the assistant takes the patient to the consult room to begin the process.

It is up to the leader of each practice to decide who is capable of performing quality consultations, but it is a huge convenience in efficiency and cross-training to have all of your staff being proficient in performing consultations. Obviously, it is paramount for whoever is leading the initial evaluation to have a proper understanding of diagnosis and surgery. I have found that surgical assistants are really adept at this since they are a part of the surgical team and totally understand the procedures. I have older staff who integrate very well with my facelift patients because they are of a similar age and it may be easier for the patient to talk someone with aging similarities. On the other hand, I have some very energetic and bubbly young staff that do just as good of a job. It is very important that the person seating the patient and initiating the first discussions is good at what they do. This is such an important position that some surgeons give bonuses to their staff on consultations that are converted to surgical procedures. I personally feel that it is important to monitor the conversion rate (consultations to surgery) of your various staff performing evaluations. Although not 100% accurate, it can give you an idea of the proficiency of the person performing the evaluation.

My practice has a dedicated employee who performs all of the scheduling for surgeries. This staff member wears dress clothes and has a formal business office to meet with the patients after the staff are finished with the clinical consultation. The scheduler is much more than a "scheduler" as she has a lot to do with the patient proceeding to the booking phase for surgery. She has the ability to further bond with the patient as well as follow up with undecided patients. The staff member also hands out formal branded material pertaining to the surgical experience as well as the formalized fee estimates.

In terms of the consultation suite, this room should be the fanciest one in your office and should have a comfortable temperature and pleasant aroma. Aromatherapy is a powerful stimulation of the senses.

It is productive to display any accolades of the surgeon such as awards, academic appointments, charity work, and so on. Patients notice this (Fig. 4.6).

The first order at hand is for the assistant to bond with the patient by making small talk and relaxing the patient (Fig. 4.7).

As a sidebar, if the patient is serious about having a large procedure or is considering multiple procedures, it is frequently helpful to have their spouse at the consult. So often, the spouse (usually the husband) may have considerable concerns about the need for surgery, the finances, and other questions. In addition, he will most likely be the caregiver, and it is important that he realize what will happen.

For many patients, meeting a new doctor makes them very nervous. With cosmetic patients, they not only have to meet a stranger, but have to tell them and show them their biggest physical insecurities. Many patients have problems with aging and do not handle it well. This apprehension can add up to a patient that is literally perspiring by the time the doctor examines them. The best thing your staff can do before the surgeon enters the room is to help relax the patient. It is also very important for the staff to compliment the surgeon. They can make the doctor look good in advance, so the doctor does not have to sound arrogant. People want to know that they are seeing a compassionate, experienced, and popular surgeon and your staff can really help with

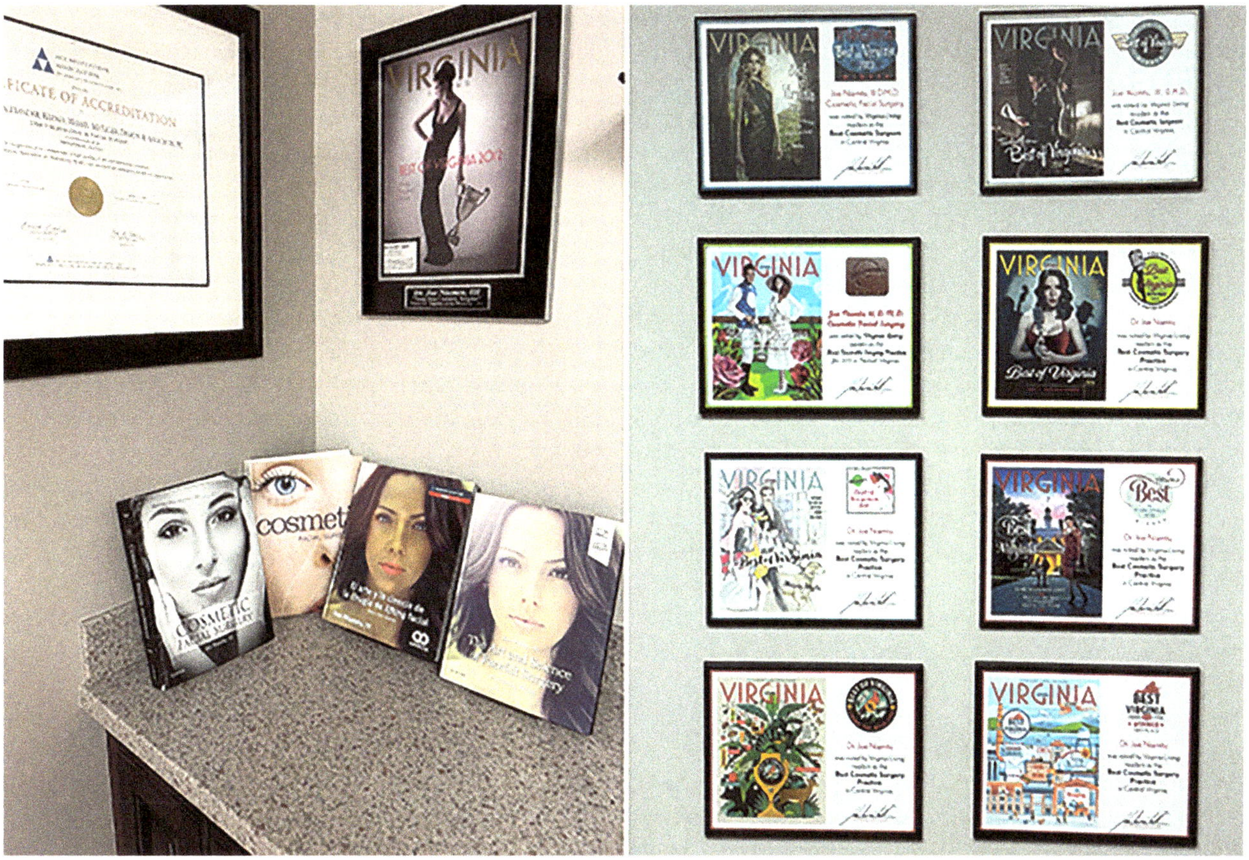

Fig. 4.6. Displaying any accolades of the surgeon or staff is a great way to let your patients know your commitment to your profession.

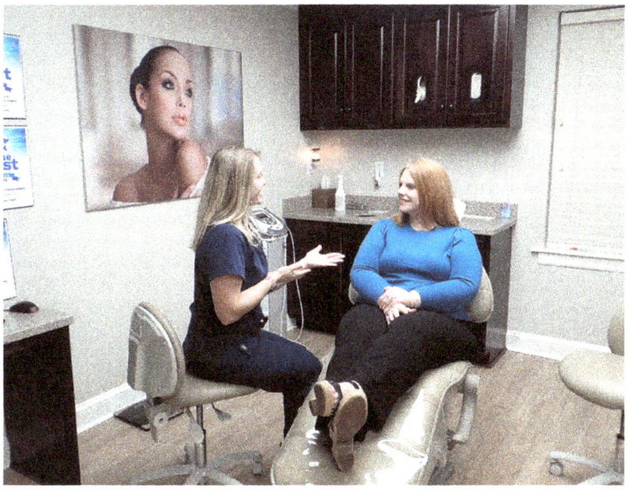

Fig. 4.7. The consultation assistant seats the patient and begins the evaluation. Experienced staff can complete most of the evaluation before the surgeon enters the room.

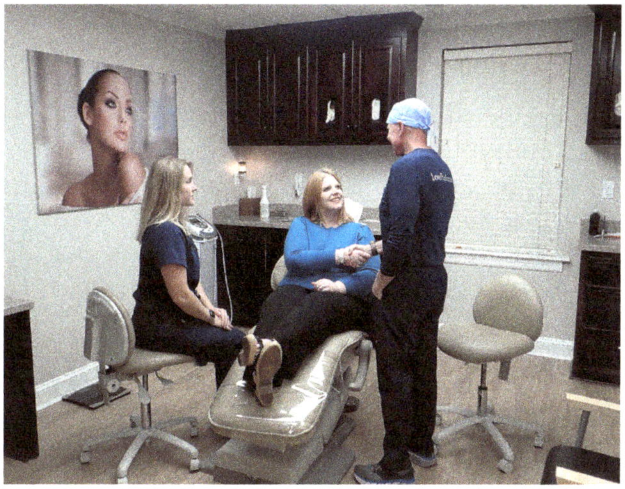

Fig. 4.8. I prefer a casual introduction and consultation. I introduce myself as "Joe" and shake the patient's hand.

this. Although patients are here to discuss cosmetic surgery, having your staff discuss pro bono or community work impresses clients and lets them know you are compassionate.

The assistant also asks the patient what they wish to discuss, and she can make cursory suggestions such as, "I believe Dr. Niamtu will want to discuss eyelid surgery, cheek implants, and a facelift with you." She then opens our website on the widescreen TV and walks the patient through the specific procedure pages to discuss what we do and how we do it. She will also show the patient before-and-after pictures of relative cases. This interaction is important as it gives the patient an idea of what the doctor will discuss and also provides them with information on the procedures and can shorten the surgeon's consultation time.

Meeting the Surgeon

When the staff consultation is completed, the surgeon enters the room and is introduced. I always shake hands with the patient and introduce myself by my first name (Fig. 4.8). I believe friendly, communicative contact puts patients at ease and subliminally enhances the doctor-patient relationship. Showcasing a friendly, smiling, and energetic persona and small talk with the patient before getting to the cosmetic problems and engaging in small talk is time well spent. As stated, patients are frequently nervous, and to relax them I may ask what they do for a living, what their hobbies are, how they heard about our office, how they are enjoying their summer, and so on. Again, putting a patient at ease is an art form. If the patient states that they love playing tennis (or whatever topic), we note that in the patient record, and next time they come, we can ask, "How is the tennis game coming?" They are always impressed we remembered. The world is full of arrogant, stuffy physicians. A smiling, energetic, down-to-earth surgeon is an attention-getter. Too many doctors are arrogant and consider themselves "too important." This is the opposite of what I want to communicate with my patients. I want them to feel that I am down-to-earth, approachable, and a nice guy.

Most of our patients register online and are asked to list their cosmetic facial concerns in advance and bring a list with them. Nervous patients often forget to ask key questions.

The most important instrument used in the consult is a hand mirror. I ask patients to tell me what bothers them when they look in the mirror at home and what they would like to change. I ask them to show me in the hand mirror. At this point I always begin with a compliment like "You have a great jawline" or noting another positive feature I can start the conversation with. Since we are going to be discussing negatives, it is best to begin with a positive. Occasionally a patient will say, "Doctor, what do you think I need?" The novice surgeon should never fall into this trap. It is imperative that the patient take ownership of what bothers them or what they would like to change. A patient that cannot communicate their cosmetic problems may have other underlying problems. Some patients are embarrassed to discuss the topic and need some prodding. The other problem with answering the question "What do you think I need?" is that the surgeon may suggest a problem that the patient doesn't see and offend the patient.

Some practice management experts say that you should not hand a woman a mirror, as it is offensive to make her look at her flaws. I do not agree with this. Every single patient looks in the mirror at home, and most of them pull their facial skin back. The mirror (and now cell phones) is where the rubber meets the road. An alternative to using a mirror is to take several pictures of the patient just before the consult and project those images on the widescreen monitor. This can have significant impact in showing patients their aging changes. Also giving the patient a copy of the pictures to take home can go a long way in having them realize their aging problems, especially in the lateral view, which no patient likes to see. A simpler means of avoiding the mirror is to use a tablet to take front, three-quarter, and side views and share it with the patient.

Although I marketed one of the original digital imaging systems in the 1990s, I am not a fan of surgical predictions. First, they are time consuming, and the doctor or staff playing around with digital surgery can waste precious patient time. At one time the cool factor of digital imaging would help promote a doctor or sell a case, but today I feel that it is passe. Second, this is simply a digital cartoon. You can make any patient look good, but you might not necessarily be able to produce that result. The accuracy is often suspect and can also give the patient a false hope of what to expect. Having said this, I have friends who love surgical predictions and feel that it truly enhances their consults.

The best way to discuss cosmetic deficiencies is to make the consult an educational experience. I explain to the patient that I am going to discuss their entire head and neck in terms of diagnosis and potential treatments—this does not mean I feel they need all the discussed procedures, but they are possible options.

The most orderly means of systematically discussing facial aging and potential treatment is to explain to the patient that the face is divided into thirds, and we will discuss the upper, middle, and lower third, then discuss the skin as a separate unit. During this discussion the surgeon should never assume, for example, that the patient understands the difference between brow aging and eyelid aging. The best thing is to stay elementary when explaining diagnosis and treatment. Many patients have never heard of cheek implants or understand what a browlift or facelift does. If patients are put off by discussion of multiple procedures, and if I sense the conversation going that way, I consider this patient more conservative and stay closer to their main concerns as opposed to additional options. As I talk to the patient, I include my assistant in the discussion. I may say, "Mrs. Smith, I think you are a great candidate for laser skin resurfacing, don't you agree, Jenny?" (Fig. 4.9). This adds a second opinion to the discussion, puts the patient at ease, and reinforces my diagnosis. This also implies a team approach. My assistant is continually recording bullet points of the consultation discussion and prepares a form to give to the patient when they leave that lists the discussed procedures and their respective fees.

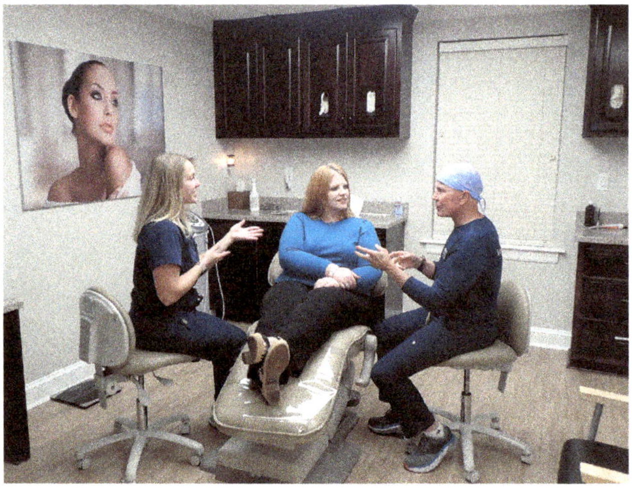

Fig. 4.9. The surgeon and staff should work together in consultation, which helps reinforce the fact that you are a team and that you value the knowledge and experience of your staff. In most cases it is the staff that will be bonding with the patient. Using the same staff member throughout the entire experience helps give the patient consistency.

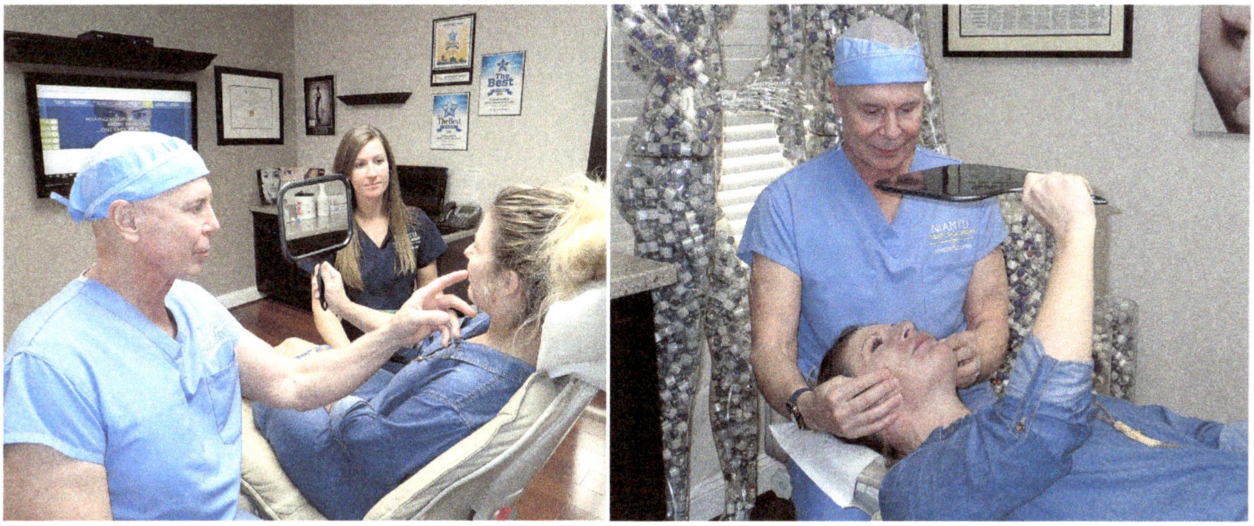

Fig. 4.10. I have the patient look in a hand mirror while we discuss what bothers them as well as elucidate other aging changes. This is an educational experience for most patients. Reclining the patient provides a predictive perspective for facelift, brow lift, or cheek implants.

I prefer to do my cosmetic facial consults in a plush, contemporary dental chair that can also double as a treatment platform for injectables or minor procedures. In every consult, I recline the chair and have the patient elevate their chin and look in the hand mirror (Fig. 4.10). This removes gravity from the equation and provides a surprisingly accurate estimation for facelift, browlift, or cheek implants. I have done this for years, and it goes a long way to help the patient understand and preview a potential result. At this point in my career, I tell them that their appearance when reclined is an accurate prediction of a facelift and neck lift.

A very important concept is not to assume that any patient really has an appreciation as to what a procedure is or does. We do surgery all day, every day, but they may do it once in their life. It is our job to clearly define the correct diagnosis and explain in an elemental way what procedures are available and what each one will and won't do. The more "props" you have on hand, the easier it is to convey how procedures are performed. In this digital age, the standard for consultations would include animations, videos, and photos. The best place in the world for me to get all of this is from my own website. Our standard protocol is to have the assistant open our website on a widescreen TV in the consult room (Fig. 4.11). Then the staff member will review the procedures that the patients are interested in. While on the web page, they can view and discuss procedural examples, animations, surgical videos, and thousands of before-and-after images. The consult should definitely be an educational experience, and I think this is a great way to do it.

I feel the best way to perform a consultation is to tell the patient, "Today we are going do a full exam and discuss what aging changes you have and what nonsurgical and surgical options are available." I further explain that cosmetic surgery is totally elective and just because I point out some aging or discuss a procedure, it does not mean that they need or want that procedure. I further explain that the list of procedures is a "menu," and they can "order" only the procedures that interest them.

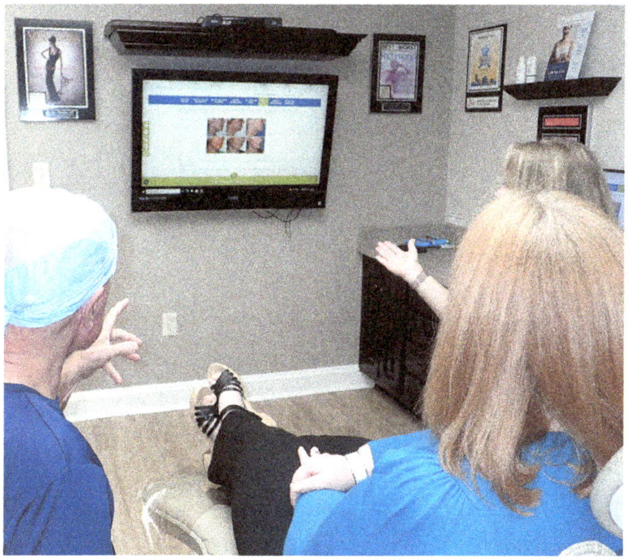

Fig. 4.11. Using my website on a wide screen TV has been the most efficient way for me and my staff to truly educate the patient during consultation.

It is very important for the staff and surgeon not to appear pushy in terms of having surgery. No patient likes a high-pressure sales pitch, and there are many aggressive offices out there that push too hard, and it is very apparent to the patient. I make a point to tell the patient that I really don't care what they do or don't do. I love doing surgery and if the procedure is good for the patient, it is good for me. I may make suggestions, but if I see that a patient is very conservative or resistant to multiple procedures, I immediately back off of discussing a comprehensive treatment plan. Of utmost importance is to address the patient's primary concern first. If a patient presents and says, "I hate my neck," then you don't want to begin the conversation about their eyelids. Stay focused on what is important to the patient and after their major concern is thoroughly discussed, other areas can be addressed. As stated, patients are frequently nervous and the office has a lot of information to present, so it is not hard to confuse the patient or skip over important details. The best way to avoid this is to do the same thing in the same order at every consult.

I frequently use myself as an example, saying, "When I look in the mirror, I see a big bald head, so I would love to have hair." That usually brings out a giggle and then they relax and tell me what bothers them. I have to say, as I have gotten older and now have some early jowling and neck skin, I can use myself as a model to discuss aging and this helps the conversation because I "feel their pain." Light, self-deprecating humor can be an icebreaker. Once I address the main problem, I tell the patient we are going to do an educational aging analysis in a specific order, addressing four distinct areas. The areas to be discussed are the upper face, the middle face, the lower face, and the skin. I then repeat that list to make sure they understand the order.

While the patient looks in the mirror or at a picture, I point out aging problems in the following areas:

- Brow and forehead complex
- Upper lids
- Lower eyelids
- Cheeks/nose
- Lower face and neck
- Skin

After I discuss each area, I present nonsurgical and surgical options, and my staff records the procedures and the appropriate fee. It is important to discuss things in the same order with every patient, so nothing is omitted. I begin with the upper face, the middle face, the lower face and neck, and the skin.

Once we discuss all the above-mentioned areas, I tell the patient that we are building their "cosmetic menu" and that every patient has a different menu and that some patients "order" everything on the menu and others may only "order" one item. I reinforce that they should only consider procedures that are important to them and not to let our list influence their decisions. By this time, we have also discussed their health history, recovery window, and budget. My average patient is a candidate for "3 L's" and a "C." That translates to lift, lids, laser and cheeks. These are the most commonly combined cosmetic procedures in my practice.

A facelift is not a one-size-fits-all operation and I feel facelifts come in three sizes: small, medium, and large (Fig. 4.12). Younger patients may benefit from a very conservative and short scar lift well, but most people in their mid to late fourth decade are not great candidates for a conservative procedure. As stated throughout this text, performing a small lift on somebody that needs a large lift will result in disappointment, lack of result, and lack of longevity.

Like any other surgical procedure, you need to pick the correct procedure for the specific problem.

Besides letting a patient know what to expect from a procedure, it is equally and sometimes more important to let them

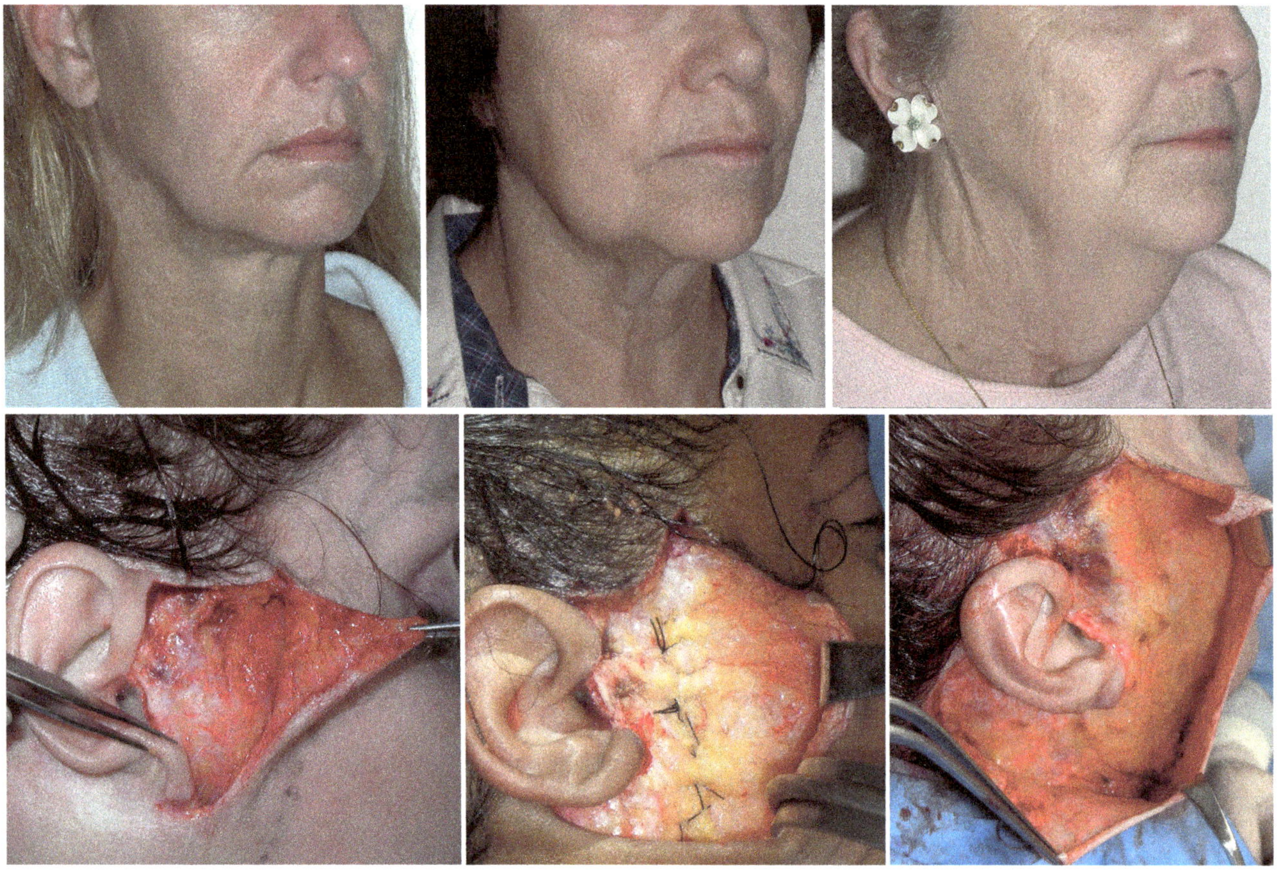

Fig. 4.12. Facelifts can be categorized into small (*left*), medium (*center*), and large (*right*). The procedural steps are very similar, if not the same, but it is the degree and extent of surgery that separates a conservative lift from a more aggressive procedure.

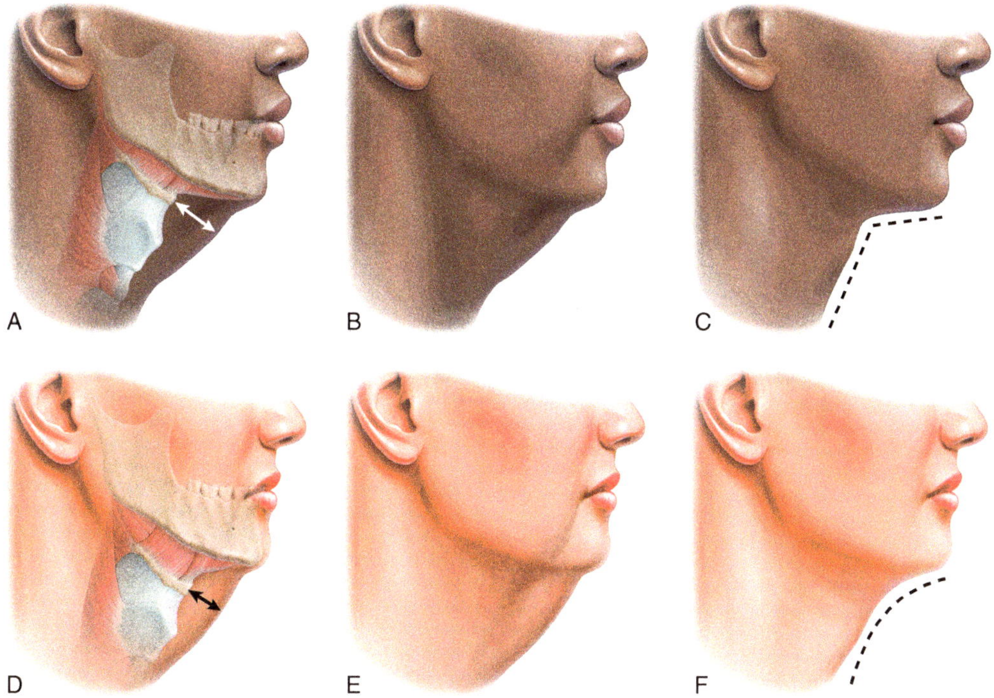

Fig. 4.13. The *top* images show a representation of a patient with normal (superior and posterior) hyoid, laryngeal and floor of the mouth anatomy. Figure A shows the anatomic position, Figure B shows a representation of the preoperative appearance and Figure C shows a representation of the possible angular result after face and neck lift surgery in the "high/posterior" neck. Figure D shows a representation of the anatomy of a patient with low and anterior hyoid, laryngeal and floor of the mouth. Figure E shows a representative preoperative appearance (similar to Figure B). Figure F shows a representation the lack of angular result after face and neck lift as a result of the "low/anterior" anatomic relationship.

know what not to expect. I always reflect back to Fig. 1.3 to explain to patients what areas of their face and neck will be improved and what areas will not. I think it is paramount for them to see this picture numerous times and understand this concept.

Also, specific patient differences can affect results. The following are situations that may need special explanation to the patient, so they understand potential problems or limitations of the procedure.

- Medical compromise (the at-risk surgical patient that may only be cleared for small procedure)
- Extreme neck skin excess
- Heavy jowling
- Obesity
- Severe facial and neck wrinkling (extreme actinic damage)
- Unfavorable anatomic neck and hyoid and laryngeal anatomy (Fig. 4.13)
- Patients that would benefit from chin or cheek implants but refuse
- Previously operated on patients with earlobe, incision, and hairline changes

Another means of evaluating submental anatomy is to use a tongue blade, suture, or long cotton-tipped applicator stick to retract the excess submental skin and/or fat and document with a picture. This can provide an idea for the surgeon and patient of the degree of submental improvement (Fig. 4.14).

What the surgeon begins with may influence what the surgeon ends with. It is impossible for a patient to have too much preoperative information. The surgeon and staff must remember that the patient will only remember a small amount of the information given to them. For the surgeon and staff, this is something that we discuss numerous times a day, but the patient may only hear it once in their life and it is our job to make sure they hear enough of it.

In my practice we generally have the patient present 2 weeks before their surgery and at that time review their history and physical, go over all of the preoperative and postoperative instructions with the patient, and discuss caregiving among other issues. By the time this appointment happens, we have been communicating with this patient on numerous events, and if they still fail to understand the finite details of their surgery and what is required of them and their caregivers, it may be prudent to delay the procedure or perhaps not operate on that patient at all. Obviously, a big part of this procedure is the verbal and written informed consent of what the procedure will do in what can happen. Equally, if not more, important is my alternate informed consent entitled "What Your Facelift Won't Do." This consent is really important and addresses areas that will not be affected by the facelift.

In concert with this discussion are patients who have small chins or a deflated midface. So many times, I have a patient that would benefit from cheek augmentation (cheek implants, filler, or fat) and or chin implant and they are resistant because they are conservative or for financial reasons. Unfortunately forgoing these augmentive procedures can have a huge negative impact on the surgical result. A chin implant can dramatically improve a retrognathic profile and tremendously enhance the facelift. Performing a facelift on a patient that needs midface augmentation but refuses makes them look tighter but not younger. In such a case, deflated cheeks make the jowls look larger. This can disable the ability to make the face tapered. In a youthful situation,

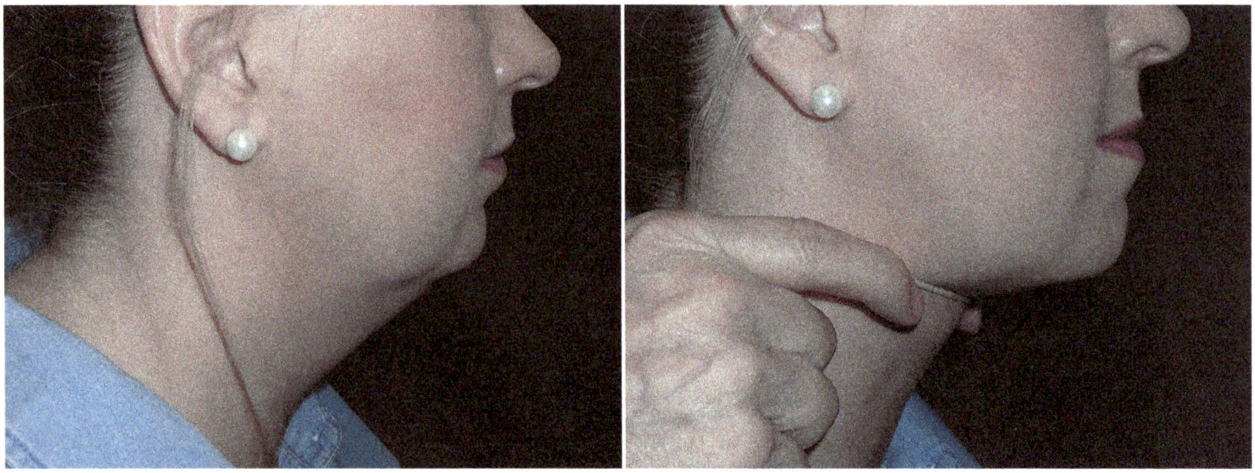

Fig. 4.14. Hyoid and other neck anatomy can portend how a patient's profile result. Retracting the submental skin can show how far posterior the soft tissues can be positioned. This patient would have a very favorable result, whereas if her hyoid and related anatomy were inferior and anterior, her result would be more obtuse.

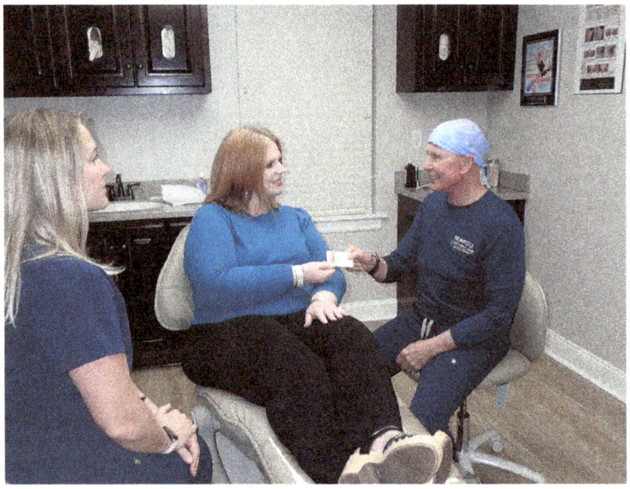

Fig. 4.15. I've always given patients my personal information, including cell phone number and e-mail address. I know many doctors would be horrified at the thought, but there's no better way to boost the patient's confidence than to know that they can call their doctor at any time. We make a big deal about concierge medicine in this day and age, but astute practitioners have been performing concierge services for a century. We have more technology now, which makes it easier.

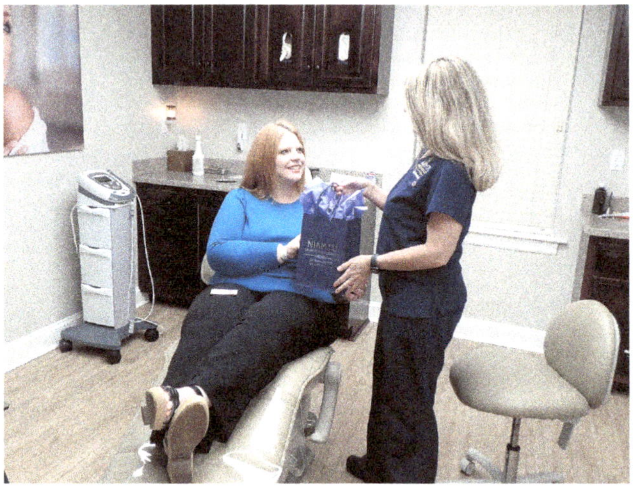

Fig. 4.16. Leaving a patient with a gift bag of skin care samples and promotional materials is a good way to stay remembered.

the face is tapered because the cheek region is fuller than the jawline. Foregoing cheek augmentation in a patient that needs it will always produce a facial imbalance. It is so important to "put something back" during facelift surgery, and patients must realize this. There are cases where the patient declines cheek or chin implants, but I feel that it is so important for my final result, reputation, and brand that I do it free of charge. To me, this is a marketing decision and not a financial one.

At this point I tell the patient that "I have done all the talking," and I ask them for their input. I sit back and listen. I, one more time, review their "menu" and tell them that I will leave them, and my staff will discuss further details (finances, scheduling, etc.). Before leaving the room, I personally hand each patient my business card with my personal cell phone number and email address (Fig. 4.15). Most patients are quite surprised by this, as many doctors hide from their patients. I tell my patients if they can't call their surgeon, then they chose wrong surgeon. This availability has a large impact on patients when choosing their surgeon. I shake the patient's hand, thank them for coming, ask them how they heard about our office, and one more time ask them if there any further questions. The average time for the consult is 45–60 minutes and the actual face time with me is about 20 minutes.

Before the patient exits, we provide them with some type of gift package that includes information about our practice, skin care samples, and promotional items. People love gifts and it's a great way to keep a patient on your radar (Fig. 4.16).

My experience shows that most people aren't using any type of professional skin care or medically based regimen. For this reason, we offer a free skin scan and skin consultation if they desire. Many patients take us up on this and purchase skin care products from our practice, which is a valuable service for them and more reason to return to our office.

When the patient leaves the evaluation room, they are taken to a more formal office and meet with my cosmetic surgical coordinator. As this is more of a business meeting than a clinical one, my coordinator wears business attire instead of scrubs. The fees, payment process, and payment options are discussed, and the patient is given a customized packet with information about the office and surgical processes (Figs. 4.17 and 4.18). This includes an overview of each step of the surgical and recovery process. Patients are also given information about caregivers, and out-of-town patients are given information about local lodging and dining. All of this information is on my website, but having a hard copy reinforces our mission and policies.

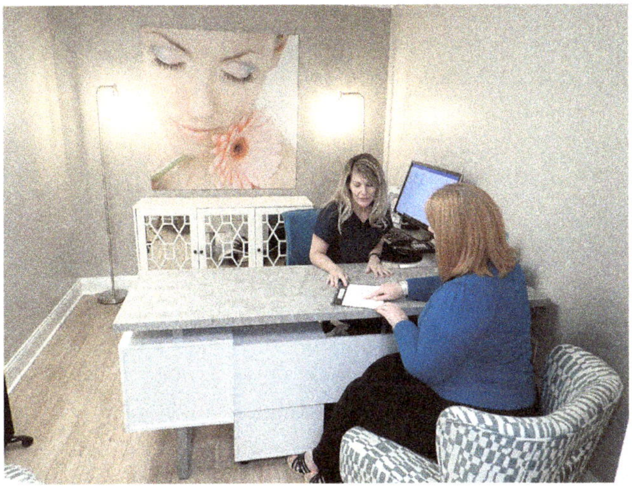

Fig. 4.17. After the clinical consultation with the doctor and surgical staff, the patient meets with our cosmetic scheduler. This is a more formal and business-oriented part of the consultation.

Finishing the Consultation

Patient Health Status: The Primary Concern

Cosmetic surgery is an elective procedure, and failure to adequately diagnose health problems could lead to severe complications, consequences, and death. The surgeon must make sure that every patient is healthy for surgery and anesthesia. Although most patients are candidates for some type of rhytidectomy procedure, it is not uncommon that they have systemic problems such as hypertension, cardiovascular disease, diabetes, hyperlipidemia, arthritis, osteoporosis, and other comorbidities. Patients are living longer and taking more medications, so their medical status may be complex. Most of these patients are candidates for cosmetic surgery if their diseases are controlled and/or medically managed. Patients taking anticoagulants or medications that affect platelet function present special problems and may require intense medical management. The more problems a patient has, the riskier the surgery and anesthesia can be. There comes a point at which the risk of surgery outweighs the benefits of looking younger. In and of itself, age is not a contraindication to facelift surgery. I have treated 85-year-old patients who were healthier than some of my 50-year-old patients. Older patients may have some component of compromise and not tolerate extended surgeries and recoveries as well as younger patients. For this reason, the treatment plan must be altered. We must always keep in mind that we are providing elective surgery. No patient has ever died because they did not have a facelift, but some have died because they did. It is not uncommon for older and

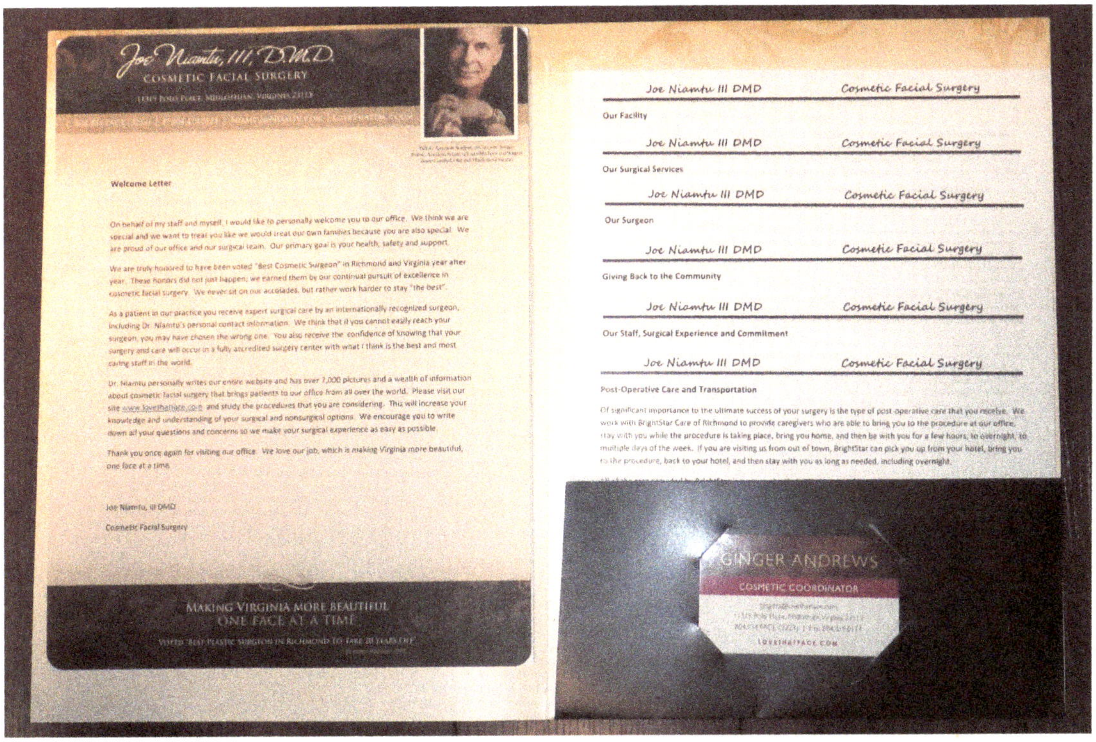

Fig. 4.18. This image shows a portion of our presurgical packet that the patient receives at the end of their consultation appointment. Having professional materials or the lack thereof can have a lot to do with a surgeon's perceived image.

sometimes sick patients to have nonelective surgical procedures such as joint replacement or cataract surgery. This instills a mindset that any senior patient can have surgery, even with multiple comorbidities. Because of this, many patients assume that they can have facelift surgery, regardless of physical condition. In an elective practice, most cosmetic facial surgery is performed in the accredited ambulatory office surgery center. An office death or severe complication can be a devastating setback that can taint the reputation of an elective surgeon, not to mention the loss for the family and related malpractice actions. I have always said that "the best surgeons are always a little bit scared." This means that many of their surgical decisions are somewhat based on what can go wrong. This can be a good limiter and ensures a double-check to stay safe with surgery and anesthesia. It is not uncommon for sick patients to want to have surgery. It is also not uncommon to have them get mad if they are turned down due to health risks. As difficult as it is to turn down a surgical patient, smart surgeons know how and when to say no.

All my facelift patients (per our accreditation) are required to have a history and physical from their physician within 30 days of their surgery. Patients with hypertension, diabetes, pulmonary dysfunction, or cardiac history will require further consultation and lab studies. One of my attendings once told me that "you want as many signatures on a patient's chart as possible," meaning you have done a through workup.

For all patients, it is imperative to have a written document from their physician stating that the patient is stable and cleared to undergo elective anesthesia and surgery. In the event of anesthesia or surgery problems, this omission is one of the first things a plaintiff's attorney would seek.

Smoking, alcohol, or drug abuse are lifestyle factors that could influence surgery and anesthesia. I have frequently operated on patients that smoke a pack or less a day and have not encountered significant problems. It is always in the best interest of everyone to have the patient stop smoking before surgery. Tobacco abuse is a very addictive habit, and many people will simply say they are not smoking and continue to do so. I have a special consent for smokers that outlines their susceptibilities to complications to surgery and anesthesia. I am also more conservative when operating on smokers and do not perform simultaneous resurfacing procedures.

Psychological Stability

Psychological imbalance or body dysmorphic disorder may not be a huge problem in a patient seeking lip filler or neurotoxin treatment, but with a facelift, it can provide extreme challenges and malpractice actions. All novice surgeons should be familiar with the warning signs of potentially problematic patients. Although some surgeons advocate a psychological evaluation of questionable patients, I do not. In my experience if a patient requires a psychological evaluation, they are not a good candidate for my office.

Choosing the correct patient can have everything to do with the success or failure of a case. A patient with a positive attitude and realistic goals and expectations can make the cosmetic facial experience a joy. Patients that do not understand the procedure, are uncooperative, and have unrealistic goals and expectations can present significant clinical and legal problems. A frequently quoted sentence is that "1% of your patients will cause 99% of your problems" and it is so true. One of the keys to happiness and balance in a surgeon's professional life is the ability to avoid the problematic patient. Unfortunately, there is no quantifiable way to do this and sometimes we all get fooled. The surgeon and staff must continually be on the lookout for patients that exhibit "red flags" for potential problems. The best reason for a patient to have cosmetic surgery is to look as good as they can for their age. When I hear this, I know I have a potentially great patient. Patients that are trying to look like someone else, trying to get a job promotion, attempting to follow social media trend, or trying to save a failing relationship may be poor surgical choices.

Surgeons should proceed with caution with patients that exhibit warning signs such as the following:

- Demand guaranteed results
- Have to be seen and have surgery immediately or as soon as possible
- Are not liked by the surgeon or staff
- Exhibit body dysmorphic disorder or psychiatric conditions
- Want to look like a celebrity
- Want to look "young" or "take 20 years off"
- Are overly narcissistic or immature
- Are unfriendly or impersonal
- Don't make eye contact
- Don't listen and do all the talking
- Don't "get it" and ask the same questions over and over
- Are too busy or important for surgery
- Don't want any pictures taken or demand unusual anonymity
- Are not telling spouse or family about their surgery or true extent of procedures
- Berate previous surgeons and compliment you
- Cannot decide on a surgical plan
- Are overly impulsive, want to book surgery immediately
- Have unrealistic expectations
- Know more about the procedure than the surgeon
- Request specific operative techniques
- Are obsessed with online cosmetic surgery patient sites and social media
- Have way too many selfies on their devices
- Are addicted to cosmetic surgery
- Overreact to small flaws or minor aging
- Complain about or want to negotiate fees
- Want surgery for the wrong reasons such as a job promotion or pending divorce
- Have a resistant spouse
- Have consulted with "all the leading specialists"
- Can't stop physical activity or exercise
- Refuse caregivers
- Send too many email questions
- Can't really afford the surgery
- Have transportation problems
- Won't come to the office for consults
- Are nice to the doctor but rude to the staff

Recovery

Patients must be able to take time away from work or play commensurate with the procedure(s) being performed. Everyone is busy, and with more women in the workplace, it is difficult to balance cosmetic surgery and work. One of the biggest mistakes a surgeon can make is to downplay a recovery. If you tell a patient they will recover in 1 week and it takes 2 weeks, they can be furious. If you tell them it takes 3 weeks and they recover in 2 weeks, you can be a hero. Many of the aspects of surgery, such as incisions, sutures, anesthesia, bandages, and so forth, can be objectively and accurately described. Recovery, on the other hand, is very subjective. I have, on several occasions, performed the same procedure on identical twins, and one twin did great while the other twin had unusual swelling and bruising. It is impossible to guarantee precise recovery, and the surgeon must rely on the mean recovery time of a procedure or procedures. I tell facelift and laser patients that the average patient can return to work or social situations at 2 weeks. I explain to them that on the bell curve, some patients may look great at 9 days and others may still be bruised at 3 weeks. The surgeon should always err on the high side; if the patient is given a range of 6–14 days, 6 days is the only number they will remember. All of this needs to be covered in the consent and presurgical material issued to the patient. I give patients the option of a Thursday surgery, which gives them a weekend, a full work week, and another weekend to recover. This is sufficient for selected surgeries, but I tell them that no surgeon can guarantee a specific recovery. If they are having a facelift before a big event, such as a child's wedding, a reunion, or an important vacation, I suggest 4–6 weeks for recovery. I also explain that the recovery process can take up to a year.

Budget

Patients must have adequate finances for the procedure(s). Cosmetic surgery is expensive, and I tell my patients it is a good long-term investment. Some patients desire cosmetic surgery but in reality cannot afford it. In normal circumstances, there is significant stress for the patient when having cosmetic surgery. Add the stress of a poor financial situation, and this may put some patients over the edge. In addition, patients who cannot afford a procedure tend to skimp on details that are important, such as not purchasing expensive antivirals or antibiotics or using private duty nurses. If the financial stress causes family problems, the experience can turn into a negative one. Some patients should simply postpone surgery until they can afford it; otherwise, they may ask the surgeon to compromise throughout the surgical experience. Offering alternate financing options to patients is helpful but occasionally can enable them to do something that at this point in their lives is impractical. Almost 60% of my facelift patients are from out of town. This adds extra expenses of travel, lodging, and private duty nursing care. Not every patient can afford this, and it underlines that cosmetic surgery is a luxury expense.

New surgeons frequently do not charge consultation fees, as they welcome any type of patient contact. Seasoned surgeons that have a very busy facelift practice may be booked out for months and beyond. In a very busy practice, every minute is extremely valuable, and most experienced surgeons will charge a consultation fee. This keeps all of their time profitable and discourages patients that aren't serious about surgery from clogging the schedule. The dynamics in a new surgical practice versus a mature practice can be very different.

When I leave the consultation room, the assistant sits back down and continues the conversation with the patient. My assistant provides the handwritten fee estimates to our cosmetic scheduler who in turn provides a formalized print out for the patient. The patient is passed from the assistant to the scheduler and meets with them in her business office, away from the clinical space (Fig. 4.14). The scheduler discusses finances and provides literature about payment plans (if asked), and gives the patient a professionally made presurgical packet that has a lot of information about our office, our doctor, and the presurgical experience (Fig. 4.15). This will also include forms for medical clearance, caregivers, and hotels and lodging (if pertinent). My practice, like many other mature practices, involves a lot of out-of-town patients, and these individuals require an increased level of communication as they will be coming from another city and staying here for a specified time after their surgery. They need not only more planning but more TLC, as many of them are going through this experience without family present.

We encourage patients to carefully study our website in relation to their anticipated procedures as it is a great educational tool. Serious patients are given information about required preoperative history and physical and lab tests so they can begin planning their surgery.

The same day as the consult, we send a personal note card thanking the patient for coming to the office and inviting them to contact us with further questions or assistance. If we do not hear back from the patient in 6 to 8 weeks, a "tickle" letter goes out reminding them we are at their service for questions or concerns, and then the staff member that attended the evaluation calls the patient to see if there are any questions that she may answer.

Preoperative Appointment

When patients schedule a surgical appointment at my office, they are required to pay a nonrefundable deposit. This screens out insincere patients and discourages broken surgical appointments. The preoperative appointment is scheduled at least 2 weeks before the surgery date. At this appointment, we conduct the informed consent process and make sure proper labs, history physical, and anesthesia information are in order. This appointment also gives the patient additional time to ask questions and the surgeon a final time to examine and document the patient. A lot of time can be saved, and repetition minimized, by having patients review postoperative instructions and signing consents online prior to this appointment. The informed consent process can be a very unnerving experience for the patient. Reviewing 4–5 lengthy consent documents that discuss significant complications can cause

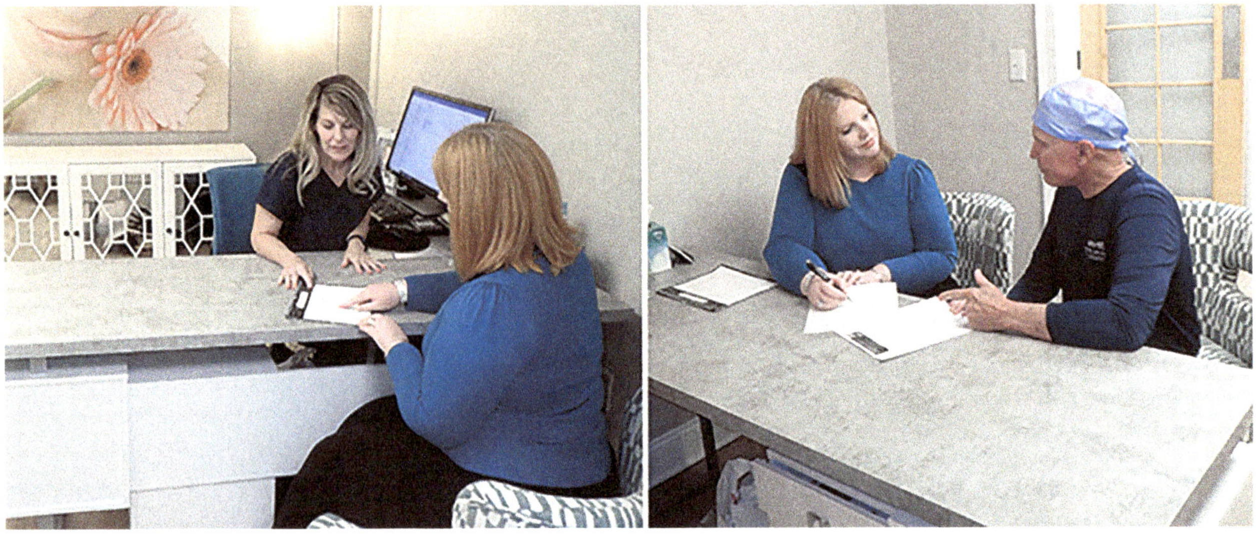

Fig. 4.19. A staff member will review the consent with the patient and begin the process as well as make sure all forms are complete and serve as a witness (*left*). I then come into the room and review the entire consent process with the patient to make sure they understand it and have no questions (*right*).

apprehension. I explain to every patient that it is perfectly normal to be worried about all the things mentioned in the consent. I also tell them that I feel that statistically they put themselves in more peril driving to my office than having surgery at my office. I never try to minimize or downplay consents but do emphasize the fact that severe complications are extremely rare and that if a patient has problems after their surgery, we will stand by them throughout the process. A surgical assistant first does a basic review of the consents and participates as a witness in the process (Fig. 4.19, *left*). I personally then review the consents and any questions the patient may have (Fig. 4.19, *right*).

Although we sometimes take presurgical photographs at this appointment, these are usually delayed until the day of surgery, where the patient will not be wearing any makeup (Fig. 4.20).

At this preoperative appointment, the remainder of the surgical and anesthetic fee is due. Many surgeons bill for the anesthesia and pass this on to the anesthesiologist. Although there is nothing wrong with this, it appears on the surgical bottom line and makes your surgical fees appear higher. By having the anesthesiologist bill separately for their services, the actual surgical fee has less impact.

We prefer to have the patient's caregiver present at this appointment. The first 20–30 minutes of the preoperative appointment are spent with the surgical coordinator or surgical nurse. They go over all of the consents and surgical details as well as the postoperative instructions. Again, the caregiver must really understand their upcoming role. At this point, I enter the room and review all the information and questions or concerns. I also perform and document a formal physical exam. I cannot stress the importance of accurate documentation at this appointment. Any problems, asymmetries, abnormal anatomy, and so on need to be documented at this time and the patient informed.

Patients are given their prescriptions and preoperative, surgical, and postoperative instructions at this appointment. Out-of-town patients or those without caregivers are offered the option of private-duty assistants or nurses and transportation if needed, although this is usually done well in advance of this appointment.

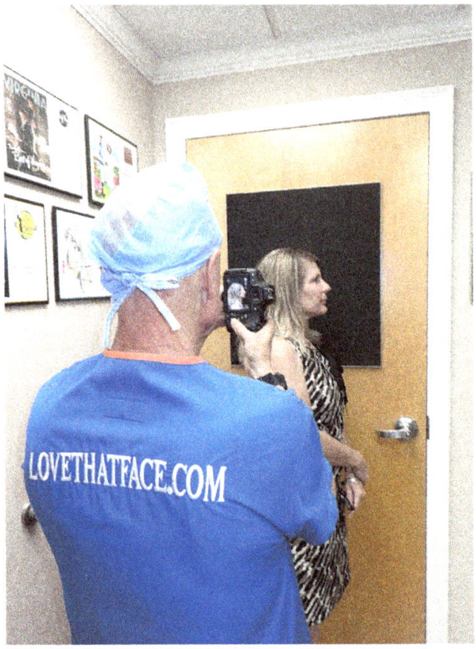

Fig. 4.20. Each room in my office has an adjustable photographic background, so we can take pictures in any room. If the patient is wearing makeup at their preoperative appointment, we take pictures with makeup, but then retake the pictures the day of surgery with no makeup. You can't have too many before pictures.

The Day of Surgery

The patient arrives at the office and nothing-by-mouth status is verified and vital signs are taken. The surgeon greets the patient, takes preoperative pictures (I actually take my own pictures), and performs the surgical markings. Patients are usually nervous, and I always maintain an upbeat bubbly attitude and tell the

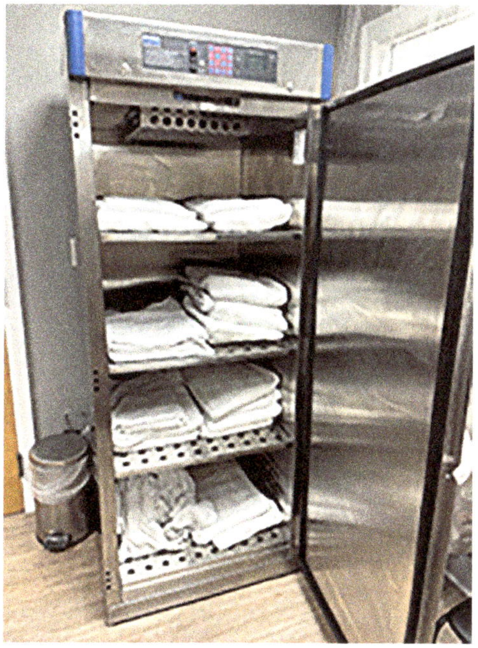

Fig. 4.21. A blanket and robe warmer is one of the best investments I've ever made in my practice. Nothing feels better in a cold surgical environment than a warm blanket or robe. It makes the patient feel comfortable and relaxed.

patient I am very excited to be their surgeon, and everything will be fine.

In our practice, the anesthesiologist meets with the patient that morning before surgery. If there are any significant medical or anesthetic concerns, a meeting would have been scheduled several weeks before, but for routine cases on healthy patients, the anesthesia evaluation is performed the morning of the surgery.

At this point the patient changes into a hospital gown. It is very important to give these patients a warm robe and to keep them out of the hustle and bustle of the office. Nervous patients in skimpy gowns and cold rooms with a lot of activity is not the environment you want. Remember, we do this every day and can be immune to the comfort and privacy required (Fig. 4.21).

The Intraoperative Period

The intraoperative period is very busy, and this is when mistakes can happen. The room is kept warm and quiet during the anesthetic induction. The very first thing that is done when the surgeon enters the operating suite is a formal time-out. A standardized form is projected on the widescreen in the room, and all personnel in the room stop. The circulating nurse reviews the patient, their medical history, allergies, specific surgical sites, and proposed procedures. Any specifics relating to the surgery such as lid ptosis, asymmetries, or previous surgeries are also mentioned (Fig. 4.22). I also personally mark the patient's cricothyroid ligament in the rare event an emergency airway would be required during the case. In 30-plus years, this has not happened, but it is a preventive intervention.

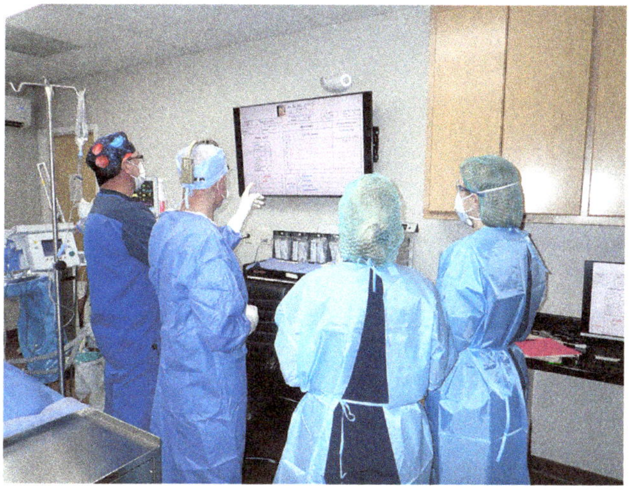

Fig. 4.22. An official timeout is taken to ensure that the entire staff is aware of procedures, surgical sites, and patient history.

Every surgeon and staff member should understand the stressful situation of waiting for a loved one who is having surgery. This is the time that family frets and fears bad things happening and they need be updated and reassured. We encourage our relatives or caregivers not to stay in the office, but if they desire to, we keep them in a segregated small family waiting room that is stocked with beverages and snacks and has a large screen TV and Internet access. The circulator also personally updates the family or caregiver in the middle of the case to let them know everything is going well. As I have progressed, I don't like having the caregiver wait in the office for the patient unless it is a shorter procedure. Sitting in an office for 3–5 hours makes the caregiver anxious, and they may also misread what else is going on in the office. We discontinued waiting in the office during COVID-19 and I now prefer that.

The Postsurgical Period

After the surgical procedure(s) is completed, the patient is transferred to the postanesthesia suite. This is also a vulnerable time for medical mistakes to occur, as a lot of things are going on. The operating room is being cleaned, instruments are being washed, and preparations are made to see afternoon patients. It is imperative that a qualified dedicated staff member stay by the side of the patient and monitor their vital signs until they leave the office (Fig. 4.23). Many tragic stories exist about unattended or poorly attended recovery patients. After the patient is coherent, the caregiver is brought back to the recovery suite. It is important that they have been prepared to see their spouse or family member bruised, battered, bleeding, and burnt. You don't want to have a fainting caregiver; they need to be strong for the patient. Although I, on rare occasions, will keep a patient in my office for 23 hours, some surgeons have in-office suites for the patient to stay, which is a huge advantage.

Ambulatory outpatient anesthesia recovery is very different from a hospital postanesthesia unit with an entire shift of nurses and ancillary staff attending. It is imperative that no patient is

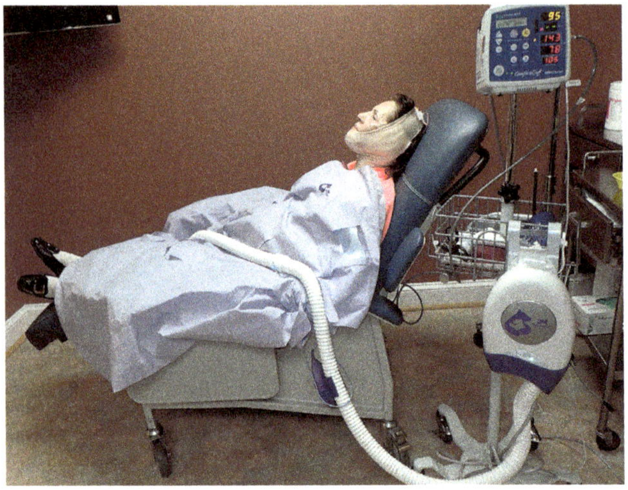

Fig. 4.23. The recovery period is a critical time for patient safety and staff communications. Proper monitoring and staff are essential. Keeping the patient comfortable, warm, pain free, and normotensive are basic goals.

ever discharged without proper stability of vital signs and mentation. I am aware of numerous lawsuits where a surgeon discharged a patient who was not stable enough to leave. A recovery scale must be used and documented. A caregiver that has previously been properly instructed is a huge asset for patient management. The caregiver is given my cell phone and told that I, or one of my staff, will check in with them later in the evening. Germain to this conversation is to be prepared in the event that the patient has a postsurgical hematoma or complication. The office has to have an emergency plan for returning to the operating room. You will need available staff, clean instruments, anesthesia support, and medications. If you are not prepared for this, you are putting your patient and yourself at risk. Be prepared!

Patient Recovery and Biopsychosocial Implications

Getting a patient "in the door," completing the preoperative phase, and finishing the surgery are generally considered to be the bulk of the surgical experience. As every surgeon is aware, this is often only the beginning, and sometimes the recovery process is the most complex of the entire doctor-patient experience. Although some patients understand, are prepared, and breeze through their recovery, others are ill prepared, are misinformed, and struggle to maintain the normal balance of life. In extreme cases, these patients may require psychological assistance or other intervention to prevent mental decompensation. Patients with a straightforward, uncomplicated recovery are a pleasure, and patients that become entwined in a web of complicating physical and mental factors can literally suck the energy and spirit out of the surgeon, staff, and the patient's family.

Why do some patients do so much better than others in healing and recovery, accepting the temporary disability, and returning to normal life than others? There is no single answer, other than the uniquely complex constitutions of each individual. Simply put, some patients have more drama than others. This does not only apply to when they undergo surgery. I would bet if one could follow a patient with a complex recovery through their life before and after surgery, they would see that these complexities extend into other psychosocial aspects of the patient's life. This may include trouble with interpersonal relationships, manipulating spouses, problems interacting with their children's teachers or neighbors, and other similar situations that categorize individuals as "high maintenance."

These individuals may create an accelerated problematic environment, having problems, symptoms, and reactions that are beyond the mean for an average patient having a given procedure. Suddenly their cosmetic recovery becomes intolerable. The patient may wallow in self-pity or experience unimaginable pain. They may fear that something is terribly wrong or become totally physically incapacitated or unable to sleep, eat, or drink. Some patients simply do not handle pain, swelling, or recovery very well and have a terrible recovery, although they are totally normal before and after they heal. It is typical for this type of patient to troll the Internet to discover scores of things that "went wrong" with their surgery. Other patients, however, may exhibit intentional problems in an effort to extract pity from doctor and or family, manipulate relationships, and induce retribution. A good example of this dichotomy is a patient who undergoes facelift, blepharoplasty, full face laser, and cheek implants. She recovers quickly in the office surgery center, goes home, and presents the following morning bruised and swollen, but smiling and joking about her appearance. She is sipping on orange juice and eating snacks from the waiting room. Her husband is supportive and has been a good caregiver. Patient A has a positive attitude and wants to make sure she does all she can do to hasten her recovery. Patient B is the same age with the same frame, health, and so on and has the same procedures as patient A. Patient B is crying from pain immediately upon anesthesia recovery and begs for pain medicine. She is worried that she may not have enough pain medicine from her preoperative prescription. She stays in recovery twice as long as normal for her procedure. Her husband begins calling the office soon after they arrive home, and she has uncontrollable pain and is crying in the background. Her husband is confused because she told him that she was just getting a little tune-up. The surgeon's cell phone rings numerous times during the night, as the patient is still in pain and does not know how to perform her recovery care despite having been given comprehensive instructions and handouts a week before. Patient B presents the next morning for follow-up and can't get out of the car without assistance. They ask for an emesis basin and ask for the room lights to be turned off. She has the demeanor of a multisystem trauma patient and will not make eye contact or engage in discussion. She still complains of severe pain and is sorry she had the procedure and states that we did not tell her it would "be like this."

The differences between patient A and B are notable. Patient A makes surgery fun, and patient B makes the surgeon wonder why he or she chose this profession. Not every patient that acts like patient B has psychological problems, some patients are merely fragile and have lower pain thresholds. More often than not, however, a distinct pattern is seen in the B type of patient. Sometimes the surgeon and staff can settle the patient down and get them back on track. Other times it may require some TLC and the surgeon explaining to the patient that what she is experiencing can happen and the doctor and staff will support her. Some patients need increased pain control and sleep medications. The mix of pain, swelling, sleep deprivation, and fear can put some patients into an acute psychosis. Even strong and "normal" patients can become emotional, especially females who may have spontaneous crying episodes, and when asked what is wrong, they honestly say "I don't know." Emotions can sometimes run rampant with the combination of surgery, swelling, bruising, and medications. Males are not exempt from such behavior, but with my practice being 85% female, I obviously see is commensurate with my gender population. To combat the problematic patient, I spend significant time in the preoperative consultation discussing the good, bad, and ugly aspects of recovery with the patient. I tell them (as does my staff) that they probably won't like me for several days and that they may ride an emotional roller coaster in the immediate and sometimes extended recovery period. The patient's affect can go from remorse, "What did I do?," to depression, and later when healed to elation. There is a wide gap between a patient saying, "Did I make the biggest mistake in my life?" to "Hey, if you ever consider a facelift, go see Dr. Niamtu, he is the best!"

Dealing with the Unhappy Patient

Most of this chapter has been about making patients happy, but every cosmetic surgeon will have unhappy patients from time to time. This may be because of a complication, an unanticipated outcome, or a patient that simply had unrealistic expectations. An angry or unhappy patient can upset your world from several aspects. First of all, most cosmetic surgeons truly care about their patients, outcomes, and their reputations and take it personally when things don't go well. Second, elective cosmetic surgery is fertile ground for lawsuits. Even though the vast majority of lawsuits are won by the doctor, it can be a humiliating, time-consuming, expensive, and stressful ordeal.The best to way to stay out of a lawsuit is to ensure that every aspect of the patient experience will protect the practice. Poor documentation is one of the frequent conditions that lead to suits.Although it is time-consuming, accurate documentation is imperative, and this is where your staff can really assist.Your informed consent process should be very broad, and these documents should be dynamic. By that I mean that informed consent forms need to be continually updated to protect the practice. Each time you feel that your consent has everything covered, some patient finds a new way to say they were not made aware of a given situation. Updating your consents helps protect you.You literally need to go out of your way to think of the most unusual situations that could arise and reflect them in your consents. As stated numerous times in this chapter, if you or your staff see red flags with a given patient, do not operate on them. Picking the right patients has a lot to do with success.

There are basically two types of unhappy patients, those that have a complication or problem and those that have a normal course or result but are unreasonable. Let's discuss the latter first. Some patients will never be happy. They may decide to have a facelift and think that it is literally going to transform their entire life and being. These are frequently patients with low self-esteem or patients with other problems such as poor interpersonal relationships, relationship stress, obesity, and so on. They go through the entire surgical process, have an acceptable outcome, and look in the mirror and still don't like themselves. This is not your problem, it is theirs, but in their mind, it is your problem. To get through this, you need to make it "your problem." Sometimes all these patients want or need is some attention. This is not a case for a coarse or defensive doctor attitude, but rather the time to bring these patients in at the end of the day and spend time with them, letting them vent. As will be discussed in this chapter, this is a time for the doctor to be small in the room. This is when a compassionate staff member is invaluable. They can bond with these patients and hold their hand, literally and figuratively. It is also important for the patient record to have a place to document if the patient is happy or unhappy at the time of their visit. I have had cases where several months down the road an unreasonable patient becomes unhappy and claims they were never satisfied with the treatment or result. It is extremely valuable (especially if the case involves legal proceedings) to be able to review the record and show the patient that the documentation shows that were happy at the last six appointments. I know some surgeons that actually have a place on the record for the patient to state their satisfaction level and actually sign the chart. This obviously would carry even more weight.

If an unreasonable patient turns sour, you must, at some point, review the informed consents with them and point out the preoperative discussions of what their surgical procedure would and would not do. I have the regular preoperative consents in my office, but for every operation, there is also a consent for "what your procedure won't do." This is important as some patients may think a facelift will lift their brows or fix wrinkles around their lips, for example. Also, if I have a case that may portend a revision, I discuss this with the patient in the presurgical period. An example may be a bariatric surgery patient that has extreme submental skin or a laser patient with extensive wrinkling or acne scars. I add a section to the consent stating that their situation is more extensive than the average patient and a secondary procedure may be necessary at the expense of the patient. I do this in writing and mention it several times in verbal conversations, preferably in the presence of their spouse. Actually, all my consents have a paragraph that clearly states that "surgery is not an exact science, and the result is subject to many variables, some beyond the control of the surgeon or patient. In these cases, a revision may be necessary and additional surgical and anesthetic fees will be applicable." This is not ironclad but does set the stage for postsurgical conversations. As stated, in cases that may need obvious retreatment, I use this paragraph and the "what your surgery won't do" section that was previously mentioned. The bottom line is to make your policy clear *before* the surgery. When dealing with an unrealistic patient, showing them this consent can back them off. Some patients may act very unhappy at first, but after significant communication and passage of time, they often settle down. The worst thing you can do with these patients in to act arrogant. Arrogant surgeons get sued; be "small" in the room. If the surgeon is not a good communicator and mediator, then they should use a staff member proficient in these skills. Some of these patients simply realize that their facelift did not "make them pretty" or change their life and they have buyer's remorse from the expenditure. This is especially true with patients that really could not afford the surgery and now have debt. Other scenarios include a spouse that is unhappy or friends of the patient that "can't see any difference." Most patients are reasonable, but every surgeon will encounter some that are not.

I think the single most important thing for the surgeon to ask this type of patient is "What can I do to make you happy?" Sometimes the answer may be "just listen to me," sometimes the answer may be to revise a part of the surgery, and sometimes the answer may be a refund of the surgical fee.

There is no universal answer here, and it is dependent on the situation. If a patient has a facelift but still has some residual submental skin or jowl, a small submental skin excision or jowl liposuction under local anesthesia may make them happy. Some will agree to pay for a revision and others may be adamant against it. Some surgeons refuse to revise anything without payment, but I always provide some options. First of all, you can have a compromised result that is the surgeon's "fault" such as skin or fat excess. There are cases where a problem may be the patient's fault, such as not taking care of laser wounds, or burning the face post rhytidectomy with a heating pad. Finally, you have postoperative problems that are no one's fault and just Mother Nature, such as infections, untoward reactions, and so on. If I truly feel that my result could have or should have been better, I am usually going to either redo it with no charge or ask the patient to cover the cost of general anesthesia if required and a "materials fee." I performed 109 facelifts last calendar year, and I probably had to perform four or five revisions, some small with local anesthesia and some larger requiring general anesthesia. I may not have charged some of these patients anything, to keep the patient happy, but others paid some revision fee if they were receptive. I am probably pretty "wimpy" when it comes to digging my heels in and requiring an unhappy patient to pay for revision. I say this even though my consent that the patient signed clearly states it is the patient's responsibility. If I feel that their problem is not a result of the surgery, I will simply have the staff tell them what our fee is for the revision and if they are unhappy, ask them, "What do you feel is fair for this extra surgery?" Sometimes they may provide a figure and sometimes they may remain insistent on paying nothing. For revision surgery, I never argue over money. In the end, all any surgeon has is their brand and reputation. You need to do your best to keep all patients happy. Sometimes it will cost you some money, but to me that is simply a form of marketing. I tell all patients numerous times in the presurgical communications that in terms of result, "It is your face, but it is my reputation and if you don't look good, I don't look good." The key is to convert this unhappy patient to a happy patient and get that negativity out of your practice and move on to happier patients.

Some patients will ask for a total refund, and this can get tricky. No surgeon wants to perform a 4-hour surgical case and end up refunding the fee. In today's social media environment, an unhappy patient can literally punish a surgeon (deserved or not) on doctor rating sites. Patients know this, and if you run across a vindictive patient, they can tarnish your great reputation quickly. Some of these patients are very unbalanced and have nothing better to do that to spend much of their time to defame you. Consumers are used to getting full refunds from many stores and services and don't think surgery should be any different. The doctor can take the hard line and if they feel that it is out of the question, they can refuse and pass the info on to their lawyer. I have seen some doctors that refused a single penny of refund, but after a week out of their office sitting in depositions, they realize that a refund was not a bad deal. Remember, it does not cost anything for a patient to sue you. Some will initiate this process knowing that it is a good bargaining chip for a settlement. If communication comes to the point of a patient requesting a refund, I will usually try to achieve a compromise. Again, I may ask them, "What do you think is fair?" Sometimes they may surprise you with a reasonable amount. If they hold out for a full refund, then a decision has to be made by the surgeon. My advice is to just get it done and move on. As I stated earlier, in cosmetic surgery, the highs are very high, and the lows can be very low.

One point of great importance is to never, ever refund any money without a legal document and release. This may vary from state to state, but my refund release states that we are making a refund in the interest of patient relations and admit no wrongdoing. It also clearly states that by accepting the refund, the patient will waive all legal actions and agree not to defame the surgeon or practice in all forms of verbal and written media. I have to say that there have been instances in my career when I was actually relieved to trade a refund for a signed patient release to dismiss a problematic patient and move on. Although a patient may sign a release, they probably could still proceed with legal action, but I have never seen that. I probably do some form of a refund every year or two in the interest of patient relations. When I go back and look at a list of these patients, 100% of them had some of the red fat flags I listed earlier in this chapter. Although it may be difficult to turn away a patient, it is really important too not accept patients that exhibit these trends are behaviors.

The second scenario is the situation where a complication occurs that may not be your fault, but it is nonetheless a bad situation. Post-facelift hematoma, skin necrosis, and infection would be examples. Complications that patients may perceive as the surgeon's fault could include nerve damage, poor scars, unnatural vectors of tension, hairline changes, or pixie earlobes. Regardless of whose fault it may be or not be, the surgeon may be faced with a significant complication. Sometimes bad things happen to good surgeons and patients. The key to handling these types of situations is to devote your complete attention to this patient and get them through their problem. The first matter of business is to maintain the patient's confidence and keep them in the practice. No surgeon wants his or her complication to end up in someone else's office, especially if it is a hostile competitor, which unfortunately is not uncommon in cosmetic surgery circles. The key to retaining the complication patient is confidence and communication. Apologizing for the problem (without admitting fault) can go a long way. "Mrs. Smith, I treated you with the same care I would provide my own family, and I am very sorry this problem occurred and has inconvenienced you. I promise you I will do everything in my power to get through this problem. I will not let you down." As long as a patient feels that you are contrite and will stand by them, they will most frequently stay the course.

There are some special considerations that need to be done with this patient experiencing complications. The foremost factors are communication and hand-holding. These patients need to be seen frequently for complication management. They need to be seen at a time when the surgeon and staff can spend an adequate amount of time with them in a calm and unrushed environment. I like to see these patients at the end of the day as the last patient. This keeps them from mixing with your other patients and gives them privacy, and since the day is over, I can spend adequate time with them. Of equal importance is not to complicate communication by having numerous staff members deal with this patient. The most understanding and compassionate staff member in the office should be the only other person that tends to this patient. I prefer to have a single staff member stick with every patient throughout their entire surgical journey as this creates bonding, which is very preferable when complications occur. In the case of a situation like skin necrosis after facelift, many wound care appointments will be required. These patients need to feel that they are your only patient. Frequent phone calls from the surgeon and staff are also helpful when appropriate, and these patients, of course, have my personal cell phone number and email address. It is also important to have the exact same level of communication with the patient's spouse. Remember, keeping these people confident that you can heal them is the key. From time to time, I have also done small things to compensate these patients for their inconvenience such as free Botox or products. If done in a sincere manner, it is not viewed by the patient as a "bribe."

If you face a complication that is not clear, a second opinion or specialty referral must be made in the early phase. Many lawsuits occur for failure to refer or failure to refer at an early enough period. A friendly consult or second opinion is a much better option than having a patient leave your practice and end up with a hostile competitor. If a referral is needed, the question of who will pay for the appointment or treatment will frequently arise. This can be a sticky situation, and there is no correct answer. Sometimes the surgeon would be best served if the already unhappy patient doesn't incur additional fees. I have done it both ways, picking up the tab or having the patient be responsible. Usually, most colleagues (who experience this with their own patients) are sensitive to this and will assist with little or no fee. In the event that a surgeon does want to pay the referral expense, I would suggest speaking with their legal counsel first.

Over my career, I have steered some typical and atypical complications through the tight straights of healing, consultation, and recovery. These patients are usually grateful for the care and attention and stay as happy patients of the practice. There will be cases that leave your care, and this will occasionally happen to all surgeons. The best thing you can do is to learn from these situations and make your practice better. Remember, all surgeons have complications, and the key is to learn from them.

When you speak with colleagues about complications, their conversation frequently starts out by saying, "I have this crazy patient," and it may be so, because at some time all doctors will have some crazy patients. We surgeons strive so much to be perfect that we sometimes get insulted or defensive when accused of doing something wrong. With complications or problematic patients, the surgeon needs to look in the mirror and examine the entire situation and be honest with themselves and their staff about what went wrong and how the doctor or staff could have avoided this situation or how it could be made averted in the future.

Management of the Difficult Patient

The goal of any elective cosmetic surgical is a happy, satisfied patient. Achieving this goal requires:

- Careful patient selection
- Well-chosen procedure(s)
- Meticulous performance of the surgery
- Empathetic postoperative care.

On the surface, completing a cosmetic surgery to improve the appearance and function of a patient seems simple. However, as any experienced plastic surgeon knows, postoperative patient satisfaction is complex and multifaceted.

The successful surgeon realizes that the goals and motivations of plastic surgical patients are complex and that understanding these goals is requisite for patient satisfaction. For this reason, the surgeon should spend time and effort on selecting patients that are likely to have proper expectations regarding surgical outcomes. The key is to deselect patient who likely are impossible to satisfy, or who present with dangerous personalities, and to learn to effectively communicate with and manage the others.

Dissatisfaction after cosmetic surgery results in distress for both the patient and surgeon. Even though a relatively small percentage of cosmetic surgery patients are truly dissatisfied with their results, these few patients usually occupy a large amount of the surgeon's time and energy. Learning to deal with patient dissatisfaction after cosmetic surgery requires significant psychological and communication skills by the surgeon.

Patient Selection

The first step to obtaining a successful outcome in facial plastic surgery is to carefully select the patient. The decision of when not to operate is rarely discussed in surgical training and requires the use of the surgeon's judgement and experience. Although patient selection may seem like an easy task, various factors can obscure the patient selection process. The surgeon's financial motivation, ego, and ineffective communication styles can contribute to poor decision-making when deciding whom to operate on and whom to avoid. Successful patient selection requires that the surgeon listen to the specific patient desires and expectations. To understand the patient's motivations for surgery, the surgeon must utilize open-ended questions and allow the patient to expose their psychological tendencies.

The key skill that the surgeon must possess is to be an *educated listener*. On the surface, the importance of being a good listener seems intuitive and easy to accomplish. However, many physicians seem intent in describing who they are and what they intend to do, rather than finding out who the patient is and what they want. Using open-ended questions during the initial consultation can help unveil the patient's psychological tendencies. For example, "How much time do you spend thinking about your appearance in a day?" or "How does your dissatisfaction with your appearance affect or disrupt the quality of your life?" Less than ideal patients are often able to hide their personality flaws to gain the surgeon's understanding of their reasons for surgery. Furthermore, the true character of the difficult patient often manifests in the postoperative healing process.

Dealing With the Difficult Patient During the Consultation

Aesthetic surgery is, in almost all instances, elective, and therefore if a patient is not a suitable candidate for medical reasons or psychological reasons, the surgeon is tasked with refusing surgery to the potential patient. The task of denying surgery to a patient who seemingly desires the procedure can seem problematic. Surgeons are wired to help people and to "fix" things, and the prospect of refusing a patient who wants your help seems contrary to natural instincts. Refusing services can be a sensitive issue, as the surgeon may be confident that a procedure will objectively improve the patient's appearance.

An additional issue that often obscures the judgment of surgeons is money. The surgeon benefits financially only when surgery is paid for and performed, and refusing the patient can be economically impactful. Although an unhappy patient often creates a large amount of economic and emotional distress to the surgeon and his practice, many surgeons are blinded by the potential positive economic impact of each patient and their bias can cloud their judgment.

If concerns regarding a patient's ability to psychologically tolerate aesthetic surgery are raised during the initial preoperative consultation, the first option for management is to schedule a second consultation. This allows both the patient and the surgeon to reevaluate the situation and address lingering questions or concerns from the initial encounter. If the surgeon's concerns are alleviated by the second consultation, then surgery can be scheduled with greater confidence that the outcome will be satisfactory to the patient. However, if the patient continues to exhibit difficult or dangerous personality characteristics, then the second consultation was of great value in that it provided additional evidence to support the decision to avoid surgery in a potentially problematic patient.

Managing Dissatisfaction in Cosmetic Surgery Patients

Despite all efforts to screen patients preoperatively for realistic surgical expectations and emotional health to withstand the psychological stresses of surgery, patients can be disappointed with the outcomes of surgery. Dissatisfaction after cosmetic surgery results in distress for both the patient and surgeon. Although the incidence of patient dissatisfaction after cosmetic surgery is low, the amount of time and energy spent on an unhappy patient is often much greater than the time required for most other patients. Learning to deal with patient dissatisfaction after cosmetic surgery requires a unique skill set by the surgeon.

To effectively manage an unhappy cosmetic surgery patient, the surgeon must have a strategic plan that involves listening to the patient and making the patient feel understood and accepted. Surgeons want happy and satisfied patients. When a patient is less than satisfied with their surgical outcome, the surgeon often feels that they have done a bad job. This can affect the surgeon's self-esteem. It is common for the surgeon to feel attacked and to become defensive about the surgical result. In general, surgeons want to help people and to be appreciated for their efforts and skill. The surgeon's self-worth is wrapped up in their perfecting (or trying to perfect) their craft and being acknowledged for their experience. Being criticized for their failings does not feel good.

It is important for the surgeon to recognize the unhappy patient, to listen to the patient, and to have a strategy geared to make the patient feel understood and accepted. It will diffuse anger from the patient, will promote or regain trust, and will provide possible remedies to achieve patient satisfaction. A strategy to manage an angry, dissatisfied is as important as making a diagnosis or performing the surgery well.

The Importance of Listening

Communication is essential in management of dissatisfaction in the postoperative cosmetic surgery patient, and the key to effective communication is *listening*. It is important that the patient feels listened to, understood, and accepted. The surgeon should avoid the temptation to rush to "fix" the problem. Providing a fix will obscure the surgeon's ability to listen and will make the patient feel unheard.

There are several techniques for optimizing listening skills to maximize the value of the physician-patient relationship. Listening with curiosity and genuine interest will help the surgeon to better understand the etiology of the patient's concerns. It is also important to give the patient adequate time and space to express their concerns freely and listening in silence provides this opportunity. *Reflective* listening, which involves paraphrasing what the patient says back to them, can help the patient understand that the surgeon is listening and understanding their points. Phrases such as "If I could summarize what I am hearing . . ." or "It sounds like you are saying . . ." followed by "Is this correct?" or "Have I properly characterized your complaints?" can be helpful in these conversations.

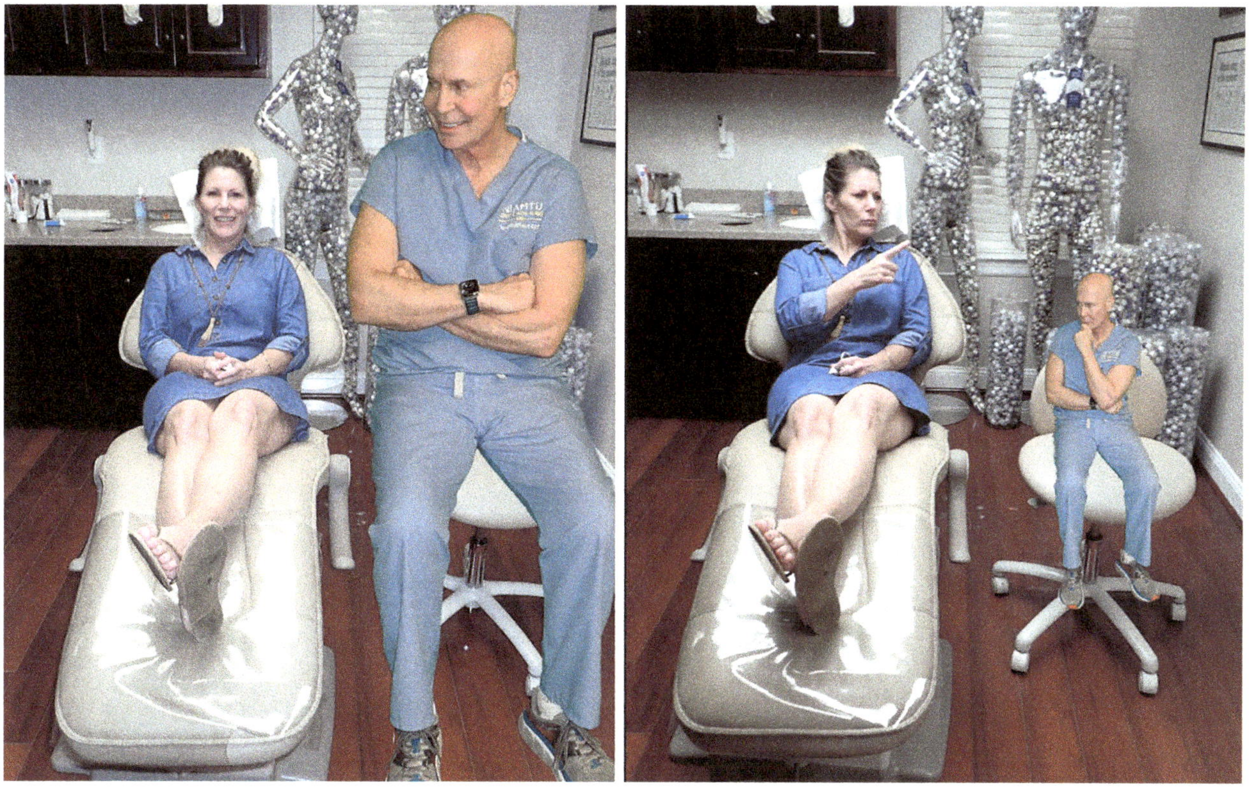

Fig. 4.24. This picture is a metaphor for the surgeon's stature, posture, and personality in the preoperative period where they are confident and self-assured (big in the room) (*left*). The *right* image conveys an unhappy patient and the surgeon's role as an empathetic, effective, and calm listener who is not defensive (small in the room).

Reflective listening should be used by the clinician to allow the patient to feel understood. Repeating what the patient says in summary phrases (e.g., "It seems what is bothering you . . ." or "If I could summarize what I'm hearing . . .") allows the patient to feel that the clinician is truly listening to their complaints. Additionally, follow-up questions such as "Have I correctly characterized your complaints?" can further demonstrate empathy and strengthen the physician-patient connection. It is difficult to a patient to hold on to anger if the patient feels as though the surgeon is listening and empathetic.

Stature and Position: "Get Small in the Room"

It requires a different skill set for the surgeon to be effective pre- vs. postoperatively. Preoperatively, the surgeon needs to be confident and to be an educator. Before any treatment, the surgeon should be self-assured and have a definitive perioperative treatment plan ("big in the room") (Fig. 4.24, *left*).

When a patient is upset about the cosmetic surgery outcome after surgery, the surgeon should not be logical and should not be confident. They should be empathetic and kind ("small in the room") (Fig. 4.24, *right*).

It is advisable that the surgeon sit low in the room (preferably in a chair lower than the chair that the patient is sitting in). It is also advisable that the surgeon does not sit near the door, so that the patient does not feel as though the surgeon is rushed or in a hurry. *Avoid the hand-on-the-door* phenomenon (Fig. 4.25). It is difficult to receive criticism for a less than optimal surgical result; the surgeon should stay calm and avoid the temptation to be defensive regarding the surgical outcome.

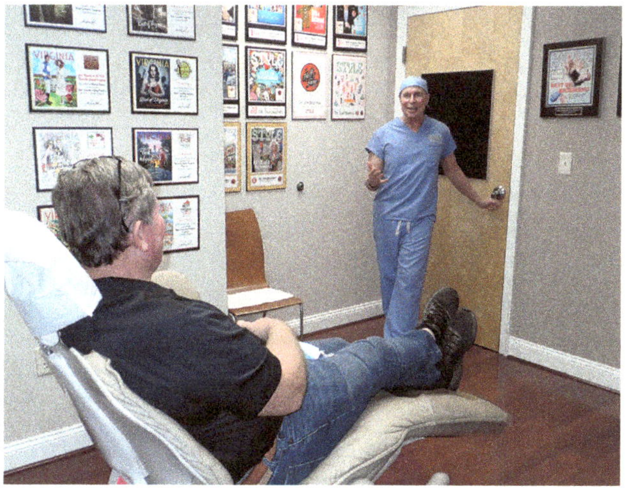

Fig. 4.25. The "hand on the door" communication is a poor way to interact with any patient but can truly offend a dissatisfied patient who feels that the arrogant doctor is in a rush to leave the conversation.

Finding a Satisfactory Solution

After carefully listening and understanding the problem, the surgeon should ask if it is reasonable to suggest a management plan. A question such as "Would it be reasonable to suggest possible solutions?" is a safe method to transition into a treatment plan.

Even though the possibilities for problem-solving are the same as with the find it–fix it method, reflective listening and request for permission from the patient to treat the problem feel different to the patient. It is also acceptable for the surgeon to express disappointment in the surgical result. This must be done without fostering any blame for the result upon the patient.

In rare cases, when the physician-patient relationship is poor and the patient dissatisfaction persists, it is appropriate to consult with risk management specialists and the physician's liability carrier. This will provide the surgeon with legal protection. If the patient asks for a refund of surgical fees, this can be performed in selective cases, but should only be done after consulting legal advice and after the patient signs a complete release of liability.

Managing patient dissatisfaction after cosmetic surgery is difficult and stressful for the surgeon. It requires a wide skill set including the ability to listen carefully to and empathize with the patient. The surgeon must have a strategic plan that includes listening first and eventually suggesting a solution. Regaining lost trust is essential.

The keys to success in plastic surgery are:

1. Careful patient selection
2. Appropriate setting of expectations
3. Honest communication of goals and limitations
4. Reflective listening
5. Get small in the room
6. Avoid the hand-on-the-door phenomenon postoperatively
7. Jointly arrive at a possible solution for the unhappy patient

If these principles are followed, patient dissatisfaction can usually be avoided or, at least, can be properly managed.

Conclusion

Cosmetic surgery is an elective upper-class luxury, and we serve a patient population that is used to having excellent service and an industry that perpetuates it. Clinical competence is obviously the biggest factor in the equation of success but can be totally overshadowed by a poorly run office or arrogant physician. It is said that excellence is a journey and not a destination. This means that you can never actually achieve excellence as even the best things can be improved. If you and your team strive to continually improve all aspect of patient care, safety, and satisfaction, you truly can have an excellent office. Cosmetic surgery is a tremendously fulfilling practice and I have a passion for it. I love going to work and love the interaction with my team and patients. Continually striving to make it all better is pleasure.

Further Reading

Bellard A, Mathew J, Sun W, Denkow L, Najm A, Michael-Grigoriou D, Trotter P, McGlone F, Fairhurst M, Cazzato V. Topography and relationship-specific social touching in individuals displaying body image disturbances. *Sci Rep.* 2023;13(1):13198.

Stevens SM, Markatia ZA, Ameli K, Bayaraa E, Lee WW. Prevalence of body dysmorphic disorder in orbital plastic surgery and its relationship with the use of social media. *Aesthetic Plast Surg.* 2023.

Ghadimi TR, Rieder EA, Phillips KA. "Zoom Dysmorphia?" language and body dysmorphic disorder in the age of social media. *Dermatol Surg.* 2023;49(7):720–721.

Richey P. Commentary on "'Zoom Dysmorphia?' language and body dysmorphic disorder in the age of social media." 2023;49(7):721–722.

Chen Z, Zhou J, He Q, Feng S, Wa Q, Chen X. Prevalence of body somatic deformities in plastic surgery patients: a systematic review with meta-analysis. *Aesthetic Plast Surg.* 2023;47(3):1217–1224.

Laughter MR, Anderson JB, Maymone MBC, Kroumpouzos G. Psychology of aesthetics: beauty, social media, and body dysmorphic disorder. *Clin Dermatol.* 2023;41(1):28–32.

Khattab NR, Abdelraouf N, Ashour T. Conflicting cultural and religious views on cosmesis: the modern women's dilemma. *Aesthetic Plast Surg.* 2022;46(4):2040–2052.

CHAPTER 5

The Surgical Facility

Joe Niamtu, III

Chapter Outline

A chef has their kitchen; a judge, their courtroom; a pilot, their cockpit. A musician has their instruments and a surgeon has their operating room. The operating room and surgical spaces are the workhorse of the practice, and everything funnels in and out of these spaces. They must be safe, comfortable, well equipped, and convenient, as this is where the surgeon "lives."

Office Accreditation

In the 1970s an uncomplicated facelift required a 4.5-day hospital stay. There have been huge paradigm shifts in hospital stays for all surgical procedures, and currently, most cosmetic surgery is not performed in the hospital environment. There are numerous reasons for this including exorbitant hospital costs, presence of nosocomial infections, lack of insurance coverage for cosmetic surgery, having cases bumped by emergencies or other surgeons running behind, and lack of privacy for elective cosmetic procedures.

Having a fully accredited surgery center in one's office offsets the need to operate in a hospital and all the negatives associated with it. It gives the surgeon total control of their operating environment. There are no other surgeons to run late or bump your case. Surgery is much more cost-effective compared with hospitals. Safety is usually enhanced due to the fact that the same people do the same job all day every day, which eliminates shift changes and related problems. There is no worry about infections from other patients. Since cosmetic procedures are usually very personal and discrete, patients can come and go without exposure to scores of employees that work in a hospital environment. Also, small offices usually have one or two anesthesia providers that work on a continual basis, and this prevents surprises that can occur with random anesthesia providers. Finally, convenience for the doctor, staff, and patient is unparalleled. I used to spend a lot of time driving back and forth from the hospital, and now my operating room is just several steps away.

Office accreditation is not a panacea and has relative drawbacks. First and foremost, the surgeon is the captain of the ship and every good and bad thing falls on their shoulders. If an emergency occurs in the hospital environment, there are dozens of trained personnel immediately available. In your office, it is you and your staff. For this reason, the surgeon must use discretion as to which cases are not suitable for the office surgery center. I never take a chance and I cancel cases five to six times per year because the patient has some medical condition that may put them at risk. As I have stated many times, a big part of having a good reputation and being safe has to do with picking the right patients. Never take a chance with a patient's health. We do not operate in our office on American Society of Anesthesiology class III patients. Significant comorbidities can ruin lives.

One of the best things I have ever done in my professional career was having my office and surgery center accredited. I have hundreds of colleagues that will echo the same remarks. Many surgeons are hesitant to pursue this because of the perceived extra work and expense. Also, many surgeons mistakenly believe they have to physically rebuild their facility. In reality, accreditation is attainable for the average practitioner and facility if the surgeon and staff are willing to rise to the requirements. The biggest misconception is that accreditation is a bricks-and-mortar undertaking when in reality it is actually more about policies and governance (Fig. 5.1). The basis of accreditation is to ensure a safe, efficient, and accountable facility to better serve patients, surgeons, and staff by meeting or exceedingly nationally recognized standards. In effect, you are making your office function as a small hospital. This definitely ups the ante for work and paperwork and is not something to be taken as casual. In short, it is a lot of work, mostly paperwork, but it unequivocally will make you a better and safer surgeon with a better and safer staff, facility, and patient experience.

The most common organizations for outpatient, office ambulatory surgery center accreditation are Accreditation Association for Ambulatory Health Care (www.AAAHC.org), Joint Commission on Accreditation of Healthcare Organizations (www.jointcommission.org), and the American Association for Accreditation of Ambulatory Surgery Facilities (www.AAAASF.org).

Some examples of changes to routine office protocols include the requirement to dictate all surgical operative reports, quality review studies for sterilization, malignant hyperthermia rehearsal, infection prevention and reporting, studies for patient waiting times, peer chart review, impaired physician and operating room fire rehearsals, and credentialing all users of the operating facility. Again, this is all very paperwork intense. Trying to become accredited on your own can be a task of awesome proportions. I highly recommend that any practice that is interested in becoming accredited seek the services of professional accreditation consultants. It is not excessively expensive, and they coach the office and staff through every step of the way, including a mock accreditation site visit. Although I know doctors that have become accredited without a consultant, I can speak from experience that the consultant route is much easier on the doctor and staff. Finally, one drawback to accreditation is the fallacy that the surgeon must do all the work. In actuality, the staff does 90% of the work and record keeping and the surgeon is the team leader. Having one nurse or exceptional employee handle all the accreditation work makes this task very straightforward. Since accreditation comes in 3-year cycles with office inspections, having a stable employee that will be there for a long time is preferable.

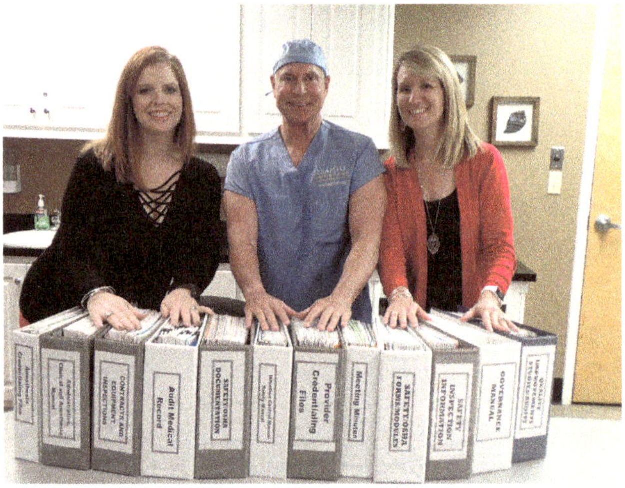

Fig. 5.1. The author, his manager, and nurse are shown with some of the numerous manuals of policies, procedures, documentation and governance for Accreditation Association for Ambulatory Health Care accreditation. In the accreditation process, the staff perform much more of the legwork than the doctor. It is imperative to have knowledgeable staff that can implement and enforce the required policies.

Facility

Financial constraints are always a consideration for the new surgeon, and it can be a challenge to set up a well-equipped operating space. New surgeons may operate in local surgery centers or hospitals. Many surgeons in large cities don't have room for an in-office ambulatory surgical space and also use surgery centers or hospitals. There is no doubt that, if possible, an in-office facility will make life easier.

If possible, having two operating rooms is a significant convenience and allows more diversity of cases and shorter turnover times. Fig. 5.2 shows the author's in-office operating suites.

Some younger surgeons, in the beginning, may choose to operate with a procedure chair, dental chair, or procedure table. If a surgeon is serious about cosmetic surgery, there is no substitute for a formal operating table, and these can be purchased refurbished. Having the ability to position patients laterally (airplane) can be of great assistance, especially with older patients with limited neck mobility, which makes intraoperative head positioning difficult (Fig. 5.3). This prevents the surgeon from bending over and working upside down. Most hospital operating tables are square and meant for body procedures; hence, when doing head-and-neck surgery, the surgeon has to

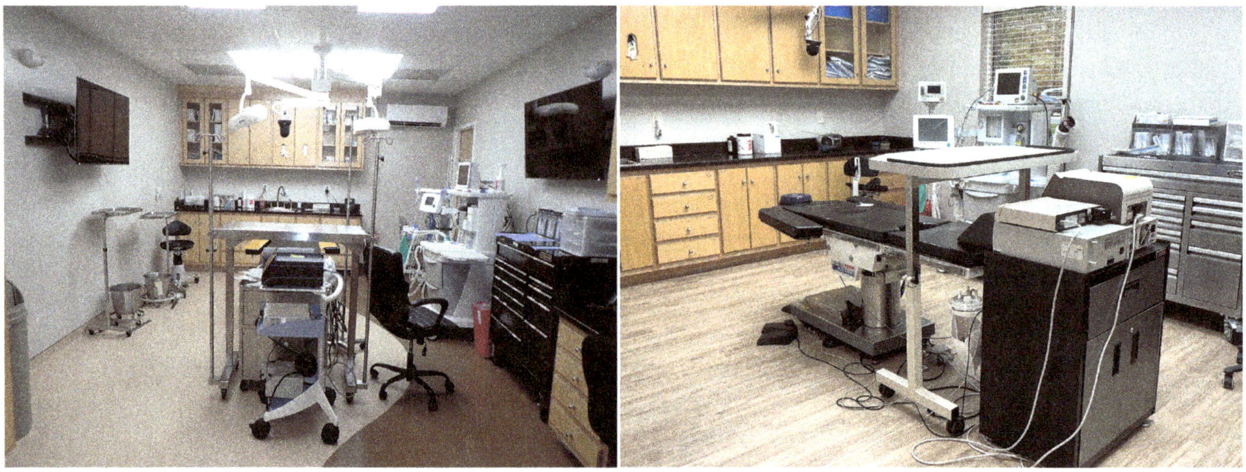

Fig. 5.2. The author's in-office ambulatory operating suites.

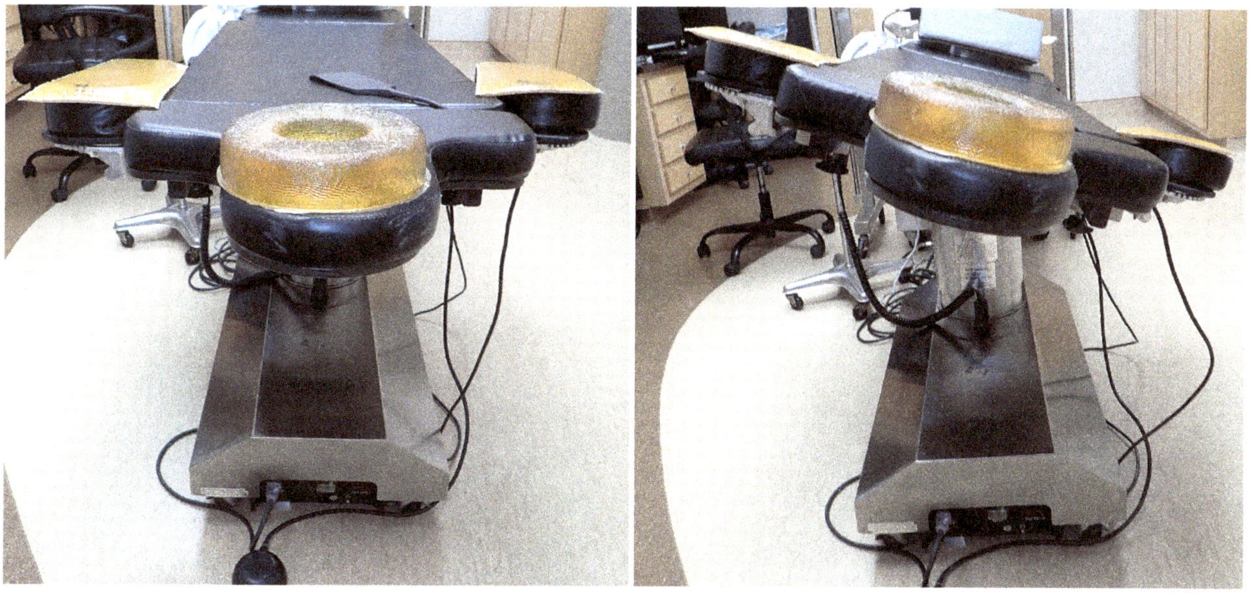

Fig. 5.3. A fully adjustable electronic hospital operating table with a head-and-neck extension can greatly facilitate surgery.

bend over, and this can be very taxing on one's posture. A head-and-neck extension sometimes called neuro-extension allows the head and neck to be extended from the table allowing closer access for the surgeon. These extensions also allow the surgeon to operate in a seated position with their thighs under the patients' head, similar to ergonomic dentistry. I perform the platysmaplasty in the standing position and sit for the remainder of the facelift procedure. The fully adjustable positions of an operating room table are important. In addition, you want your operating room to look like an operating room.

An additional item that has become personally indispensable is an operator stool that can be vertically repositioned (Fig. 5.4). Cosmetic facial surgery and especially facelift surgery require much repositioning of the patient, and hence the surgeon must change his or her position throughout the procedure. I begin in an elevated position but frequently "drop down" to look under the preauricular flaps and other structures. Having an easily adjustable and comfortable stool can facilitate long procedures. As previously stated, surgery can produce a lot of wear and tear on the surgeon, and paying attention to these details early in one's career can extend one's longevity.

The sterilization room should be in close approximation to the operating rooms as well as the nonsurgical treatment rooms. Although a steam autoclave is most common, having a gas sterilizer allows the ability to sterilize virtually any type of instrument or material that would not be compatible with steam heat (Fig. 5.5). An in-office surgery center requires specialized instrumentation such as an anesthesia machine and hospital-grade emergency cart (Fig. 5.6). Whether accredited or not, every in-office surgery center requires some power backup system. This is usually in the form of a generator or battery backup system.

With the affordability of wide-screen televisions, equipping the operating suite with several monitors can be useful for many purposes (Fig. 5.7). For surgeons interested in teaching or recording, an overhead operating room camera can record or broadcast to monitors for educational purposes (Fig. 5.8). I would like to discuss some other useful items for the surgical area. One thing that is also important for staff and patient comfort is an ancillary room conditioner for heat and cooling. Operating rooms can get uncomfortably hot or cold and the ability to augment the ambient HVAC system is useful (Fig. 5.9).

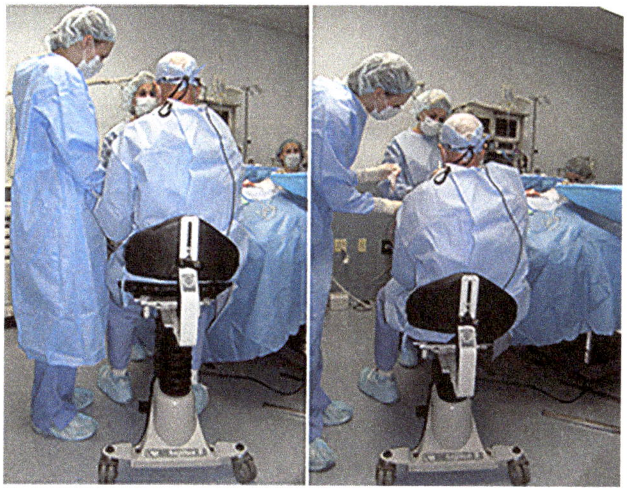

Fig. 5.4. A high-quality adjustable operating stool is well worth the investment and can last a lifetime and extends the surgeon's career.

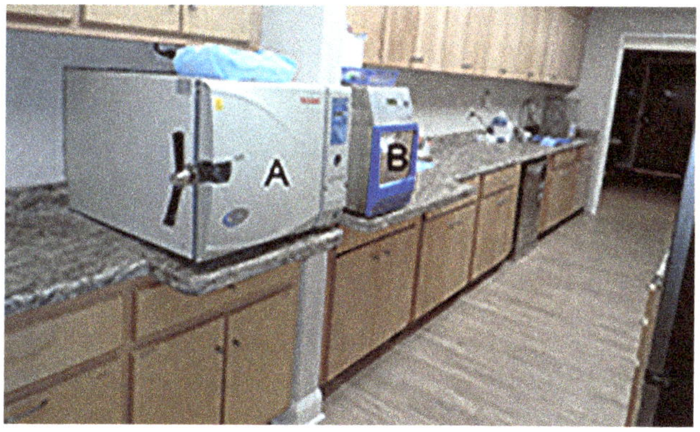

Fig. 5.5. The author's sterilization room with a steam autoclave (A) and a gas sterilizer (B).

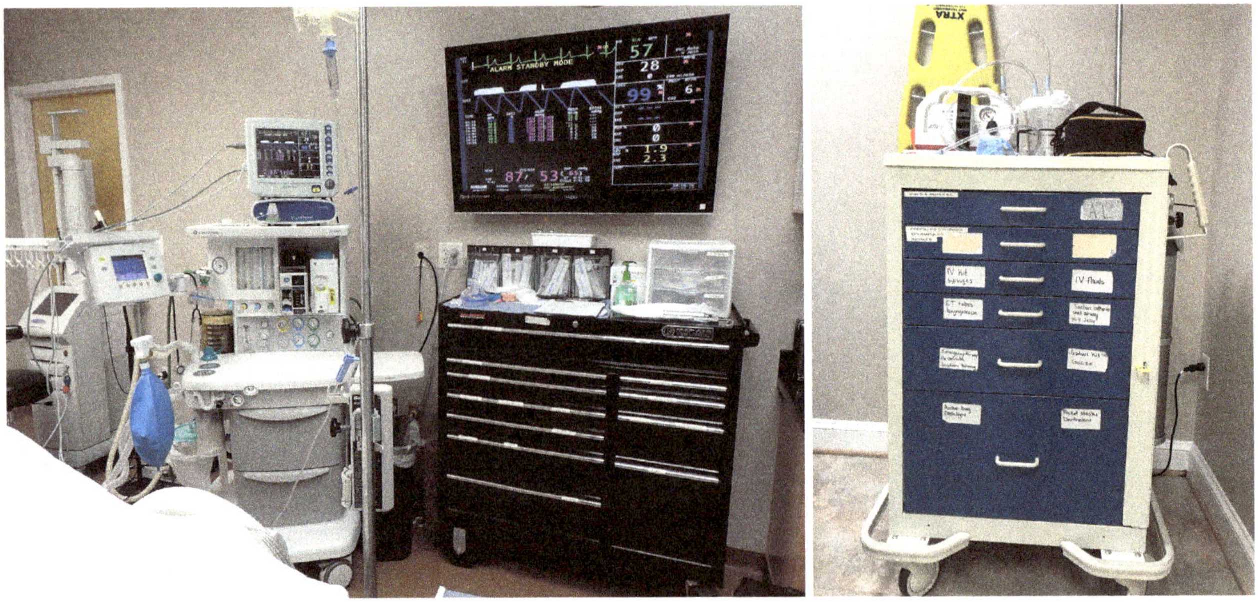

Fig. 5.6. An in-office surgery center requires hospital-grade anesthesia and emergency equipment.

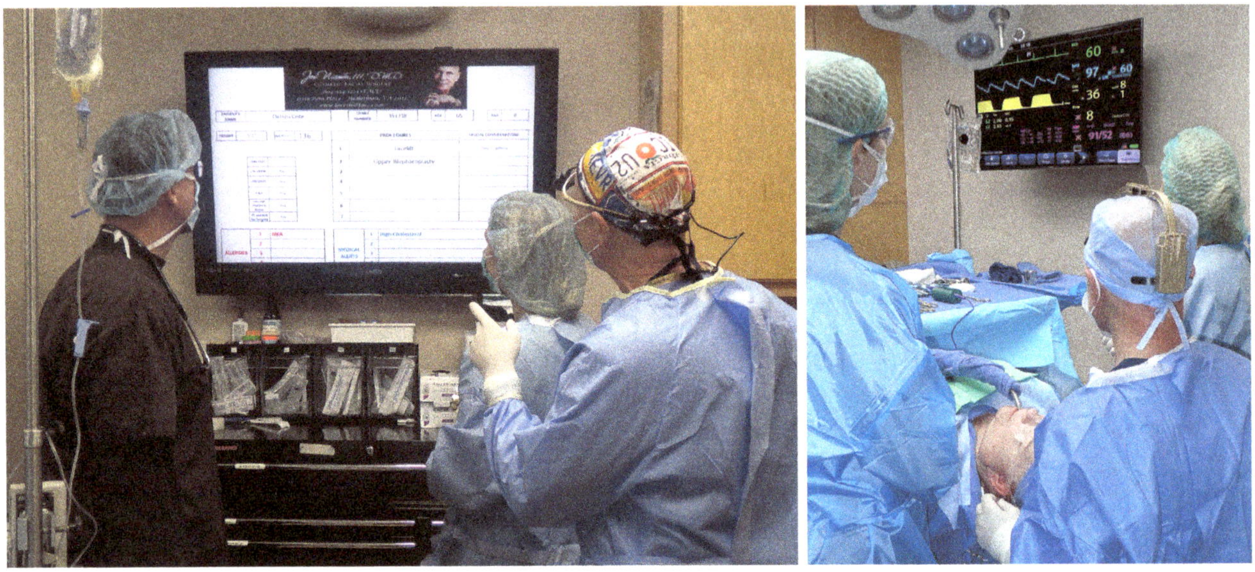

Fig. 5.7. Wide-screen TV monitors can be very useful in the operating room. The *left* image shows the team performing a "time-out" in preparation for surgery. Having the anesthesia vital signs displayed on a monitor for the entire team to see is also a valuable tool.

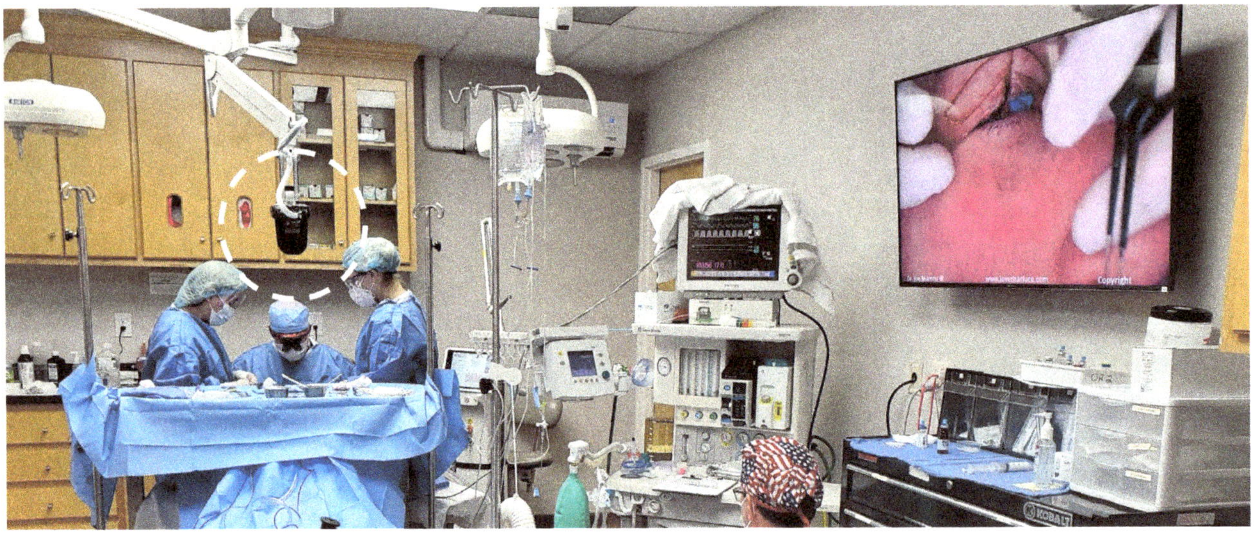

Fig. 5.8. An overhead camera can broadcast to monitors for educational purposes or recording surgeries.

Although many operating rooms use large overhead lights, I personally believe they are falling out of favor for numerous reasons. Number one, they can be very hot and cumbersome, and they have to be continually adjusted. Although we have standard operating room lights in our office, we rarely use them as I favor headlights. I have used all popular headlights over the years and recently purchased a Mamang shadowless dual-beam headlight. Although pricey, this particular light and loupe system has proven comfortable and versatile (Fig. 5.10).

Instrumentation

Instrumentation is largely a personal choice, as we all have special things we like to use. Over the years, a surgeon can accrue a vast array of instruments that they don't use. They went to a meeting, saw an instrument, brought it home, and then never used it again! I personally have gone to an exhibit hall and purchased a "new" instrument, only to bring it to work and have my staff laugh as I already had two!

Anyhow, instruments are part of the fun and precision of surgery. Although many specialized instruments exist specifically for rhytidectomy, the procedure can be performed with relatively basic surgical instruments that most surgeons already have in their offices (Figs. 5.11 and 5.12).

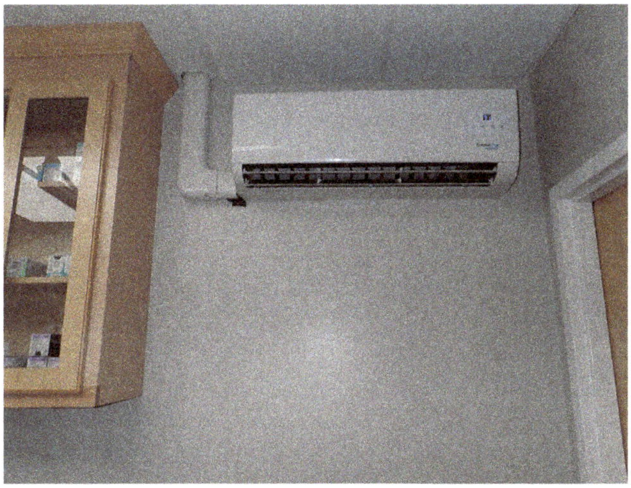

Fig. 5.9. An ancillary heat and cooling system can be a welcome addition to the operating room. Lengthy cases can be made more comfortable with the ability to control the operating room environment above and beyond the building HVAC system.

A basic list follows:

1. Operating table
2. Headlight and loupes, fiber-optic retractors
3. Marking pen, surgical ruler, measuring caliper
4. Surgical prep
5. Tissue dissector cannulas (https://www.kmiimigroup.com/)
6. Liposuction cannulas (2 mm, 3 mm, and 5 mm)
7. Retractors
   a. One pair of Senn retractors
   b. One pair of Army Navy retractors
   c. One pair of 6-inch small skin hooks
   d. One pair of double-ended skin hooks
   e. One Aufricht nasal retractor for generalized soft tissue retraction
8. Periosteal elevator
9. Round-handle scalpel
10. Padgett Gorney facelift scissors (www.miltex.com)
11. Pickup forceps (two of each)
    a. Medium
    b. Small
    c. Long bayonet
12. Radiowave or electrosurgery system for coagulation
13. Mosquito hemostats of various sizes, including long, thin tonsil clamp for placing cheek implants
14. Needle holders, various sizes
15. Micro skin stapler and staple remover
16. Suture scissors
17. Sutures (www.ethicon.com)
    a. 2-0 Vicryl
    b. 4-0 gut
    c. 5-0 gut
    d. 4-0 Vicryl
    e. 6-0 gut
18. 4 × 4 radiographically marked gauze
19. Hair comb
20. Suctions, various size Frazier-tipped and tonsil suction
21. Local anesthetic (2% lidocaine with 1:100,000 epinephrine) and syringes with 1.5-inch 25-gauge needles (or 32-gauge needles for eyelid injections)
22. 1 L of tumescent local anesthesia mixture (0.1% lidocaine with 1:1 million epinephrine)
    a. 1 g of lidocaine
    b. 1 mg of 1:1,000 epinephrine

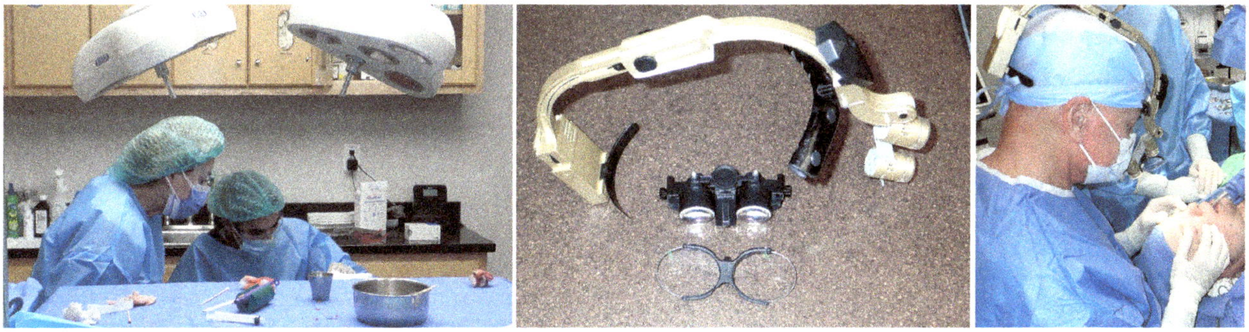

Fig. 5.10. Many surgeons use overhead lighting (*left* image), which can be hot and cumbersome. I prefer working with a headlight, and the new style of dual lamp "shadowless" lights are very effective and convenient. Loupes are easily attached and removed and the light can be flipped up during surgery when not in use. This headlight from Hayden Medical (haydemmedical.com) is lightweight and comfortable (*right image*).

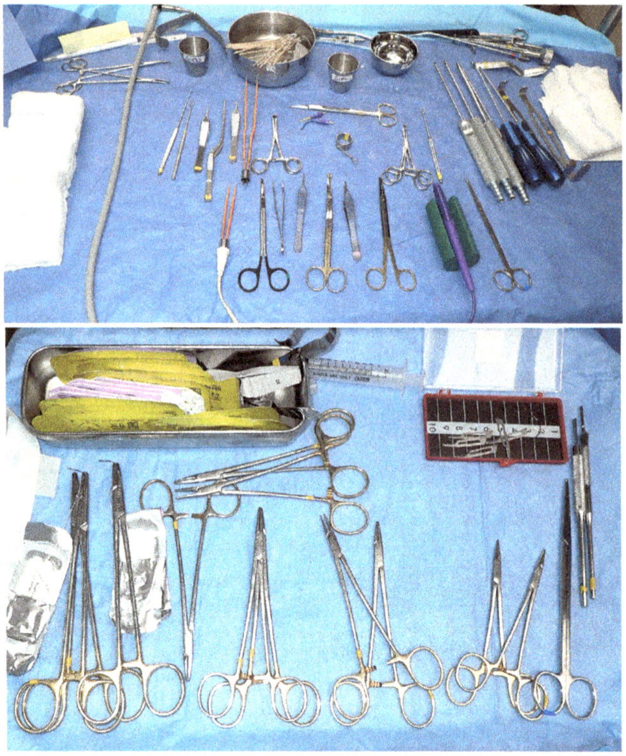

Fig. 5.11. The author's basic facelift tray is pictured.

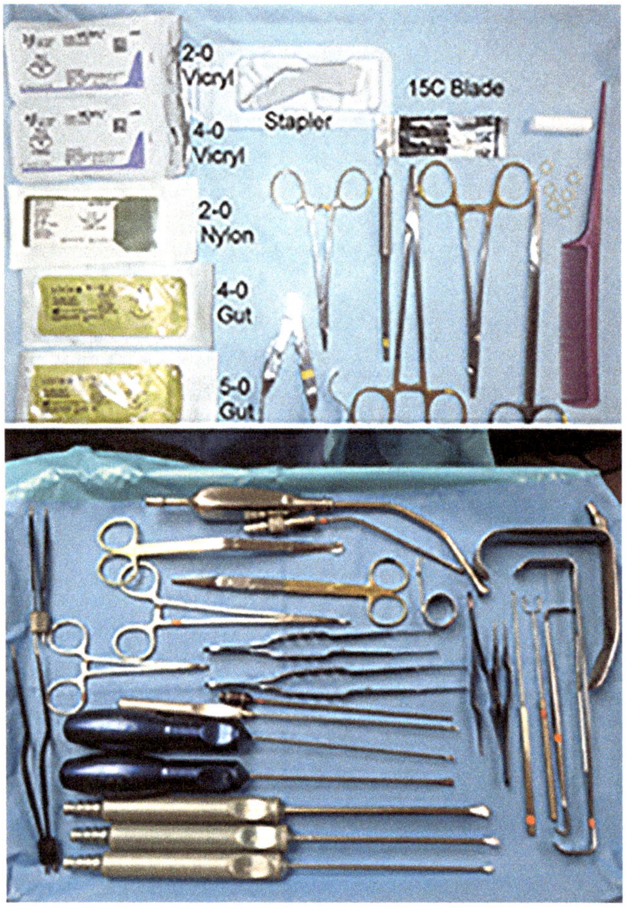

Fig. 5.12. A close-up of various facelift instruments showing sutures and related instruments.

   - **c.** 1 g of tranexamic acid
   - **d.** As only 500 mL is used on the average facelift patient, the formulation can be split in half with 500 mL normal saline

23. Tumescent pump or 60-mL syringe, and 18- or 22-gauge spinal needle or blunt infiltration cannula

24. Hair wash
   - **a.** Hydrogen peroxide (H_2O_2)
   - **b.** Sterile water
   - **c.** Large plastic trash bag to catch run off when washing hair

25. Dressings (for traditional facelift dressing)
   - **a.** Triple antibiotic ointment
   - **b.** Xeroform gauze
   - **c.** 3-inch Kling
   - **d.** 3-inch Coban bandage
   - **e.** Gauze "fluffs"

26. "Niamtu facelift dressing"
   - **a.** 4 × 4 gauze
   - **b.** Elastic head and neck compression bandage (jaw bra)
   - **c.** Jackson-Pratt drains for selected patients (#10 for females, #15 for males)

Fiber-optic lighted retractors are also an extremely useful adjunct for facelift surgery (Fig. 5.13). They are specifically useful for platysmaplasty, flap dissection, and superficial musculoaponeurotic system work, as they provide the ability to simultaneously retract and light the field. This is a great investment and also allows the surgeon to see the bottom of deep flaps without placing their neck in extreme bent over positions.

Some of the selected equipment that is mandatory or has improved our facility is discussed below.

Any surgeon that performs surgery anywhere on the body requires a means of hemostasis. Although there are numerous types of devices on the market, electrosurgery, and or radiowave generators most commonly used (Fig. 5.14).

Although syringes and needle can be used to deliver tumescent anesthesia, a dedicated tumescent pump is a great timesaver and improves efficiency (Fig. 5.15).

Sequential compression devices are standard of care in ambulatory office operating facilities (Fig. 5.16).

The recovery space is very important as the patient is still under the effects of anesthesia and must be monitored closely. The recovery space should be close to the operating room(s) and close to an exit for patient discharge. Group practices that are running multiple operating rooms with multiple surgeons need multibay recovery spaces. Single-surgeon recovery space is more simplified (Fig. 5.17).

Although a recovery bed can be useful for longer recovery stays, it also implies "sleep" and this is not what is desirable in an ambulatory office surgery center. We want patients to be discharges as soon as they are stable and have a competent caregiver. Fig. 5.18 shows a Stryker recovery chair, which is very useful for numerous reasons. First and foremost, it has wheels and can be easily moved between the surgery and recovery spaces. Second, it is fully

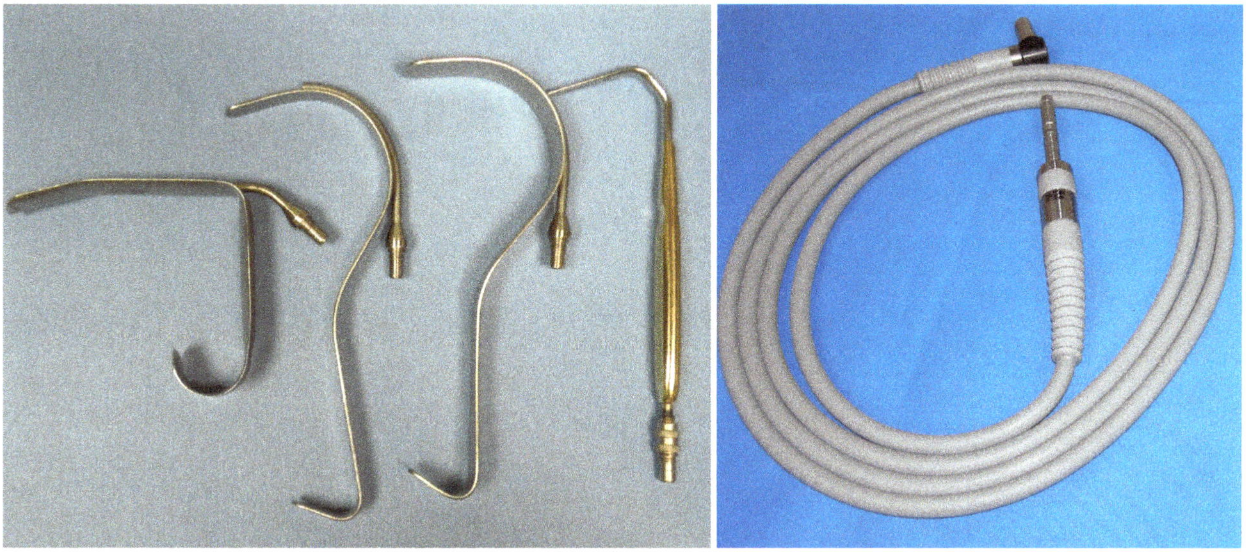

Fig. 5.13. A set of fiber-optic retractors are a sound investment and last for years. Having the right amount of light in tight places greatly facilitates facelift and other cosmetic surgery procedures.

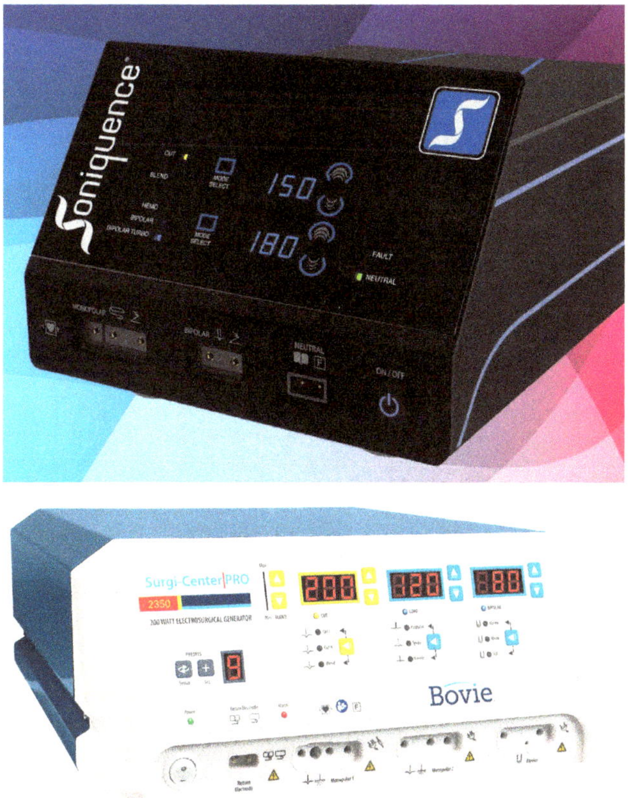

Fig. 5.14. A hemostatic device is a requirement for all surgery rooms. Cauterization and/or incision makes these devices indispensable. The *top* image shows the Soniquence Radiowave System and the *bottom* image shows a Bovie electrosurgical device.

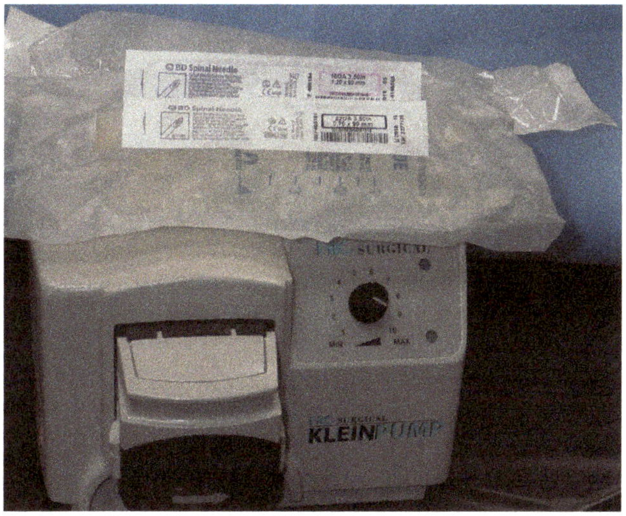

Fig. 5.15. A tumescent anesthesia pump, which greatly simplifies the delivery of tumescent anesthesia.

adjustable from anywhere between sitting, lying, and reverse Trendelenburg positions. It is also imperative to have suction and vital sign monitors in the postanesthesia care suite.

Postanesthesia patients must remain warm for comfort and safety. A forced air-warming system is an affordable option to maintain patient temperature in the operating room and recovery suite (Fig. 5.19).

A blanket warmer is also a good investment for warming patients (Fig. 5.20). Surgical spaces are usually cold and nothing feels better than a warm blanket.

A recent purchase that has truly simplified our instrument washing and sterilization is the Hydrim L110 automated instrument washer (www.scican.com). This device performs washes, ultrasonic cleaning, and drying much like a home dishwasher. Instruments go in contaminated and come out ready for the sterilizer. Not only has this been a great time-saver for my staff, but it also decreases their exposure to blood and surgical debris.

Another useful device in any cosmetic office is a commercial ice machine. I have tried "affordable" tabletop devices with

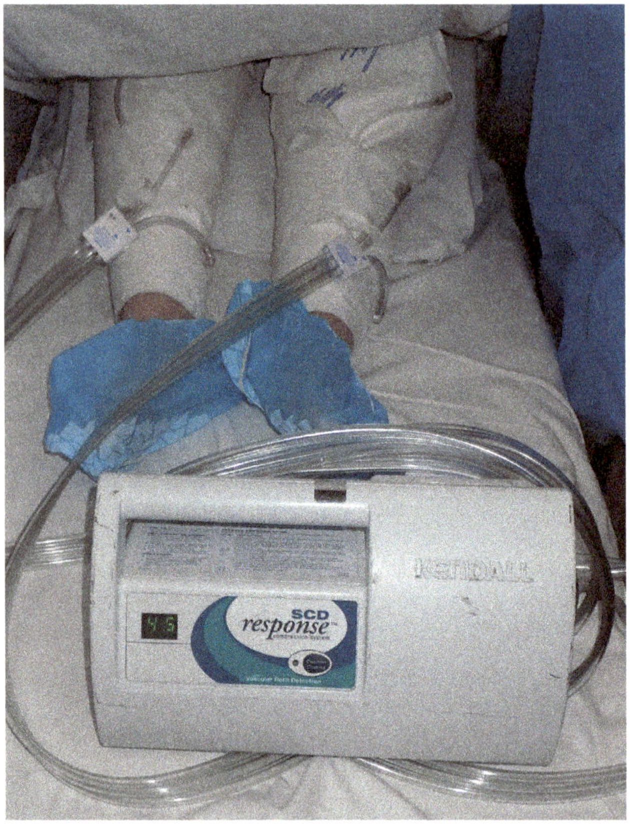

Fig. 5.16. A sequential compression device is used an all patients in addition to compression hosiery. Deep vein thrombosis prophylaxis and prevention is a critical part of surgery and anesthesia.

disappointment. Purchasing a true commercial-grade machine provides the availability of unlimited ice cubes or crushed ice Fig. 5.21. Ice is used all day long for injectable and surgical patients.

During the consideration of privacy, surgical patients should have a dedicated restroom and secure lockers to store their personal effects (Fig. 5.22). Undressing and dressing in a public place is unnerving, so providing convenient, comfortable, and secure spaces is essential.

Conclusion

Equipping an in-office surgical facility can be a task of awesome proportion and is frequently limited by the financial constraints of the practitioner. Patient safety and predictable outcomes should always be the goal of any office setup. Younger surgeons may have to build their ultimate surgery center over a number of years. This is where you will spend much of your life so you want it to be a nice and safe facility.

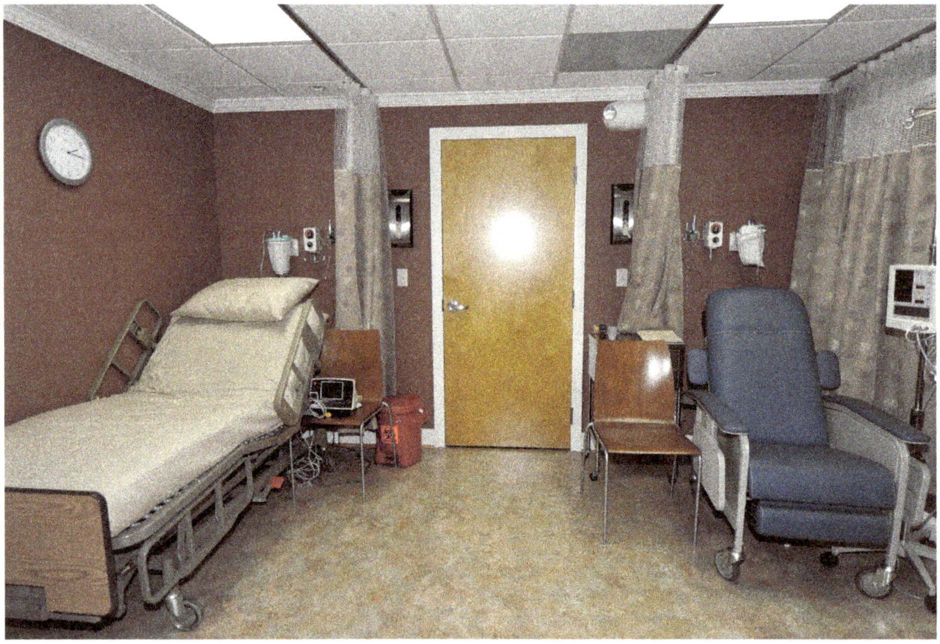

Fig. 5.17. The author's recovery space is shown. Having a hospital-type bed for longer recoveries is convenient, and a simple ambulatory recovery chair is also useful.

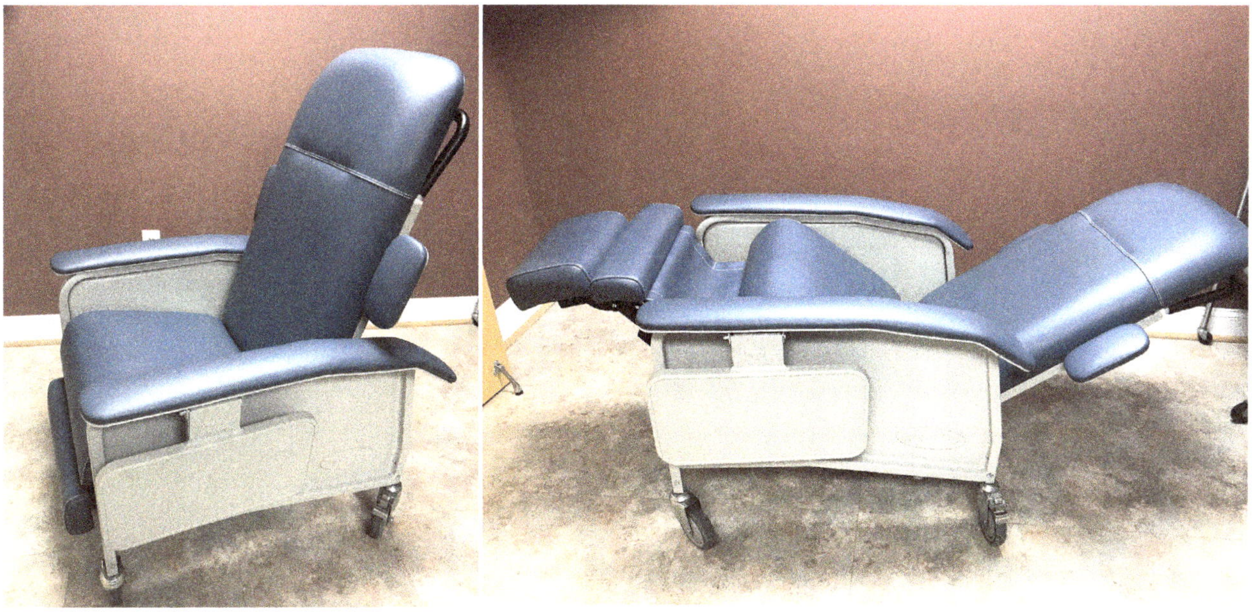

Fig. 5.18. An extra-wide clinical care recliner with drop arms has proven very effective for the author's ambulatory in-office surgery facility.

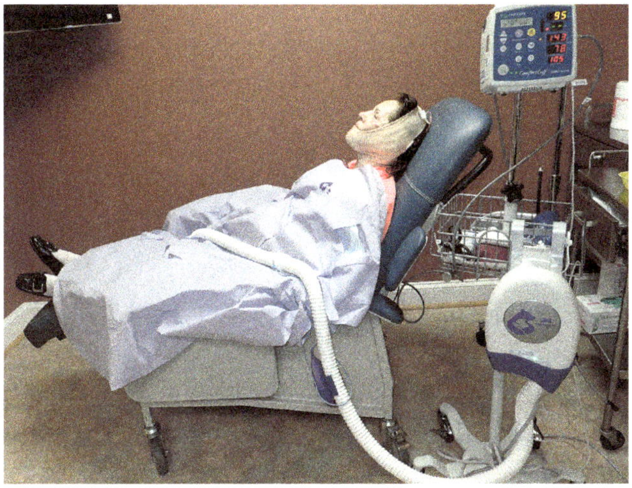

Fig. 5.19. A forced air-warming system is an affordable and essential part of an in-office surgery center.

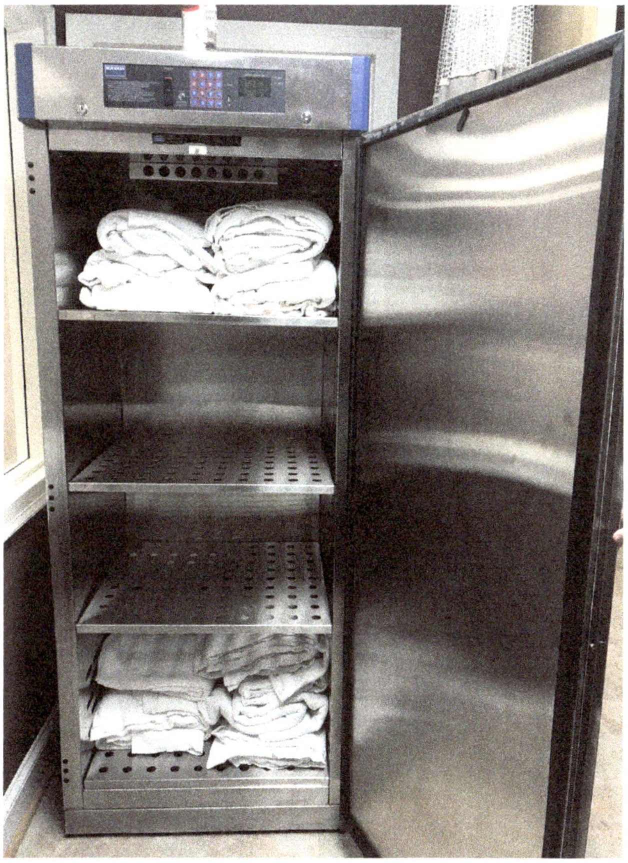

Fig. 5.20. The author's blanket warming cabinet is a great comfort to pre- and postsurgical patients.

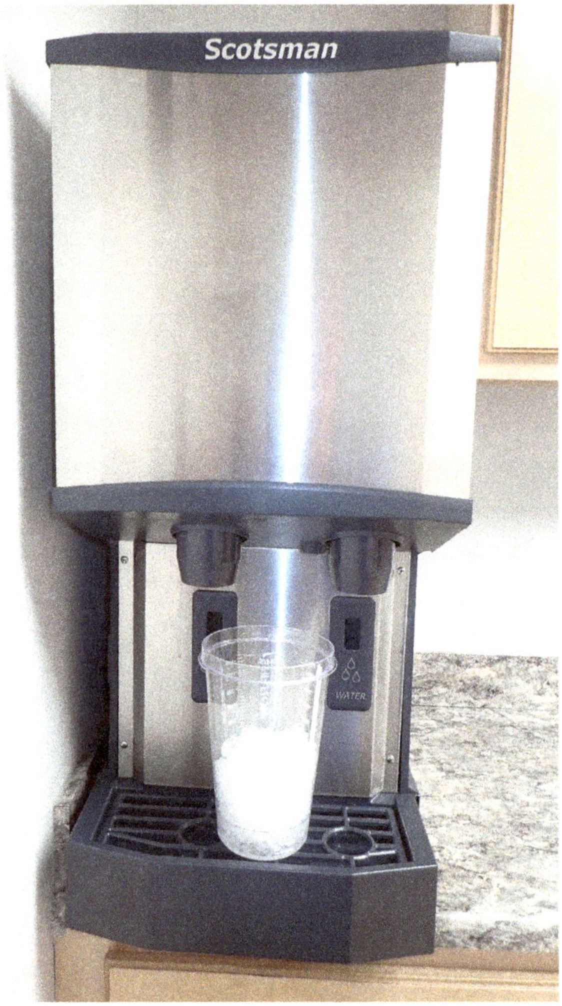

Fig. 5.21. A commercial ice machine is an appreciated benefit in any cosmetic office as many types of surgical and nonsurgical patients require ice for comfort or swelling.

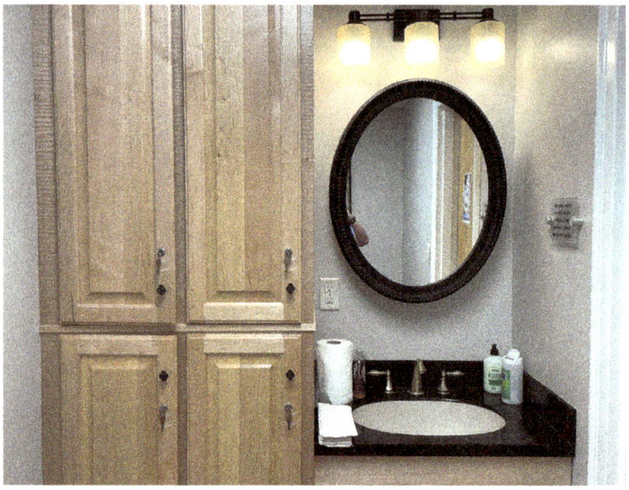

Fig. 5.22. A dedicated patient bathroom and secure storage area is incorporated into our recovery suite. This allows privacy for changing, using the restroom, and storing personal effects.

CHAPTER 6

Facelift and Neck Lift: The Procedure

Joe Niamtu, III

Chapter Outline

This is one of my favorite chapters because I get to discuss my evolution and current technique for cervical facial rhytidectomy. If 100 authors wrote the same book, you would probably have 100 different ways to perform these procedures. Despite all the customization and specialization that various surgeons do, most facelifts boil down to extremely similar techniques.

I do not profess that this is the only way to perform a facelift and neck lift, simply because this is the way I do it. The following is an evolution of almost 1700 facelifts at the time of this writing leading to my current technique. What is important is the fact that this has provided extreme patient safety and predictability and longevity in my practice.

I would like to comment on surgeons and their facelift numbers. As stated, at the time of this writing, I have performed almost 1700 lifts as the only surgeon. I hear some surgeons brag about performing over 7000 cases. First of all, surgeons have a tendency to inflate statistics. Also, many surgeons may have several residents or fellows that perform much of the procedure, which allows numerous cases in a day with much less time of the attending surgeon. Finally, some surgeons only perform minilifts or short scar lifts, which take a fraction of the time of larger lifts. In my situation, I am the only surgeon, and I perform everything from incision to closure. I can document all of my cases with pictures, so my number is accurate and real. I feel that it takes over 500 lifts to truly understand facelift surgery and over 1000 lifts to master it. Having said that, facelift surgery is a journey and not a destination. I still learn and strive to improve my technique on every single case.

Following this chapter, other expert facelift surgeons will present their techniques in detail.

Since much about patients and diagnosis has been previously discussed, this chapter outline will be as follows:

- Preoperating room
  - Photographing and marking the patient
  - Finalizing diagnosis, procedures, and health history
  - Final anesthesia exam, history, and physical
  - Patient taken to operating room
- In the operating room
  - Anesthesia induction
  - Prepping and draping the patient
  - Delivery of tumescent anesthesia
  - Ancillary procedures
  - Platysmaplasty
  - Periauricular incisions
  - Skin undermining and dissection
  - Liposculpture
  - Superficial musculoaponeurotic system (SMAS) management
  - Key sutures
  - Skin excision and tailoring
  - Earlobe tailoring and position
  - Postsurgical washing and preparation
  - Drains and dressings
  - Anesthesia emergence
  - Transfer to postanesthetic care unit

The preoperative time spent is important for both the surgeon and the patient. Patients are always anxious about the procedure and it helps to reassure them and calm them. This is the last time that the surgeon can examine the patient and ask questions and the last time the last time the patient can do the same. At this point, the surgeon wants to make sure that all communication is complete, all consents are signed, and there are no surprises from this point on. The surgical procedures and operative sites are confirmed.

Patients should be comfortable and a warm blanket is standard for my practice. This is also the time for them to use the restroom prior to going to the operating room. Finally, the caregiver and transportation are verified.

Marking the Patient and Incision Design

I personally feel that marking incisions are just as important as a blueprint for construction of a house. I also feel that it is paramount to mark the patient in the upright seated position before any anesthetic is injected. I have already discussed the importance of surgical markers, and if your markings rub off before you are ready to make your incisions, it can be very confusing, especially if tumescent anesthesia has already been injected. There is absolutely no place for inaccuracy when it comes to incision design. I firmly believe that you can look at any given surgeon's patients and determine the surgeon's ability by looking at the incision scars, the earlobe position, and the natural appearance of the hairline. All surgeons must understand that although we perform aggressive and extreme procedures inside the flap and with the SMAS, the only thing that the patient ever sees after their surgery is their incision. Becoming known for great postoperative incision scars can greatly increase the referrals in a facelift practice. Although the patient may not be able to see most of their scars, they are certainly visible to hairdressers, friends, and other medical practitioners. I have received many referrals over the years due to my commitment to excellent postoperative incisions.

Facelift incision markings include:

- Marking of ancillary procedures such as blepharoplasty, brow lift, and so on
  - Preauricular and sideburn incision
  - Postauricular and hairline incision
  - Submental incision for platysmaplasty
  - Markings made around the jowls, the platysmal bands, and region of anticipated submental liposuction

A facelift marking video accompanies this text.

Preauricular Incision

Each time I write another edition of my text, I research the literature about the subjects on which I write. Incisions can be one of the most controversial topics from article to article and textbook to textbook. There are so many types of surgical incisions, approaches, and modifications thereof. This dogma from author to author that can really be confusing for the novice surgeon. When I read some of the descriptions for facelift incisions, it would lead me to think that I am operating incorrectly. My surgical results, however, are not consistent with this. I, like many surgeons, incorporate various techniques to match the anatomy, hairline, and size of lift on the given patient. Experience provides diversity in surgical technique.

Some authors would lead one to think that a pretragal facelift incision is doomed for poor scarring and is simply improper technique. I could not disagree more with this. I use it on all males and most of my female patients. I have performed almost 1700 facelifts at this writing with 3400 incisions (two sides for each patient). For the first decade I used retrotragal incisions (on females), which healed well but occasionally led to tragal blunting. A blunted tragus is just too much of a stigma for an established facelift surgeon (Fig. 6.1). For the past decade I have used primarily pretragal incisions and have experienced great results and aesthetic scars. My decision to use pre- or posttragal incisions has to do with patient preference, local anatomy, and previous procedures. If a patient has a very petite tragus, I feel that it is more prone to blunting and I will usually employ a pretragal approach. Some patients have tragal anatomy where the tragus turns outward. Placing a

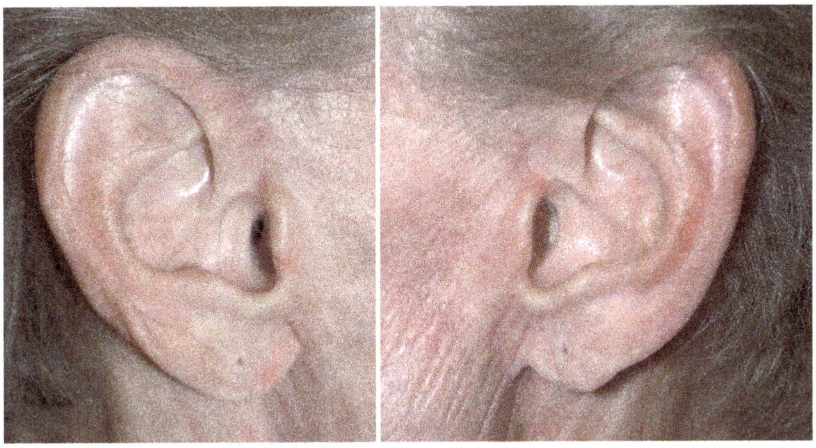

Fig. 6.1. Blunted tragi scream "I had a bad facelift" and should be avoided at all costs.

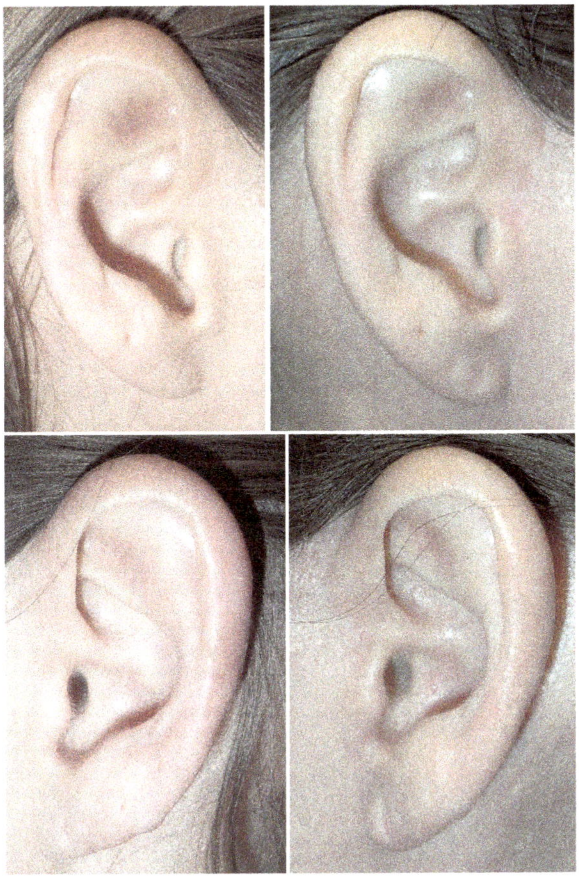

Fig. 6.2. The *left* images are before and the *right* images are after facelift using a pretragal incision by the author.

posttragal incision on this type of patient can cause it to be more visible. If a patient has well-developed rhytids in the pretragal region, then my usual incision is pretragal. In cases of revision facelift where the tragus has already been compromised or I feel may be compromised, I use a pretragal incision. If the patient has a well-developed tragus, I frequently choose a posttragal approach. Discussion with patients about incision placement is also considered. Each surgeon needs to find out what works best in their hands, realizing that it may vary from patient to patient. Remember, the scar is your signature and in part how your skills will be judged.

I feel that a valid way to judge the proficiency of a facelift surgeon is to look at their incisions, their sideburn conservation, the conservation of their posterior hairline in their earlobe position. Even in the hands of an experienced surgeon, cartilage healing can be unpredictable and result in tragal blunting. By incising anterior to the tragus, it will always be preserved (Figs. 6.2 and 6.3). Fig. 6.4 shows a pretragal and a posttragal incision, respectively. For males, pretragal incisions are utilized almost exclusively. The reason for this is that using a posttragal incision can pull the bearded cheek skin over the new tragus. This looks unnatural and is hard to shave. Pre- or posttragal incisions can be used on female patients.

When making traditional posttragal incisions, a right-angle horizontal cut at the incisura just below the tragus allows for a natural-looking scar (Fig. 6.5). Again, all surgeons should use the type of incision (pre- or posttragal) that produces the best postoperative scars in their own experience. Fig. 6.6 shows excellent postoperative scars using posttragal incisions.

When drawing the pretragal incision, the assistant puts traction on the cheek and the surgeon uses some downward pressure on the marking pen (Fig. 6.7).

This allows the tip of the pen to fall into the natural crease between the ear and cheek skin. It is very important to place this incision in the junction between the cheek and ear skin, or it will be visible postoperatively (Fig. 6.8, p. 72).

To best accommodate the delicate preauricular anatomy, I use a "triarcuate" incision, which as the name indicates produces three separate arcs at the helical attachment, the pretragal region, and the earlobe (Fig. 6.9, p. 72).

The next step is marking the sideburn incision, and there are many ways to do it. One of the major commandments of facelift surgery is not to elevate or otherwise displace the sideburn. Preauricular and sideburn incisions with aggressive temporal extension are well described in various textbooks and can result in major hair loss in the temporal region, which is one of the worst stigmata of facelift surgery (Fig. 6.10, p. 73).

Some surgeons make their incision at the junction of the temporal tuft and the skin. This is a guaranteed way not to displace the temporal tuft but is problematic if the incision becomes hypopigmented, which in not uncommon in this area. This can be extremely visible and difficult to correct (Fig. 6.11, p. 73).

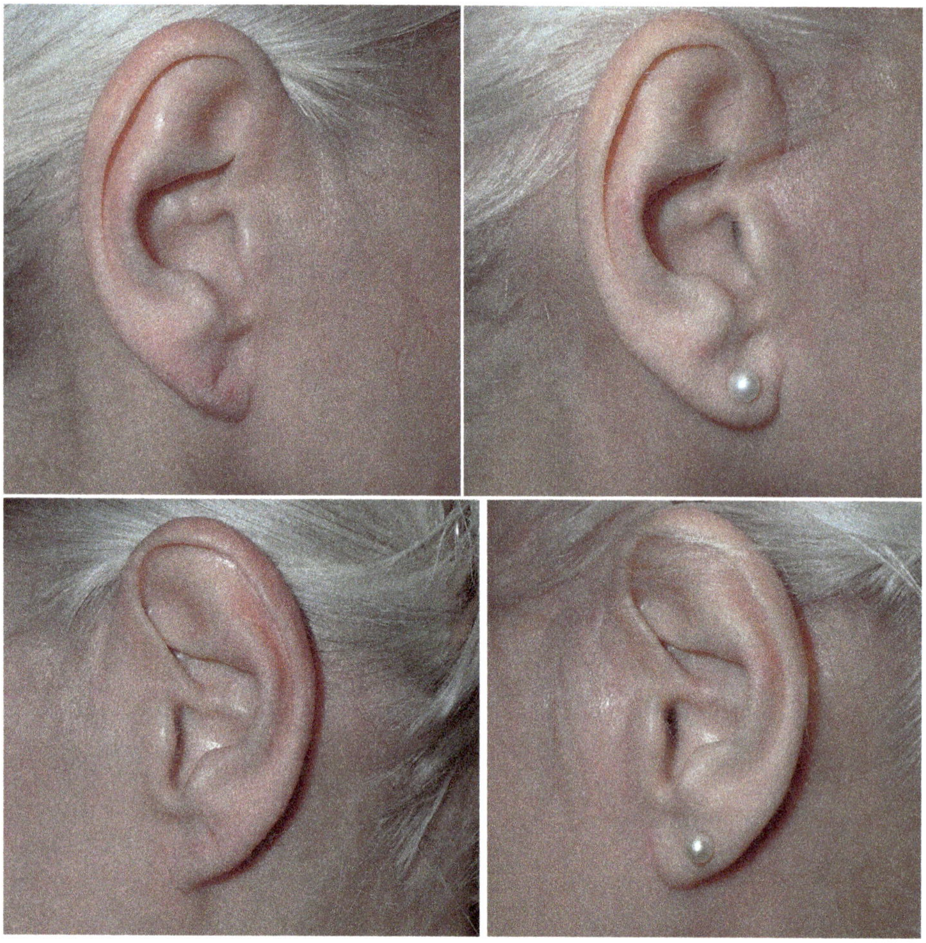

Fig. 6.3. The *left* images are before and the *right* images are after facelift using a pretragal incision by the author.

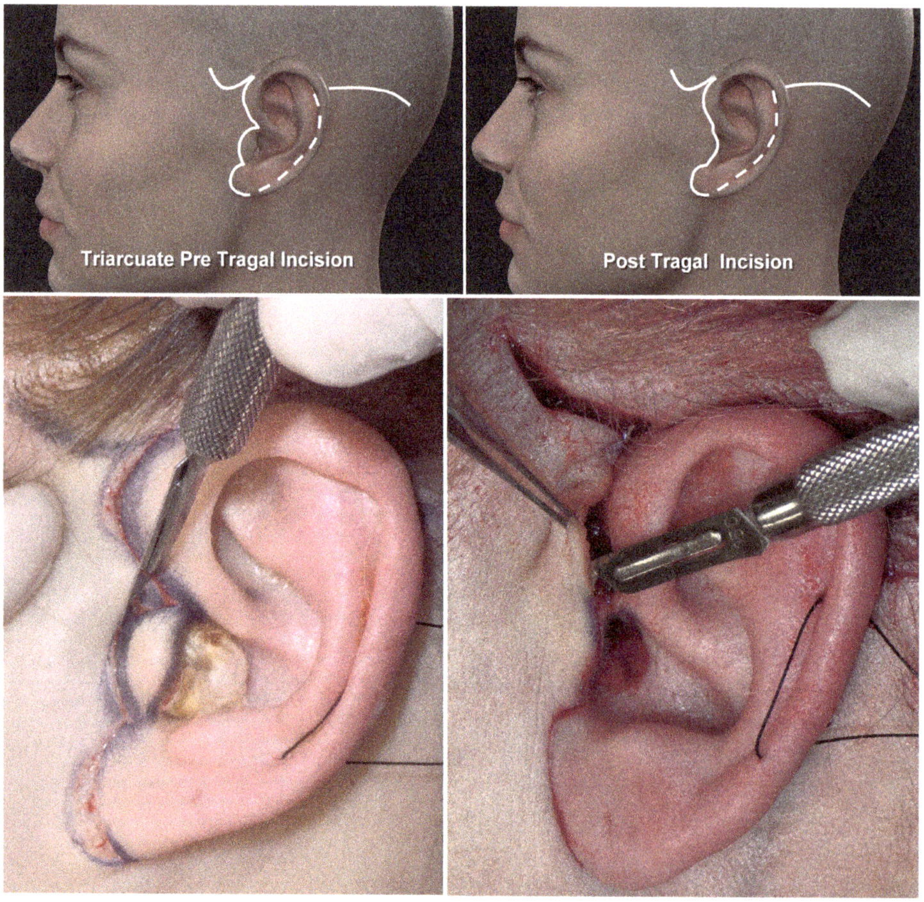

Fig. 6.4. The *left* image illustrates a post tragal incision and the *right* image shows a pretragal triarcuate incision.

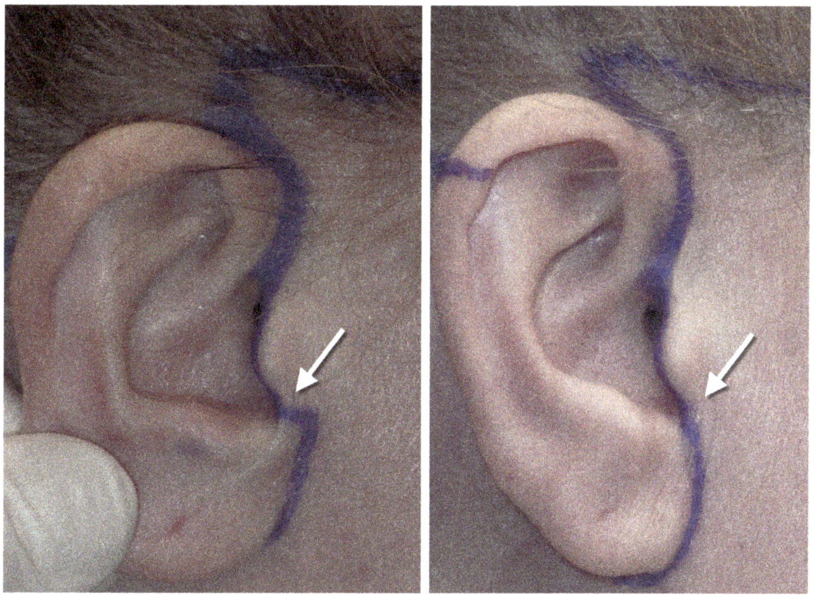

Fig. 6.5. These images show typical pretragal incision patterns. The *arrow* in the *left* image shows the incision extended horizontally at a right angle at the tragal incisura, which produces a natural scar line. The *right* image shows a contiguous posttragal incision. Both techniques are commonly utilized.

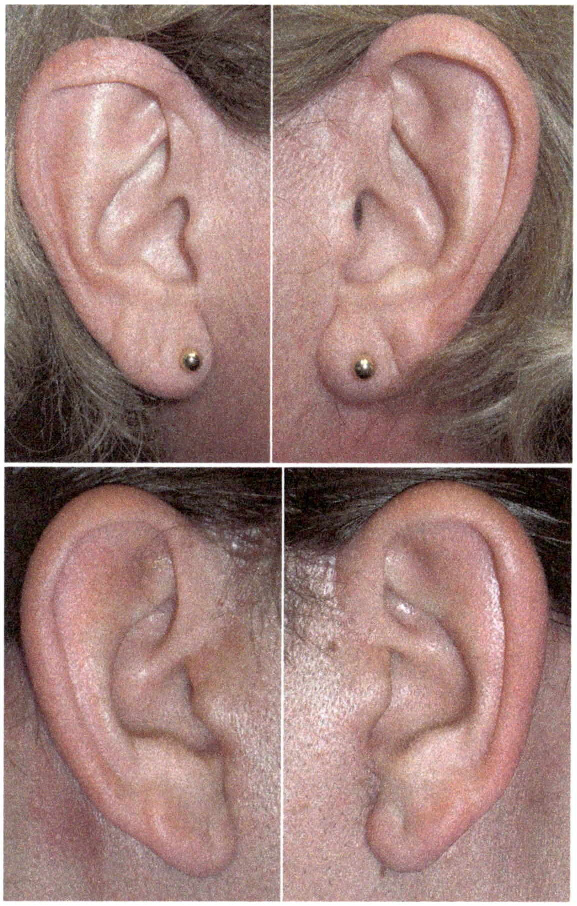

Fig. 6.6. The images show excellent posttragal incision after facelift surgery in a female (*top*) and male (*bottom*). I could show hundreds of before-and-after pics with either pre- or posttragal incisions. I use them both based on the aforementioned factors.

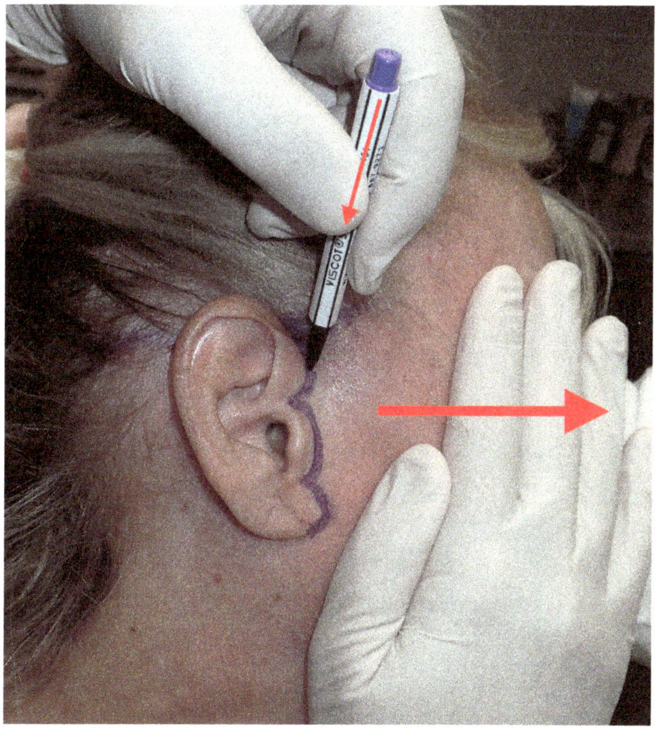

Fig. 6.7. It is imperative to place the incision in the natural transition between the ear and cheek skin. Forward traction with downward pressure on the marking pen assists correct placement.

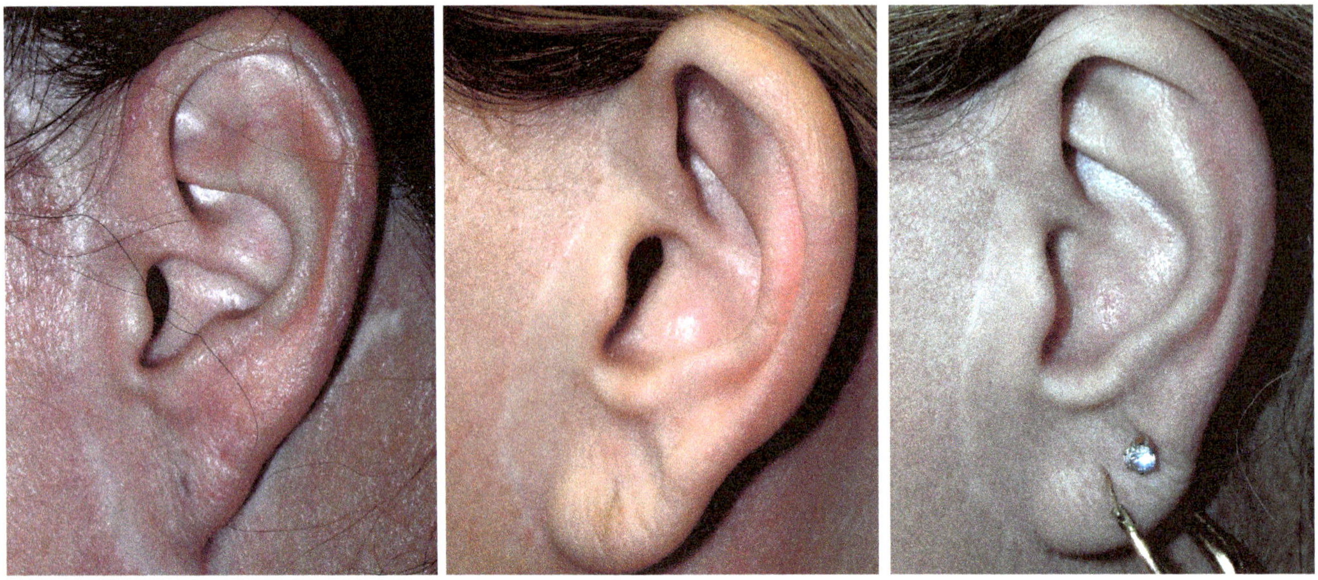

Fig. 6.8. These images from other surgeons show the problematic scars from placing the preauricular incision too anteriorly.

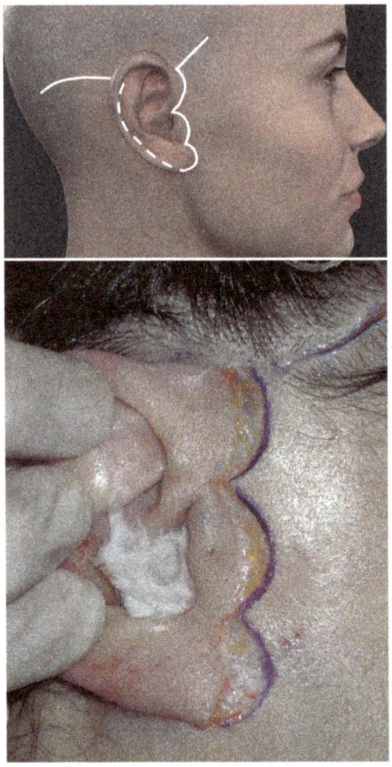

Fig. 6.9. The triarcuate pretragal incision frequently used by the author.

As stated, many surgeons place the temporal incision at the junction of the temporal tuft and the skin (*line 1*, Fig. 6.12). When at all possible, my goal is to have the sideburn incision fall within the temporal tuft so it is hidden (*line 2*, Fig. 6.12). On smaller cases, I may use an incision that comes off the helical attachment at a 45-degree angle (*line 3*, Fig. 6.12). If this 45-degree incision is used in larger cases, it can leave a hairless notch in front of the sideburn. With any sideburn incision I have the best results when I retract the helical rim and hide the incision junction behind the pinna, where it then extends into the temporal tuft (Fig. 6.12, *right*). Cases with minor to moderate skin excess will allow placement of higher incisions hidden in the temporal tuft (Fig. 6.12, *incisions 2* and *3*). Cases of large neck skin excess are better treated with a low sideburn (Fig. 6.12, *incision 1*) incision as excising large amounts of skin excess can elevate the temporal tuft (sideburn). All these pictured configurations allow vertical adjustment of the preauricular flap, which is a necessity.

Any incision made in the anterior or posterior hairline is made in a transfollicular (also called trichophytic) manner. This type of transfollicular incision is described in great length in the open brow and forehead lift section of this text. Basically, the incision is made in an extreme hyperbeveled manner with the scalpel almost horizontal to the skin. This produces a transection of some of the follicles, which remain viable and grow back through the incision to camouflage the scar (Figs. 6.13 and 6.14).

In addition to the hyperbeveled incision, I prefer to keep my sideburn incision within the temporal tuft, when possible, as it will be totally camouflaged by the patient's hair. I also make my incisions irregular and undulating as these incidental geographic incisions heal superiorly to straight-line, nonbeveled incisions (Fig. 6.14).

As stated earlier, there are many ways to craft the anterior incision, and every surgeon needs for find what works best in his or her hands. The main things for success are a well-healed scar, no elevation of the temporal tuft, a natural tragus, and a normal earlobe position.

Posterior Facelift Incision

Just like the anterior incision, there are numerous ways to create the postauricular incision during facelift surgery. I will describe the postauricular incision beginning from the earlobe, superiorly in the postauricular crease and horizontally into the posterior hairline.

I extend the preauricular incision around the earlobe, which is marked previously to surgery. It is important to follow the natural attachment of the lobe. I also release the earlobe to its attachment with this incision (Fig. 6.15). As the incision meets the postauricular crease, numerous texts recommend placing the posterior auricular incision several millimeters superiorly to

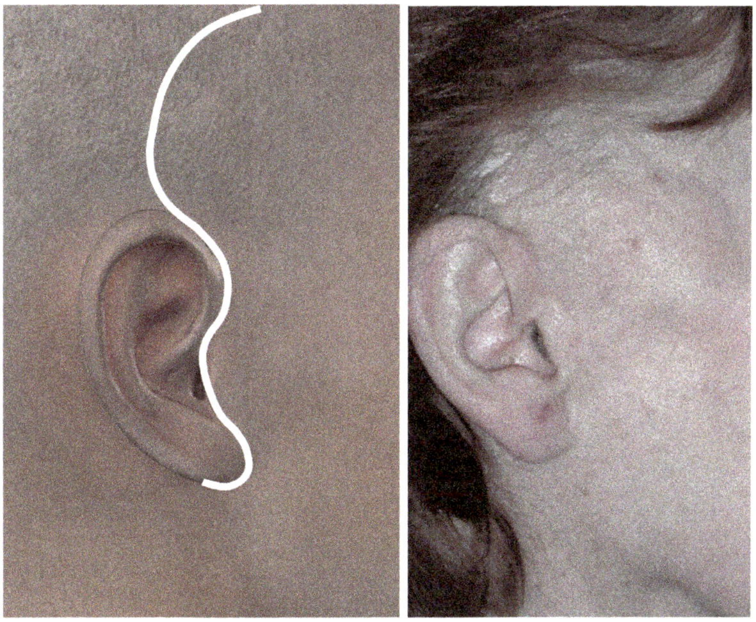

Fig. 6.10. Some surgeons employ aggressive temporal extension of the temporal tuff. This may be done in an attempt to elevate portions of the upper or midface, but can be disastrous as shown in this facelift patient from another office.

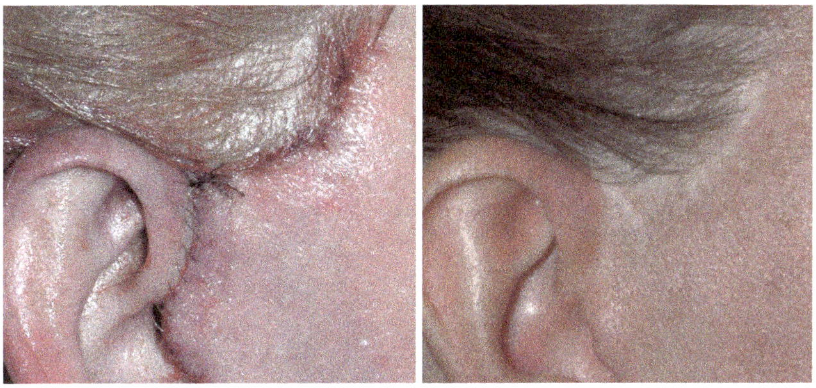

Fig. 6.11. Incisions made just below the hairline will not raise the sideburn, but if they hypopigment, they can be extremely visible. This same problem can occur when postauricular incisions are made at the occipital hairline.

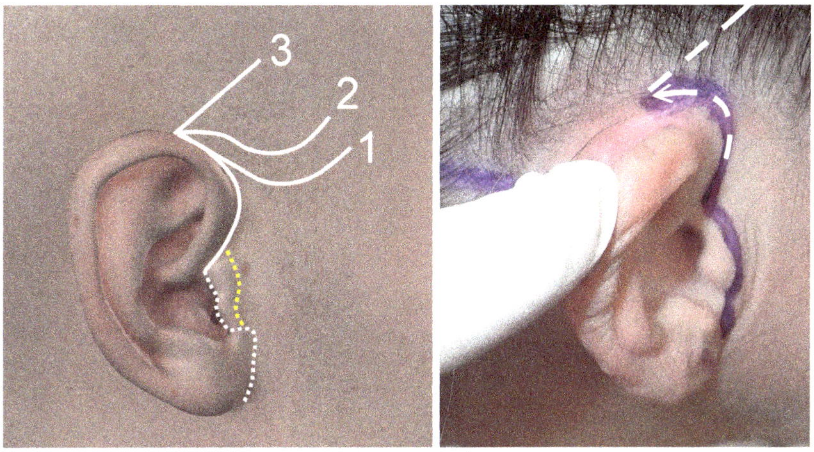

Fig. 6.12. The *left* image shows my three common options for the placement of the sideburn incision. The *white dotted line* shows a posttragal incision, and the *yellow dotted line* shows a pretragal incision. Regardless of which incision is used on the temporal tuft, it meets the helical attachment incision (*arrow*) at an acute angle hidden behind the pinna (*right* image). I may use any combination of all these pictured incisions based on the gender, size of the lift, and existing hairline. I prefer incision location 2 when possible, as it remains hidden in the hairline.

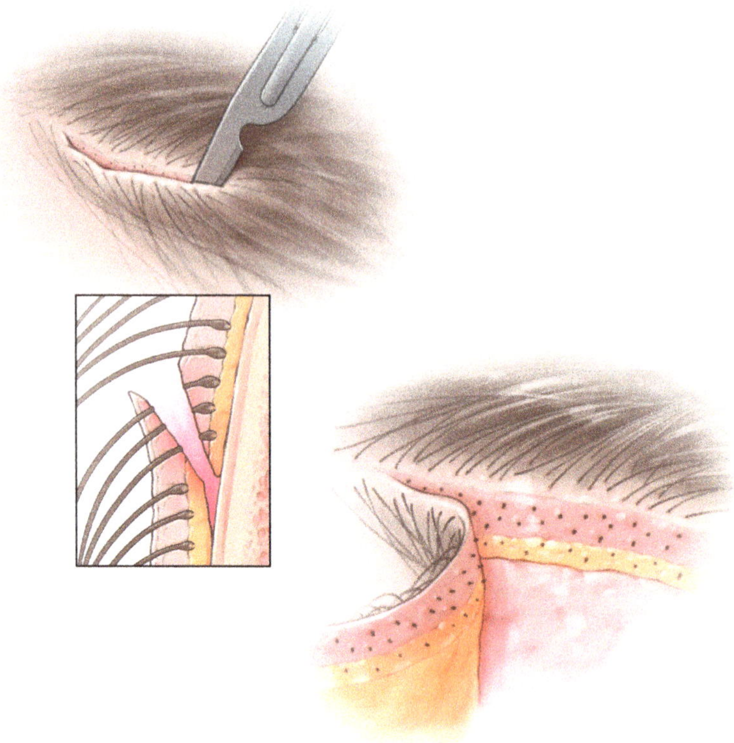

Fig. 6.13. The author employs transfollicular hyperbeveled incisions in any hair-bearing area. The *right* image shows transected hair follicles on the dissected flap. The bulbs of these hairs are still intact on the fixed part of the scalp and will regrow through the flap.

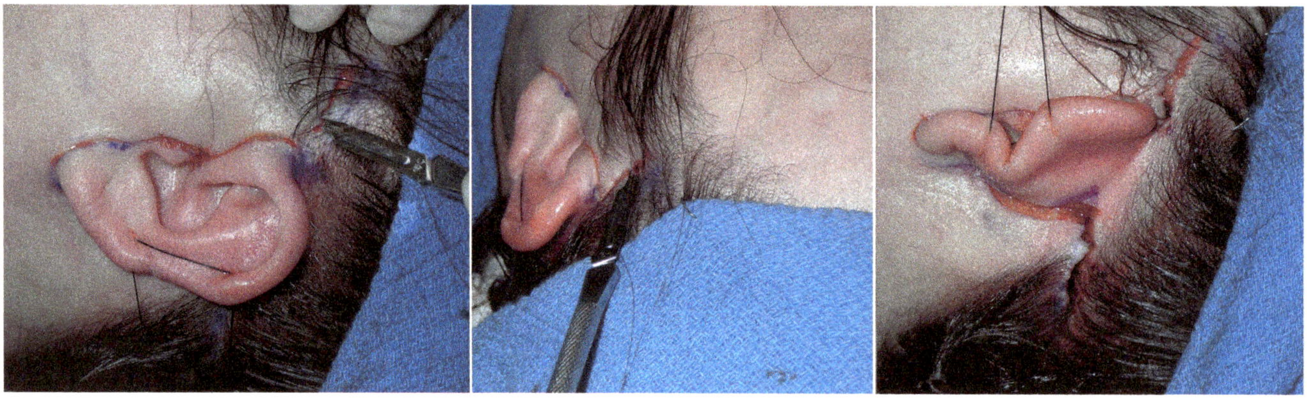

Fig. 6.14. My best postoperative hair-bearing scars involve hyperbeveled transfollicular incisions made in an irregular pattern within the hairlines. The *left* and *middle* images show the extreme bevel angle of the scalpel. The *right* image illustrates how the intentional jagged or irregular pattern makes a less noticeable scar than a straight-line incision. Note that the sideburn incision will remain hidden in the hair.

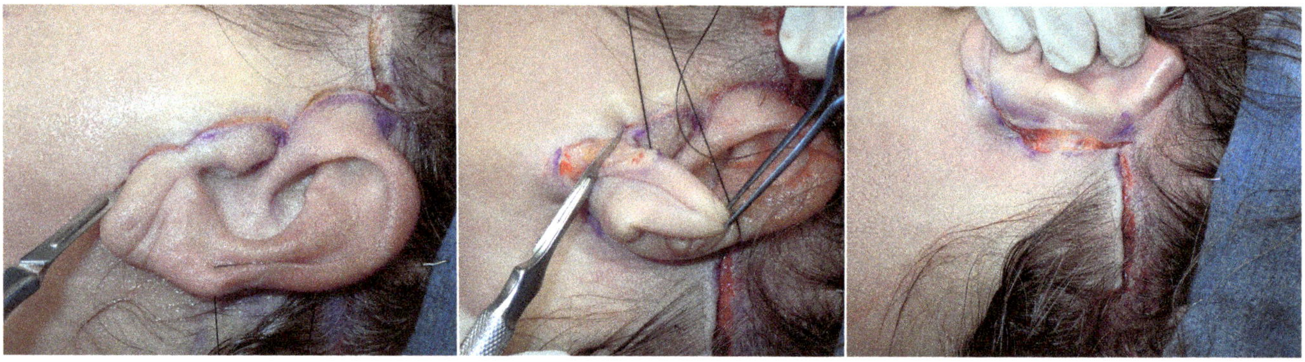

Fig. 6.15. The *left* image shows the triarcuate incision extending along the natural attachment of the earlobe. The *center* image shows lobe being detached, and the *right* image shows the posterior sulcus incision and the hairline incision.

the posterior auricular crease with the suggestion that the scar will contract into the crease and be hidden. This is something that is not consistent with my personal experience as I have found the scar to remain where it was placed. I, therefore, place the incision in the center of the posterior auricular crease where it is most hidden (Figs. 6.15 and 6.16).

At the greatest width of the pinna, the sulcular incision transitions to the posterior hairline incision (Fig. 6.17, *left*). Making the incision at the widest part of the pinna hides the skin incision as it enters the hairline (Fig. 6.17, *right*). Once the incision transitions the posterior auricular skin, it can enter the hairline in several positions (Fig. 6.17, *right*). I prefer the higher, solid blue line shown in Fig. 6.17 (*right*). Placing the incision high into the hairline will always hide the scar within the hair. Placing this incision high does make a longer flap and requires more dissection and potential dead space, but hiding the scar is worth the extra work in my experience. The higher hairline incision (Fig. 6.17, *left*) works well with mild to moderate skin access. With cases involving large amounts of neck skin excess, the occipital hairline incision (*dashed line* in Fig. 6.17, *right*) may be preferred as gross skin excision can raise or distort the posterior hairline when using a higher incision.

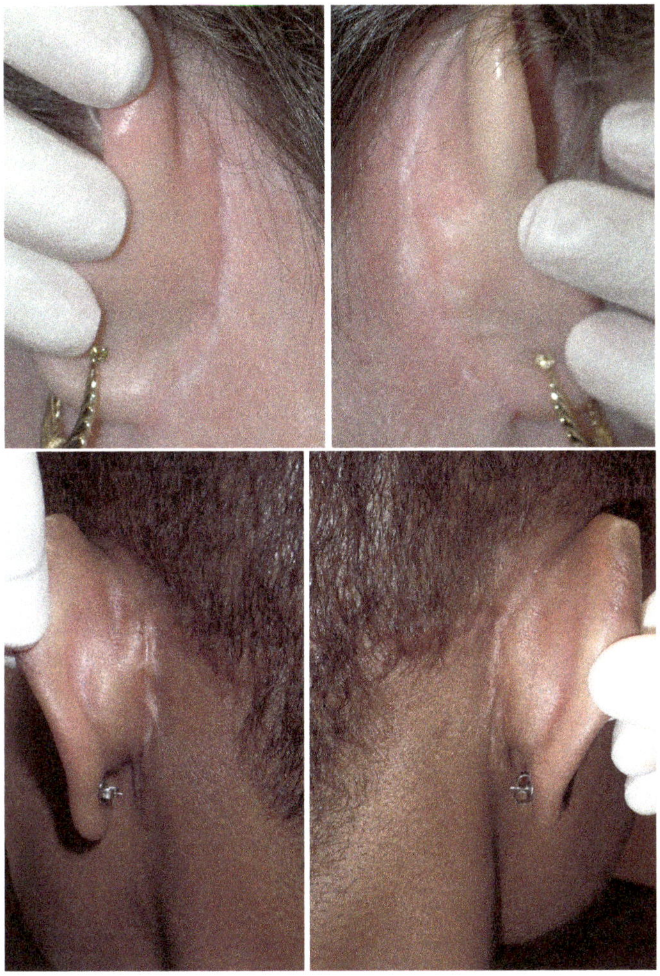

Fig. 6.16. Making the posterior auricular incision directly in the sulcus has provided excellent aesthetics in my experience.

One of the "incisional travesties" that I see from other surgeons is a low-placed mastoid postauricular incision (Fig. 6.18). Placing an incision in this low and highly visible region is "lazy" and guarantees a noticeable scar.

Many surgeons favor the occipital hairline incision. Again, this makes a smaller flap with less dissection and is an acceptable incision assuming normal healing. If this incision, for any reason, heals with hypopigmentation or hypertrophic scar, it is extremely noticeable and prevents women from wearing their hair up and is visible on men (Fig. 6.19). For this reason, I prefer the more superior hairline incision at the greatest width of the pinna as shown in Fig. 6.17 (*left*), unless the patient has a large amount of neck skin excess. Keeping the incision at the occipital hairline will not raise the hairline in these cases.

Over almost 1700 facelifts, I have had my best postauricular hairline incisions with the extremely beveled, high-hairline incision (Fig. 6.20).

The type of posterior auricular incision will also be important when performing skin cutbacks and will be discussed later in this chapter.

Of almost 1700 at the time of this writing, I have only personally operated a handful of bald patients. I explain to them that there will be some visible incision scar and note that in the consent. Using a hyperbeveled, transfollicular incision, even on bald skin, has produced acceptable scarring (Figs. 6.21 and 6.22). A summary is provided if incision placement involves the amount of neck skin excess (and skin to be excised), the

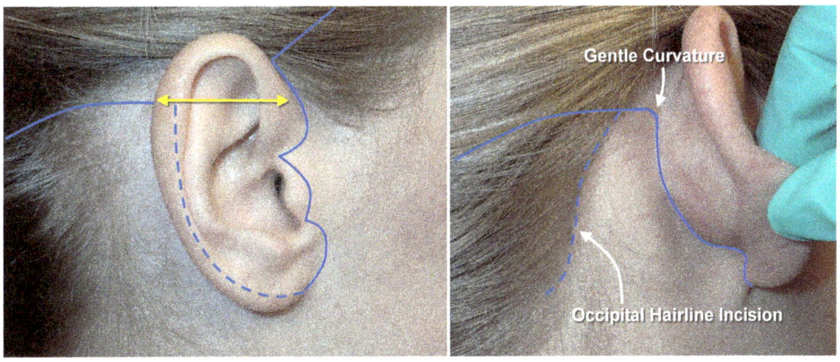

Fig. 6.17. The *left* image shows the author's preferred posterior incision, which transitions from the sulcular incision horizontally. The *right* image again shows the author's preferred posterior hairline incision (*solid blue line*) and an alternate occipital incision (*dotted blue line*). Note that the sulcular incision transitions to the other incisions with a gentle curvature.

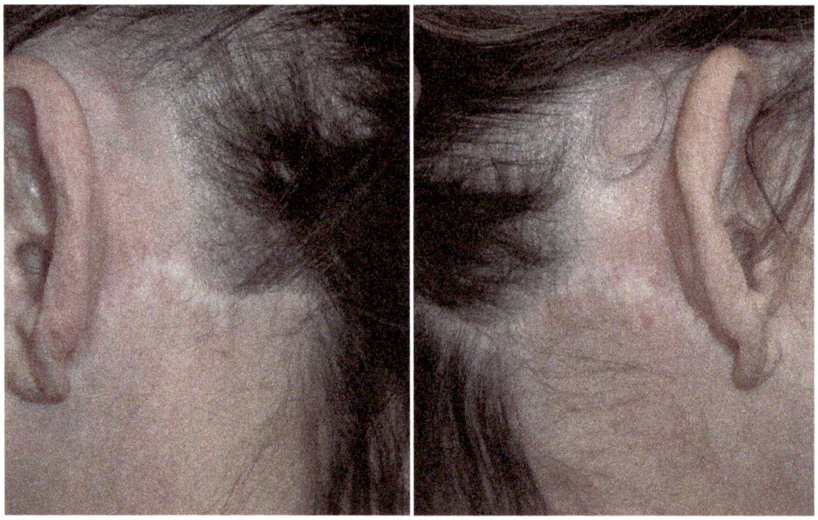

Fig. 6.18. Placing the postauricular incision low on the mastoid region is poor technique in the author's opinion.

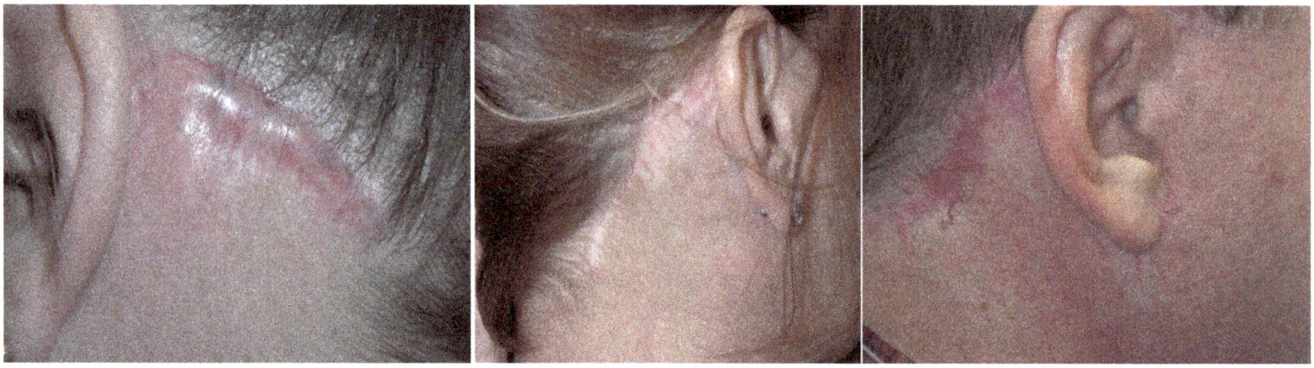

Fig. 6.19. Although occipital hairline incisions usually heal gracefully, if they have problematic healing the result is extremely noticeable.

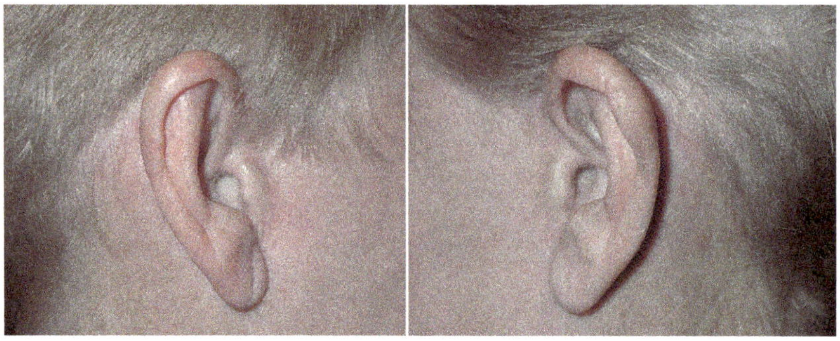

Fig. 6.20. This patient is shown 90 days after comprehensive facelift with the author's preferred high posterior hairline incision placement.

patient's hairline, and the experience of the surgeon. I modify all of my pre- and postauricular incisions to suit the specific case. My front incision may be pretragal in some patients and posttragal in others, and my posterior incision may be high in the hairline at the greatest width of the pinna or follow the occipital hairline, again depending on the specifics of the patient. There is no right or wrong, just good or bad scars and hairlines. Young surgeons should find what produces their best results.

After the pre- and postauricular incisions are marked, I mark the jowls, the submental incision, platysmal bands if present, and submental structures. For the submental incision, the patient extends their neck and a mirror is held under the patient to illuminate the area and the incision is placed several millimeters below the submental crease (Fig. 6.23).

The submental incision is not as noticeable as the other incisions, but it is still very important to make this incision in the correct area and to make it symmetric (Fig. 6.24, *left*). Many patients have a deep submental crease, and making an incision in this crease as described in many textbooks can actually deepen the crease (Fig. 6.24, *right*). I generally make this incision several millimeters below the submental crease. In the case of a very deep submental crease, I make the incision even lower and undermine the deep crease to improve it. If a chin implant is planned, the crease is placed lower as the implant can move it forward and cause it to be more visible.

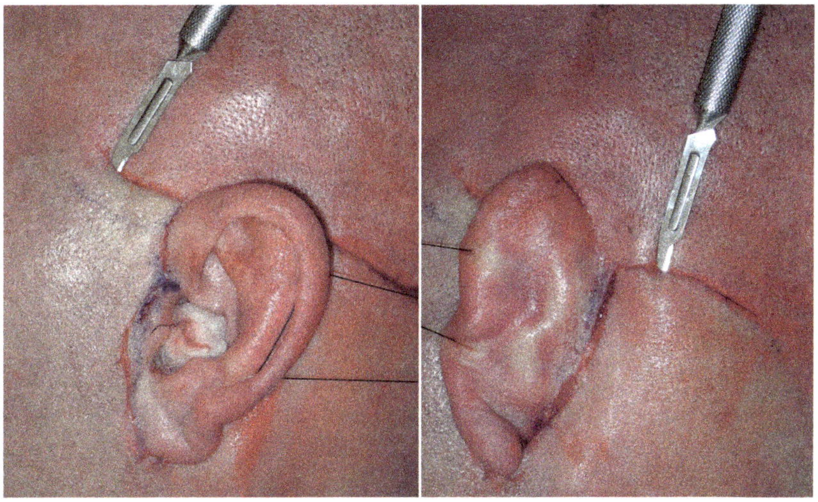

Fig. 6.21. Transfollicular, hyperbeveled incisions have the potential to heal well, even in the case of baldness.

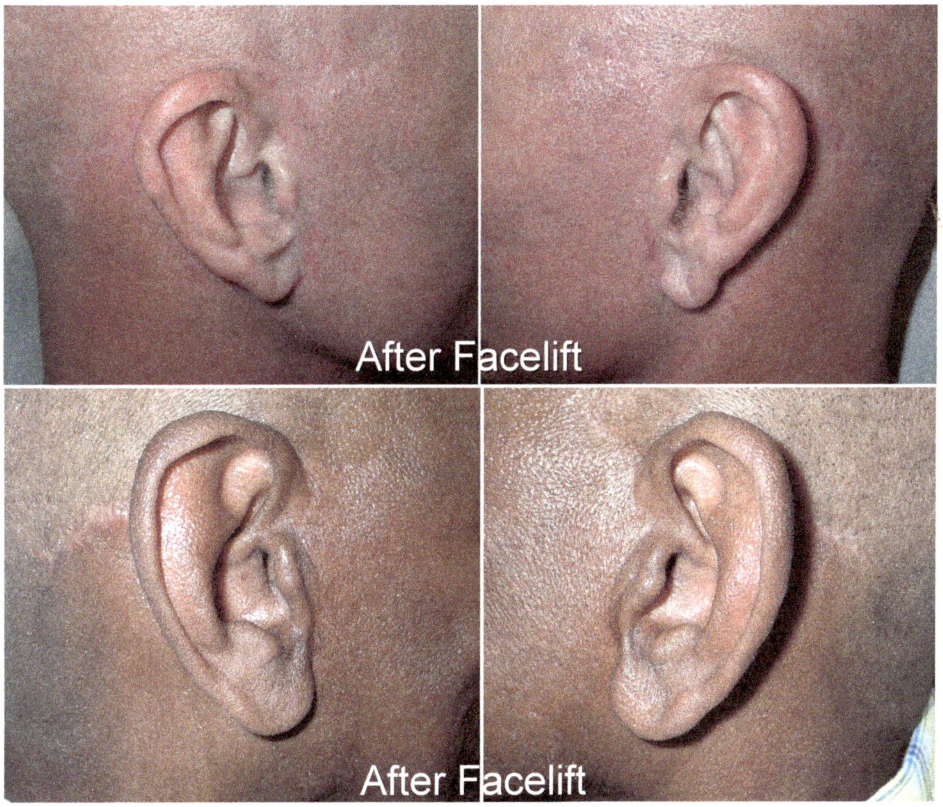

Fig. 6.22. The *top* image is the same patient shown in Fig. 6.21. The *lower* image shows healed facelift incisions in a bald African American patient.

Although this crease is somewhat hidden, a crooked or depressed scar in this area is still extremely noticeable. It is important to keep the incision on equal sides of the midline and to keep the incision as small as possible when performing platysmaplasty.

Like so many other facets of surgery, some well-known surgeons advocate placing the incision in the crease and don't feel that it accentuates it. Always remember that different techniques work better for different surgeons. My advice to new surgeons is to figure out what gives you the best result and stay with it.

Off to the Operating Room

Although the facelift incisions are actually a part of the surgery that takes place when the patient is asleep, I described them in detail because the incision planning is paramount for an aesthetic incision.

I will describe in detail how I perform facelift and neck lift surgery in this chapter. Following chapters will show techniques of other busy facelift surgeons.

When the patient is taken into the operating room, some of the most vulnerable times are at the very beginning of the case and at the very end of the case because the staff is frequently preoccupied with their initial duties. Especially in the beginning of the case, when everyone is trying to get their tasks started, medication, wrong procedure, and wrong surgery site errors can occur. The surgical staff undergoes a team timeout, at which point we review any pertinent medical or anesthetic information, medications, drug allergies, surgical sites, consents, and any other pertinent information. This is a critical time in our office, and everyone must stop and pay full attention during the timeout (Fig. 6.25). If the surgeon takes a break during the case for any reason, an additional timeout is performed before resuming surgery.

One of the main goals of facelift anesthesia is to prevent hypertension, which is one of the major contributors to postoperative hematoma. A bloody field also complicates and obscures the surgery and can lead to postoperative hematoma. Rigid preoperative control of any medication or preparation that affects platelet function and attention to blood pressure are imperative for successful surgery.

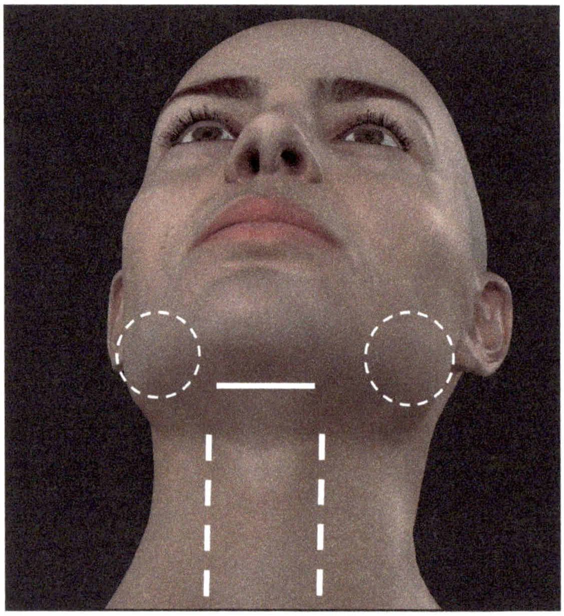

Fig. 6.23. The jowls (*circles*), submental incision (*solid line*), and platysmal bands (if present, *dotted lines*) are marked with the patient in the upright position. (Base image, courtesy *Complete Anatomy*, Elsevier.)

Controlling blood pressure pre- and intraoperatively is also essential for successful surgery with low complication rates. The majority of our patients are given 0.1 to 0.2 mg of clonidine with a sip of water just before surgery. This is because many patients have borderline hypertension and it also makes it easier for anesthesia to control intraoperative blood pressure and use less medication for blood pressure spikes. I also prefer to operate with a systolic blood pressure less than 100 mm Hg. I can tell a significant difference in oozing when the systolic blood pressure exceeds 100 mm Hg. It is important to keep the mean blood pressure at 60 or above. Mean blood pressure is calculated by the following formula: median blood pressure = diastolic blood pressure + $\frac{1}{3}$ (systolic blood pressure − diastolic blood pressure).

All offices have different setups and vary with the amount of time a surgeon has been in practice, their facility, and their method of anesthesia. In my office-based Accreditation Association for Ambulatory Health Care–accredited surgery center, we operate in a sterile hospital-type environment, employing intubated general anesthesia (Fig. 6.26).

Some surgeons operate in a "clean," but not sterile, environment and use local anesthesia for facelifts. In my experience, most surgeons with high-volume facelift practices operate in sterile environments with general anesthesia. I also have friends that use IV sedation instead of general anesthesia and prefer to do their facelifts in that manner. All surgeons must find the method that works best for them for safety and predictable outcomes.

The surgeon and surgical staff can assist the anesthesia provider during anesthetic induction an intubation. Once the endotracheal tube is placed and confirmed, the tube is sutured around the upper teeth to maintain stability throughout the case. As part of our deep vein thrombosis prevention, the patient wears compression hose, and we also use sequential compression devices on the lower extremities, as shown in Fig. 6.27.

After anesthesia is induced, the surgical staff begins prepping the patient for surgery. Using a surgical marker, I make a mark

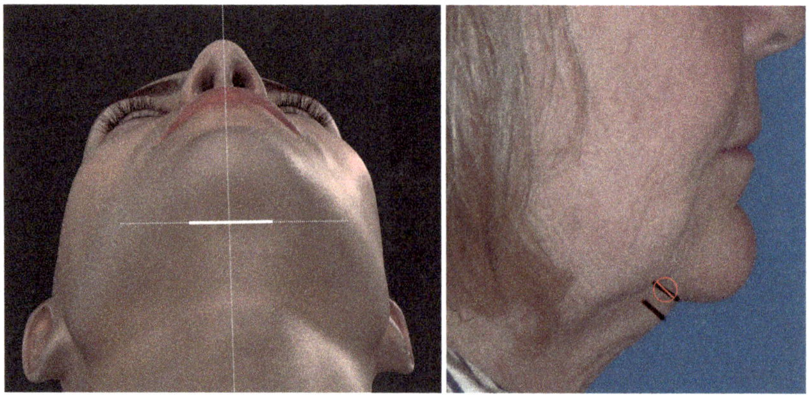

Fig. 6.24. Although the submental incision is generally not noticeable, it should be placed very symmetrically to hide it (*left*). A crooked, angled, or oversized submental incision should always be avoided. In the case of a deep submental crease (*right* image), the incision is not placed in the crease, which could actually deepen it. In this type of deep crease, I place the incision even lower (*bottom line*) and undermine the crease to improve it (*Left base* image, courtesy *Complete Anatomy*, Elsevier.)

over the region of the carotid pulse and the cricothyroid ligament. I have never had to resort to a surgical airway but in the event of emergency, it would be helpful to have landmarks in an otherwise tumesced neck. Having a similar mark for the carotid pulse has the same reasoning in the event of the necessity of resuscitation.

The hair is then washed with a surgical scrub, and the entire head, ears, nose, and upper shoulders are also prepped with an appropriate surgical scrub that is not oculotoxic (Fig. 6.28). We use Techni-Care (Care Tech Laboratories, St. Louis, Missouri).

The hair on either side of the hair-bearing incisions is braided with orthodontic rubber bands. This isolates the incisions and in general, keeps the remainder of the hair contained and out of the operative field (Figs. 6.29–6.31).

After the surgical prep is completed, the patient is draped with cloth and paper drapes. The cloth headwrap is attached with staples to keep it in place during the procedure and keep the hair out of the operative field (Figs. 6.31 and 6.32).

One chore for the surgeon and the assistants in facelift surgery is continually picking up and putting down instruments to retract the ear during surgery. To facilitate this, I place a 3-0 silk suture through the lateral helical rim and attach it to a hemostat. This allows us to have retraction present the entire case (Fig. 6.33)

One prime job of the surgical team is to protect the patient during surgery. To keep debris and blood out of the external auditory canal, we pack the canal with a cotton ball and change it

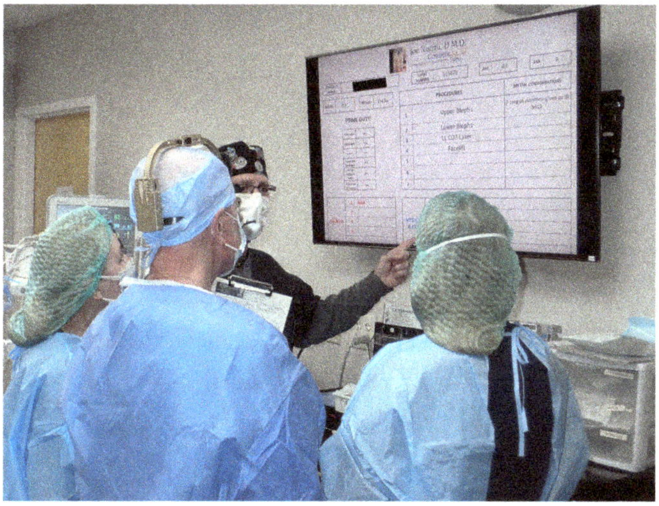

Fig. 6.25. The formal timeout is taken with the entire operating room team to discuss pertinent medical information, consents, surgical site, and so on. This is perhaps the most important 60 seconds of the case.

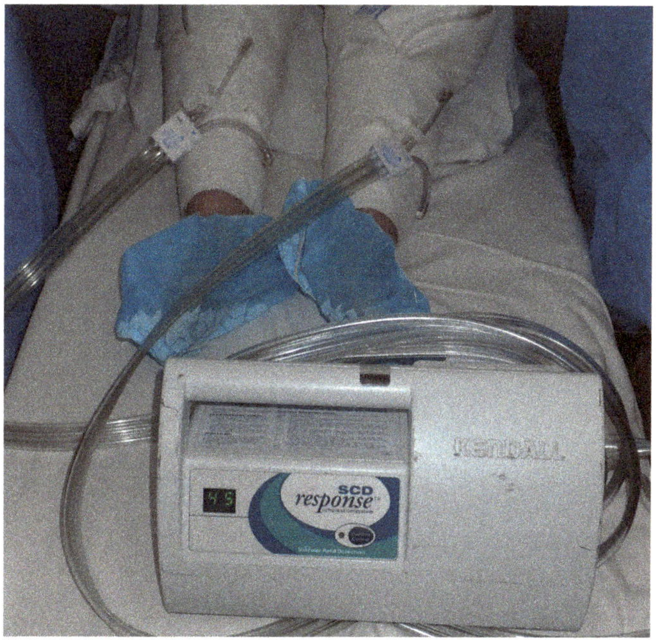

Fig. 6.27. Intraoperatively, the patient wears compression hose, and sequential compression devices are used on the lower extremities.

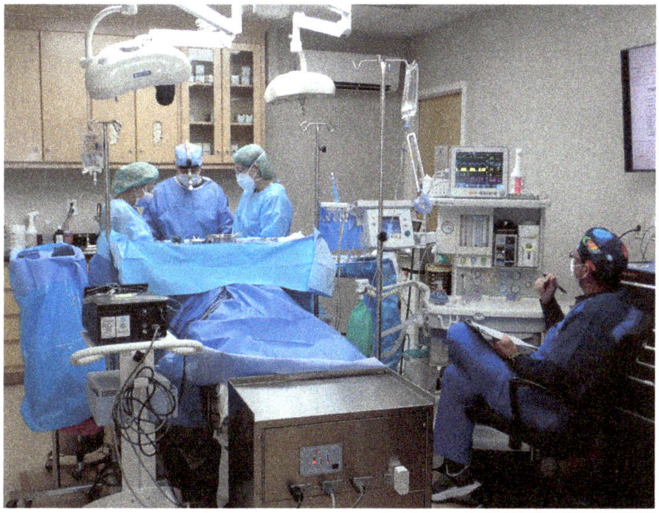

Fig. 6.26. All the authors' surgeries are performed in a sterile operating room environment with intubated general anesthesia support from a qualified anesthetic provider. As shown earlier, we have two accredited operating suites.

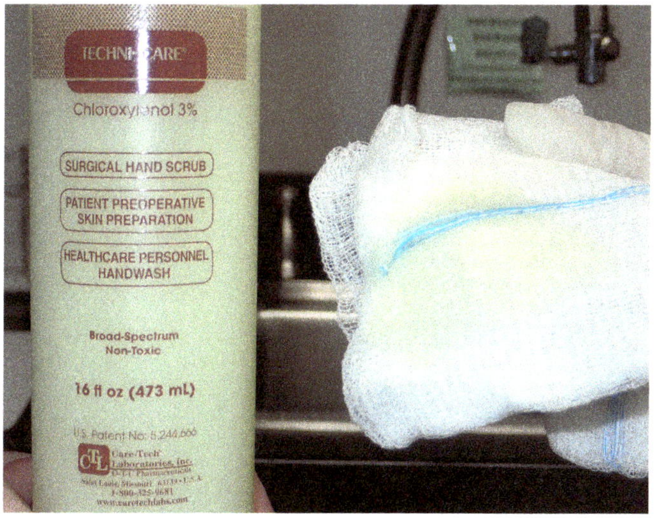

Fig. 6.28. A 3% chloroxylenol surgical scrub is used for the skin and hair. This preparation is alcohol free and safe to use around the eyes and on mucous membranes.

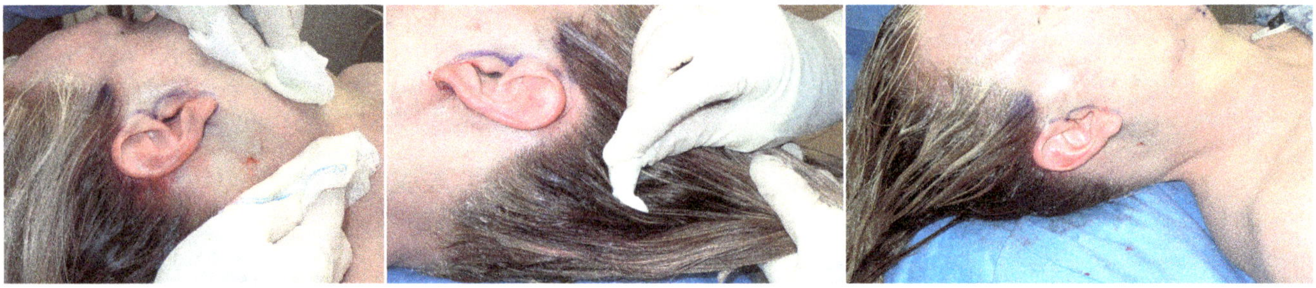

Fig. 6.29. All the exposed regions of the entire head, neck, and upper shoulders are prepped as well as the nostrils and ear with a suitable and safe skin preparation.

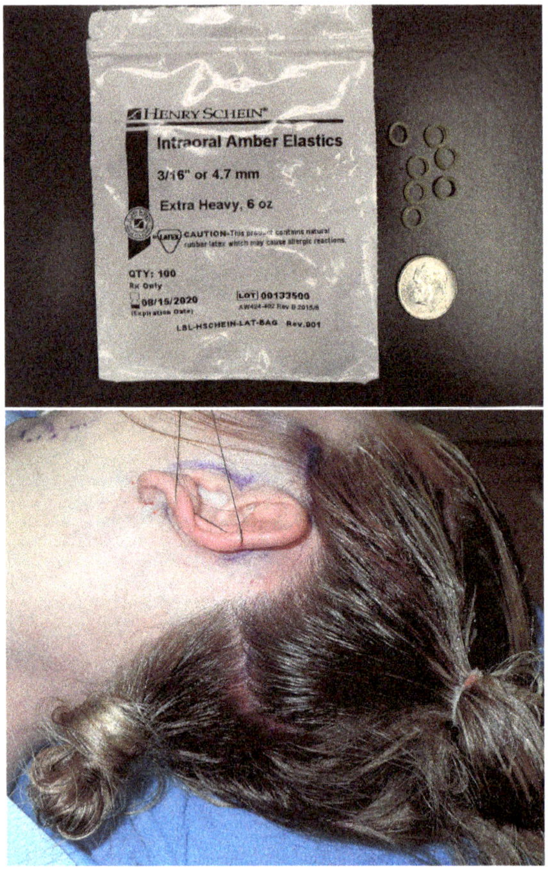

Fig. 6.30. Orthodontic rubber bands are used to braid the hair to better isolate incisions and keep the hair out of the operative field.

if needed during surgery. It is important to remember to remove this after surgery, otherwise as it can become compacted and left in place (Fig. 6.34). Keeping the ear canal free of blood is important, as allowing blood to clot can impair hearing and is painful when the clot contracts on the tympanic membrane.

The eyes must also be protected to prevent corneal abrasion. There is a lot of activity, and it is not uncommon for a surgical drape, gown cuff, surgical tubing, and so on to inadvertently rub against the eye, causing injury. Protection can be performed with corneal shields, tape, barrier membrane, or a tarsorrhaphy suture. This is frequently managed at the beginning of the case by the anesthesia team. I prefer a simple strip of tape for cases without blepharoplasty. Since I usually laser the lower lids with my blepharoplasties, the tape does not stick on the lasered skin, so we use a 6-0 gut tarsorrhaphy suture (Fig. 6.35).

Tumescent Anesthesia

One of the major innovations in facelift surgery over the last 3 decades has been the development of tumescent anesthesia. In the past, surgeons used local anesthetic injections or sometimes no local anesthetic at all. Having local anesthetic and epinephrine in the tumescent anesthesia produces a threefold advantage. Number one, it serves to hydrodissect the tissue planes to make the facelift dissection easier. Number two, it serves as a local anesthetic, which reduces perceived pain and allows the anesthesia team to use fewer drugs and agents. Number three, the epinephrine and transexamic acid promote hemostasis. I

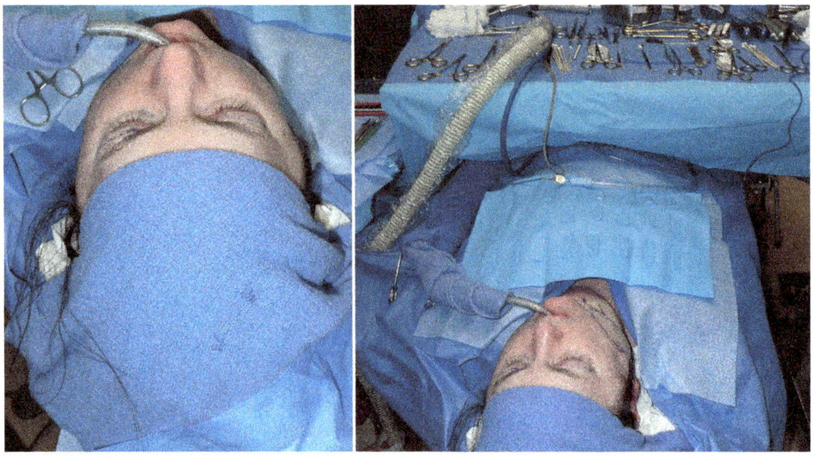

Fig. 6.31. The patient with sterile cloth and paper drapes and a magnetic chest pad placed to retain instruments from falling off the sterile field.

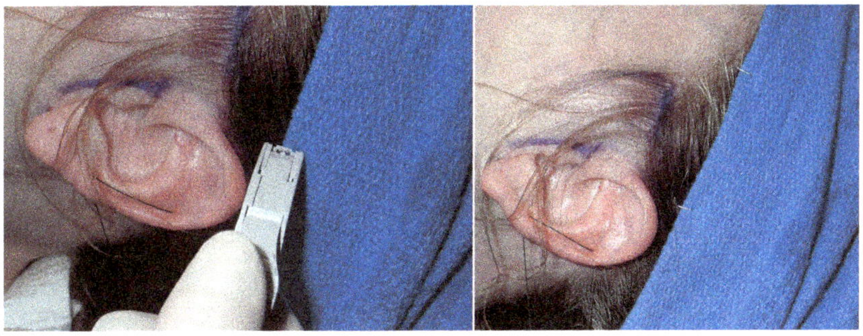

Fig. 6.32. The cloth head drape is secured with staples to maintain position throughout the case and to prevent the hair from entering the surgical field.

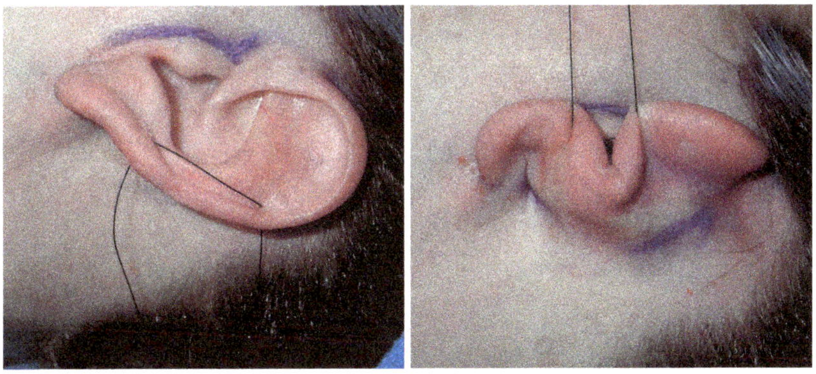

Fig. 6.33. A suture can serve as a simple ear retractor for the entire case. This saves time from not having to continually reach for and replace retractors on the surgical tray.

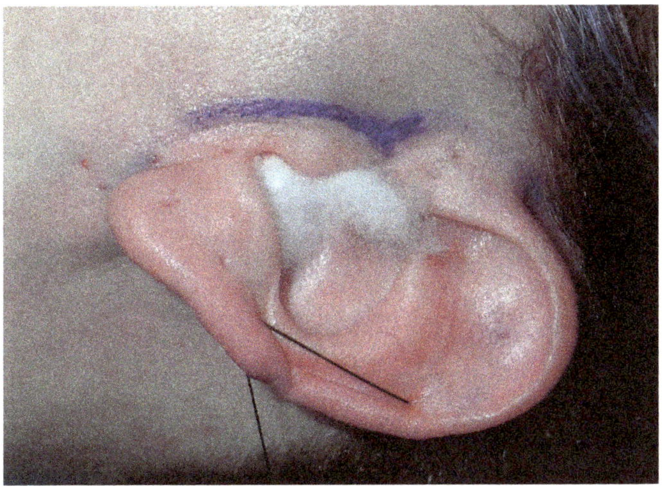

Fig. 6.34. A cotton ball or similar material is used to keep blood and foreign material out of the external auditory canal.

feel that tumescent anesthesia is a critical part of facelift surgery.

There are many recipes for tumescent anesthesia and I generally use 500 mL of tumescent solution for a typical facelift and neck lift. My mixture contains (Fig. 6.36):

- 500 mL of normal saline
- 50 mL of 1% lidocaine (0.5 g)
- 0.5 mL of 1:1000 epinephrine (0.5 g)
- 1 g of tranexamic acid

This produces 500 mL of 0.1% lidocaine with 1:1 million epinephrine. The tranexamic acid has produced a noticeable effect on hemostasis. In the 6 years that I have been using transexamic acid in my tumescent solution and during anesthesia, I have not had a single incidence of returning to the office the night of surgery for an emergent expanding hematoma. We also routinely give every patient 1 g (single vial) of tranexamic acid IV at the beginning of the case. Tranexamic acid can also be used topically by diluting a 1-g vial in 250 mL of normal saline. Soaking gauze with this topical preparation can be used to pack the flap to control oozing.

I generally inject the tumescent solution with a Klein pump before the patient is totally prepped and draped for surgery. The injection points are prepped with the surgical scrub, and using an 18-gauge spinal needle or blunt infiltration cannula (best choice for novice surgeons), the solution is infiltrated in the pre- and postauricular regions on each side and the submental region. All areas that will be undermined or dissected are infiltrated with the tumescent anesthesia (Figs. 6.37 and 6.38). All tumescent injection is performed in the subcutaneous plane.

When tumescent anesthesia is used for body liposuction, it is frequently taught to inject the solution until the tissues are "rock hard." I do not feel this is necessary in facelift surgery and feel that overinjection of tumescent anesthesia can balloon the tissues to a point that it may affect the skin tightening. Mild ballooning of the tissues is usually adequate for local anesthesia hemostasis and hydrodissection.

I find it most convenient to perform tumescent infiltration before the patient is prepped and draped. This allows sufficient time for the tumescent solution to take effect while the patient

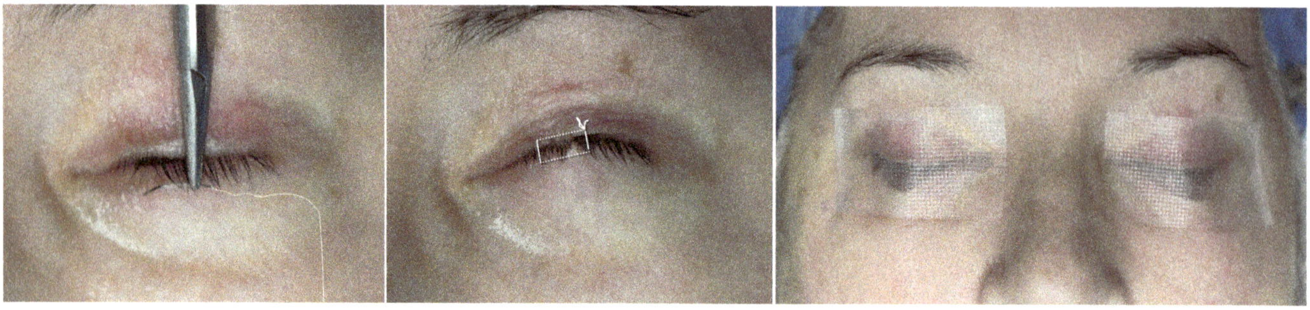

Fig. 6.35. A tarsorrhaphy suture (*left* image) keep the corneas moist and protects them from abrasion during the case (*left* and *center* images). Sterile surgical tape can also be used for eye protection (*right* image).

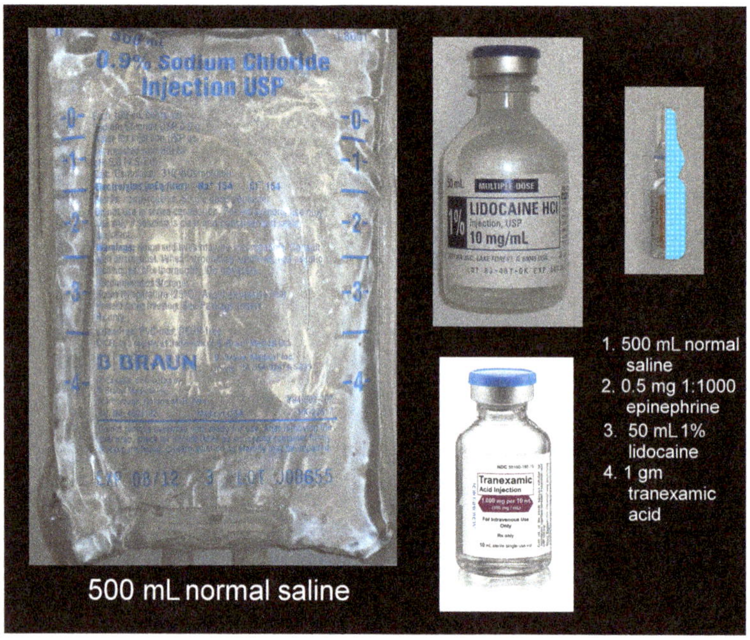

Fig. 6.36. The tumescent mixture includes saline, lidocaine, epinephrine, and tranexamic acid. A total volume of 500 mL is usually adequate for the average facelift and neck lift.

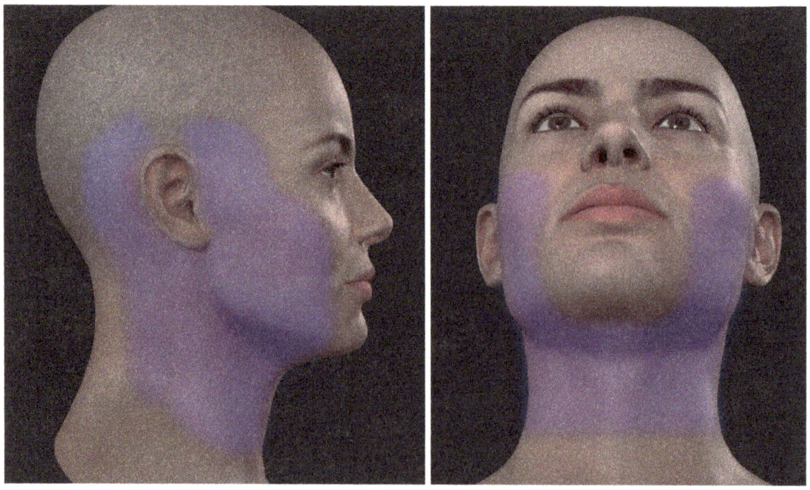

Fig. 6.37. The average facelift and neck lift patient is tumesced with 500 mL of solution. The shaded regions illustrate the approximate placement of the tumescent solution. This may vary with the size of the facelift, but the average patient is injected with 500 mL. (Base image, courtesy *Complete Anatomy*, Elsevier.)

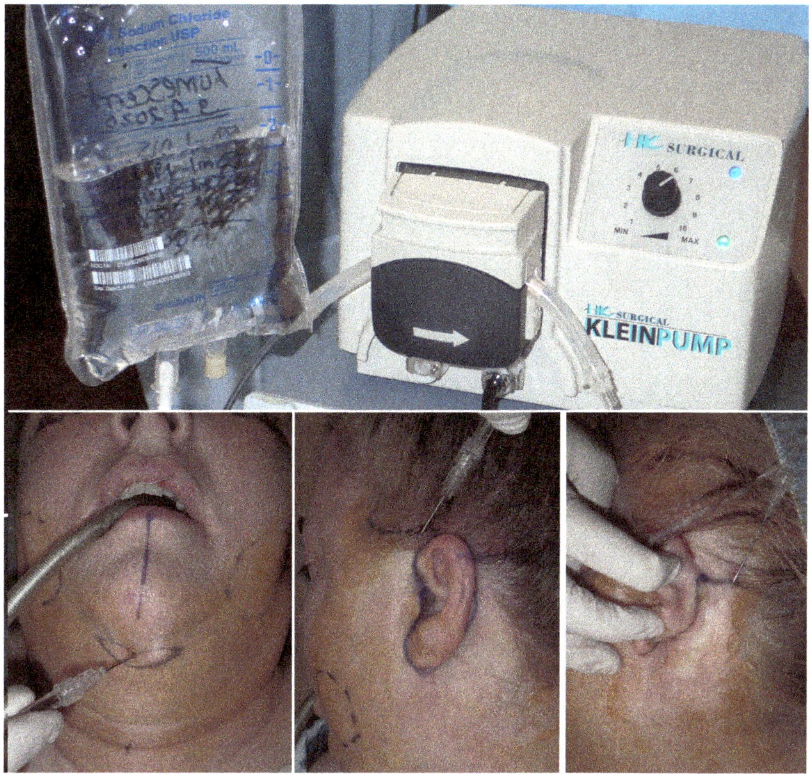

Fig. 6.38. The *top* image shows a Klein pump used for facilitating rapid infiltration, and the *bottom* images show the various infiltration sites using an 18-gauge spinal needle. Novice surgeons should use a blunt infiltration cannula, which is safer around vessels and other structures.

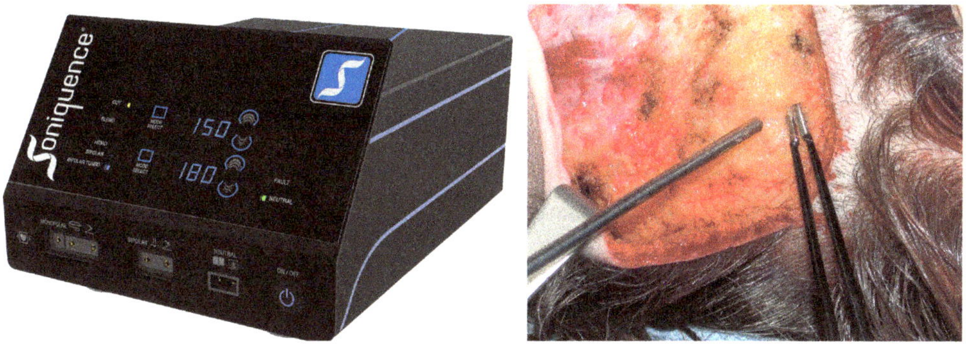

Fig. 6.39. Any surgeon performing facelift surgery must have some means of hemostasis. Many surgeons use hospital-grade electrosurgery Bovie unit (symmetrysurgical.com), or a radiowave machine such as the Soniquence device (pictured) (soniquence.com) works well for coagulation and incisions. Many surgeons also have an Ellman Surgitron (ellman.com), which likewise can be used.

is prepped and draped for surgery. Alternately, the tumescent anesthesia can be injected after the patient is prepped and draped at the beginning of the case. We do this when we are performing eyelid surgery, brow lift, or other ancillary procedures, so the tumescent anesthesia has time to work while we are performing those procedures.

While discussing hemostasis, it is imperative for any surgeon attempting facelift surgery (or most cosmetic procedures) to have some type of coagulation modality. The most common devices are traditional electrosurgery units or radiofrequency machines. Although rare, significant, and serious bleeding can occur during facelift surgery, it is important to not only have the skill to be able to control the bleeding but to have devices to use for large or small hemostatic applications. I have significant experience with the Ellman and Soniquence Radiowave System (Fig. 6.39).

Step-by-Step Facelift Technique

Part I: Platysmaplasty/Submentoplasty

After the patient is anesthetized, prepped, and draped, the surgical team is ready for surgery. My team consists of the surgeon, two surgical assistants, one circulator and one anesthetic provider (Fig. 6.26).

Before getting into the actual step-by-step facelift technique, it is important to mention that most facelift patients have other procedures performed at the same time as their facelift. In my practice, the most popular simultaneous procedures are cosmetic blepharoplasty cheek or chin implants, brow lift, buccal fat reduction, and CO_2 laser resurfacing.

It is personal preference as to which procedures are performed in what order. Personally, I prefer to perform upper face procedures such as blepharoplasty and brow lift before the facelift. Cheek implants can be placed at the beginning or the end of the procedure (I prefer to place before facelift), and chin implant is placed during the platysmaplasty procedure. For years, I performed aggressive simultaneous full-face CO_2 laser resurfacing with my facelifts, but I no longer do that because of the intensity of the recovery of these combined procedures. If I do perform simultaneous laser resurfacing, I will aggressively treat the central oval of the face but treat the undermined flaps and a much lower fluence. Again, I've gotten away from this as a routine procedure. I have found it better for the patient to perform full face laser resurfacing as a secondary procedure. Another reason not to perform simultaneous laser is that the facelift flaps cannot be treated as aggressively as the central oval of the face. For this reason, the skin over the flaps may be a different color and texture than the central oval of the face. If this happens, a secondary laser procedure may be required. This is just another good reason to separate the procedures on patients with significant wrinkling or dyschromia.

Another reason not to perform simultaneous laser is that the facelift flaps cannot be treated as aggressively as the central oval of the face. For this reason, the skin over the flaps may be a different color and texture than the central oval of the face. If this happens, a secondary laser procedure may be required. This is just another good reason to separate the procedures on patients with significant wrinkling or dyschromia.

The next part of this chapter will deal with a step-by-step description and pictures (supplemented by accompanying videos) of various facelift and neck lift procedures and approaches. These will vary from the simplest short scar facelifts to the more complex deep plane lifts. For novice surgeons, the short scar facelift is an important starting point, and for midlevel or experienced surgeons, the comprehensive facelift and neck lift is probably the most common procedure performed today. Other descriptions of various types of lifts from expert practitioners will also be described for reference and for surgeons with significant expertise and experience. As stated in the introduction of this textbook, no doctor should ever attempt to perform procedures for which they are not trained or cannot manage the common complications associated with those procedures. Facelift and neck lift surgery takes years to master and my advice too new surgeons is to "walk before you run"; start with the smaller procedures and progress to the larger procedures when you have mastered the common techniques.

The intraoperative surgical discussion will begin with what I call the "comprehensive deep plane facelift and neck lift." Deep plane facelift dissections have become very popular, but this is more of an advanced technique and I will discuss my modified approach to the deep plane technique and other authors will discuss their "classic" approaches to deep plane facelift and neck lift.

My "comprehensive" facelift consists of an SMASectomy procedure while my "comprehensive deep plane technique" involves SMASectomy with deep plane dissection. The former is what most people think about when they discuss "facelift." It consists of pre- and postauricular incisions, platysmaplasty, flap elevation, liposuction, treatment of this SMAS, and removal of excess skin. In a nutshell that is the basic facelift technique. The latter is more of an advanced approach for experienced surgeons.

The skin incisions have been described in the previous section, and my preferred technique is the triarcuate incision preauricularly and keeping the posterior and sideburn incisions in the hair-bearing regions as shown in Fig. 6.4.

Every surgeon has a preference for what they do first or last. My personal order of face and neck steps are as follows:

1. Tumescent anesthesia
2. Submental dissection, liposuction, platysmaplasty
3. First side pre- and postauricular incisions
4. Flap dissections
5. Jowl liposuction
6. SMAS treatment
7. Skin cutbacks/key sutures
8. Posterior auricular flap tailoring and closure
9. Anterior auricular flap tailoring and closure
10. Temporal tuft tailoring and closure
11. Earlobe tailoring, positioning, and closure
12. Repeat on second side
13. Submental incision closure

Submental and Anterior Cervical Treatment: Dissection, Liposuction, and Platysmaplasty

Treatment in the submental area for the average facelift surgery includes subcutaneous dissection, liposuction (if required), and platysmaplasty and for advanced surgeons, may include deep platysma fat reduction, digastric muscle reduction, and submandibular gland reduction. I'm aware of some surgeons that may perform the platysmaplasty procedure at the end of the case, but I have always performed it as the beginning procedure.

I prefer round scalpel handles for all my cosmetic procedures. I feel they are simply more artistic and have the feel of a pen or paintbrush and can be rolled with the fingers to change direction and just provide better control. Flat scalpel handles are fine for body incisions but are not as well suited for the curvilinear facelift incisions. To make a level, horizontal scar in the submental, the surgeon can use their index and second finger to make an inverted "peace sign" and stretch the tissue laterally on each side (Fig. 6.40, *left*). Once the incision is made, two bleeders are usually encountered (one on each lateral side) and need to be coagulated (Fig. 6.40, *right*) or they may bleed the entire case. For aesthetic reasons, this incision should be kept to the smallest length needed to allow the surgeon to perform the surgery, which is usually around 3 to 4 cm. A caveat for novice surgeons is not to make too long of an incision, as closure can produce bilateral dog-ears on each side of the

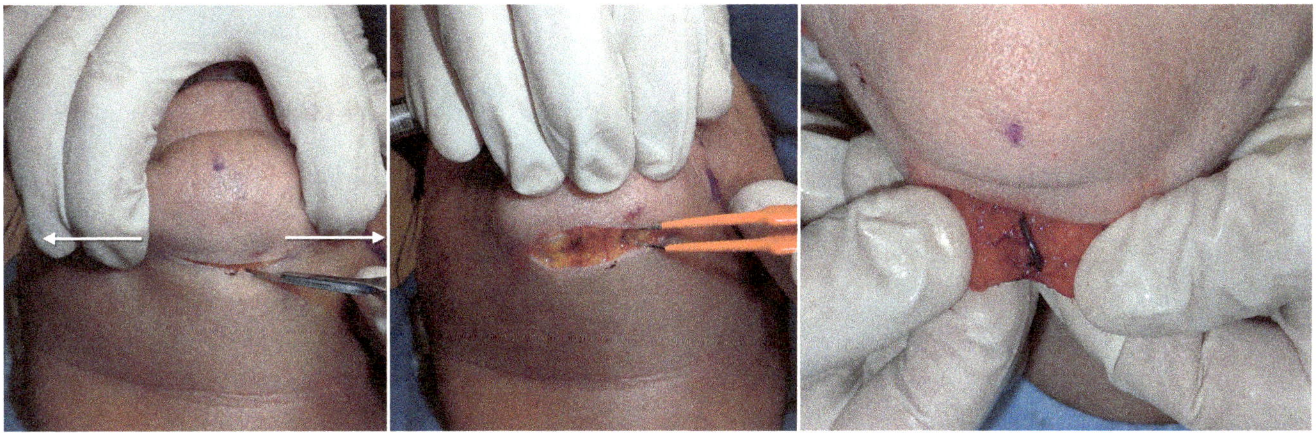

Fig. 6.40. Putting the submental incision on stretch before incising helps create a level and straight incision (*left* image). The *middle* image shows Soniquence bipolar coagulation of small but persistent bleeding vessels found in each side of the incision. The *right* image shows larger-caliber vessels that can occur in this area.

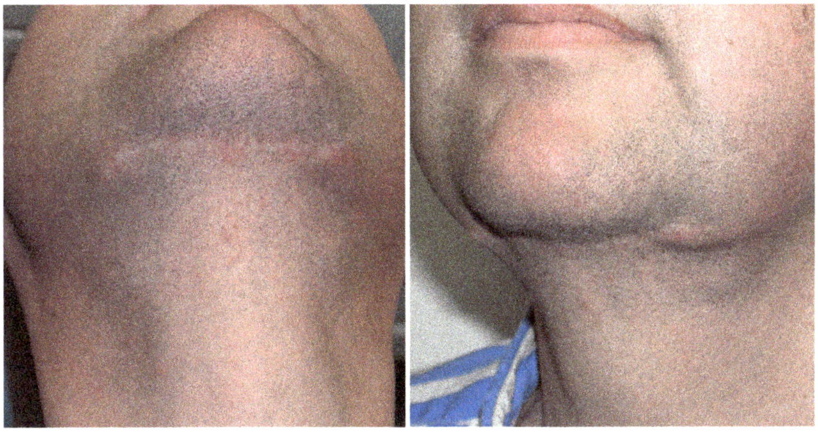

Fig. 6.41. This patient was treated by another surgeon and shows the problem associated with excessively long submental incisions and resultant dog-ear deformities. This is a difficult situation to improve, so prevention is critical. Limiting incision length and staying within the inner border of the mandible will keep the scar manageable.

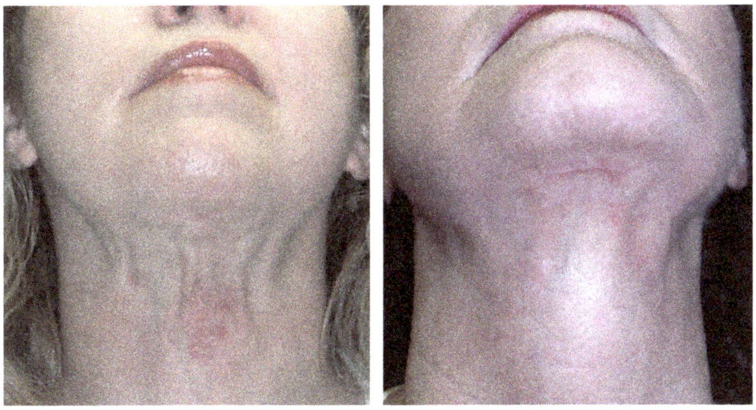

Fig. 6.42. These images from other surgeons show deformities from overzealous fat removal causing the dermis to scar to the underlying muscle. These situations are very difficult to improve.

incision that are difficult to deal with postoperatively (Fig. 6.40). To prevent this, the incision should not extend past the inner table of the mandible on each side.

After the incision is made, the next step is to begin the subcutaneous dissection. It is important to leave an adequate layer of fat on the dermal side of this flap. Not leaving enough fat and having a thin flap with exposed dermis are problematic for several reasons. It can show underlying irregularities very easily because of the thinness, and the dermis may be traumatized during dissection when making a very thin flap. This can cause the dermis to scar with the underlying muscle and create deformities that are quite visible postoperatively and are difficult to improve (Figs. 6.41 and 6.42). A 5-mm-thick flap is a reasonable thickness.

The submental incision is retracted inferiorly by the surgeon using the Cottle ring retractor and superiorly, by the assistant, using the forked skin hook (Fig. 6.43).

I feel that a large part of performing competent surgery is having great assistants who understand how to help the surgeon navigate the various tissues. Placing the tissues on vertical and horizontal stretch help dissection in this area by making a curvilinear structure flatter during the dissection. This allows the scissors to advance more easily with less trauma or chance of perforation of the flap.

Subcutaneous dissection of anterior neck is also facilitated by superior/inferior and lateral retraction by the assistant. As stated, this stretches this curved anatomy into a straighter anatomical unit therefore facilitating dissection (Fig. 6.44).

Another means of facilitating dissection in this area is using the curve Pagett facelift scissors. The angle on this instrument is perfect to ergonomically negotiate this area (Figs. 6.45 and 6.46).

As the surgeon begins the dissection, there are several methods of performing this task. Many surgeons will use sharp scissors and simply advance (push) the scissors with the tips open to cleave the tissue plane. Other surgeons will do more of an alternating snipping and spreading action where they are snipping the tissue, then advancing the scissors and spreading the tips. The cut/spread method works well because many facelift scissors have cutting edges on both sides of each blade. Whatever the surgeon's preference, the important thing is to leave enough fat on the dermal side of the flap without traumatizing the dermis and to extend the dissection adequately for the specific patient. Smaller facelifts may only require inferior dissection to the hyoid region, medium facelifts may require dissection to the thyroid prominence, and large facelifts may require dissection to the sternal notch. The extension of any dissection should be commensurate with the amount of release needed for that patient. Overdissection creates more dead space and bleeding and can promote hematoma, seroma, or other complications. The inferior extent of dissection is determined when the neck tissues are released and there is no dimpling or adhesions at the base of the flap.

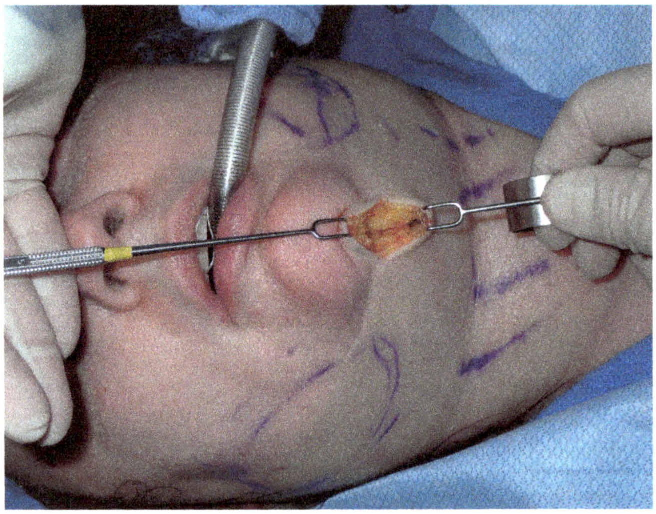

Fig. 6.43. Superior and inferior retraction of the incision will facilitate dissection. Although the author prefers the pictured instruments, surgeons can choose the instrumentation of their choice.

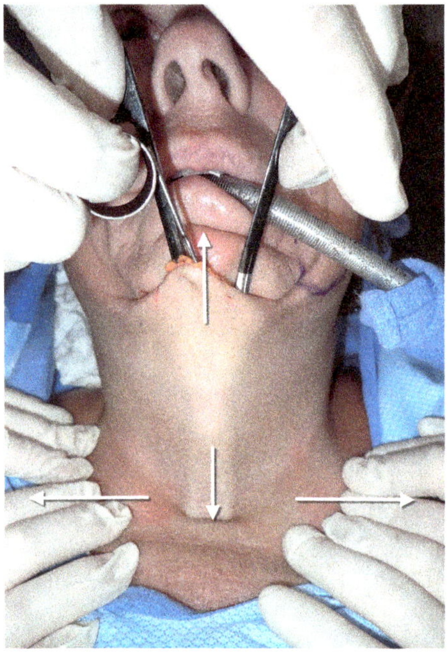

Fig. 6.44. Stretching the tissues in this area facilitates dissection. The surgeon is shown retracting the skin superiorly with the Cottle retractor, and the scissors are pushing inferiorly. The assistant's hands are stretching inferior and laterally. The stretching makes this curvilinear structure flat and facilitates dissection.

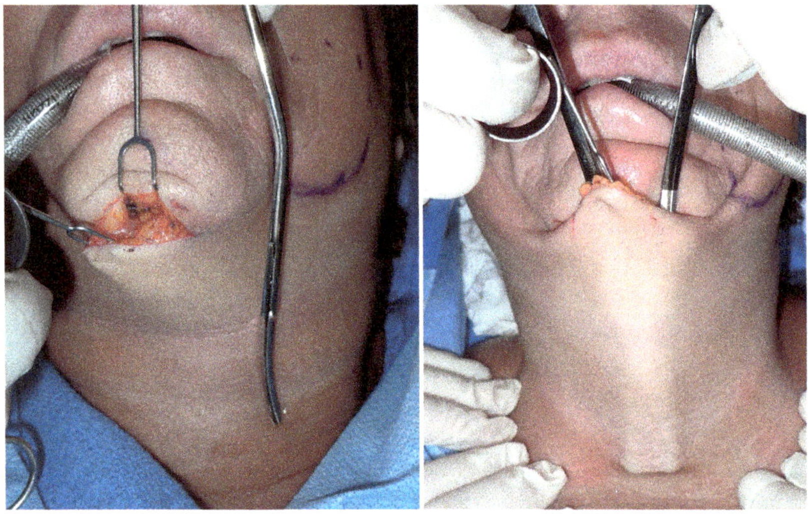

Fig. 6.45. The curved Padgett facelift scissors are ergonomically angled to facilitate dissection in the submental and cervical region (*left* image). The *right* image shows inferior dissection in the anterior neck and lateral dissection of the inferior border of the mandible.

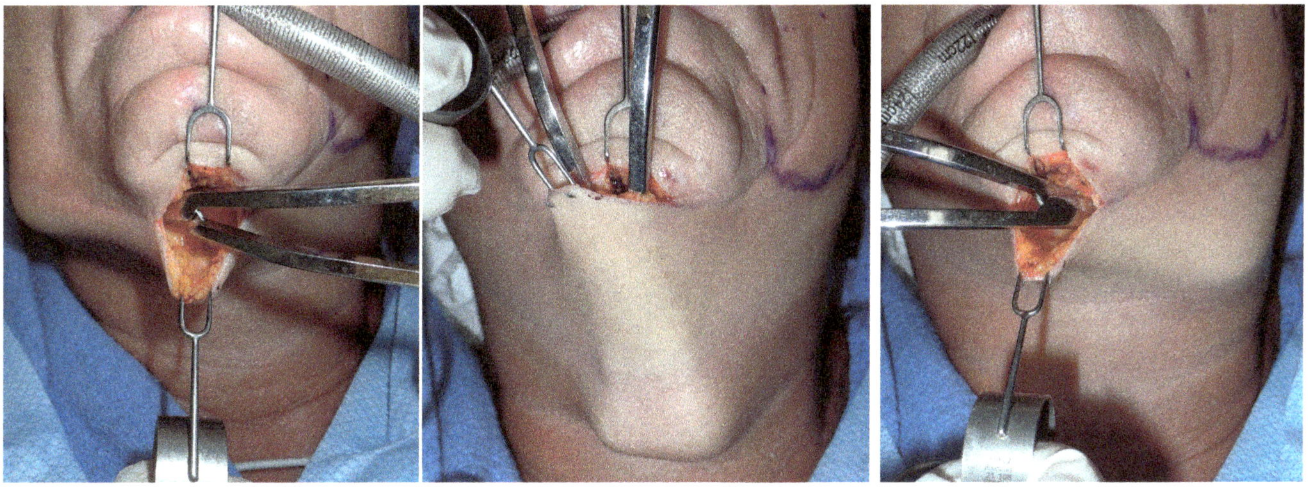

Fig. 6.46. Using facelift scissors, the anterior and lateral submental dissection is performed.

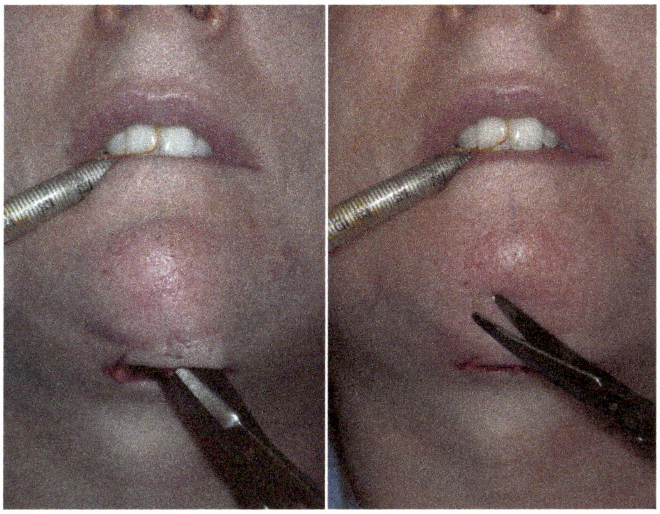

Fig. 6.47. Dissecting superiorly from the submental incision can free up a bound down, ptotic chin or release a deep submental crease. This is an advantage of placing the incision inferior to the crease, otherwise the crease itself cannot be undermined.

Ptotic chin anatomy with a deep cervical mental crease has been discussed previously. This "witch's chin" deformity can be addressed by superior dissection from the submental incision as shown in Fig. 6.47. This superior dissection coupled with sectioning of the mandibular ligaments will release much of the tethering on the chin. Placing a chin implant in these patients can also greatly improve the chin and profile aesthetics and normalize chin ptosis (Figs. 6.48 and 6.49).

A curved, lighted retractor is extremely useful in this region. It is difficult to aim overhead lights or headlights in this area, and the angled fiber-optic retractor not only retracts the issue but provides light directly on the surgical field to enhance precision (Fig. 6.50).

The average facelift patient is at an age where increased body mass index, obesity, and generalized aging are responsible for increased cervical facial fat deposits. Usually, only the thinnest patients that present for facelift and neck lift do not need any fat reduction.

Some surgeons prefer to perform the submental liposuction through a small stab incision (closed liposuction). This allows more of a vacuum and is somewhat more efficient, but it also does not allow the operator to view the surgical field. Since facelift surgery with platysmaplasty will involve an open incision, it is my personal preference to make this incision perform the skin undermining and then liposuction the fat with direct vision. I refer to this as open liposuction. If I were performing a submental procedure that did not require platysmaplasty and only required liposuction, I would not make the wide incision but rather perform the liposuction through a small puncture.

When operating in the submental region, the surgeon is potentially treating two different fat layers. The more superficial subcutaneous fat is the layer immediately beneath the dermis and above the platysma muscle. In the superior part of the neck in jaw/hyoid region, the deeper subplatysmal fat pad lies between the two anterior bellies of the digastric muscle (Fig. 6.51). It is rare that I would remove deep fat on thinner patients, but patients with thick necks or increased adipose tissue or body mass index are usually candidates for some deep fat reduction. This is not done with liposuction, but rather direct lipectomy.

Although many surgeons use dedicated liposuction aspirators as a suction source, these machines are large, expensive, noisy, and not necessary when limiting liposuction to the face and/or neck. I use a standard wall suction unit with a collection bucket as shown in Fig. 6.52. The amount of suction flowing through the average wall unit is more than adequate for the amounts of fat encountered in facial surgery.

After I make my submental incision, I generally begin with a 4- to 6-mm cannula to efficiently reduce the cervical, submental, and inframandibular fat (Fig. 6.53).

As the liposuction is performed under direct vision, it allows me to gauge how much fat I am removing. "Liposculpting" is the word sometimes used to describe this type of fat reduction. Instead of thinking of the situation as a total removal of fat, it is better to think of it as sculpting, or terracing the fat, to allow fullness where you want it and reduction where you need it. Again, I cannot mention too many times the importance of not

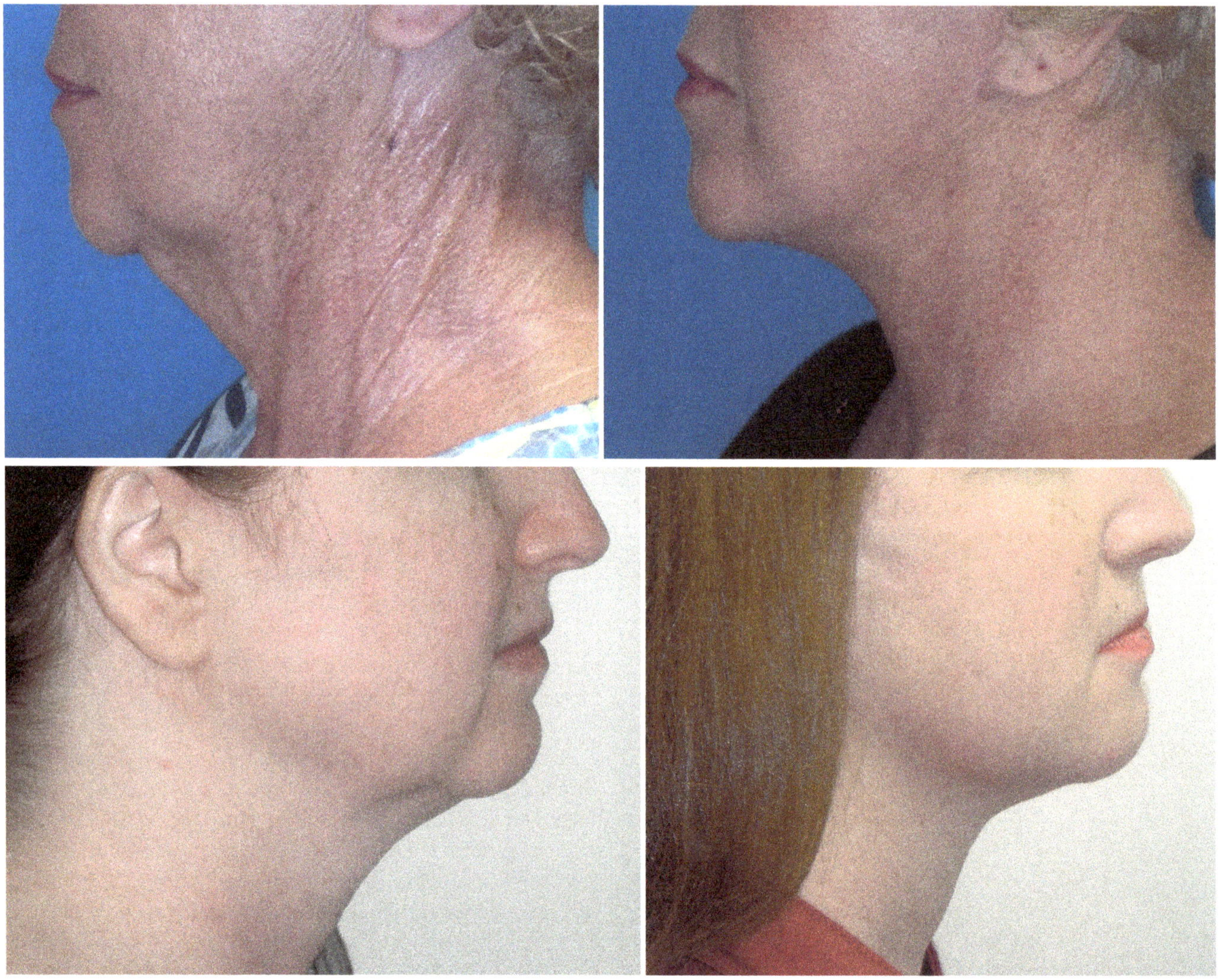

Fig. 6.48. The *top* patient presented with a witch's chin deformity. This was improved by making the submental incision lower than her existing crease, undermining the superior portion of the submental crease, and placing a silicone chin implant at the time of the facelift. The *bottom* patient had a deep submental crease, which was undermined.

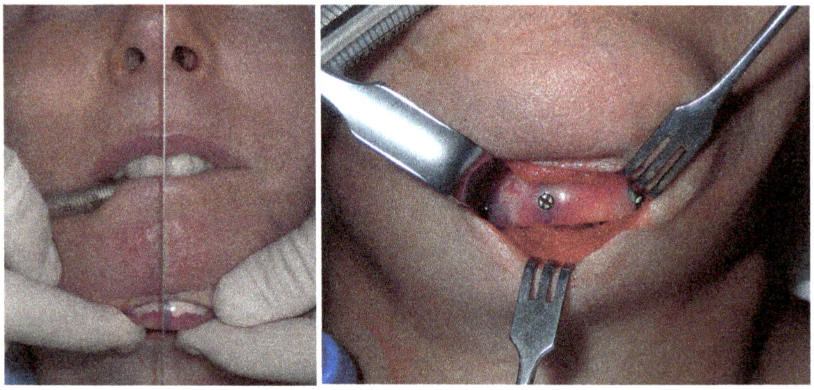

Fig. 6.49. Placing a chin implant is performed through the submental incision prior to platysmaplasty. The *left* image shows the importance of centering the chin to the patient's midline, and the *right* image shows the implant in place with three 10 to 12 mm titanium 2.0 mm screws. Placing three screws not only retains the implant but prevents rotation.

overtreating fat in the neck. Over the years, I have become less aggressive with submental and anterior cervical fat reduction as this layer is necessary for a soft, smooth result. As stated, overtreatment of these tissues can show subdermal irregularities. The key is to remove excess fat and leave enough "good" fat. This is especially important in facelift surgery to leave enough fat when dissecting the flaps. A thicker flap can hide a lot of irregularities.

After dissection and liposculpting, the next step is addressing the platysma muscle and possibly the deeper fat compartments.

As I have stated, I perform platysmaplasty in about 99% of my patients. Exceptions are younger patients without platysma banding, undergoing short scar lifts or elderly patients that may have some level of medical compromise requiring a less detailed and shorter procedure. The prime reason is that most patients despise platysma neck banding, and if a facelift is performed without some component of addressing the anterior platysma borders, then the banding may not be improved or may return in the early postoperative period. One of the most disconcerting factors for postfacelift patients are residual platysmal bands. In addition, I think platysmaplasty is important because it enables more undermining of neck skin. By mobilizing the skin from the subcutaneous structures, more free skin is available in the cervicomental region. I feel this translates into an increased amount of freed skin that will be available to be removed from the auricular flaps (Fig. 6.54). Finally, patients that have a midline and posterior "plication" will have an anatomic platysmal sling, which tightens the entire neck, sometimes noticeably reducing the neck size in patients.

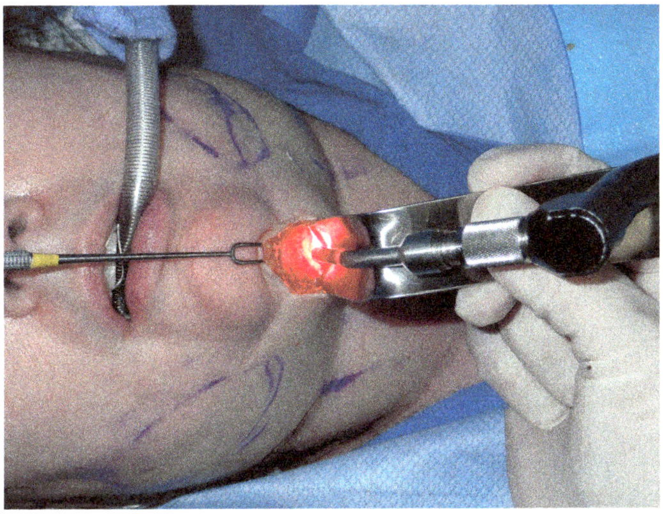

Fig. 6.50. An angled fiber-optic retractor is invaluable under flaps in tight spaces. It provides both the simultaneous retraction and visibility required for precision surgery in these areas.

At this point, the platysma muscles are addressed. Many patients have a significant mass of fibrofatty tissue overlying the submental region and anterior neck. Sometimes this is difficult to see in the supine position as gravity flattens it, but easy to see when it is picked up with forceps as shown in Fig. 6.55. When this tissue mass is lifted, it can be excised, and this excision can extend inferiorly for as low as necessary. Generally, I remove a rectangle of this overlying tissue on the anterior neck that extends from the inferior border of the mandible to the level of the thyroid cartilage. Smaller lifts may only extend to the hyoid level and may extend more inferiorly. I elevate this tissue with a bayonet forcep and use a facelift scissor to reduce the elevated excess tissue and continue inferior dissection in this plane.

This excision involves a reduction of the medial platysmal border bilaterally. Patients with significant platysmal banding generally have ptotic and atrophic medial platysmal borders. Excising several centimeters of this tissue in a lateral direction

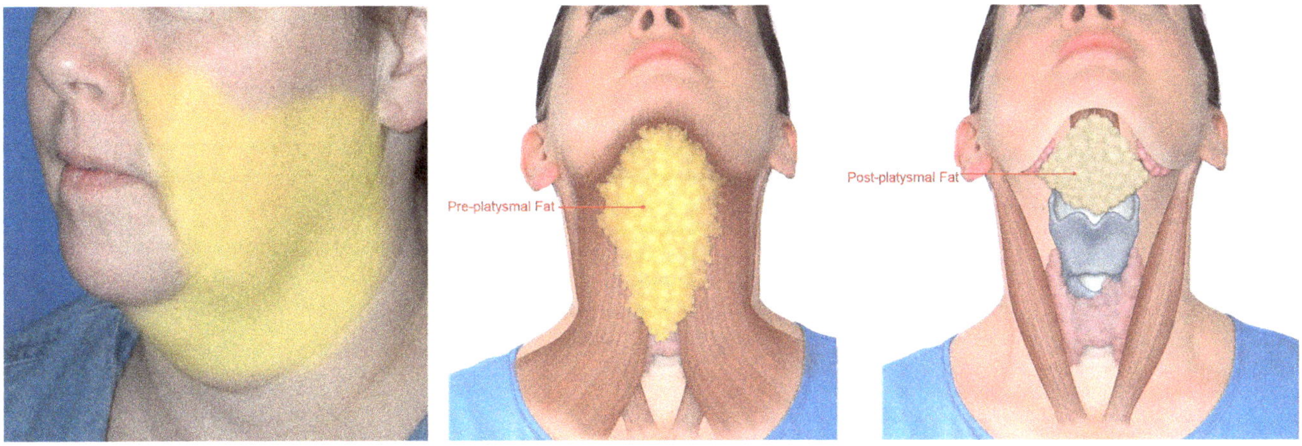

Fig. 6.51. The *left* image shows common areas of facial and neck adipose excess. The *middle* image illustrates the subcutaneous (preplatysmal) fat, and the *right* image illustrates the deeper subplatysmal fat collection.

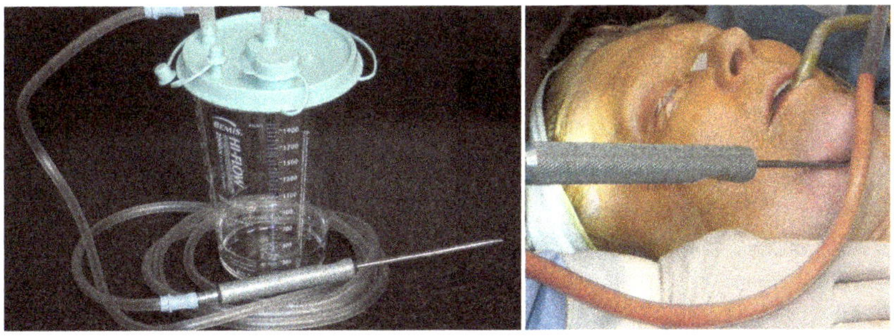

Fig. 6.52. The *left* image shows a typical surgical wall suction collection bucket, which serves as an adequate liposuction source for face and neck procedures. This type of suction is very efficient at fat removal (*right* image).

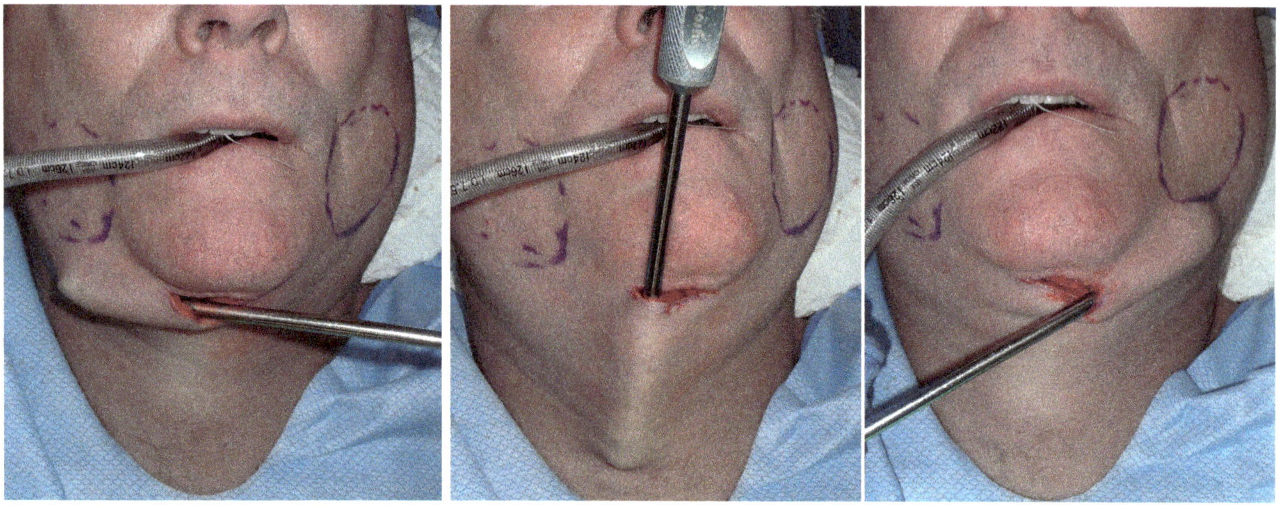

Fig. 6.53. A 6 mm spatulate liposuction cannula is used for the submental, anterior cervical, and inframandibular regions.

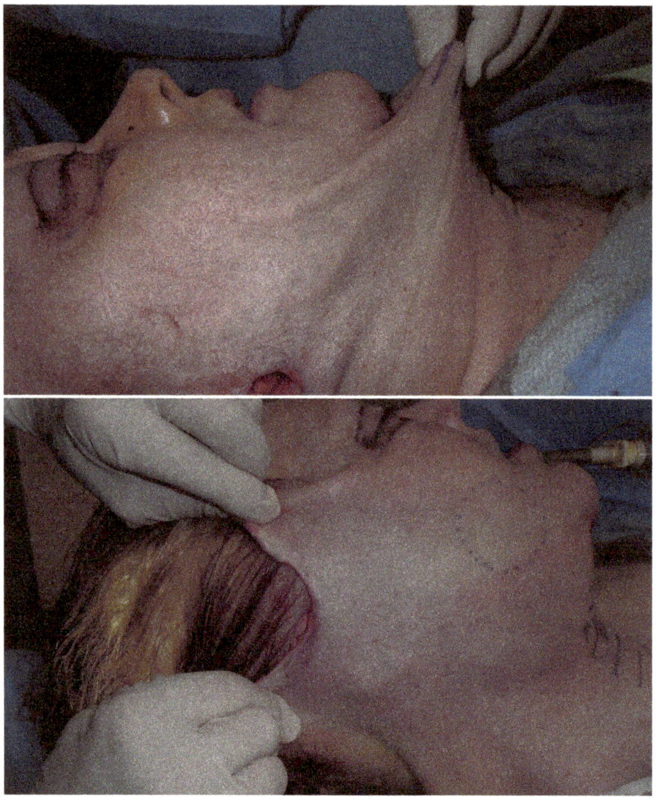

Fig. 6.54. It is the author's opinion that the increased surface area from skin mobilization on the submental and cervical regions translates into increased skin to be excised and therefore a more comprehensive lift.

removes the ptotic tissue back to a level where the platysma is more substantial.

After this excision, the surgeon can view the deep platysmal fat and deeper structures of the neck. The paired anterior jugular veins can be occasionally encountered in this deeper plane and produce brisk bleeding that can be controlled with cautery. In patients with extreme submental fullness, the deep platysmal fat can be debulked and reduced (Fig. 6.56). The deep fat lies between the anterior bellies of the digastric muscles (Fig. 6.56). Some surgeons will also resect part of the anterior digastric muscles as well as portions of the submandibular gland. This is not something I do on the average patient but the topic will be addressed several times throughout this text. Although patients with thick necks benefit from profile enhancement from deep fat reduction, thinner patients do not need deep fat recontouring, which can lead to a hollow depression on the submental region referred to as a "cobra deformity."

If there is a single technique that has improved my cervicomental aesthetic outcomes over the past decade, I would attribute that to being more aggressive with my submental tissue excision, which I refer to as "deep neck lift" (Figs. 6.57 and 6.58). This usually applies more to heavy-necked patients, but some thinner patients may require more aggressive reduction in selected cases. The key to treating heavy-necked patients is first to make sure the submental skin flap is thick. By this, I mean that adequate subcutaneous fat is left in place on the skin flap. This is important, as the thicker flap will hide irregularities from deep dissection.

In my experience, the direct midline platysma plication (corset platysmaplasty) is the most common procedure performed to address the bands and tighten the neck. Although this is frequently referred to as a plication, the Latin word *plica* means "fold" and generally is not an open repair. There are numerous ways to treat this area. Some surgeons use crisscross sutures that attach to the mastoid fascia (Giampapa suture). Some surgeons resect a portion of platysma on each side instead of placating it (platysectomy). The prevents recurrent platysmal banding but can also expose the submandibular glands, which may protrude into the lateral submental area. In this case, a partial submandibular gland resection can be performed. This will also be discussed in the deep plane facelift section and is a procedure for advanced surgeons.

Some surgeons do not treat the midline platysma at all. I personally have had my best results with a simple midline platysma repair, which I refer to as a "shoestring" repair Fig. 6.59 (*center*). This is also called a corset platysmaplasty as it resembles the stitching on a woman's corset.

I always trim the medial platysmal borders before they are sutured together in the midline. This reduces some of the ptosis and allows for a tighter repair, and the raw borders will heal

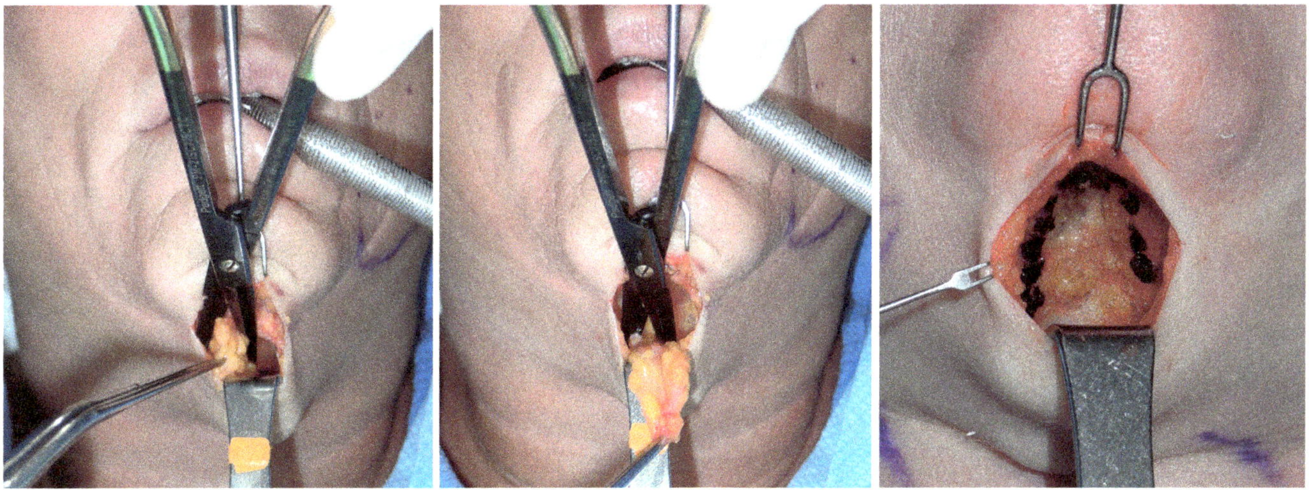

Fig. 6.55. The *left* image shows elevation of the fibrofatty muscular tissue in the midline of the neck. The *center* picture shows inferior excision of this tissue, and the *right* image shows the area after excision. The medial platysmal borders are shown after excision by the blue markings.

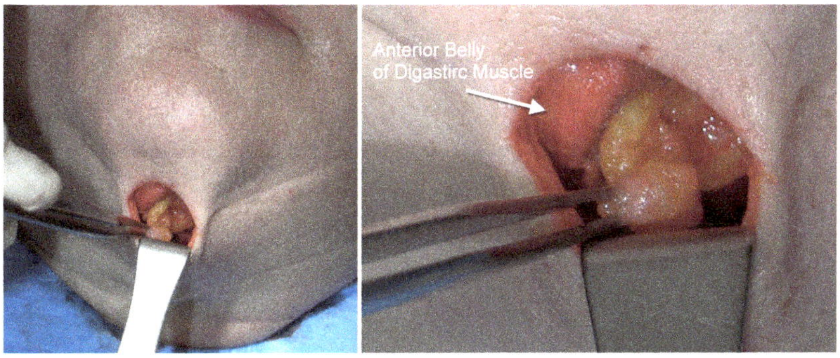

Fig. 6.56. Deep fat resection is performed on selected patients with heavy necks. The subplatysmal fat (deep fat) lies between the anterior bellies of the digastric muscle and extends inferiorly. The *left* image shows the deep fat being elevated. The *right* image shows a close-up with the right anterior belly of the digastric (*arrow*).

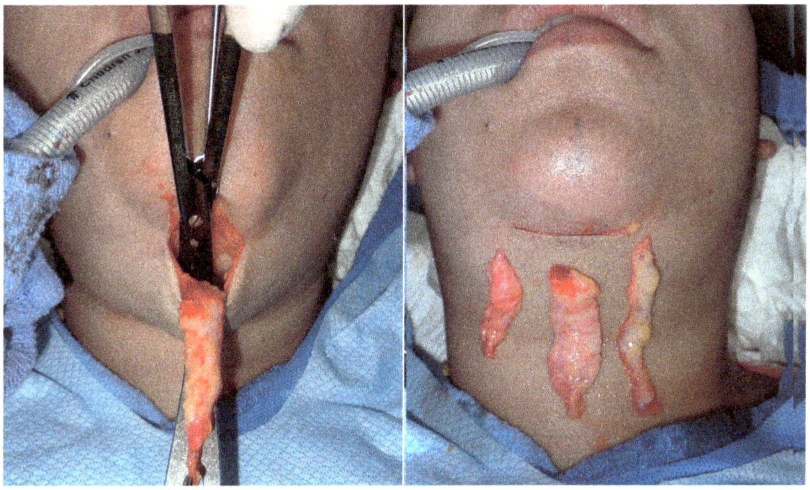

Fig. 6.57. The *left* image shows a midline section of the platysma and associated tissues being resected with scissors. The *right* image shows further lateral reduction of excess tissue. On patients with extremely heavy necks, a portion of the platysma may be resected and ptotic submandibular glands can be reduced.

together. If the medial platysmal borders are extremely ptotic, it is important to excise the edges back to normal muscle. Performing a midline repair with ptotic platysmal borders detracts from the result and can produce visible bunching under the overlying neck skin. In some patients the platysma is a very visible thick red muscle, and in some patients, it is very thin and wispy. It is easy to place midline sutures in patients with the thicker platysma structure as you are simply picking up the muscle and sewing it to the contralateral muscle. On the occasional patient with a less defined platysma border, the surgeon may be

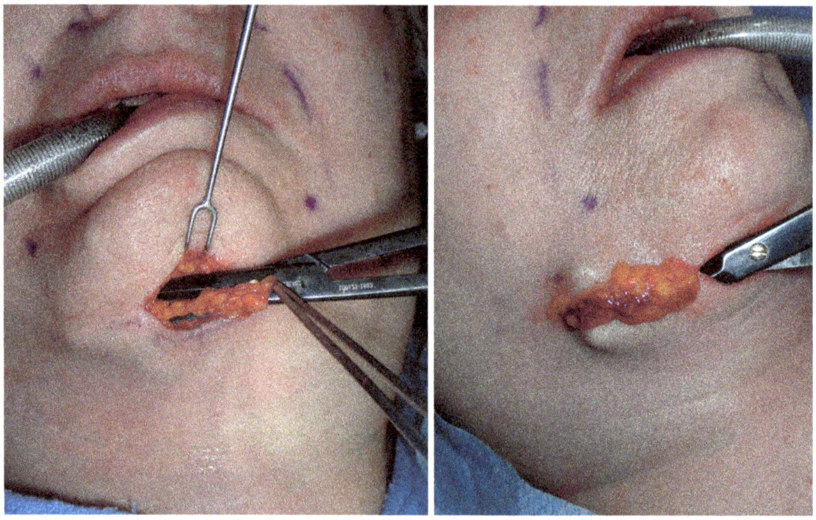

Fig. 6.58. These images show resection of lateral excess adipose tissue at the mandibular border. This is performed in patients with extremely thick or heavy necks to help define the anatomy of the inferior border and infra mandibular region.

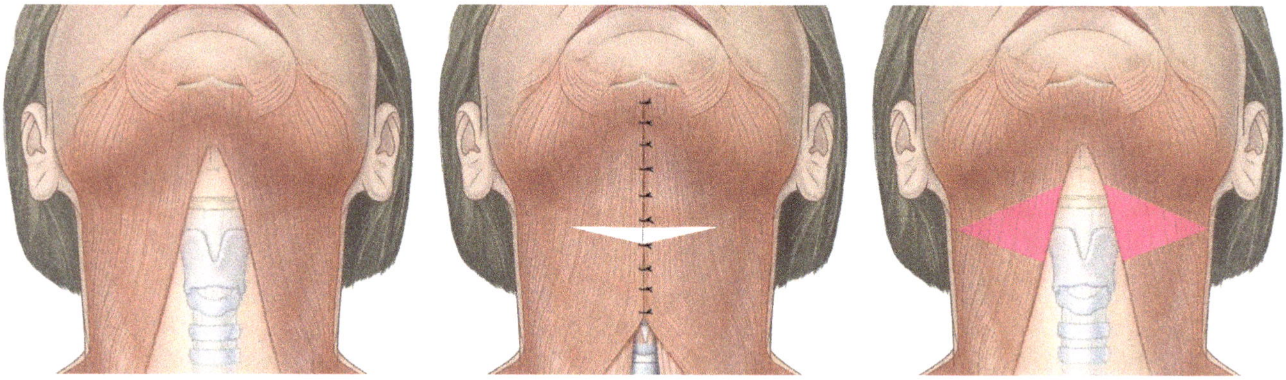

Fig. 6.59. The *left* image shows the dehisced medial platysmal borders. The *center* image shows a shoestring or corset repair. The *white triangles* show where cutbacks are made, if indicated. The *right* image illustrates a platysectomy where a wedge of platysma is removed on each side.

securing other tissues associated with the platysma border and bringing those to the midline on each side. This has the same effect, and the point is that the platysma is well defined in some patients and poorly defined in others.

I prefer a 2-0 Vicryl absorbable suture for the platysma repair. Some surgeons use bigger or smaller sutures and some surgeons also use permanent sutures. Resorbable sutures are my choice because the sutures that hold tissues together are only important until the dissected tissue planes scar together. It is this scarification during healing that maintains the result. After this healing occurs (usually within 4 to 6 weeks), internal sutures are not necessary. Experienced surgeons are aware of the fact that during revision facelift surgery previously placed permanent sutures are frequently seen loose in the tissues, serving no function. Secondary to that, (although rare) permanent sutures can become a source foreign body reaction or infection. I choose the 2-0 Vicryl suture because it ties easily, has adequate friction to keep the knot together, is a strong suture, and again is resorbable.

The platysma repair is begun by using the lighted retractor to retract the anterior cervical skin and illuminate the deeper tissues. I place the first platysma suture at the cervicomental angle, which is the junction of the neck and submental region that corresponds to the hyoid region (Figs. 6.60–6.62). By placing the first suture in the region, the loose tissues are tucked superiorly and posteriorly and "set" the platysmal position for the remaining sutures. I feel this first suture defines the cervicomental angle. I place approximately six or seven interrupted sutures above and below this first holding suture. These midline sutures run from the inferior border of the mandible to either the hyoid region or the thyroid region, depending on the amount of platysma dehiscence. Generally smaller facelifts only require dissection to the hyoid region, where larger lifts may require dissection to the thyroid cartilage area or beyond.

As previously stated, sutures are placed from the mandibular border superiorly and extend to the hyoid or thyroid region inferiorly, depending on the magnitude of the facelift. Fig. 6.61 shows a representation of the 2-0 Vicryl midline sutures.

Many surgeons advocate performing a releasing "cutback" at the hyoid region to prevent a "bowstring" effect of the sutured platysma border seen as a longitudinal ridge under the skin. A bowstring deformity produces a thick palpable and visible band postoperatively and is especially visible during neck extension.

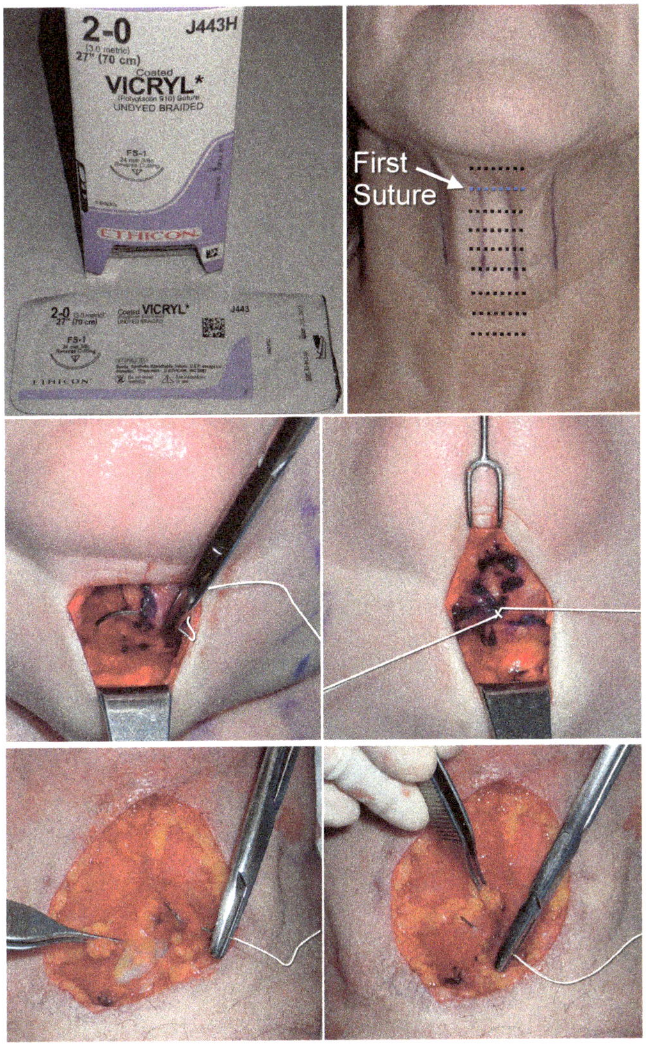

Fig. 6.60. The *top left* image shows the 2-0 Vicryl suture used by the author for platysmaplasty. After the platysma borders are trimmed, the first Vicryl suture is placed at the cervicomental junction (blue line *upper right* image). Burying the knot will prevent a visible and palpable bump in patients with thin tissues. Additional sutures are also shown by the *dotted lines in the upper right image*. The *middle* images show an intraoperative picture of the first suture being placed, and the *lower* images show an additional suture placed inferiorly.

For smaller lifts where my platysmaplasty only extends to the hyoid region, I rarely perform a cutback. For larger lifts that extend to the thyroid region or beyond, I do make cutbacks at the cervicomental region in selected cases to release the tension or bowstring. The contour of the neck and submental regions are curved, and a long midline platysma repair can tighten the borders to the point where the platysma becomes a straight line instead of negotiating the curvilinear contour of the neck and submental regions. Making the releasing cutback allows the tissues to relax at that junction, thus preventing a straight-line ridge that can show through the skin (Fig. 6.62). The cutback allows a more normal skin drape.

It is notable that numerous texts describe various positions of the cut back on the platysma. Some texts recommend the platysma be cut back to be as low as possible in the neck to allow better skin drape. When I utilize a cutback (and I do not always), I try to place it at the level where the neck and submental contours merge. This seems generally to be in the region somewhere between the hyoid and the thyroid, but technically can differ from patient to patient based on their specific anatomy. It makes sense to me that taking the straight-line repair in releasing it at the region where the normal anatomy converges from vertical (the neck) and approaches horizontal (the submental region) would be the most likely place for optimum skin redraping and prevention of a visible ridge deformity through the skin.

The way I determine the need for a cutback is to extend the patient's head after the midline repair. If I can see or feel a thick band of tissue on extension, I perform a cutback at the greatest part of the tension band to relax the tissues. This is frequently at the cervicomental junction (Fig. 6.62). By making a cutback, the surgeon is splitting a single midline repair into two segments with a separation between the submental and neck tissues.

Some surgeons perform a secondary plication by adding additional rows of midline sutures, going laterally with each plication (Feldman platysmaplasty). I have not found this necessary.

Once the platysma flap is dissected and bleeding is encountered, the pocket can be packed with peroxide gauze using

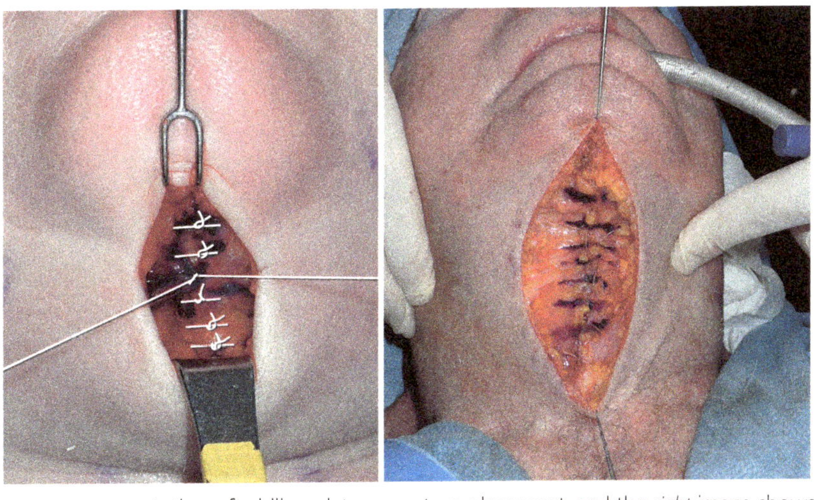

Fig. 6.61. The *left* image shows a representation of midline platysma suture placement, and the *right* image shows an actual midline platysmaplasty performed on a direct skin excision neck lift. (Note: This longitudinal incision is not made with a routine facelift and neck lift and is shown to illustrate midline platysmaplasty repair.)

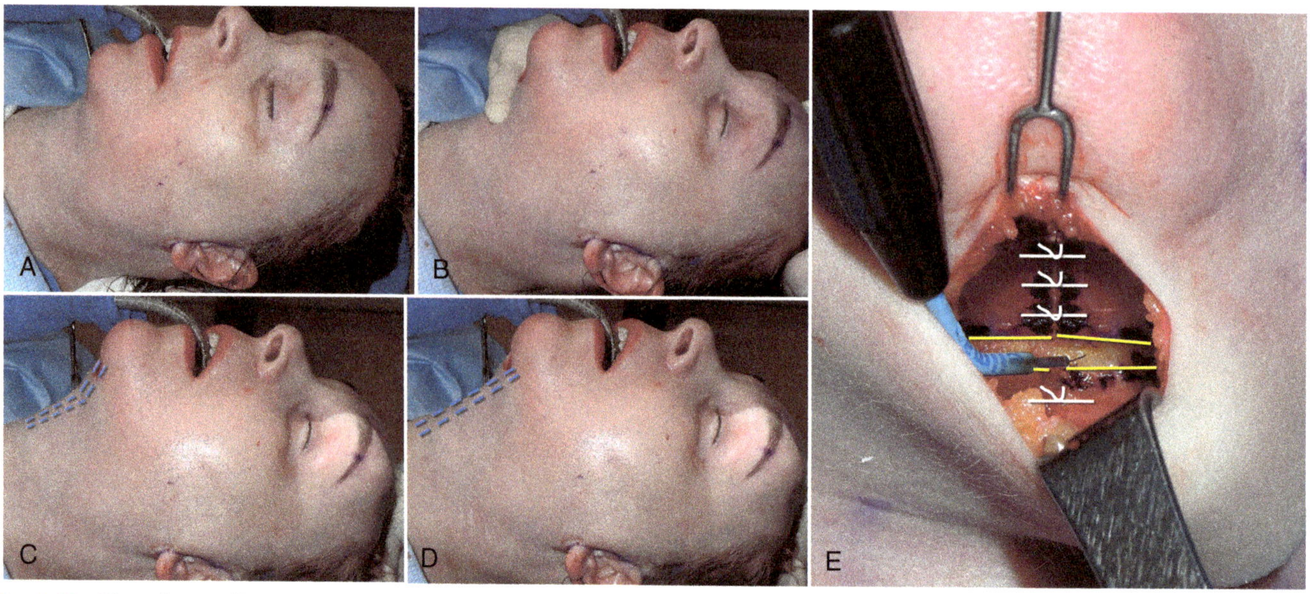

Fig. 6.62. These images illustrate how I determine the need for a skin cutback with midline platysmaplasty. (A) The patient in the neutral position immediately after platysma plication. Image (B) shows the author extending the neck and palpating for a discernable thick band. If no band is present (C), the procedure is complete. If a band is present (D), a cutback is made at the region of the band with the greatest tension. Basically, I view the band with the neck extended and transect it at the region that will allow the most relaxation. Image E shows an actual intraoperative cut back to release a bowstring.

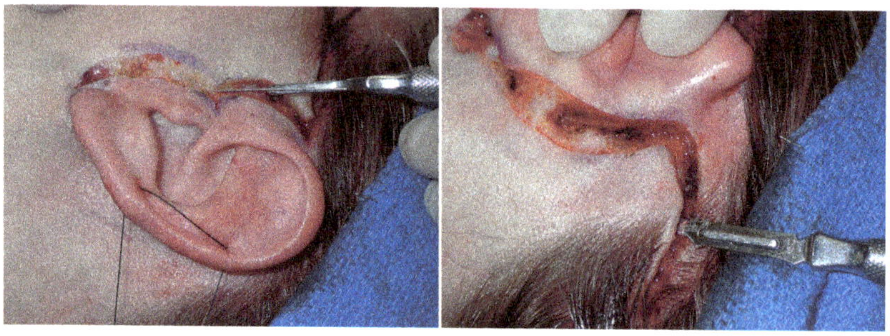

Fig. 6.63. The *left* image demonstrates the author's triarcuate incision pattern. The scalpel position in the *left* image overlies the area where the superficial temporal vein is frequently encountered and can cause brisk bleeding. The *right*-hand image shows the authors' typically high posterior irregular incision.

standard 3% hydrogen peroxide. This has an excellent hemostatic affect, and it will help clear the field. Conversely, at the end of the procedure when the platysmaplasty is completed and there is mild bleeding, the same treatment can be done. This can be done in any flap where there is bleeding and will be discussed later in the text.

Part 2: Facelift and Neck Lift Dissection

After the platysmaplasty is completed, attention is then focused to the first side of a facelift. In my experience, right-handed surgeons usually begin on the right side and left-handed surgeons, like myself, begin on the left side. This makes no difference and is simply a matter of convention. Incision design has been discussed at length in the previous portion of this chapter. I begin using a round scalpel handle with a 15c blade. On the average case, I begin with the transfollicular sideburn incision and the triarcuate preauricular (and pretragal) incision, which continues into the temporal tuft and around the base of the earlobe. The posterior auricular incision is then continued superiorly in the depth of the postauricular sulcus to the greatest width of the pinna. At this point, the incision is extended horizontally with an inferior taper into the posterior hairline. Small facelifts may only require 3–4 cm of horizontal extension into the hairline, and larger lifts may extend 8–10 cm into the posterior hairline (Fig. 6.63).

One of the most challenging parts of facelift dissection for beginning surgeons is staying in the correct plane. The initial plane for most facelift and neck lift surgery is the subcutaneous plane. Failure to dissect deep enough can thin the lipocutaneous flap and cause problems with perforation or viability. Dissecting at too deep of a level can damage significant neurovascular structures, but a too superficial dissection can damage the dermis and blood supply to the skin. One of the first skills to be mastered in facelift surgery is finding and staying in the proper surgical plane. For novice surgeons I recommend a predissection technique (also referred to as pretunneling). This is performed after tumescent infiltration and before any flap dissection. Small stab incisions are made in the sideburn, at the earlobe, and behind the ear. This can be performed before or after the preauricular incisions. Using blunt dissection cannulas specifically designed for this (or a spatulate liposuction cannula without a suction source) the cannula is rapidly passed back and forth in a reciprocal manner to undermine the subcutaneous plane from the deeper tissues (Fig. 6.64). The pretunneling makes "Swiss cheese" tunnels in the subcutaneous plane, and performing this maneuver for several minutes makes hundreds of these perforations under the flaps (Fig. 6.65).

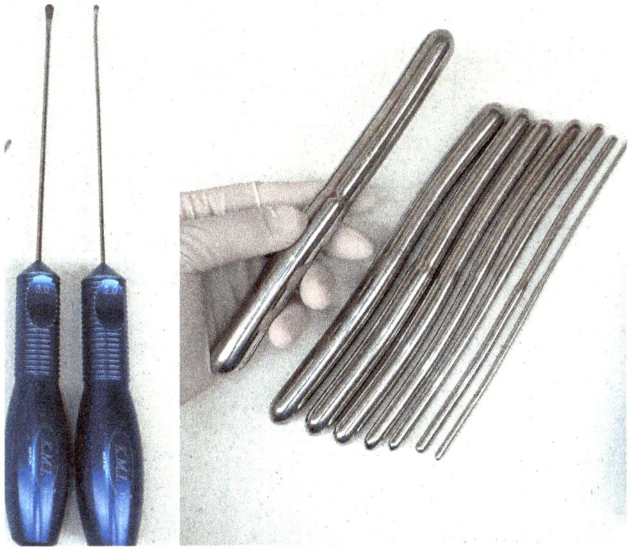

Fig. 6.64. Specialized dissection cannulas can be used to "pretunnel" the lipocutaneous flaps. The *left* image shows dissectors from KMI Surgical, and the *right* image shows inexpensive Hegar Uterine Cannulas that can be purchased online for around 20 dollars.

If this procedure is performed, it is easier for novice surgeons to find and stay in the subcutaneous plane. It also greatly facilitates scissor dissection, because of the predissection (Figs. 6.66 and 6.67, *right*). When the scissors are inserted, cutting is much easier, as you are simply joining the "Swiss cheese" tunnels. In many cases the scissors do not even need to be opened and closed (for snipping) and can just be held in an open position and advanced through the tissue to dissect.

The pretunneling is especially useful in the mastoid region. The posterior auricular flap is normally very thick, but as the mastoid region is approached, there is little or no subcutaneous tissue. In this region, the dermis can be bound down to the fascia of the sternocleidomastoid muscle (SCM). This is a trying area for both novice and experienced surgeons as it is easy to perforate the flap. Alternately, if the dissection is carried deeper and follows the SCM muscle inferiorly, the external jugular vein and greater auricular are at risk. Pretunneling is an effective procedure in patients that are easy to dissect. By this I mean that some patients have tissues that offer very

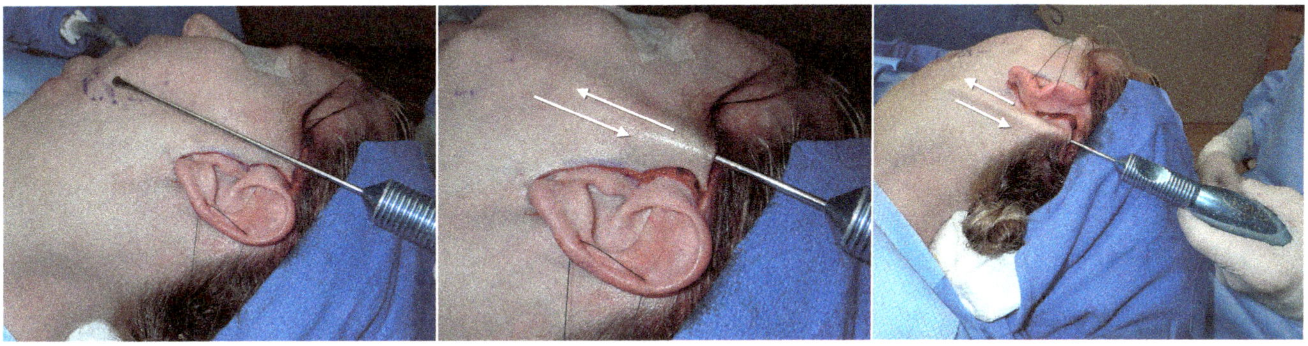

Fig. 6.65. The pretunneling (also called predissection) cannula is placed through small stab incisions and moved under the skin, in the subcutaneous plane, with rapid reciprocal motions to create small dissection tunnels.

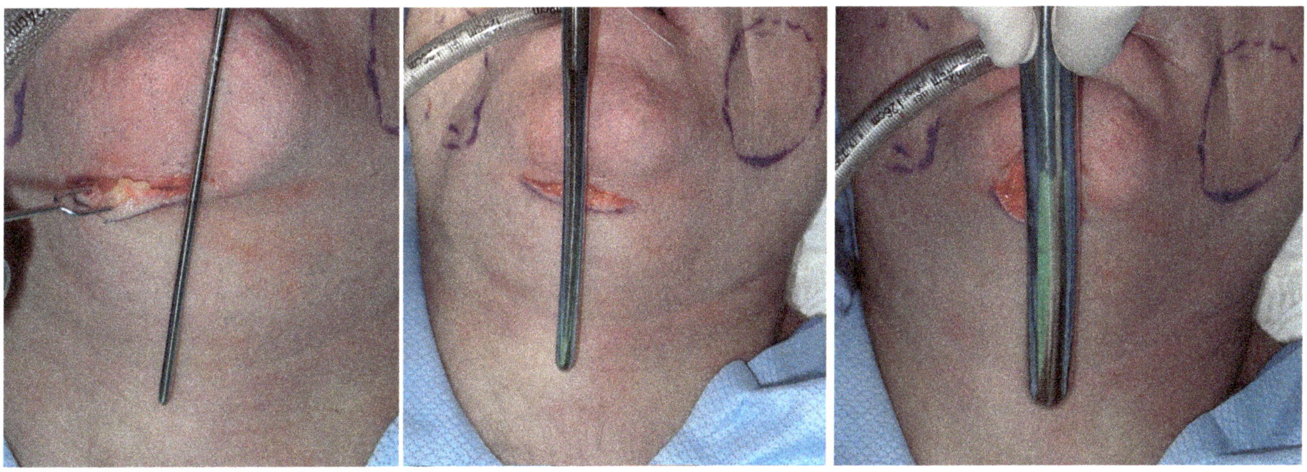

Fig. 6.66. Hegar uterine dissectors are inexpensive progressive cannulas used for predissection. If the larger dilators are used, very little scissors dissection is required.

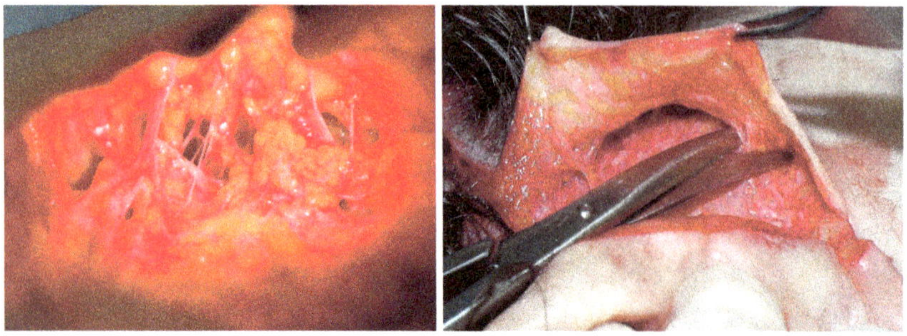

Fig. 6.67. Pretunneling with a dissection cannula creates tunnels in the subcutaneous plane (*left*) that assist the surgeon in staying in the correct plane and greatly facilitate scissor dissection (*right*).

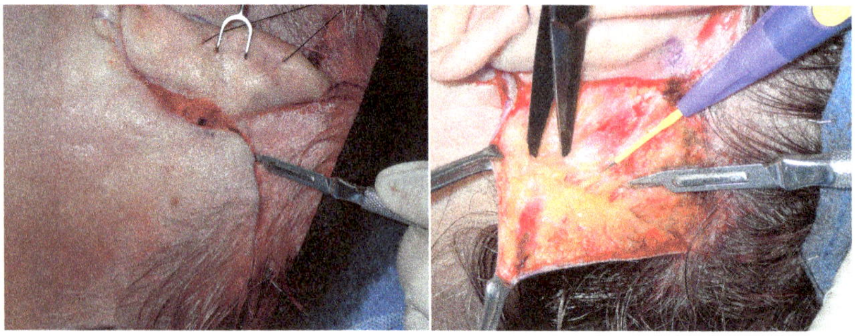

Fig. 6.68. The *left* image shows the initial flap incision with a #15c scalpel blade, and the *right* image shows that the dissection can proceed with scissors, electrosurgery, or scalpel blade.

little resistance to pretunneling or scissor dissection. Alternatively, some patients have extremely tight tissues, and the surgeon must fight for every centimeter of dissection. Some patients dissect easily, and some are more fibrotic and it takes much more effort to dissect. Pretunneling is not as easy in the latter.

Flap Dissection

The crux of facelift surgery is creating lipocutaneous flaps on the anterior neck and pre- and postauricular areas. My dissections are contiguous, so all the flaps and dissections connect with one another. Some surgeons do not connect the anterior cervical and submental flaps with the pre- and postauricular flaps. I believe that connecting all the flaps will mobilize more skin and result in a better drape with a more comprehensive result. A possible negative feature of having all the flaps connected is that a hematoma in one region could involve all dissected regions, but I believe the advantages outweigh this possible disadvantage.

After the initial incisions are made, behind the ear the lipocutaneous flaps are developed. As previously stated, a sufficient layer of fat should be left on the dermal side of the flap as well as this SMAS side of the flap. As also previously stated, these flaps should be treated in a gentle manner as loss of viability can result in horrific circumstances. Excessive traction or compression can affect flap viability, so it is important that the staff understand to handle the flap gently.

Flap dissection can be performed with scissors, scalpel, or cautery depending on the preference of the surgeon (Fig. 6.68). Cautery dissection should only be used in experienced hands as excessive lateral thermal damage can be problematic. Scalpel dissection also takes experience as it is easy to dissect too thin or too deep during the dissection. I personally believe that scissor dissection is the easiest method to learn and control for beginning surgeons.

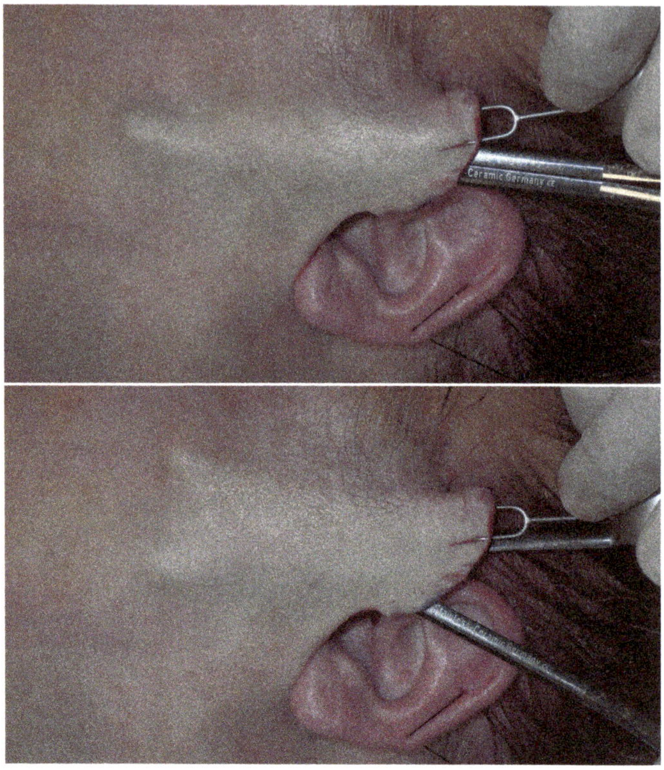

Fig. 6.69. Many facelift scissors are sharp on the inside and outside of the blades and will cut when closing or spreading for effective dissection.

Once the scissor dissection is started, the facelift scissors can be advanced by several methods. On patients with thicker and more tenacious tissues, opening and closing the tips in a snipping motion as well as spreading the tips is required to advance (Fig. 6.69).

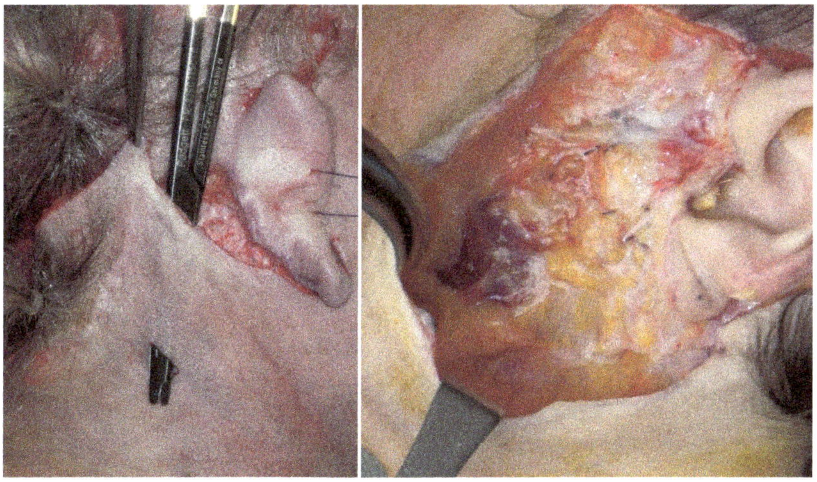

Fig. 6.70. Dissecting too superficially can result in dermal damage or perforation (*left* image), and dissecting too deeply can damage neurovascular structures. The *right* image shows the masseter muscle and facial nerve branches exposed with overaggressive dissection. Generally, a small rent in the tissue as shown in the *left* picture can be closed with 5-0 or 6-0 gut and usually does not present a problem.

On patients with less fibrotic tissue, leaving the tips in a semi-open position in advancing the scissors without opening and closing is effective. This depends on the preference of the surgeon and the resilience of the tissue being dissected. Some patients have extremely thick and fibrous tissues that require a cutting motion, and other patients have less robust tissues that can be separated with a gliding motion of the open scissors. As stated many times in this chapter, controlling the level of dissection is paramount to avoid perforation or unintended tissue depth (Fig. 6.70).

The extent of flap dissection is commensurate with the amount of aging and tissue excess. In general, a 45-year-old patient would have smaller flaps than a 65-year-old patient. I previously mentioned that facelifts come in three sizes: small, medium, and large (Fig. 6.71). The bottom line is that the flap dissection needs to extend enough to free the excess tissues so that they can be retracted and redraped in a passive manner without dimpling or puckering (Fig. 6.72). The extent of the flap dissection is essentially what defines the size of a facelift. It is important to remember that this lipocutaneous flap is delicate, as shown in the figure, and should always be protected from excessive retraction, compression, heat, and other physical insults that occur during surgery.

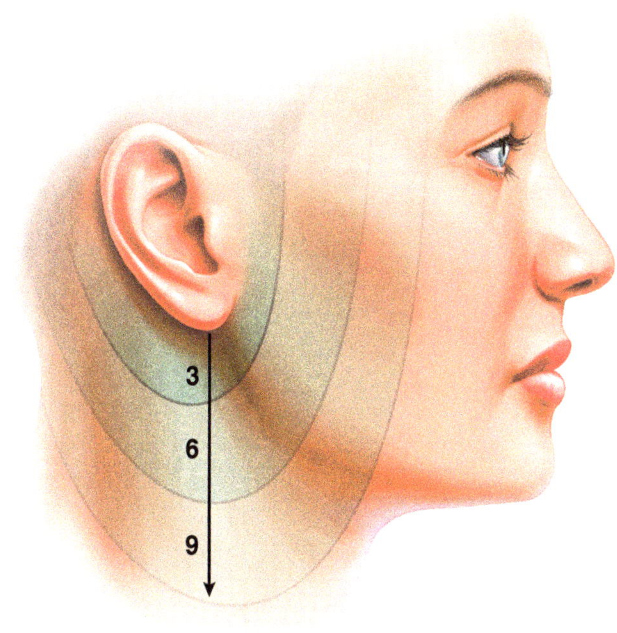

Fig. 6.71. The author describes facelift sizes based on the amount of flap dissection circumferential to the ear, in this case measured in centimeters.

"When do you stop dissecting the flap?" is a common question from beginning surgeons. The answer is multifactorial, but when the surgeon has freed enough tissue without dimpling or visible adhesion (Fig. 6.72). Also remember that the patient will be standing upright and this will cause inferior traction on the anatomy. It is this reason that a "pixie earlobe" may not be as noticeable when the patient is supine, but with gravity and wound contraction, it may become more severe.

Before any dissection, pretunneling can be performed as described in Fig. 6.65. Some surgeons begin with dissection of the preauricular flap, and other surgeons begin with the postauricular flap, which is a matter of preference. I generally begin with the posterior. The goal of flap dissection is to extend the subcutaneous undermining in the correct plane while protecting dermis and underlying anatomy. After the initial scalpel incision, the remainder of the flap can be secured with Allis clamps for backward traction and dissected with scissors, scalpel, or electrosurgery/radiofrequency (Fig. 6.73).

If the flap dissected is excessively thin, the hair follicles may be exposed (Fig. 6.74). Care must be taken to preserve these follicles, or a large bald spot could ensue in the occipital area. This is especially true when dissecting with electrosurgery, which can destroy the follicles. I have heard surgeons say that "if you see the follicles, they won't survive" (meaning they are already damaged). I disagree with this as I have seen them many times without problems. Respect the hair follicles!

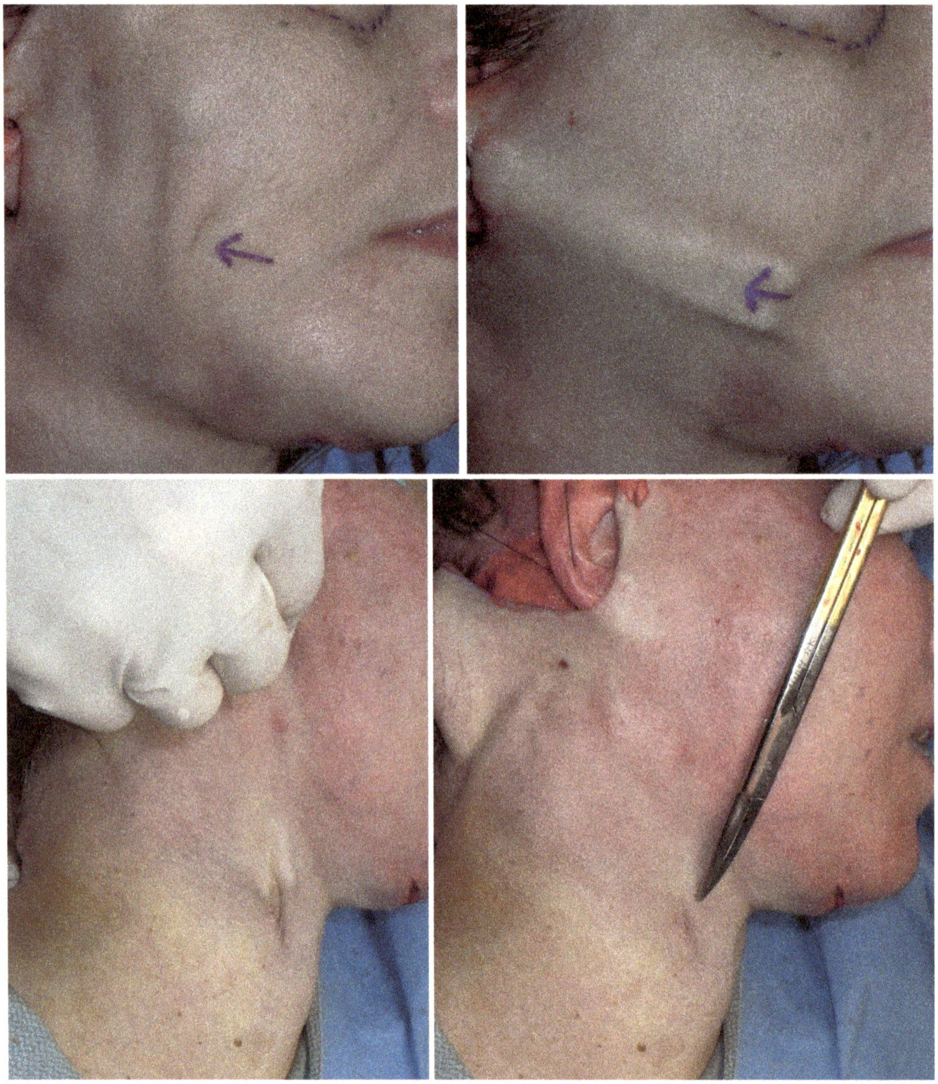

Fig. 6.72. Tissue dissection is adequate when the amount of tissue excess can be passively retracted and redraped without dimpling or puckering. When dimpling or puckering exists, the flap dissection usually needs to be advanced to undermine these areas.

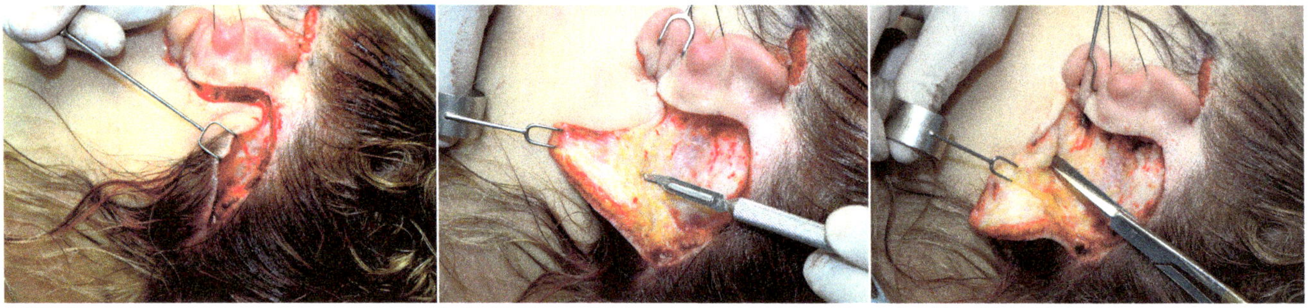

Fig. 6.73. The *left* image shows the flap retracted during initial dissection. The *middle* image shows the beginning dissection using a scalpel. The *right* image shows the scissors completing the remainder of the dissection.

To facilitate monoplane dissection, the skin is retracted with Allis clamps or a Cottle retractor. As the skin is retracted away from the dissection, the scissors (or other dissection instruments) are advanced toward the dissection. Pulling the flap away while advancing the dissection inferiorly helps the surgeon stay in the same plane (Fig. 6.75).

The posterior flap dissection can extend to the midoccipital region, and as stated, the incision can vary from 4 to 10 cm in length. The inferior extent of the pre- and postauricular flaps is usually contiguous with the cervical dissection and becomes a single unit (Fig. 6.71). During the posterior incision, it is critical to understand the anatomy of this region. Taking into consideration the significant anatomy described earlier in Chapter 3, close attention and direct vision is necessary when proceeding inferiorly with this dissection. The first complexity encountered with this dissection is the thin tissue over the mastoid region. Careful

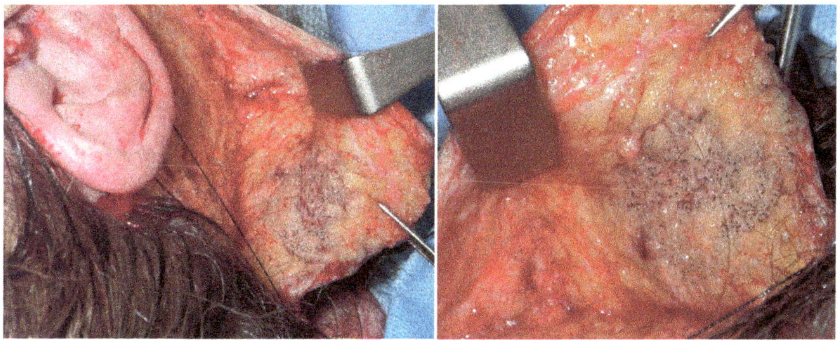

Fig. 6.74. These images show exposed hair follicles while dissecting the postauricular flap. Although the operator may see follicles, this does not necessarily mean they are damaged, but it means that caution should be used. This is especially significant when using electrosurgery or radio frequency due to the heat generated.

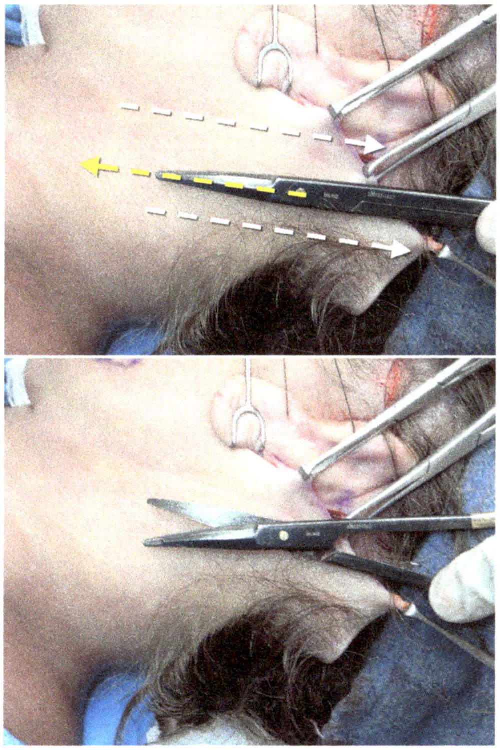

Fig. 6.75. The *upper* image shows the flap retracted with Allis clamps in the opposite direction of the scissor dissection. The *lower* image shows the scissor opened. By advancing and snipping or spreading the tissue by opening the scissor tips and pushing, the posterior dissection is advanced.

dissection is required to stay in the correct plane. Dissecting too superficially can result in damage to the dermis or skin perforation (Fig. 6.70, *left*). As the posterior dissection extends inferiorly, overly deep dissection can lead to injury of the greater auricular nerve and external jugular vein as they cross the SCM (Fig. 6.76). Erb's point is a reference for this area which is 6.5 cm inferior to the external auditory canal and is shown by the *X* in Fig. 6.76 (*left*). Fig. 6.76 (*right*) shows the external jugular vein (*blue*) and the greater auricular nerve (*arrow*) at Erb's point. It will benefit the surgeon to dissect with direct vision and a lighted source in this region to avoid this significant anatomy. It is of note that although rare, the spinal accessory nerve may be damaged during rhytidectomy, resulting in shoulder pain and movement deficit. The spinal accessory nerve crosses under posterior SCM and is superficial in this region as it traverses to the trapezius muscle. Dramatic movement disorders of the shoulder girdle can result from damage to this nerve. Fig. 6.77 illustrates vulnerable nerves encountered in lateral neck dissection.

As the posterior dissection advances around the earlobe, the lobe is incised to its base and mobilized (Fig. 6.78). I prefer to make a releasing incision at the base of the lobe so it can be manipulated to a natural position when trimming the flap later in the operation.

As the cervical dissection proceeds inferiorly, the surgeon will frequently encounter adhesions from incomplete release of the platysmaplasty flap. These are separated, and care must be

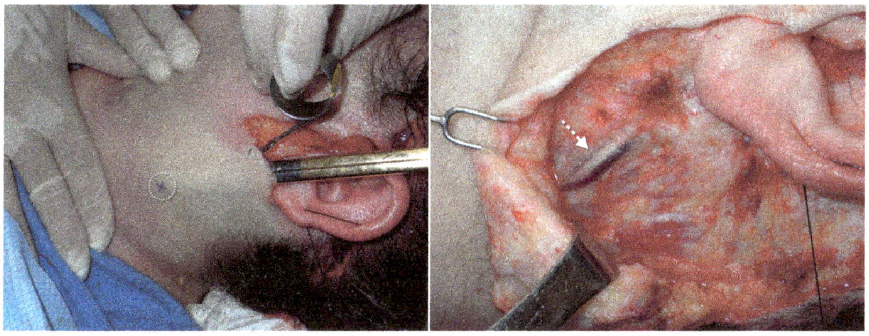

Fig. 6.76. Erb's point is shown by the *X* in the *left* image, and the greater auricular nerve and external jugular vein are also shown. If the external jugular vein is nicked, punctured, or lacerated, it must be tied off with ligature suture.

taken to ensure no visible skin dimple or adhesions exist. These are visible from outside of the flap, and dissecting past the adhesion will free the tether.

As the final portion of the cervical dissection progress medially, I perform two functions. The first is to make sure the mandibular ligament is released (Fig. 6.79, *left*). Just like the zygomatic ligament, failure to release the mandibular ligament can result in incomplete dissection. The second maneuver is to connect the posterior flap with the submental and anterior cervical dissection (Fig. 6.79, *right*). When the preauricular flap is dissected, all three of the flaps will be contiguous.

At this point, the submental and cervical flaps have been dissected, a platysmaplasty has been performed, the posterior flap has been dissected, the mandibular ligament sectioned, and the flaps made contiguous.

At this juncture, experienced surgeons may reduce the submandibular gland in the case of gland ptosis (Fig. 6.80). In my experience, this is not something that the average facelift surgeon routinely performs. Some surgeons may perform gland reduction routinely, but I only do it in cases of significant submandibular gland ptosis. Since I perform aggressive deep neck lift in many of my heavy-necked patients (and I do seem to attract these patients), I frequently encounter the submandibular glands. When I encounter the glands, it frequently means that they are ptotic, and I therefore reduce them. Extreme bleeding, nerve damage, and sialocele can occur, so experience is paramount. Although submandibular gland reduction may enhance the inframandibular aesthetics in some patients, it can also produce a skeletal look. It is up to the surgeon, based on their level of experience, to decide how much glandular tissue is removed. Generally, the removal is superficial and enough gland is removed to enhance the aesthetics. The excess glandular

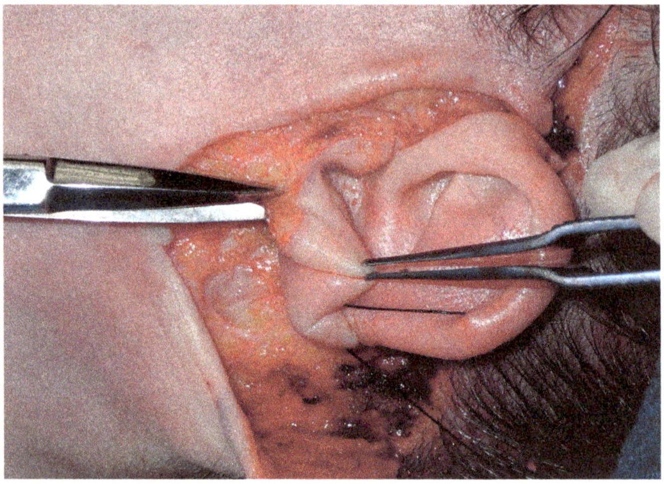

Fig. 6.78. The earlobe is incised and mobilized to its base so it can be properly positioned later in the operation.

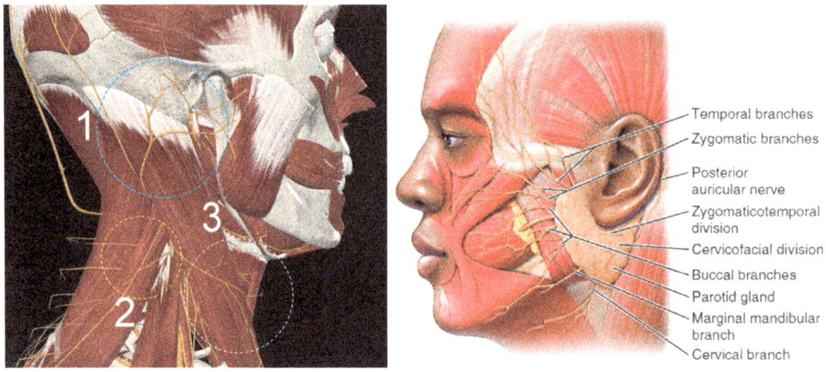

Fig. 6.77. The *left* image shows vulnerable nerves that may be encountered when dissecting the posterior auricular and cervical portions of the facelift. Circle *1* shows the greater auricular nerve (which in reality extends further down the sternocleidomastoid muscle), circle *2* shows the spinal accessory nerve (which exits from under the posterior sternocleidomastoid muscle), and circle *3* shows the transverse cervical nerves. (Base image, courtesy *Complete Anatomy*, Elsevier.) The *right* image shows the facial nerve branches. These branches are protected by the parotid gland but become superficial and more superficial as they cross the masseter muscle.

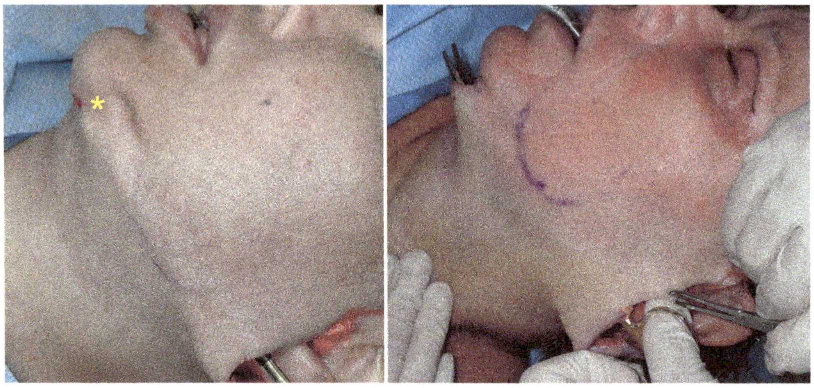

Fig. 6.79. The *left* image shows the mandibular ligament (*yellow asterisk*) being released, and the *right* image show the connection of the posterior and cervical flaps using scissors.

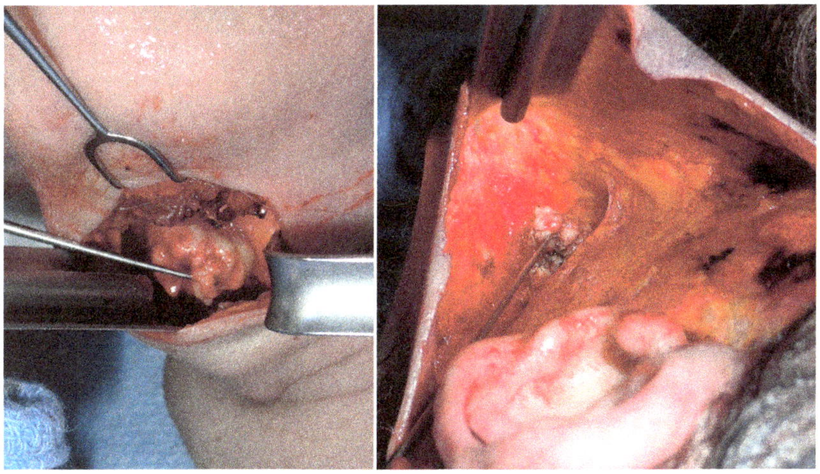

Fig. 6.80. Some surgeons will reduce ptotic submandibular glands to enhance the submandibular aesthetics. The gland may be reduced through the submental incision or from the anterior facelift flap.

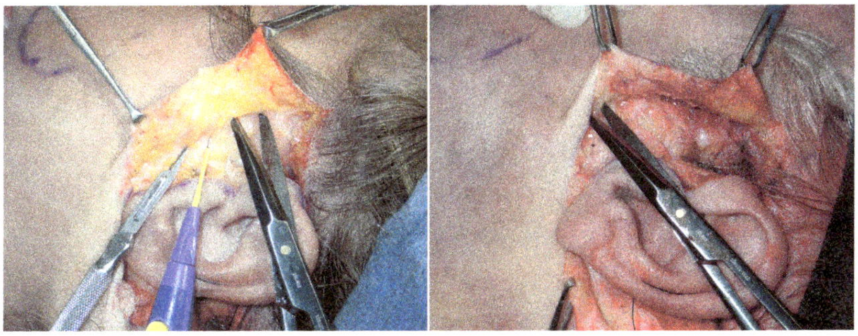

Fig. 6.81. The initial flap dissection is made with the surgeon's preferred instruments. I personally begin with a scalpel and progress to facelift scissors.

tissue is reduced by electrosurgery needle electrode or specialized energized tissue snares. I also close the gland capsule or the deep cervical fascia with 4-0 Vicryl suture to prevent further ptosis and possibly reduce the chance of post operative sialocele. Dissecting deep into the gland can be invasive and problematic. Some surgeons also inject 20 units of Botox into the gland at the time of surgery to suppress salivation via autonomic action.

Preauricular Flap Dissection

As stated earlier, some surgeons begin with the preauricular dissection and others begin with the postauricular dissection. It is purely the surgeon's preference.

The preauricular dissection is started with scissors, scalpel, or electrosurgery, depending upon the surgeon's preference. I usually begin with a scalpel for 3–4 cm and then switch to facelift scissors (Fig. 6.81).

As the preauricular flap is developed anteriorly in the subcutaneous plane, various structures may be observed. First and foremost is the attachment of the zygomatic ligaments, also referred to as McGregor's patch. This ligamentous structure anchors the skin of the cheek to the inferior border of the zygoma and is found just posterior to the origin of the zygomaticus minor muscle (Fig. 6.82). In the average patient the surgeon will recognize that this is a tenacious connection between the dermis in the deeper tissues. It frequently presents as an obstacle to dissection, and if it is not transected, a visible skin dimple will result intraoperatively and possibly postoperatively (Fig. 6.82, *top*). The anterior dissection cannot proceed without transecting this area of

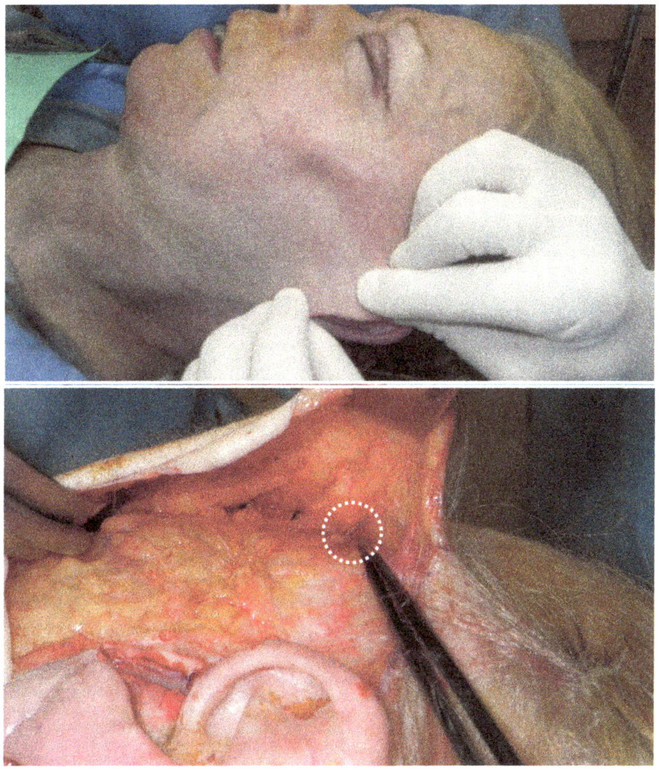

Fig. 6.82. McGregor's patch is a name given to the zygomatic ligaments that anchor the dermis to the zygomatic region in the midcheek region. This is usually an easily identifiable region during dissecting, and it is imperative to transect these fibers for complete dissection in this area. Failure to do so can cause permanent dimpling as well as limit the effectiveness of the facelift procedure.

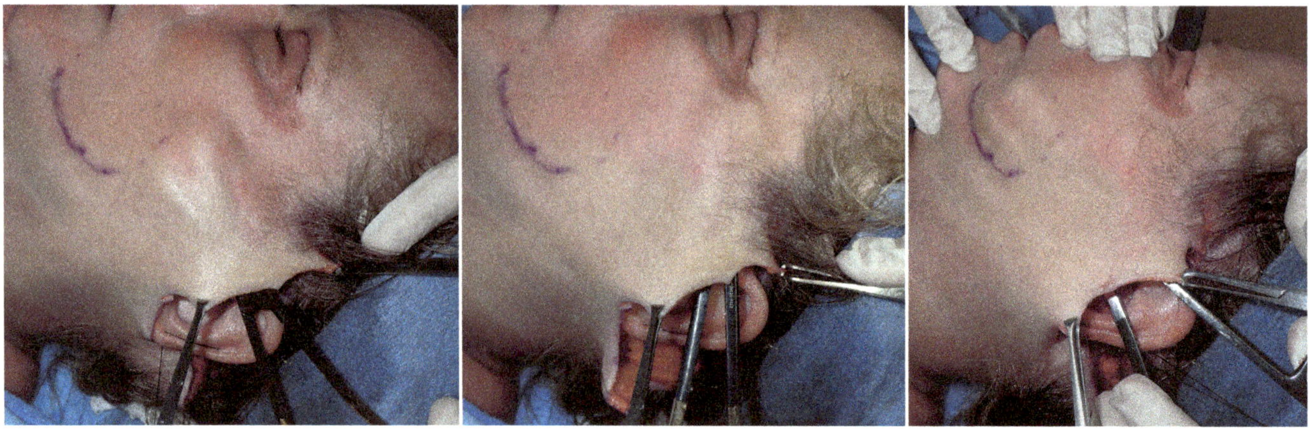

Fig. 6.83. The initial subcutaneous scissor dissection extends anterior to McGregor's patch (*left*) and in larger lifts can extend to the orbital rim (*center*). I personally dissect over the premarked jowl, and I perform significant work over this area to treat the jowl (*right*).

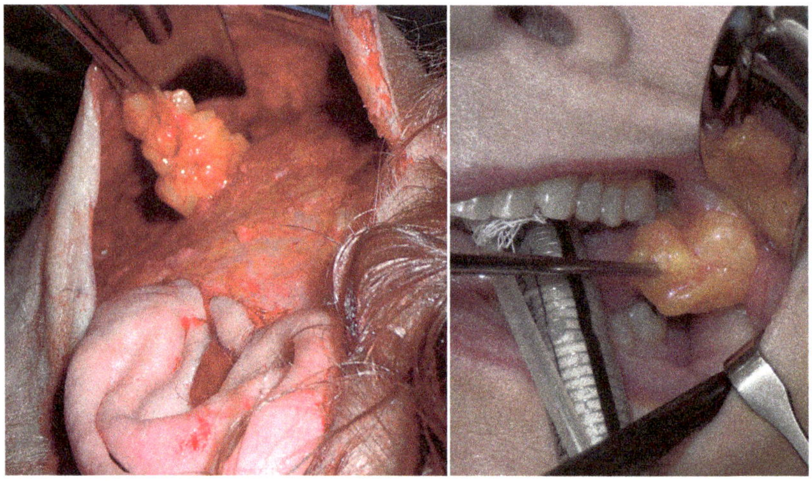

Fig. 6.84. The *left* image shows a significant buccal fat pad herniation under the preauricular flap. If a surgeon does not feel comfortable addressing the buccal fat pad from this approach, it can also be effectively reduced into orally (*right* image). If reduction is part of the diagnosis and treatment, then I usually reduce the buccal fat pads from an intraoral approach at the beginning of the case.

adhesion. As stated earlier, many surgeons who perform deep plane lifts utilize a short skin flap and transect the zygomatic ligament under the SMAS. As I have discussed, my particular deep plane technique utilizes a larger area of skin undermining, and I am transecting the zygomatic ligament in the subcutaneous and subSMAS planes.

The extent of undermining, as previously described, is commensurate with the amount of aging and skin excess. It is not uncommon for the preauricular flap to extend to the orbicularis oculi muscle, the midcheek, the midjowl region, and the mandibular border as shown in Figs. 6.71, 6.72, and 6.83.

In many patients, the buccal fat pad may be prominent or herniated, and is identifiable under the anterior flap during dissection. Failure to address a full or herniated buccal fat pad can detract from an otherwise great facelift due to residual cheek and jowl prominence. If this structure has significant bulging, then it should be treated at this point. In the case of minor prominence, the buccal fat pad can be reduced by placing horizontal mattress sutures over the fascial to flatten the area. In the case of significant herniation, I enter this space with blunt dissection to prevent damage to facial nerves and tease the buccal fat pad out of its capsule and reduce it intraoperatively (Fig. 6.84, *left*). After this reduction is performed, the fascia is closed with 4-0 Vicryl sutures. The buccal fat can alternately be reduced via an intraoral incision at the preference of the surgeon (Fig. 6.84, *right*). Treating the buccal fat pad can slim the face; ignoring a full buccal fat pad can detract from a result. Generally, the decision whether to reduce the buccal fat pads is made preoperatively in patients with fullness in that area.

During the entire dissection of all flaps, close observation is required by the surgical assistants as well as the surgeon. As stated, this is a fragile anatomic entity and nourished by the dermal plexus and should be handled in a gentle manner (Fig. 6.85). As dissection proceeds, any facial muscular twitching or evidence of stimulation of facial nerve branches that may run superficial in that region must be monitored for safety.

Throughout the entire case hemostasis is critical and bleeding must be controlled as the surgeon progresses, otherwise it may be impossible to "catch up" at the end of the case. Periodically packing the surgical site with 3% hydrogen peroxide and waiting a few minutes is a good way to further control hemostasis and identify existing bleeders (Fig. 6.86).

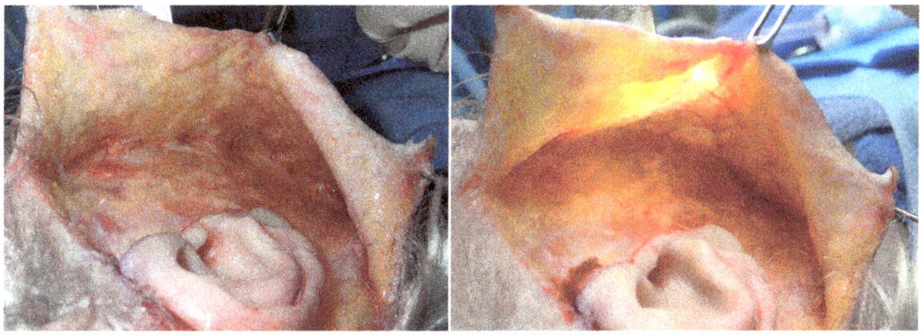

Fig. 6.85. These pictures show an anterior facelift flap without (*left*) and with (*right*) transillumination, which show the delicate and intricate nature of the tissue and blood vessels. Excessive tension, heat, or pressure on this flap can cause devitalization with significant negative consequences. Always respect your flaps!

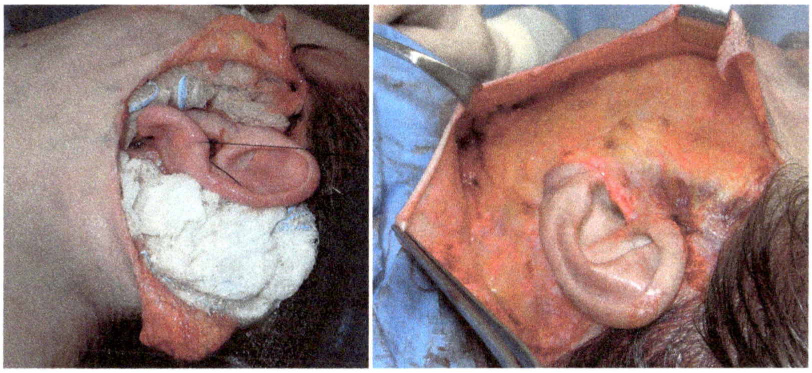

Fig. 6.86. Periodically taking a break to allow the staff to reorganize and perform gauze counts and packing the surgical site with chilled saline gauze or 3% hydrogen peroxide (*left* image) is an additional way to control hemostasis and identify malingering bleeders. The *right* image shows a clean, hemostatic surgical field. Hemostatic "combat" gauze can also be used. A dry field is essential for successful outcomes.

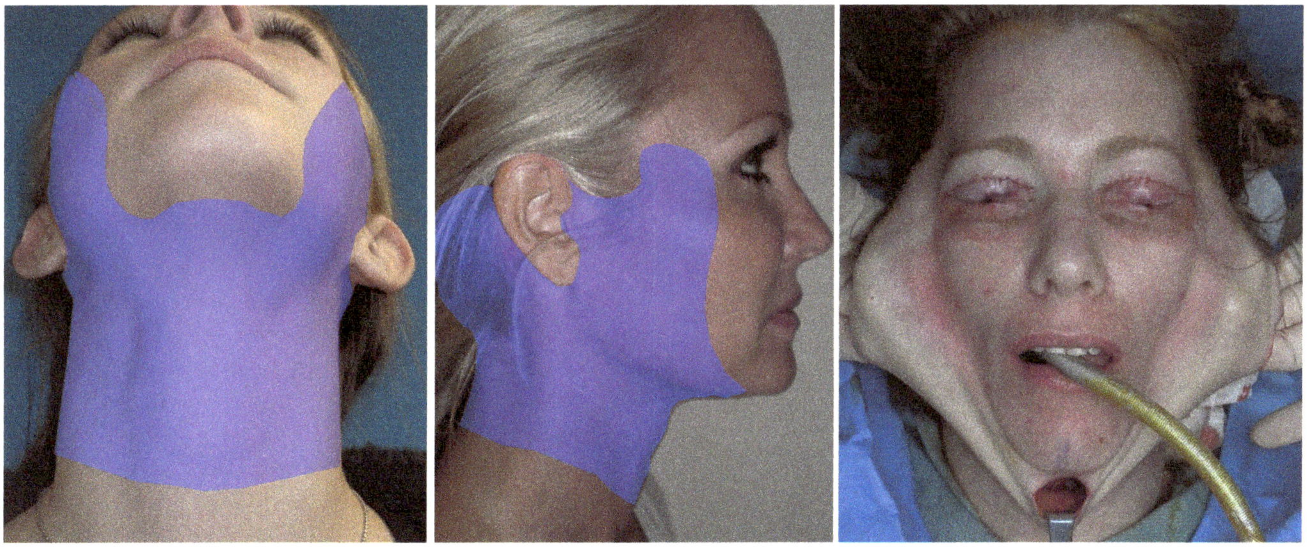

Fig. 6.87. The approximate extent of a typical dissection for a facelift (*left* and *middle* images), and a patient shown with all flaps dissected (*right* image). The extent of dissections will be less in smaller lifts.

I am describing my technique in a step-by-step manner, beginning with the submental region, progressing to the left side and then to the right. At the end of the case, if all flaps were dissected, the result would look like Fig. 6.87. Some surgeons prefer to dissect all the flaps at one time before addressing this skin. I have done this at certain stages of my career and published this technique, but currently I perform the steps I have described in this order (Fig. 6.88).

Now that all flaps are dissected, the platysmaplasty completed, and hemostasis achieved, further liposculpting may be performed. Since this is done with direct vision, I refer to it as open liposuction. This may involve areas of the lateral neck but is focused especially on the jowl region. Fig. 6.89 shows the areas of jowling above and below the mandibular border that were marked in the upright position before surgery. Fig. 6.90 shows actual liposuction of these areas with aspirated fat in the

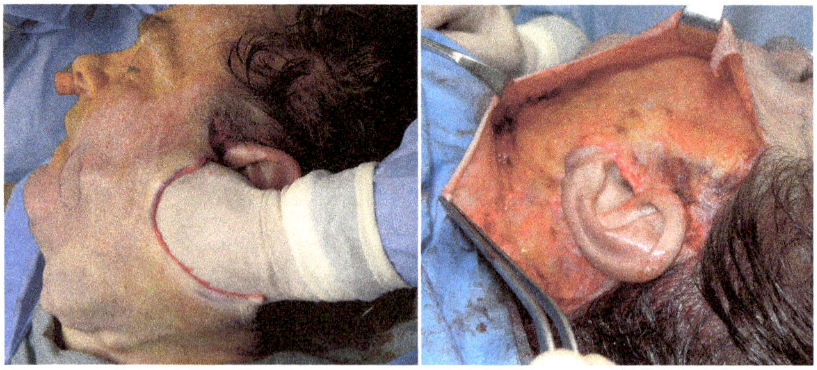

Fig. 6.88. The extent of the author's average facelift and neck lift dissection. Smaller lifts will have less dissection.

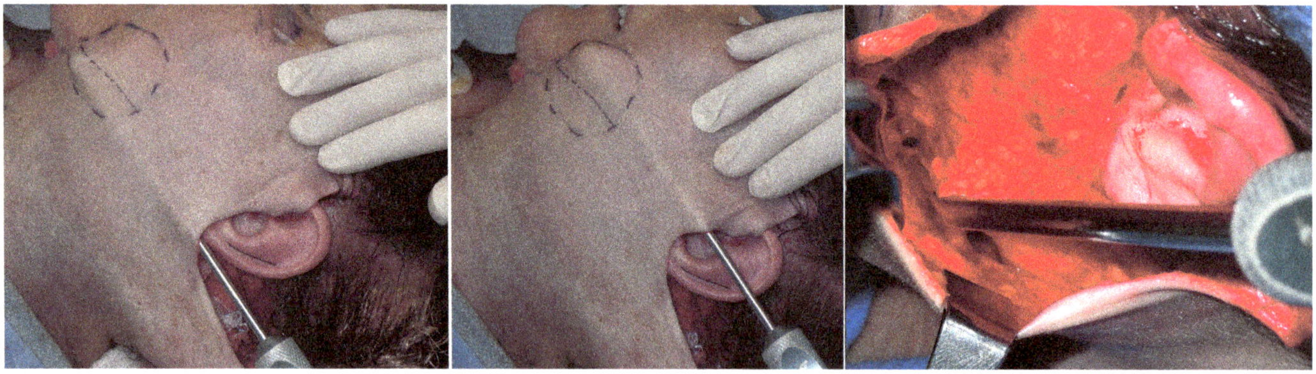

Fig. 6.89. The *left* and *middle* images show "open" liposuction on supra- and inframandibular jowl regions, and the *right* image show the intraoperative view.

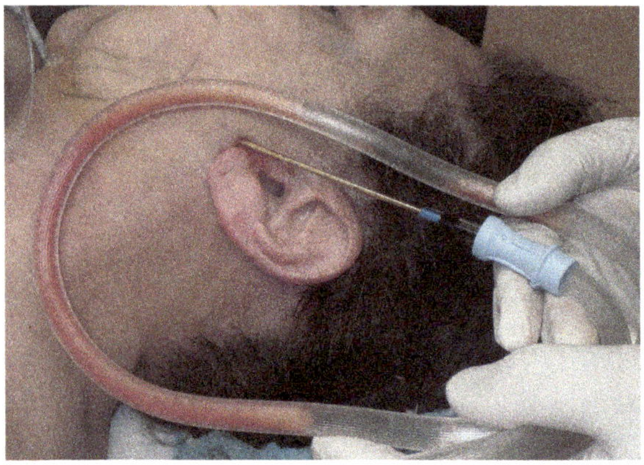

Fig. 6.90. This image shows aspirated fat from jowl liposuction in the tubing. This was performed with wall suction only.

suction tubing. Almost every patient, with the exception of thin or atrophic individuals, is a candidate for some component of jowl liposuction. As will be discussed in the later part of this chapter, two of the most common complaints after facelift and neck lift surgery are residual jowling and submental skin excess. I have modified my facelift technique over the years to specifically address these deficiencies. One of the most important parts of addressing this situation is extra attention to the jowl region during liposuction and SMAS treatment. With all the flaps open and optimum lighting and visualization, the surgeon may discover areas of fat there that were overlooked during the liposuction at the beginning of the case. Liposuction may also be performed in the lateral neck at this point. It may be especially helpful for patients with extremely heavy necks. The surgeon must be careful to never overliposuction any area that may allow dermis to contact muscle because of the postoperative deformities that can occur.

Addressing the SMAS

The more a person studies facelift and neck lift surgery, the more differences they see performed by various practitioners. One common denominator is that every accomplished facelift surgeon addresses the SMAS layer in some manner. Experience over the past century has shown that only treating the skin and ignoring the deeper structures will have significant implications on longevity results. There are many surgical descriptions of how to treat the SMAS and more than I list here.

Some of the more common means of treating the SMAS layer include:

- SMAS plication
- SMAS flap
- SMASectomy
- Deep plane SMAS
- Energy-based SMAS tightening

Various SMAS techniques will be shown in the video section of this text.

The SMAS is described in more detail in the earlier part of this chapter but is a dynamic layer in the structure of the face. The SMAS layer can be difficult as it is described differently in many different texts and articles. Some surgeons really don't believe there is a such thing as the "SMAS" and that it can't be picked up, can't be cut, and so on. In this text I am defining the SMAS as the fibrofatty layer beneath the dermis and above the parotidomasseteric fascia (PMF) in the cheek (Figs. 3.1–3.7). This layer can also extend into the neck under the dermis and above the deep cervical fascia and throughout the anterior face. As stated, it allows an entire group of facial muscles to be animated in vivo or surgically repositioned without addressing the individual structures. In short, the surgeon is repositioning the "sheet of SMAS," which will in turn reposition the entire middle layer of the face.

Closed SMAS Treatment (SMAS Plication)

The most basic techniques for management of the SMAS begin with suture plication. These may be in the form of purse-string sutures, which as the name implies, gather a circular portion of the SMAS and produce tightening. I have never been a fan of this type of suturing technique. Although it may be effective in a degree of tightening, if for any reason the suture breaks, the entire repair is jeopardized. When used, several purse-string sutures are placed at different angles and positions to achieve the desired SMAS repositioning (Fig. 6.91).

The facelift literature is not only full of controversy about the actual structure and histology of the SMAS, but also is full of the nomenclature of SMAS treatment, namely SMAS plication and SMAS imbrication. In this text I would like to simplify things as "closed SMAS" procedures and "open SMAS" procedures.

Plication is a "closed SMAS" procedure and is defined as "folded, crumpled, or corrugated." The word is derived from the Latin "plicātus folded, from plicāre to fold." The term "plica" commonly describes a fold in the orthopedic surgery and ophthalmology literature. In this text, plication will describe a bunching or folding of the SMAS. This would be achieved by passing the needle and suture through the SMAS (distally), pulling it in a given direction, and taking another bite (proximally) and securing with a knot (Figs. 6.92–6.94).

There is no absolute common position for plications sutures. It is, however, quite common to place the first suture at a distal position on an imaginary line from the corner of the mouth and then secure it in a proximal position to an area in front of the tragus (Fig. 6.92). It is imperative when placing sutures through the SMAS to maintain a level above the PMF so as not to ensnare deeper structures such as the parotid gland or branches of the facial nerve with the suture. Care of suture depth is also observed over the parotid gland as suturing through the gland could contribute to a sialocele.

SMAS plication is very effective and I would suggest this technique of SMAS management for beginning surgeons. Having said this, I know many accomplished surgeons that perform SMAS plication as their only SMAS procedure and have a long track record of excellent and long-lasting results. One relative drawback of this technique is the fact that the bunching or folding can create a thickening that may be visible under the skin. This is usually not significant, and if there is visible thickening, it resolves with healing. It is also important to understand that as

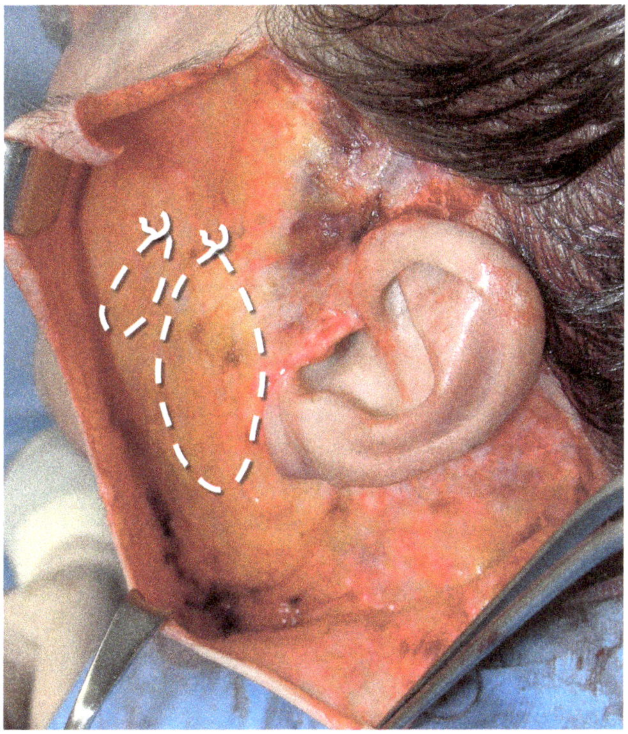

Fig. 6.91. This illustration shows a representation of purse-string suspension of the SMAS. Like the name implies, the suture tightens by synching the sutures as the loop is tightened.

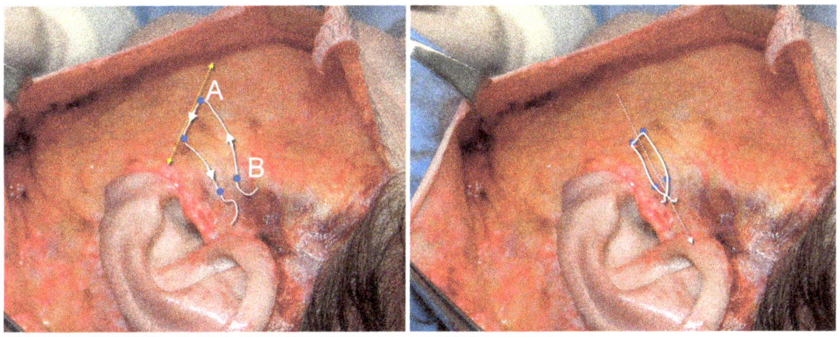

Fig. 6.92. A representation of a SMAS plication is shown where the distal suturing (A) pulls the ptotic tissues toward the proximal (B) position, thus creating a bunching or fold. The *yellow line* represents an imaginary line from the corner of the mouth.

many SMAS sutures can be placed as desired by the surgeon until the ptotic SMAS tissue tightened.

Open SMAS Treatment (SMASectomy)

Another means of SMAS treatment is also referred to as "imbrication." The actual definition is from the Latin root word "imbricare" is to overlap as in scales, plates, tiles, etc. Applied to SMAS treatment this means excising a section and joining the resultant edges together. I have never seen this done with any form of overlap, so I truly feel that this is a misnomer. In reading various facelift texts I have seen plication and imbrication described incorrectly. As stated earlier, I have always felt that it makes more sense to describe SMAS treatment as closed treatment or open treatment. An example of closed treatment would be purse-string and placation sutures and an example of open treatment would be SMASectomy.

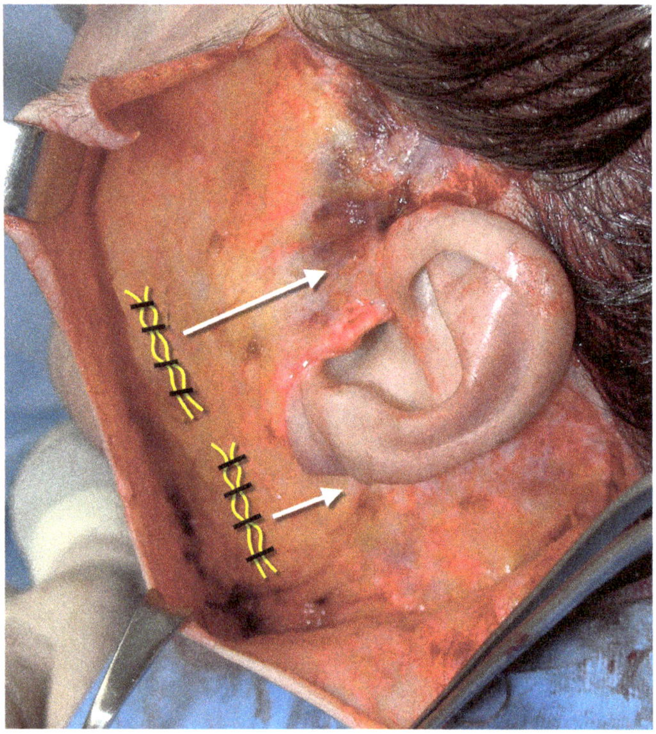

Fig. 6.93. Another representation of SMAS plication is shown. The sutures are positioned to address the main regions of SMAS laxity.

SMASectomy

Over my 25-year experience with facelift surgery, I would say that SMASectomy has been the most common SMAS treatment among all the specialties that are performed in cosmetic facial surgery. The technical definition of SMASectomy is to cut and remove a section of SMAS (ectomy) and tighten the SMAS layer by sewing the edges of the excision together. As with other procedures in any other type of surgery, many variations exist. I believe that SMASectomy is an intermediate technique and that novice surgeons will have safer and more predictable outcomes beginning with SMAS plication. Once a surgeon is comfortable navigating the various anatomic layers of the face, then they can proceed to the SMASectomy procedure.

The most basic SMASectomy procedure involves the excision of a strip of SMAS that is parallel with the nasolabial fold. The confines of this excision are from the zygomatic area to the angle of the mandible (Fig. 6.95). The width of the SMAS excision varies from 1.5 to 3 cm (one to two fingerbreadths) and is commensurate with the amount of ptosis in the SMAS layer and the desired amount of desired traction and tightening anterior to excision. For inexperienced surgeons, it is best to

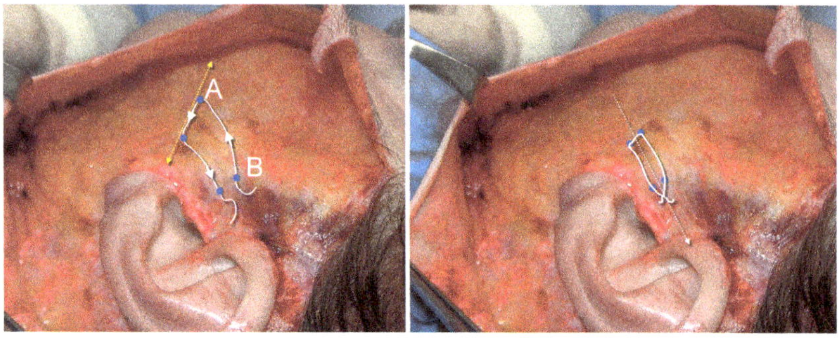

Fig. 6.94. Clinical intraoperative images are shown illustrating the mechanics of SMAS plication. The distal suture bite is frequently on an imaginary line extending from the commissure (A) and sutured to the SMAS anterior to the tragal region (B).

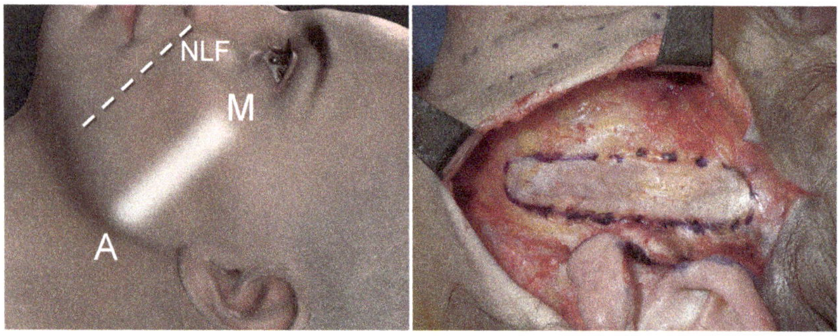

Fig. 6.95. The basic SMASectomy involves excising a 1.5 to 3.0 cm strip of SMAS, parallel to the nasolabial fold (*NLF*), from the malar region (*M*) to the angle of the mandible (*A*). The excision remains superior to the parotidomasseteric fascia (*right* image). (*Left* base image, courtesy *Complete Anatomy*, Elsevier.)

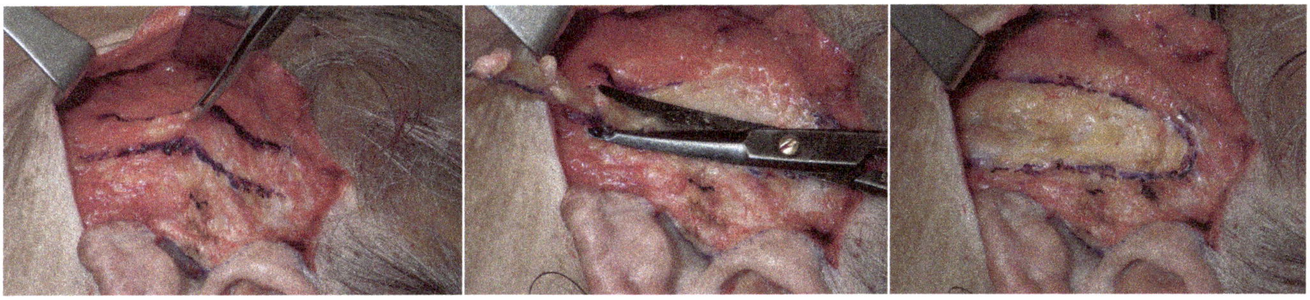

Fig. 6.96. The *left* image shows "tenting" of the SMAS to safely elevate it from the underlying parotidomasseteric fascia. The *middle* image shows the area of SMAS being excised, and the *right* image shows the SMASectomy defect.

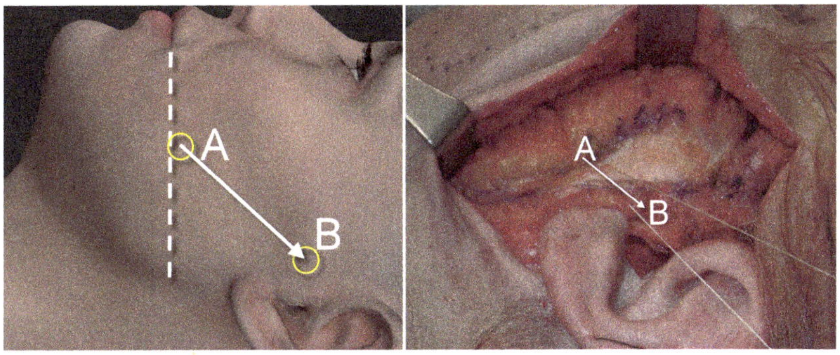

Fig. 6.97. The initial SMASectomy suture is placed on the distal margin of this SMAS on an imaginary line lateral to the corner of the mouth (*left* image). This is secured with a strong suture bite, pulled in a superior and lateral vector, and secured to the proximal SMAS in the region of the inferior tragus (*right* image). In both images, the *A* point is pulled to the *B* point. (Left base image, courtesy *Complete Anatomy*, Elsevier.)

perform this excision over the substance of the parotid gland to remain posterior to the facial nerve branches as they become exposed when they exit the anterior border of the gland and cross the masseter muscle. It is important to keep the excision out of the glandular tissue, which can cause a postoperative sialocele. Regardless of where this excision is placed, it always remains superficial to the PMF. Tenting the SMAS by elevating with a forcep during excision will assist in excessive depth (Fig. 6.96).

This described technique is the most basic SMASectomy procedure, and the excision is not undermined or carried into the cervical tissues. In this case the lateral platysma in the neck is treated as a secondary procedure. It is also important to state that some patients have a very wispy or friable SMAS layer, and it may not be thick enough or strong enough to hold suture tension. In these cases, the technique is reverted to SMAS plication. The situation is not unusual in revision facelift surgery where the layers are scarred and there is no definitive SMAS to excise and suture.

In theory, the strip of SMAS is removed to the level of the PMF. In reality, not every bit of SMAS tissue needs to be excised nor does it need to be excised 100% to the level of the PMF. Only enough SMAS needs to be removed to allow mobility of the approximated tissues and have thick enough SMAS margins to hold sutures. Too thin of an SMAS resection may not be effective for elevating the distal tissues and may be friable, allowing sutures to pull through. The section of excised SMAS should be an ellipse with tapered ends to allow closure without bunching. In some cases, the SMAS is too friable to hold sutures, and an SMAS plication is performed instead.

To close the SMASectomy, I prefer a 2-0 Vicryl suture. They are easy to tie, resorbable, strong enough to withstand tension, and small enough to not be visible through the skin. One of the main reasons for performing SMASectomy is to allow the surgeon to control various vectors. There is no set order of placement of the SMAS sutures, but I prefer to place the initial SMASectomy suture lateral to the jowl on an imaginary horizontal line from the corner of the mouth. The suture is then secured to the proximal border of this SMAS in a superolateral vector as shown in Fig. 6.97.

Before placing the first SMASectomy suture, the surgeon should explore various positions on the inferior and anterior portion of this SMASectomy. A bayonet forcep is used to elevate the ptotic tissue in a superolateral direction. This location is not the same in every patient, and it may take several attempts to pick up the most mobile tissue. When the surgeon finds a position that elevates the neck, the mandibular border, the jowl, and the corner, the suture is placed in that spot. I refer to this as the sweet spot, where elevation of this area will improve the appearance of the neck, mandibular border, jowl, and the corner of the mouth. This will be obvious in the video section that accompanies this textbook. The surgeon will find that above or below the sweet spot, the vector of pull only elevates the lower face or jawline. The surgeon should be persistent in finding that single spot that elevates the neck, jowl, and corner of the mouth. After the sweet spot is anchored, sutures are placed above and below the first suture to continue to elevate the ptotic SMAS in the desired vectors. The end point is when all the mobile SMAS from the mandibular border to the midface is elevated and tight. This may take six to eight additional sutures.

Extending the inferior portion of the SMASectomy below the inferior border of the mandible (*dashed white line* in Fig. 6.98) allows more ability to control the ptotic SMAS in the upper cervical and mandibular regions.

Fig. 6.99 shows the sutured SMASectomy site (*left*) and the excised strip of SMAS overlying the skin in its approximate position. Some surgeons will use the excised SMAS as grafting material in the lips, nasolabial folds, or other areas.

The basic SMASectomy technique I have evolved using several personal modifications is effective. As surgeons advance in their knowledge, experience, and ability, they will understand that modifying the SMASectomy procedure can provide more flexibility in controlling vectors and improving and stabilizing results. The second modification of the SMASectomy I have used is a right-angled SMASectomy that I call a hockey stick, inverted L, or a 7 SMASectomy. The nomenclature is not standard and simply describes the geometry of the excision. In addition to the previously described vertical member, a horizontal SMAS strip is removed at or above the zygomatic arch (Figs. 6.100 and 6.101). Staying above the PMF layer protects the frontal branch of the facial nerve. The combination of this vertical and horizontal member allows for greater control of vectors especially in the superior and lateral direction. If this right-angled flap were undermined in a sub-SMAS dissection, the procedure would be similar to that of an SMAS flap or a deep plane facelift sub-SMAS dissection.

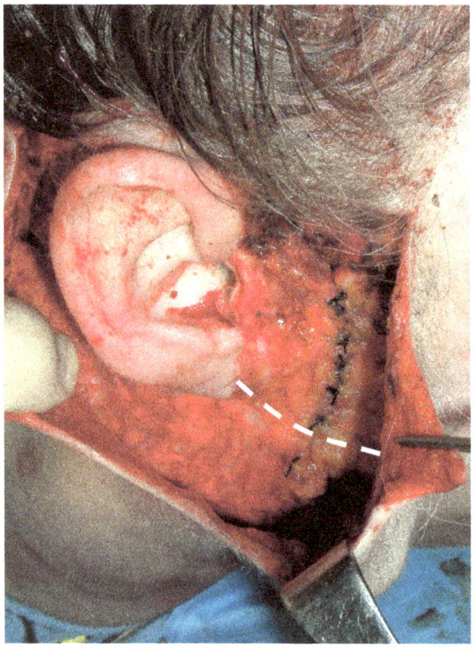

Fig. 6.98. The basic SMASectomy is shown closed with sutures. The *dashed line* approximates the mandibular border. Carrying the incision inferior to the mandibular border provides more definition of the mandibular border and neck. Larger SMASectomy techniques extend much more inferiorly down the neck.

The right-angled SMASectomy can be extended inferiorly on the neck on patients with SMAS tissue that is thick enough to cut and sew. The cervical portion of the SMASectomy can be continued down as far as the surgeon desires assuming the SMAS is thick enough to excise and suture (Figs. 6.102 and 6.103). In addition, the angle of the cervical SMASectomy can be manipulated for the most optimum lifting vectors. Having extended degrees of vector manipulation in the deep layers enables a more natural and less windswept look when the skin is redraped. The importance of SMAS treatment can never be overstated.

My personal SMAS experience mirrors that of many surgeons beginning with plication techniques and moving on to the hockey stick configuration, then to the cervical extension, and finally to deep plane SMAS techniques. Again, surgeons need to walk before they run and run before they fly. Getting too far ahead of a surgeon's experience can cause significant problems that can hurt patients and affect one's career.

Over the years, the two main things that I was seeing after facelift surgery were residual jowling and submental skin excess. Although revisions are a small percentage of my facelifts, they will be required of all surgeons. One of my goals has been to continually improve my facelift technique, especially to better control the jowl and the minor submental skin excess that can occur.

In previous books I've described what I called the "C" SMASectomy, where I removed a horizontal strip of jowl as just described and then closed it with sutures. The reference to the

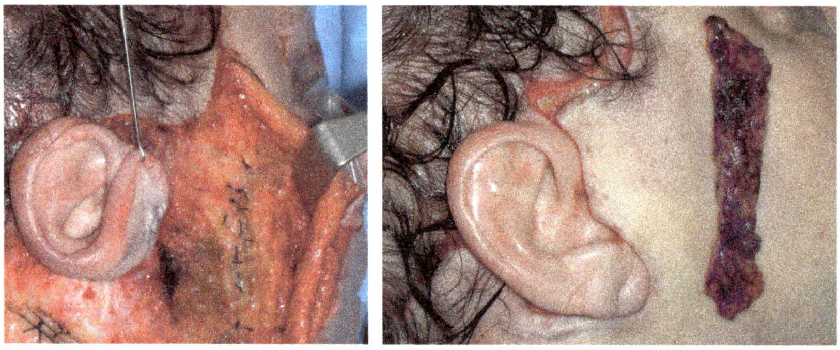

Fig. 6.99. The *left* image shows the sutured SMASectomy site. The *right* image shows the excised SMAS strip sitting on the skin in its approximate anatomic position, which extends from the zygomatic region to or past the mandibular border and is parallel to the nasolabial fold.

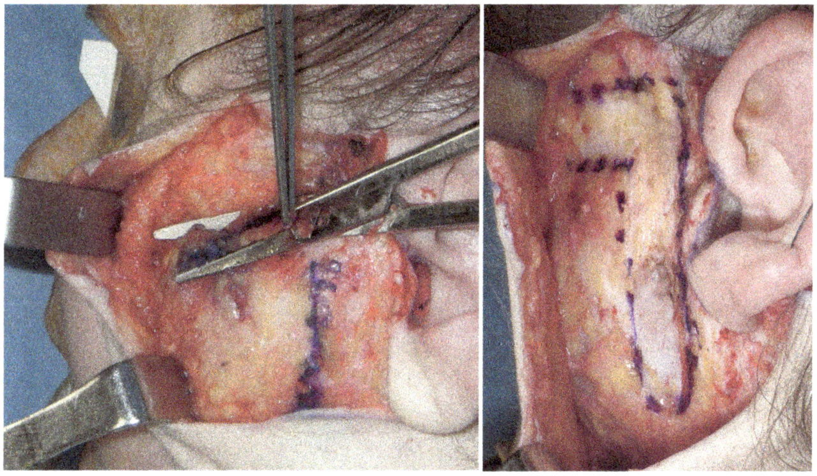

Fig. 6.100. The authors' "7 SMASectomy" pattern is illustrated with the vertical and horizontal SMAS excision.

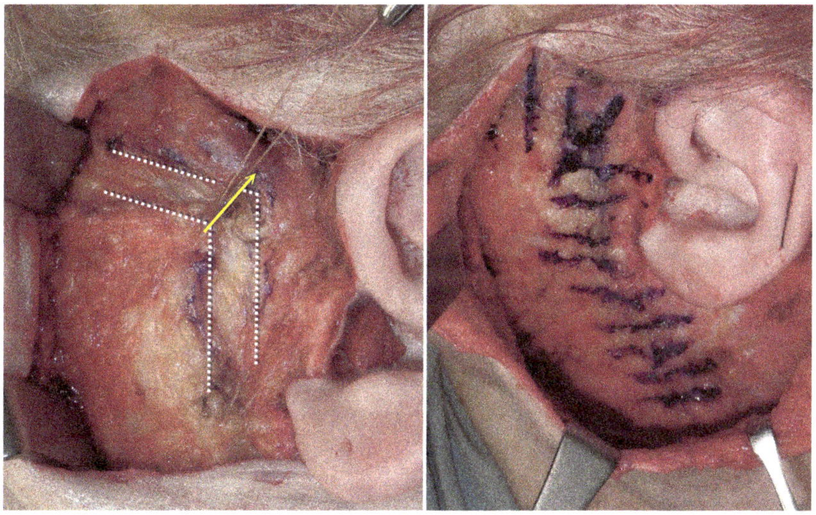

Fig. 6.101. Closing the "7 SMASectomy" begins with a key suture at the junction of the angles (*yellow arrow*, *left* image). Numerous additional sutures are placed in the horizontal and vertical dimensions when closing the SMASectomy and allow adjustment in multiple vectors directions (*right* image). As the *dotted line* shows in the *left* image, the horizontal limb can be angled at the preference of the surgeon.

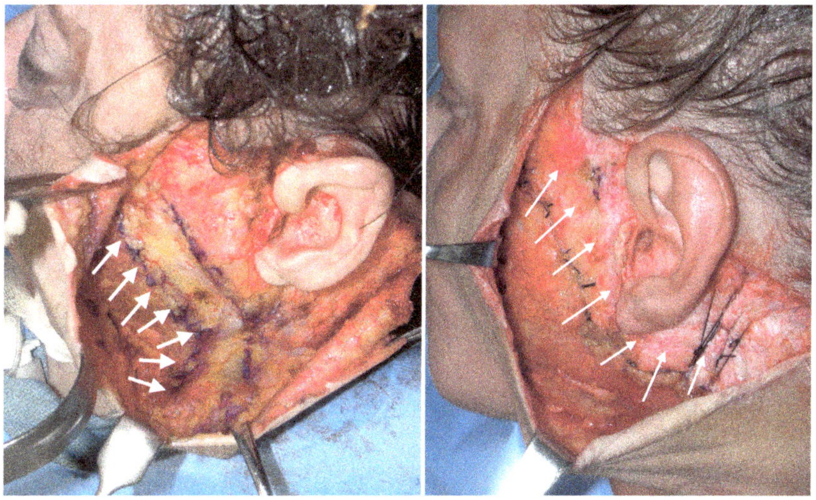

Fig. 6.102. These images show a SMASectomy performed in the facial region and extended well into the neck. As the *arrows* show, this allows numerous vectors to be used to tighten the deep layers with this extended SMASectomy technique. Excising SMAS in the neck may require more surgical experience than the basic SMASectomy as the external jugular vein and greater auricular nerves reside in the lateral neck as described in Chapter 3.

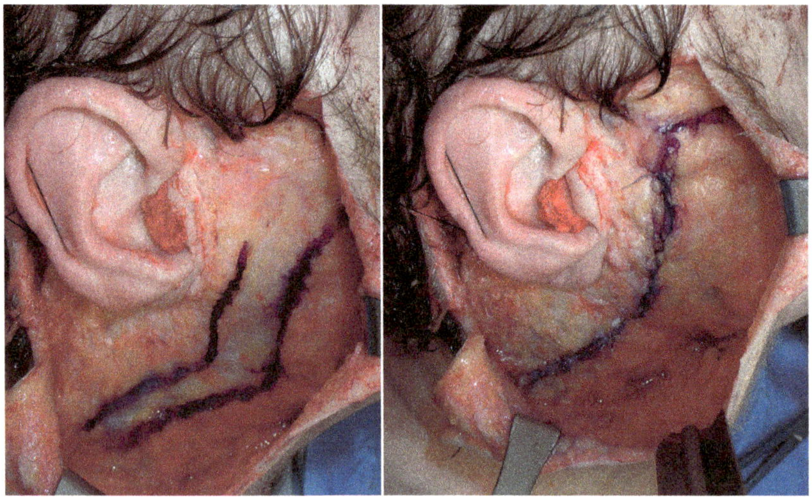

Fig. 6.103. An extended face/neck SMASectomy is shown after excision (*left*) and after closure (*right*).

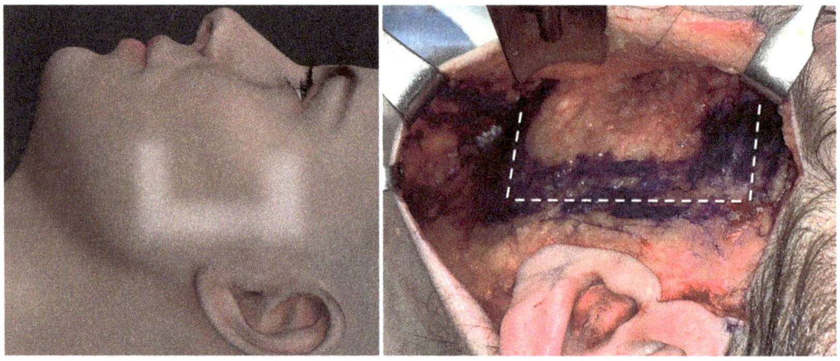

Fig. 6.104. In previous texts I described a "C" SMASectomy, which consisted of an upper horizontal limb over the zygomatic arch, a vertical limb over the parotid gland, and a lower horizontal limb over the jowl. I would resect this configuration of SMAS and suture the excised regions. (Left base image, courtesy *Complete Anatomy*, Elsevier.)

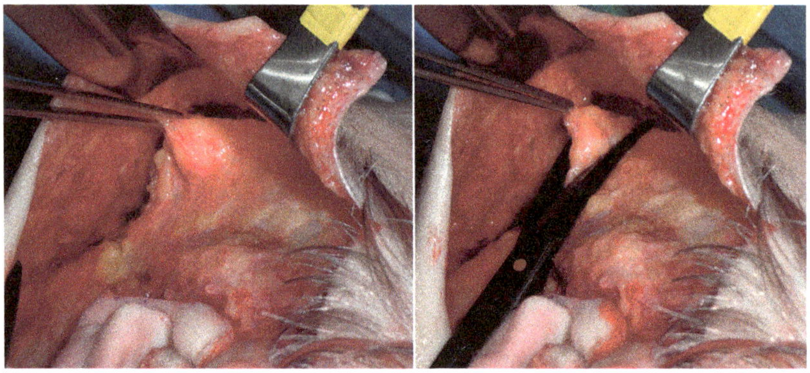

Fig. 6.105. Although not always apparent in a supine patient, most facelift patients have significant jowl tissue that is not apparent in the supine position. The *left* image shows the excess jowl present after the SMAS procedure, and the *right* image shows the excess being trimmed with care to stay superior to the platysma muscle to protect the marginal mandibular nerve.

letter "C" was from the upper horizontal, vertical, and lower horizontal SMASectomy resembling a "C" (Fig. 6.104).

Although still a viable technique for jowl improvement, I no longer excise and suture the lower horizontal limb, but merely lift the jowl area (Fig. 6.105) to expose any ptotic or excess jowl and directly trim the region without any suture closure.

I have modified my SMASectomy technique to have better control of the jowl tissue. It is important for the surgeon to understand when the patient is asleep and or recumbent, it may be difficult to judge the actual amount of jowl tissue excess because the area collapses due to gravity (Fig. 6.105, *left*). After any SMAS treatment, regardless of basic or deep plane, I test for residual jowl by grasping the jowl region of the SMAS (which was marked on the skin preoperatively) and trimming the excess with scissors. This again is an advanced technique as one must stay above the platysma muscle to not injure the marginal

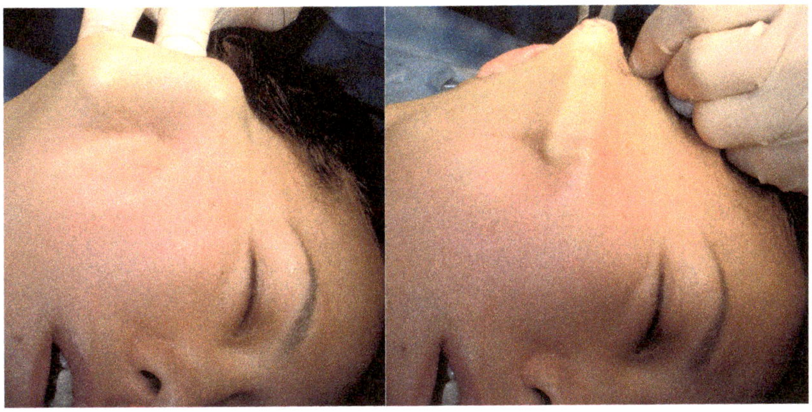

Fig. 6.106. The *left* image shows dimpling that has occurred after SMASectomy and suture fixation. These adhesions must be released before proceeding (*right* image).

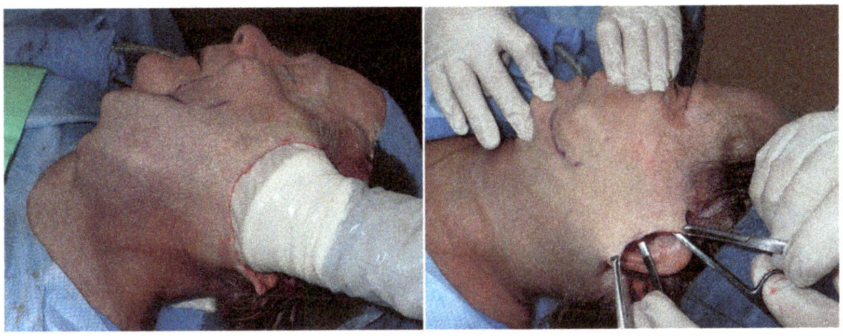

Fig. 6.107. My personal deep plane technique involves and more aggressive skin undermining, which may differ from others that espouse the superiority of traditional deep plane technique. This larger dissection allows me to directly access the jowl and increases release of ligaments and adhesions.

mandibular nerve. The jowl region is elevated and strips of excess SMAS are removed with scissors until the surgeon is satisfied with the reduction. As a review, to this point in the facelift, I have treated the jowl region with buccal fat reduction (if indicated), liposuction, SMASectomy, and direct excision. This combination of techniques has greatly reduced my revision procedure for remnant jowl.

After this SMASectomy is performed, it is important to recheck the skin surface for residual dimpling. It is not uncommon to have a smooth contour of the dissected facelift flap before the SMAS procedure but dimpling or contour irregularities after the SMAS sutures are placed. This may require further dissection to release any dimpling or contour irregularities (Fig. 6.106).

Niamtu Deep Plane Technique

Since the publication of the first edition of this book, deep plane facelifts have become very popular. This technique is not new and was described by Hamrah over 40 years ago. In my 20-plus years' tenure with facelifts, deep plane techniques have fallen in and out of favor about every decade. I feel that this technique has been rapidly popularized by social media. Social media has popularized deep plane techniques to the point where one may think that deep plane techniques are the only safe and effective technique of facelift surgery. Although this is a good and dependable technique in experienced hands, there is no evidence that it is superior to other types of SMAS treatment. One thing is certain, it is not a novice technique as the surgeon will be in close proximity to the facial nerve branches. In addition, many people that perform this technique also reduce significant anatomy in the neck that can include subplatysmal fat, digastric muscle, and submandibular glands. Again, not a novice technique. One thing that I feel is of the utmost importance is not to get ahead of one's experience and be influenced by social media or what others are doing. There are many successful surgeons that have performed thousands of facelifts using tried and true SMAS techniques and never perform a deep plane procedure. The main thing to focus on is "what works well in your hands and provides patient safety and predictable outcomes." That is truly the goal of any surgical procedure, and there are numerous ways to get there.

My personal path to facelift surgery began with SMAS plication followed by basic SMASectomy, followed by more geometric SMASectomy that extended into the cervical region; all which have been explained previously.

I have modified my SMAS techniques into my current deep plane technique. This is not the purist's deep plane technique that will described by Dr. Nayak later in this book, as it differs in several ways. Deep plane purists desire a more conservative skin dissection for reasons that will be described in that chapter 7. I, on the other hand, intentionally utilize a more aggressive skin dissection (Fig. 6.107) to allow me to have direct access to the jowl as shown in Fig. 6.105. Again, deep plane purists may decry the extensive dissection and claim that shorter skin

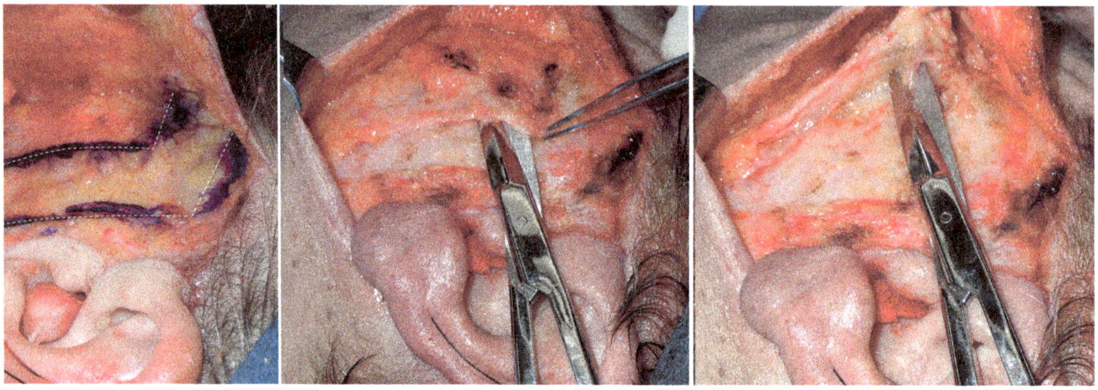

Fig. 6.108. One way to begin the deep plane SMAS dissection is to perform a right-angled SMASectomy and then undermine the deep plane.

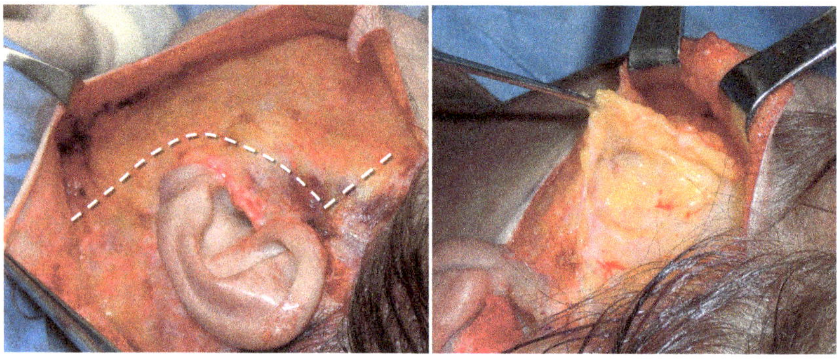

Fig. 6.109. The *left* image and *dashed line* show the region of SMAS incision, and the *right* image shows the SMAS dissection beginning in the zygomatic region. This incision and dissection can be performed with scalpel, scissors, or electrosurgery.

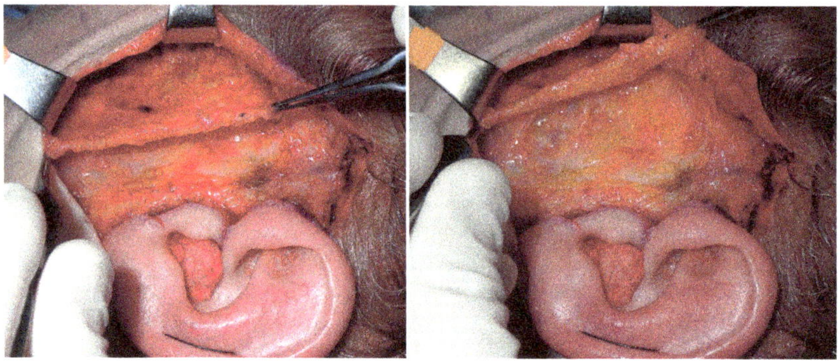

Fig. 6.110. These images show the SMAS plane being developed.

dissection has advantages (that will be described). As I stated, it is important to tune out the noise and focus on techniques that provide you with the best patient safety and predictable outcomes and improve longevity. In my hands, the technique that I am describing works well, and no one can argue that it is not a deep plain procedure. For the purposes of description, I will call it the Niamtu deep plane facelift and neck lift.

My modification of the traditional deep plane technique involves the same incisions and dissections as previously described. The SMAS can be approached in two ways. One way is to perform the right-angled SMASectomy (7 or hockey stick configuration) and begin a sub-SMAS deep plane dissection (Fig. 6.108). The other way, which more closely mirrors the traditional deep plane technique, involves entering and dissecting the SMAS and performing any SMAS excision at the end of the procedure (Fig. 6.109).

As the sub-SMAS plane is entered, the surgeon stays superior to the PMF for the entire dissection. As the facial nerve branches exit the parotid gland and cross the masseter muscle, they can frequently be visualized. This region is "tiger territory" and care must be taken to protect the facial nerve branches. Figs. 6.110 and 6.111 show further dissection in the sub-SMAS plane.

After the midface and lower facial SMAS are undermined, it is important to extend this sub-SMAS layer well into the cervical region (Figs. 6.112–6.115).

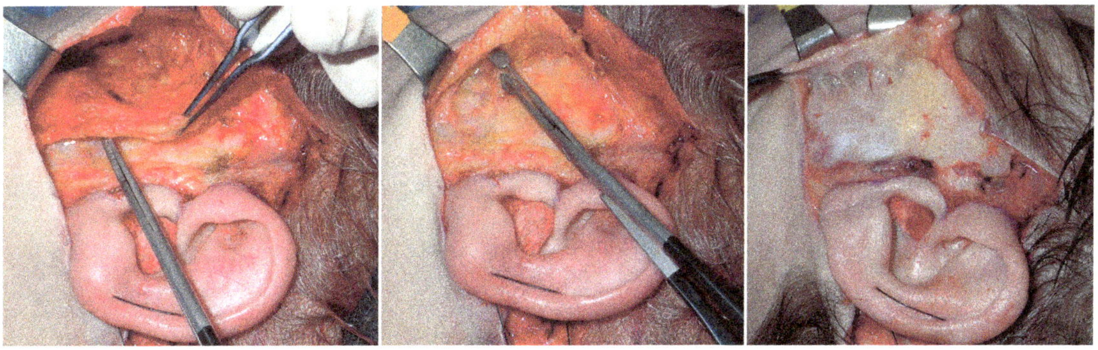

Fig. 6.111. The *left* and *center* images show the SMAS dissection assisted with a Trepsat elevator. This plane is more easily dissected than the SMAS plane and can be assisted with scissors, Trepsat type elevator, or even the surgeon's finger. The *right* image shows the SMAS elevated after deep plane dissection.

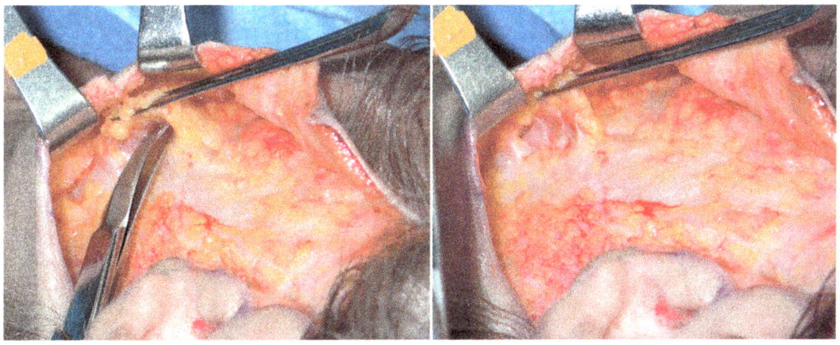

Fig. 6.112. These images show the subplatysmal plane being developed with scissors at the mandibular angle.

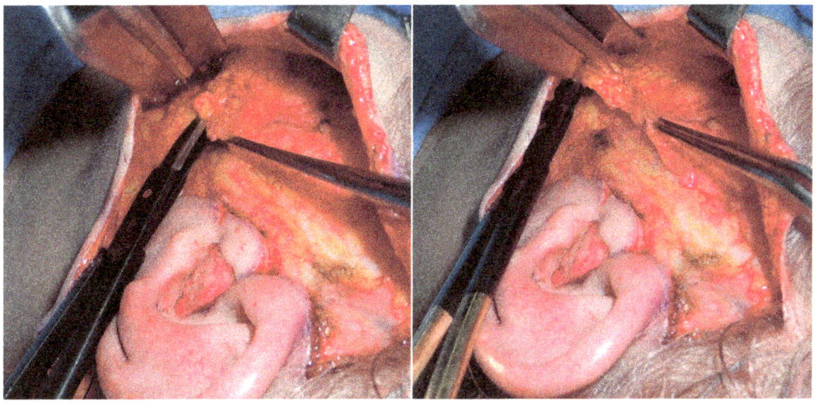

Fig. 6.113. The subplatysmal plane is extended into the neck to the desired level, which is usually at the thyroid cartilage region but may be more superior or inferior depending on the amount of aging of the patient and the size of the lift.

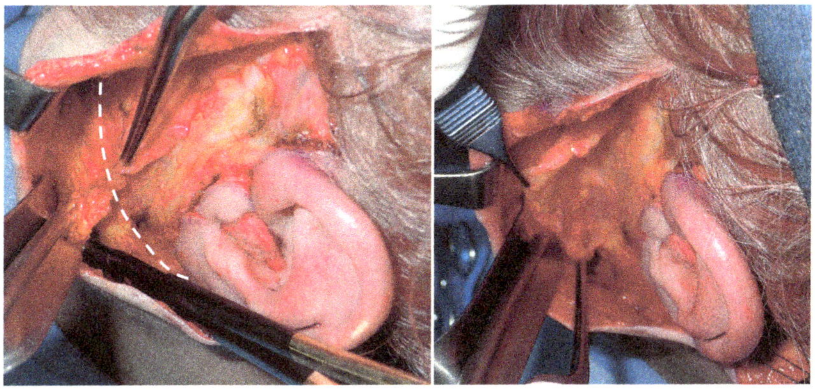

Fig. 6.114. The *left* image shows the undermined SMAS above and below the mandibular angle (*dashed line*). The *right* image shows the progressive deep dissection of the midface and cervical SMAS.

At this point, this SMAS is retracted to the desired vector in the midface, lower face, and neck and overlapping excess SMAS is trimmed (Figs. 6.116 and 6.117).

Once again, I prefer to use 2-0 Vicryl sutures as the sutures are placed. For the first suture, I look for the previously described sweet spot. This is the region that, when secured with a suture and pulled in the desired vector, exhibits the area of tension that best tightens the neck, jawline, and the jowl regions (Fig. 6.118). This is determined by securing SMAS at different locations and pulling it posterolateral for the most effective tension that lifts multiple areas.

Additional suspension sutures are placed over the entire SMAS incision from cephalad to caudad, which is generally from the zygomatic region to the inferior cervical region using 2-0 Vicryl sutures (Fig. 6.119).

Similar to the SMASectomy procedure described earlier, I perform liposuction after the skin dissection and before addressing the SMAS. Then, after the deep plane SMAS dissection and SMAS closure, I return to the jowl area and tent the tissue to determine excess. Usually there is redundant jowl tissue and I will directly excise the excess SMAS and fibrofatty tissue that contributes to the jowl. This is a safe procedure as long as the surgeon stays above the platysma muscle where the marginal mandibular nerve is protected (Fig. 6.120).

My occasional postfacelift residual jowl problem has been eliminated by the four procedures addressing the jowl, which

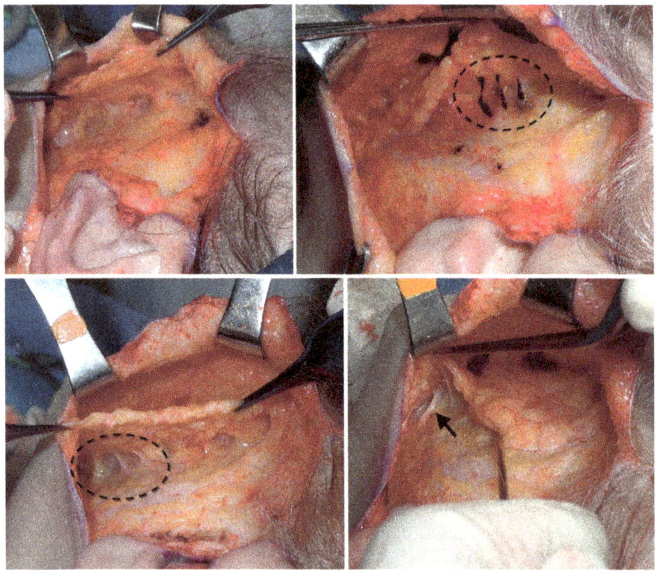

Fig. 6.115. These images illustrate excellent subSMAS anatomy. The *upper left* image shows the deep plane dissection with the SMAS retracted. The *upper right* image shows the zygomatic ligaments (*circle*) in another patient. The *lower left* image shows the masseteric ligaments (*circle*) in another patient, and the *lower right* image shows the marginal mandibular nerve in the dissection, which underlines the anatomic vulnerability and complexity of deep plane procedures.

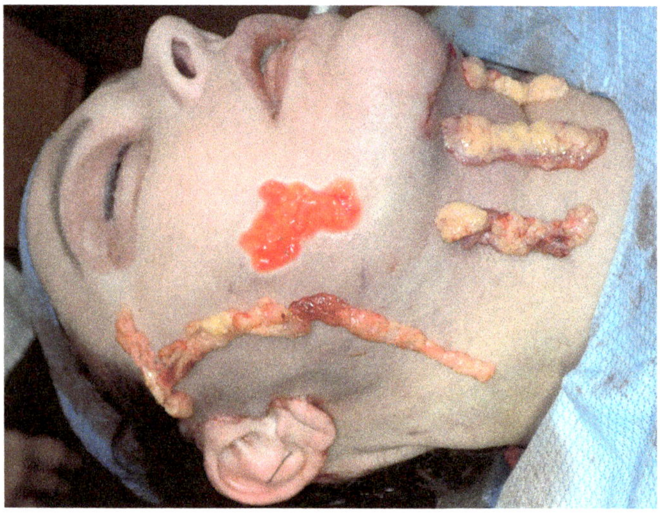

Fig. 6.117. The author shows a patient after deep plane facelift and neck lift with buccal fat reduction. The excised tissue is arranged on the overlying anatomy.

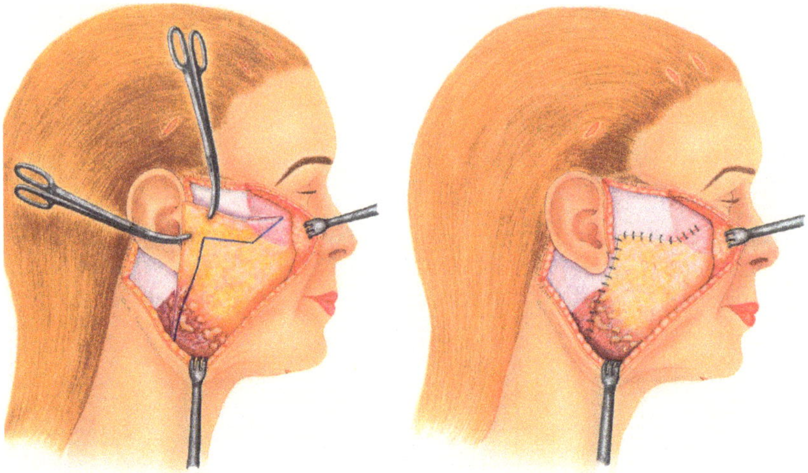

Fig. 6.116. The *left* image shows the excess overlap of SMAS retracted after the deep plane dissection. The *right* image shows the area after the excess SMAS is excised and sutured. (Courtesy Bill Evans, MD, with permission.)

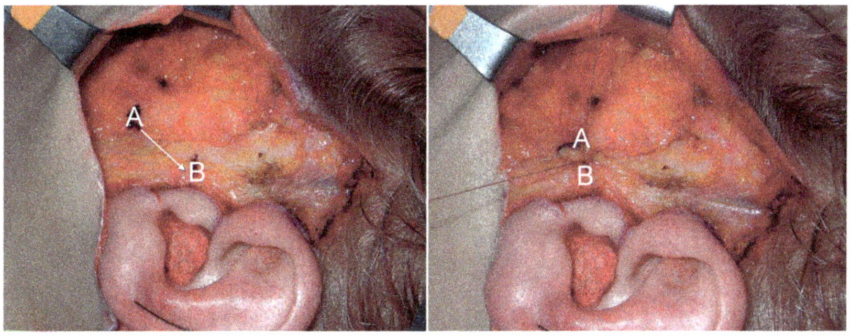

Fig. 6.118. Securing this SMAS in the deep plane technique is similar to the SMASectomy where the most efficient area (the sweet spot) is secured, so that when elevated posterolateral, the jowl, the mandibular border, and the neckline are all improved. The first 2-0 Vicryl suture is placed here. Point *A* is lower than point *B*, and when sutured, tightens the described structures.

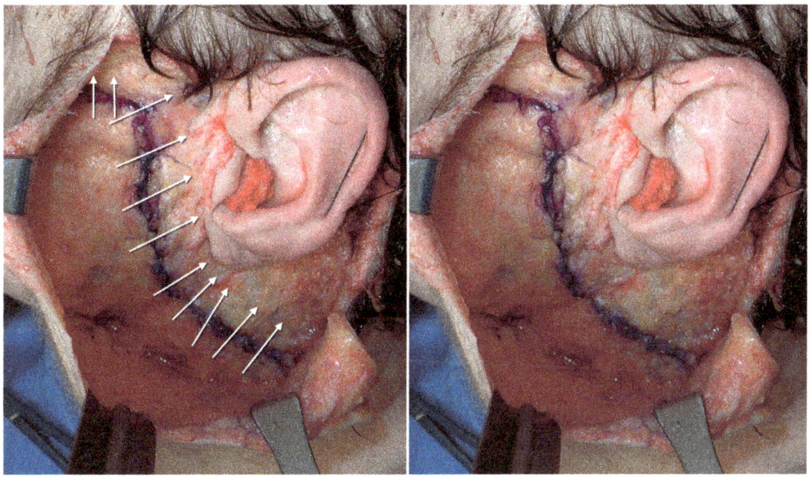

Fig. 6.119. These images show the completed suture line after deep plane SMAS procedure. Numerous sutures (10–12 is my average) are placed from the zygomatic region cephalad to the lower cervical region caudad. The *left* image shows the approximate vectors of the sutures, and the *right* image shows the completed suture line.

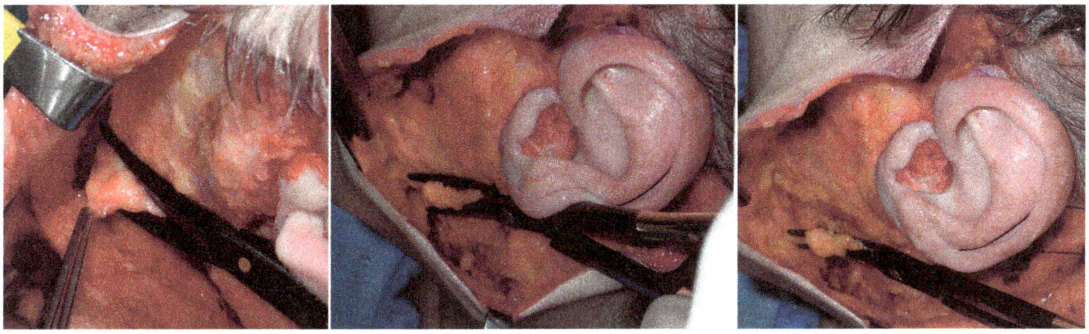

Fig. 6.120. The *left* image shows the redundant tissue in the jowl region being elevated. The *center* image shows direct trimming of that region, and the *right* image shows further trimming with the platysma muscle visible under the resection.

include buccal fat reduction (when indicated), jowl liposuction, jowl suspension, and direct jowl excision (Fig. 6.121).

The circle of contemporary deep plane surgeons may criticize points of this technique compared with their technique that has less skin flap elevation. The saying goes "the proof is in the pudding," meaning that the final result says it all. When I look at the best cases of deep plane purist surgeons and look at my best cases or other experienced surgeon's best cases, the technique does not seem to make a difference. Again, regardless of who is doing what or what the procedure du jour may be, all surgeons should figure out what works best in their hands and stick with it. For advanced surgeons, there is no problem in applying new techniques, but many commonly go back to what has worked for decades. The fine points of deep plane technique can be argued all day long. I have friends who have performed a series of deep plane facelifts on one side of the face and an SMASectomy on the other side of the face, with no observable differences. Do what works well for you and your patients. My deep plane technique works well for me!

Dr. Bill Evans, a very successful facelift surgeon from Columbus, Ohio, performs a similar approach to mine with a larger skin dissection before the deep SMAS undermining (Fig. 6.122). Deep plane technique with a smaller skin dissection will be discussed in a later chapter.

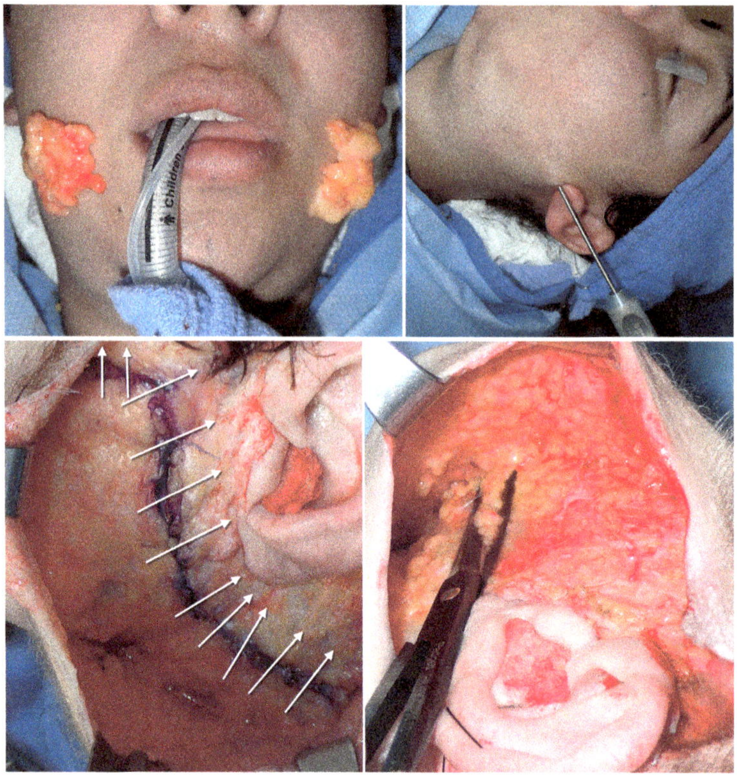

Fig. 6.121. My four pillars of jowl improvement include buccal fat reduction (when indicated) (*upper left*), jowl liposuction (*upper right*). Jowl suspension (*lower left*) and direct jowl excision (*lower right*).

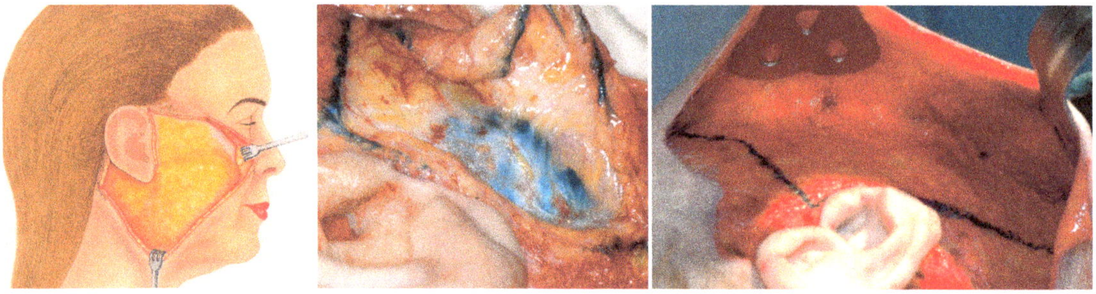

Fig. 6.122. Dr Bill Evans performs a larger subcutaneous dissection in the same manner I do (*left* image) He also injects methylene blue dye intraorally into the parotid duct (blue tissue in *center* picture) to confirm the proper deep plane so the surgeon does not dissect below the parotidomasseteric fascia. The *right* image shows his longer skin flap and markings for the SMAS deep plane dissection. (Courtesy Bill Evans, MD, with permission.)

Treating the Posterior (Lateral) Platysma

As stated previously, most surgeons perform some type of midline platysmaplasty procedure. I personally believe that it is important to also address the posterior platysma as well, regardless of the type of facelift. Addressing the lateral or posterior platysma is important because I believe that when combined with the midline platysma treatment, it creates a sling that helps tighten, support, and elevate the submental and cervical regions (Fig. 6.123).

I personally perform this lateral platysmal suspension on each side before final skin closure. The lateral (or posterior) platysma is addressed through the postauricular flap. In the SMASectomy procedures described earlier in this chapter, the lateral platysma may or may not be undermined before suspension depending on the surgeon. In many patients the lateral platysmal border is very identifiable with significant thickness of the muscle. In this case it is simple to secure the lateral border and suspended it in the proper vector. Many patients do not have an extremely visible lateral platysmal border. If the lateral platysmal border is not visibly evident, the lateral platysmal suspension can still be performed by securing the associated tissues that overlay the lateral platysma border. This usually involves fibrofatty tissue, and the suture passes through the overlying tissue and platysma and is fixated posteriorly or posterolateral. The lateral platysma is suspended in the proper vector and anchored to the mastoid region or the sternocleidomastoid fascia (Fig. 6.124). Many surgeons use long suspension spanning sutures that extend from the lateral platysmal border to the mastoid region. I prefer to

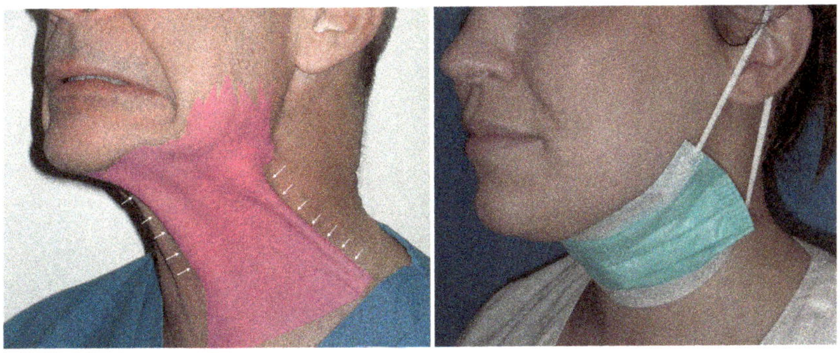

Fig. 6.123. The average patient has visible anterior and posterior platysma borders as shown in the *left* image. The *right* image shows a representation of the effect of medial and lateral platysmaplasty to create a supportive sling in the submental and cervical regions as illustrated with a face mask.

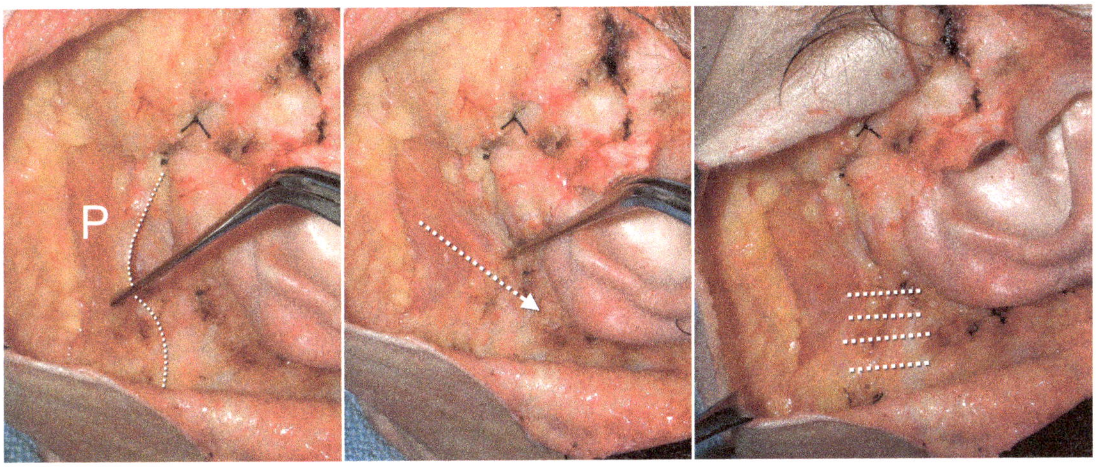

Fig. 6.124. The *left* image shows a well-defined and identifiable lateral platysmal border (*P*). The *middle* image shows forceps placing traction on the lateral platysma. The *right* image shows a representation of where suspension sutures will be placed.

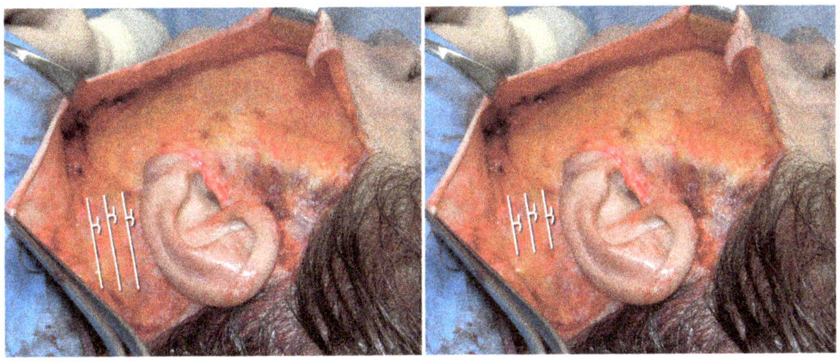

Fig. 6.125. Many textbooks describe placing long spanning sutures from the lateral platysma border to the posterior mastoid region as shown in the *left* figure. Although I performed this type of suture position in my earlier career, I have transitioned to performing the same suspension and vectors, but suture to stable tissue more anteriorly and with shorter sutures (*right* image).

use shorter sutures and suspend them to the sternocleidomastoid fascia. As long as the sutures are attached to tissue that is robust enough to hold and not pull through, I feel there is no reason for the long spanning sutures. I prefer to use a much shorter 2-0 Vicryl suture and secure the platysma to the SCM region (Fig. 6.125). I generally place two to three mattress sutures from superior to inferior.

As the surgical team prepares for the skin management phase of the procedure, it is the last chance to monitor what is happening "under the flap." Obviously, the main concern is any uncontrolled bleeding. Experienced surgeons can differentiate minor soft tissue oozing from significant bleeding that can accumulate and contribute to hematoma formation. The surgical field should be dry before proceeding to the skin closing steps. Gently packing any undermined flaps with standard 3% hydrogen peroxide and leaving them in place for several minutes greatly aids the ability to ascertain hemostasis. I routinely use this to control bleeding as well as to identify active bleeding, which will foam on contact with blood (Fig. 6.126).

Residual contour irregularities are also a concern and must be addressed before the skin closure. These irregularities can include lumps and bumps of fat from the adipose layer, bulging

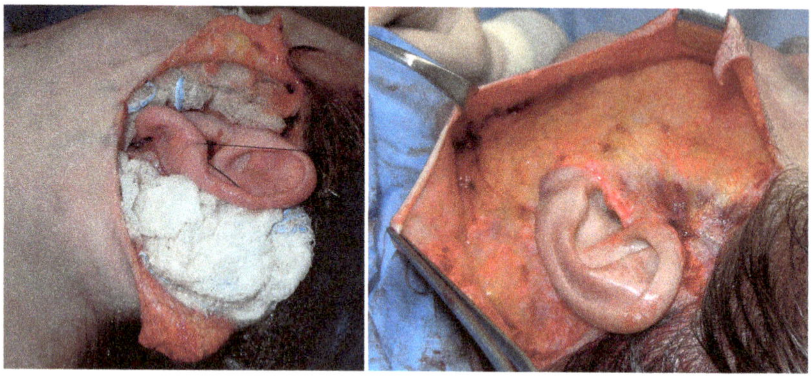

Fig. 6.126. Precise control of any bleeding is imperative before closing the face left flaps. Packing the wound with 3% hydrogen peroxide–soaked gauze is an efficient way to control minor hemostasis and identify bleeding vessels by the foaming effect of the peroxide. The *left* image shows the wound packed with 3% hydrogen peroxide–soaked gauze. This is left in place for approximately 5 minutes. The *right* image shows hemostatic control without obvious bleeding and ready for skin closure.

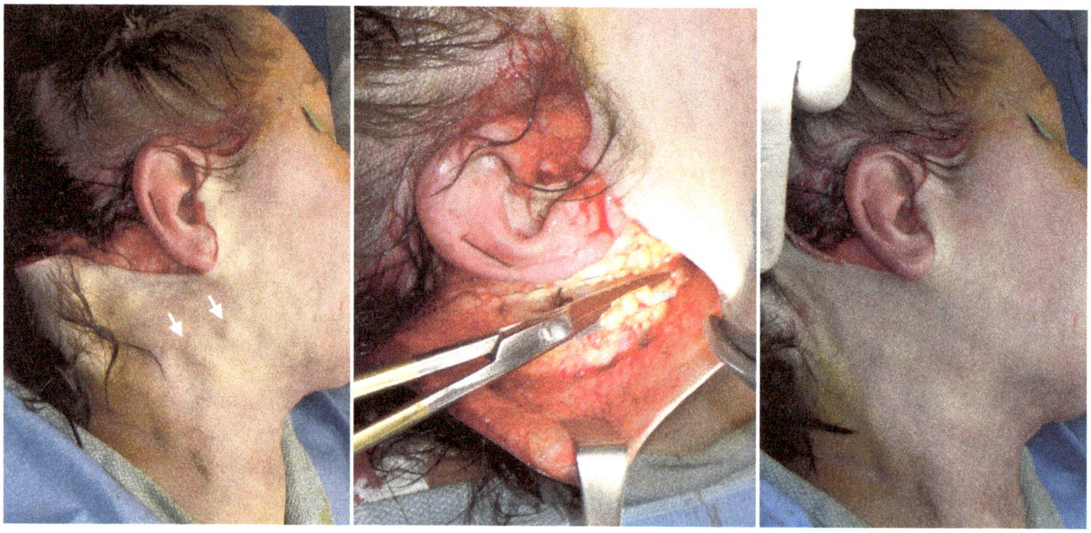

Fig. 6.127. The *left* image shows several visible bumps when the skin is draped over the deeper tissues. In this case these lumps were a result of adipose tissue bulging between the long spanning sutures. When these sutures are tightened over adipose tissue, the tension can cause the tissue between the sutures to bulge. The *middle* image shows these irregularities being trimmed and flattened with facelift scissors. The *right* image shows the smooth contour after these irregularities were addressed.

tissue that occurs between sutures, and areas of muscle or tissue irregularities over tight suture lines. Smoothing these irregularities is important as they may otherwise be visible through the skin. Although many irregularities will dissipate with healing, some may remain and be visible and permanent. It is amazing that a surgeon can do a complete facial rejuvenation with excellent outcomes and the first thing the patient notices is a small bump on the cheek or neck (Fig. 6.127). It is very important to make sure that when the skin is draped over the underlying anatomy, there are no lumps, bumps, or uneven contours. This is important to address in every portion of the dissected region.

Skin Management

The next part of the procedure deals with the management of excess skin. Facelift surgery is like many things in life where a small mistake at one point can be amplified in the final result. As previously stressed, it is important to have a smooth contour under the skin so there are no visible irregularities. Anyone that has ever seen or done upholstering understands the fact that the bottom layers must be perfectly smooth before the top covering is placed or irregularities will be visible. Again, all bleeding must be controlled at this point. Before any closure is begun, it is beneficial for the staff to take a short timeout to make sure that no previous steps have been omitted and no foreign bodies remain under the flaps. It is not impossible to leave a gauze pad within a facelift flap, and for this reason I only use surgical gauze with radiographic markers on them. My team always performs a gauze count before any skin closure is started. During the procedure, distractions can lead to omissions, where a part of the procedure is not completed. This is usually some minor part of the procedure, but for beginning surgeons I think it's a great idea to have a laminated paper in the operating room, enumerating each step of the facelift procedure. This is a great way to train the staff to make sure that all the proper steps have been completed before moving on.

Managing the skin is one of the most important parts of the case—the only thing the patient really sees. A well-done facelift can be ruined by failure to effectively manage the skin, specifically the incisions, earlobe, and hairlines. In my several-decades

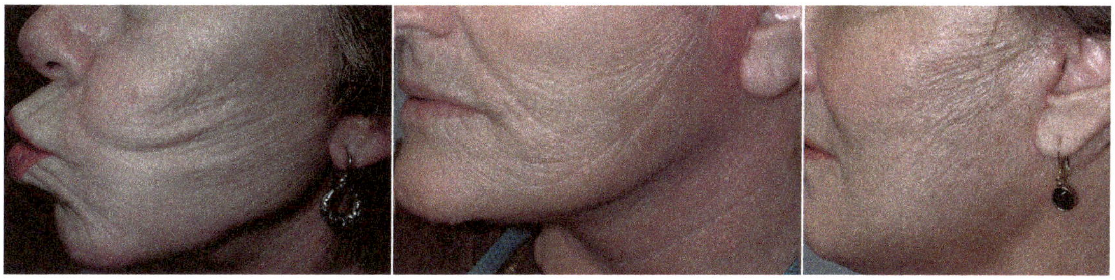

Fig. 6.128. The pictured patients with significant rhytids underwent facelift surgery and sustained an "upswept" appearance due to the skin repositioning. I would prefer to laser patients with deep wrinkles prior to their facelift. Careful attention to the skin pull vectors is also critical in patients with wrinkled skin, but sometimes not totally controllable. It is imperative to discuss these factors with the patient prior to surgery.

experience with facelift and neck lift surgery, I can attest that the main fear of every single patient is the fear of the windblown or "done" look. Some of what happens at this point must be discussed well in advance of the actual surgical procedure. First and foremost, the patient must understand that a facelift is not a procedure for skin wrinkles. Some wrinkling will be improved by the mere fact that the skin will be stretched; however, having the correct patient expectations is paramount. I've had patients who have complained that the facelift did not correct their wrinkles, even though this was addressed in numerous preoperative conversations, verbal and written consents, as well as my videos and web pages in other literature that the patient reviews before surgery. Because a facelift is considered such a big procedure, patients expect a big outcome. I stated numerous times at the beginning of this chapter they must have an accurate understanding for not only what the procedure will do but what it won't do. I spend a significant amount of extra time with patients that have significant skin wrinkling. Patients with skin wrinkling must understand that if they do not address their skin wrinkling, the vectors of the facelift reposition the wrinkles into an unnatural pattern with the feared "upswept" appearance. For these patients, laser resurfacing is an important adjunct to the facelift procedure. Although I have performed over 450 facelifts with simultaneous CO_2 laser resurfacing, I no longer routinely combine full-face laser and simultaneous facelift for several reasons. First and foremost, it truly increases the amount of recovery and postoperative care for the patient and their family. Secondly, I never laser the skin overlying the undermined flaps at the same fluence as I do on the central oval of the face. This can be problematic postoperatively because the undermined flaps can heal after laser with a different texture and color from the more aggressively lasered central oval of the face. Oftentimes this can be very noticeable and may require a secondary laser treatment over the flaps to blend with the more aggressively lasered skin. If the skin over the undermined flaps does have significant wrinkling, the lighter laser will not properly address it. For all these reasons, I now only perform more superficial simultaneous laser skin resurfacing or chemical peeling on facelift patients with minimal skin rhytids. I do, however, perform subunit resurfacing, mainly perioral and periorbital, on a majority of my facelift patients. With this rationale, patients who have skin excess and skin wrinkling will generally require two separate procedures in my office. Sometimes the patient may wish to opt for the facelift first, in the hope that it will address their wrinkling. Performing the facelift first may reposition the skin wrinkles to an unnatural appearance, which can affect the result for the patient and the reputation of the surgeon. For the small subset of patients with both severe skin wrinkling and skin excess, I prefer to perform the laser resurfacing first and the facelift procedure at a later date. This decreases the chance of unnatural repositioning of skin wrinkles with skin pull vectors (Fig. 6.128).

Additional caveats that can produce unnatural postoperative results are patients with significant volume loss or patients who have had numerous facelifts in the past. The hypovolumized patient that refuses some type of volume enhancement such as facial implants, fat injection, or filler treatment must understand that their result may be compromised. This discussion needs to be part of written consent because patients can have very short memories when it comes to their refusing a suggested treatment plan. The multiply operated on patient can also be problematic as the surgeon may perform a perfect facelift, but the problems or limitations of previous surgeries can affect the final outcome. Preoperative communication is everything in elective cosmetic surgery procedures.

Setting the skin flaps begins with grasping the pre- and postauricular skin and elevating with careful assessment the natural antiaging vectors. Any number of instruments can be used to grasp the flap edges. Hemostats, Allis clamps, or Pitanguy flap-grasping forceps—all work well. I prefer smaller Allis clamps for skin retraction (Fig. 6.129). At this stage I always take a photograph to show the patient because they frequently are interested in how much skin was removed or sometimes may challenge their result, stating that not enough skin was removed.

As stated earlier, mismanagement of skin vector traction can turn an otherwise successful case into a failure. A review of various textbooks and surgeons from the podium presents a confusing situation for any standardization on how the skin is to be retracted. Some surgeons advocate strictly vertical traction, and other surgeons advocate different vectors. I personally believe that the correct antiaging vector is a little bit different on each patient but very similar for most. Although one could try to strictly quantify the direction of skin traction, there are many variables, and I think the easiest thing to do is simply retract the skin until you have a tightening of all the desired areas with a natural appearance. In past writings I have attempted to approximate these vectors to a clock face for simplification for the novice surgeon, but I feel that it was somewhat confusing. I currently illustrate my traction vectors as shown in Fig. 6.130. As

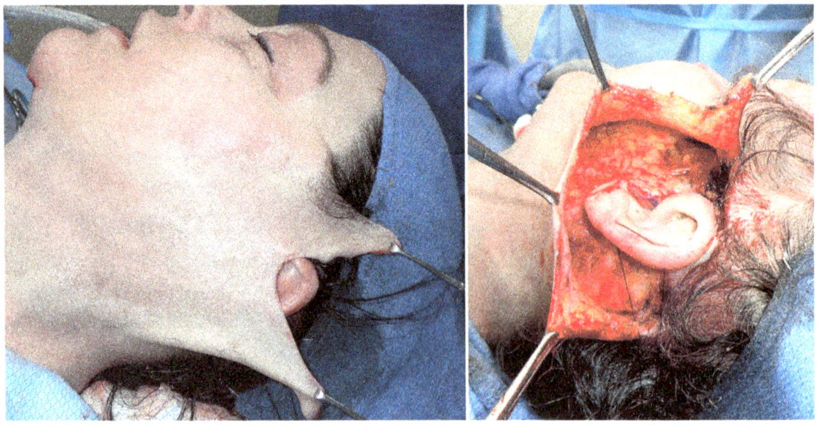

Fig. 6.129. Allis clamps are well suited for atraumatically grasping and managing flaps.

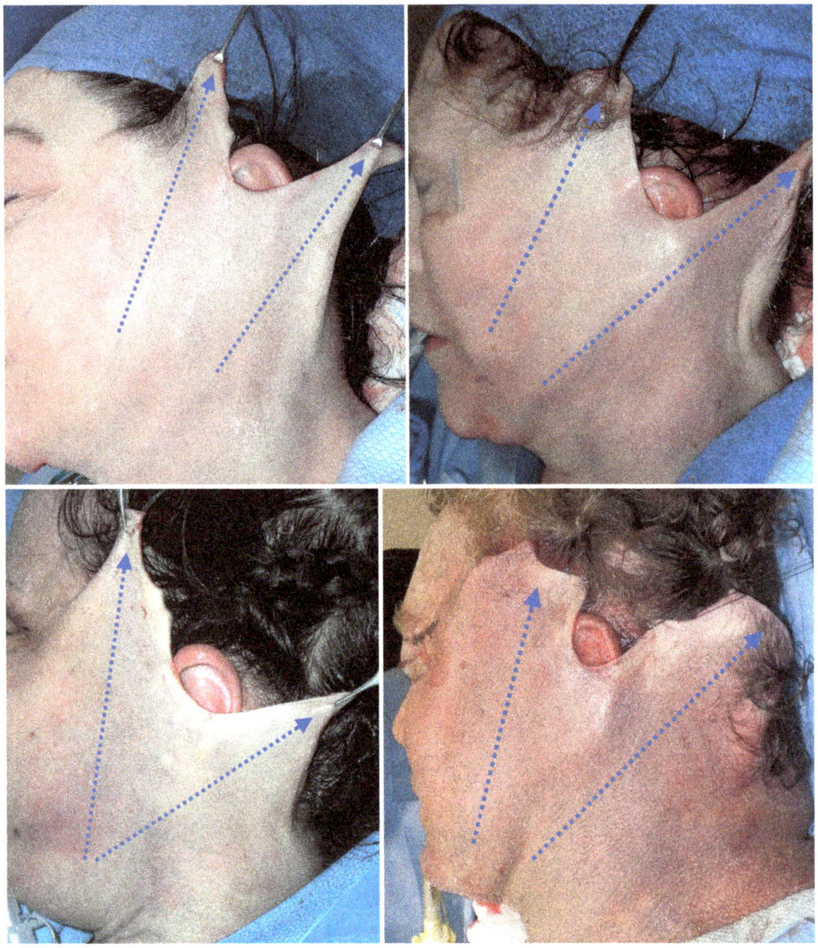

Fig. 6.130. These images show skin retraction vectors in different patients illustrating that although they are all similar, each one is a little different. Descriptions such as these merely provide the novice surgeon with an idea of how to reposition the skin.

the reader can see these vectors are not exact in these four pictures. If I showed pictures of traction vectors on 10 patients, one would see that each one is a little different. For this reason, I will not attempt to "standardize" the direction of pull. It is a little different on every case and is subject to the patient's skeletal structure, amount of skin excess, location of skin excess and elasticity of skin among other factors. In general, on the upright aging face, the vector of skin sagging is inferiorly and anteriorly (down and forward), it makes sense that in redraping the skin, it will be (a similarly opposite direction) positioned superiorly and posteriorly. Looking at the vectors separately, the preauricular flap is positioned in a superiolateral direction, while the postauricular flap is positioned in a posteriolateral vector.

One very important point to consider when retracting the posterior flap is the alignment of the hairline. It would actually be most efficient to retract the posterior flap in an exaggerated posterolateral direction as this direction of tension would provide the tightest jawline and jowl region. The problem is that pulling the skin in this direction will also create a significant discontinuity of the posterior hairline, which is highly problematic for a esthetics and especially for females who wear their hair up (Figs. 6.131 and 6.132).

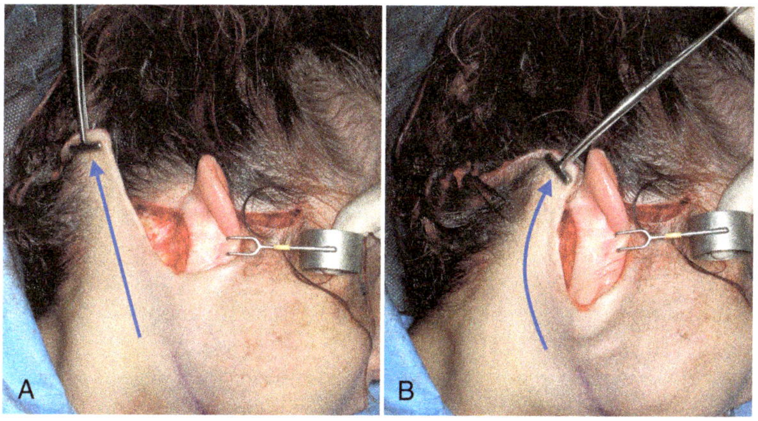

Fig. 6.131. The *left* image shows a tension vector that would ideally tighten the lower face but would also cause a discontinuity defect of the posterior hairline. The *right* image illustrates how the flap is rotated forward to match up the hairline.

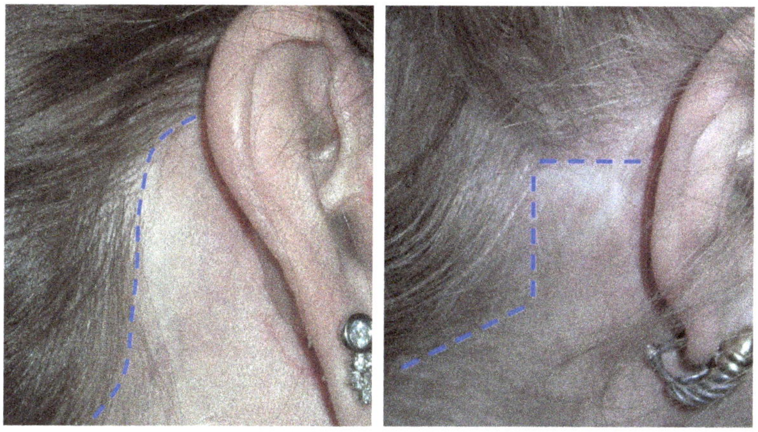

Fig. 6.132. The *left* image shows the normal contiguous occipital hairline. The *right* image illustrates a discontinuity defect from improper flap vector positioning. Rotating the flap forward will insure proper alignment.

As a little author's sidebar, when teaching any techniques, I must temper the description for beginners that have never performed facelift surgery to experts that have performed thousands of cases. This is a difficult gap to fill, and I can imagine some surgeons reading these descriptions and being so thankful to have a starting point while other experienced surgeons shake their head and saying, "I would never do it that way." This is the conundrum of writing a textbook. As I have said many times in this text, the way I describe techniques are not meant to imply "the only way," but it is the way that has provided safe, long-lasting, and natural results in my personal experience.

The described vectors provide the novice surgeon with some direction to retract the skin flaps. The surgeon must inspect the neck, submental region, corner of the mouth, jowl, midface, and temple regions to truly assess the proper direction of skin "pull" (tension). All of these areas must be improved and have a natural appearance, as the final result equals the sum of the parts. An excessive transverse vector can distort and stretch the corner of the mouth and produce the "joker"-type appearance in the lower face. An unnatural vector more superiorly can slant of the eyelids causing a "fox eye" appearance and also distort the cheeks. These are some of the most feared stigmata for patients. It is interesting that at the time of this writing, social media has popularized the fox eye look for younger patients and it is a commonly requested procedure. I never perform this type of disfiguring surgery on young patients, as it is a fad now and they may be sorry later in life.

Retracting the skin in an incorrect vector can not only change the position of the patient's wrinkles (Fig. 6.128) but also produce a distortion of the face.

While I have the skin distracted with the Allis clamps, I begin my preliminary earlobe cutback. As the earlobe has already been released from its attachment (Fig. 6.78), the flap is tucked under the lobe to give the surgeon an estimate of the amount of skin excess and required flap incision to accommodate the earlobe. At this point, I make a small (5–10 mm) cutback at the base of the retracted skin and allow the lobe to partially extend out from under the retracted skin (Fig. 6.133). This is an area where novice surgeons can overextend the cut and end up with a pixie earlobe (Fig. 6.134). This is one area where the surgeon should always "measure twice and cut once" (Fig. 6.135). I only make this cut to about one-third of what I think is necessary to release the lobe and will perform the final lobe delivery later in the procedure, which will be shown.

I prefer to "pretrim" the base of the flap to release the lobe before I place the key sutures. Some surgeons place the key sutures first and then release the lobe. It is a matter of convention if the flap is not overcut.

The next step is to place the "key" sutures (also referred to as cardinal sutures). This is a critical step, as the sutures set and hold the final vector of the skin flaps.

Neutral head positioning is something I have done for decades, and I have not seen it described in other texts. I feel this simple maneuver provides more accurate skin excision and decreases postsurgical residual skin. As I write this text, I try to remember conundrums, questions, or problems that I had in my own facelift journey that may have contributed to lessened results and/or the need for revision surgery. Neutral head position is an example of one of these pearls.

Many surgeons have the head turned away from them during surgery for better visualization. If the head is *turned away from the surgeon* while suspending and trimming the skin flaps, there will be less skin available for trimming, which affects the accuracy of the procedure. Turning the head to the neutral position (face to the ceiling) will enable more skin access on the operated side, and reducing this "extra" skin will provide a tighter result and reduce postsurgery skin excess. The take-home pearl is that more skin is available for excision when the head is in the neutral position (Figs. 6.136 and 6.137). As a hypothetical example, if there is 5 mm of available skin for the key suture and skin trimming with the head turned away from the surgeon and 10 mm of available skin when the head is neutrally positioned, this allows more skin to be trimmed and tightened. Multiply this inaccuracy by two sides of a facelift and it adds up to enough skin to compromise the result if not addressed.

The amount of available excess skin is largely dependent upon age and the degree of aging; however, skin elasticity or lack thereof is also major contributor. Fig. 6.138 shows varying degrees of skin excess, which can vary from millimeters to centimeters. In small or medium lifts, the position for anterior and posterior key sutures is obvious but can be more involved in larger lifts.

The next step in the procedure is to suspend the flaps in their final position. This is a very important part of the procedure and in some respects the only part of the procedure that the patient will see.

Once the surgeon decides on the correct vector, a skin cutback is made in the pre- and postauricular regions and secured with a suture. This is frequently referred to as the key or cardinal suture because it sets the stage for the final flap position. These are the only sutures in the entire case that will be placed under tension. I would call this "moderate tension" and the amount of

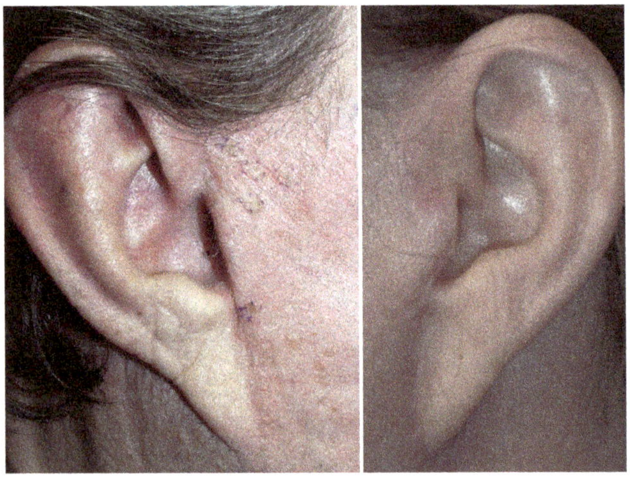

Fig. 6.134. The main cause of the "pixie ear" deformity is overresection of the skin when delivering the lobe. The patient on the *left* has a pixie ear and a blunted tragus. The *right* image shows another case of a pixie ear deformity.

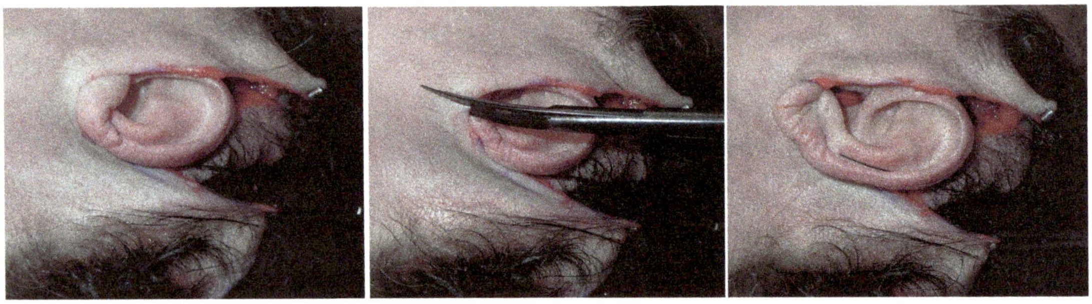

Fig. 6.133. These images show the initial release of the earlobe. The *left* image shows skin covering the earlobe while the flap is retracted. The *center* image shows a very conservative skin cutback to deliver the lobe, and the *right* image shows the lobe partially delivered. This is one of the most important and precise steps of the case. Overcutting this skin is one of the biggest novice mistakes causing a "pixie earlobe."

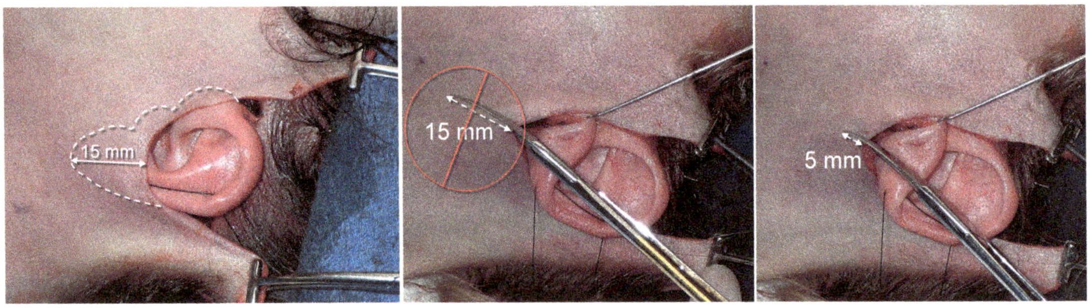

Fig. 6.135. The *left* image shows a hypothetical situation where 15 mm of excess skin overlap the earlobe. The *middle* picture shows an overestimated, excessive cutback (most commonly made by novice surgeons). The *right* image shows a conservative cutback to ensure the lobe is not tensioned. More release can always be performed later in the case.

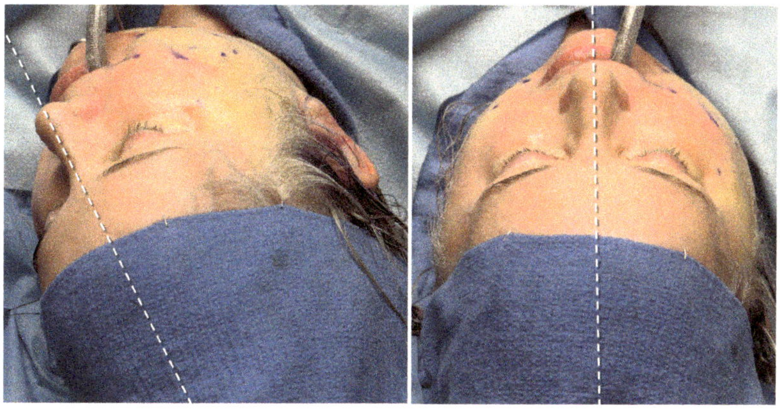

Fig. 6.136. Most surgeons have the patient turned away from them (*right* image) when placing key sutures and trimming excess skin. This can produce an inaccuracy, as it there is less available skin when the head is turned away from the surgeon. Placing the head in the neutral position enables more skin excess which will translate into a more accurate result (*left* image).

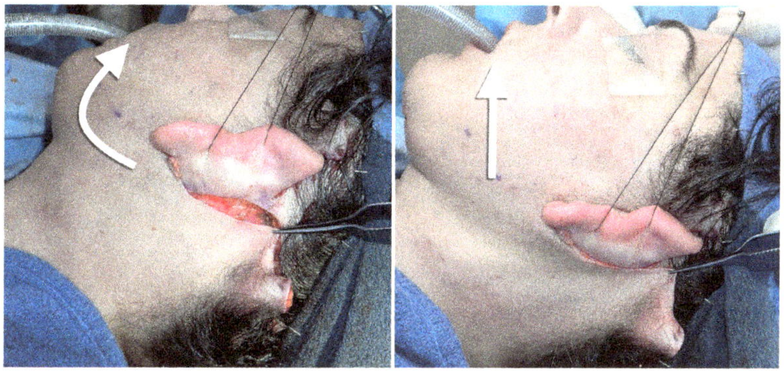

Fig. 6.137. The *left* image shows the amount of available skin with the patient turned away from the surgeon. The *right* image shows more available skin when the patient is in the neutral position (face toward ceiling).

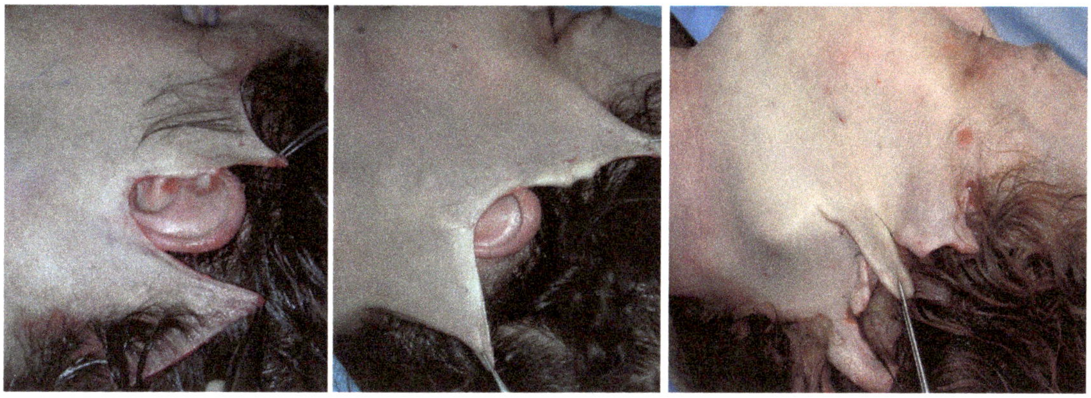

Fig. 6.138. These images show variable amounts of skin excess in facelift patients prior to trimming. Skin excess can be minor and hardly cover the ear, moderate and cover much of the ear, or major and cover the entire ear. Most facelifts have skin excess similar to the *left* and *center* pictures.

pull is enough to maintain the flap in the correct position with the head in the neutral position. Close attention is required to not overcut the skin cutback as it cannot be reversed. As with any skin incision or excision, use the adage "measure twice, cut once.". Conversely, undercutting the skin cutback can build in laxity that will be apparent postoperatively. The angle of the skin cut back is also important and should follow vector of the skin pull. I prefer a 4-0 Vicryl for the key sutures. Most surgeons simply retract this skin to the desired vector make a cutback and place a suture to hold the flap in place. Over the years I have developed a protocol that is predictable and efficient and is my current technique.

This protocol is as follows and is illustrated on the patient's left side; the contralateral side would be in reverse of the picture in terms of turning the head. As this initial description may seem confusing, closely looking at the accompanying pictures and the related videos will facilitate this process.

Step 1. Placement of Temporary Key Sutures

With the patient turned away from the surgeon, an initial posterior skin cutback is made and a suture or staple (we will also call this the posterior temporary key suture) is placed in the postauricular area to temporarily suspend the flap. Also, with the head turned away from the surgeon, the preauricular flap is positioned

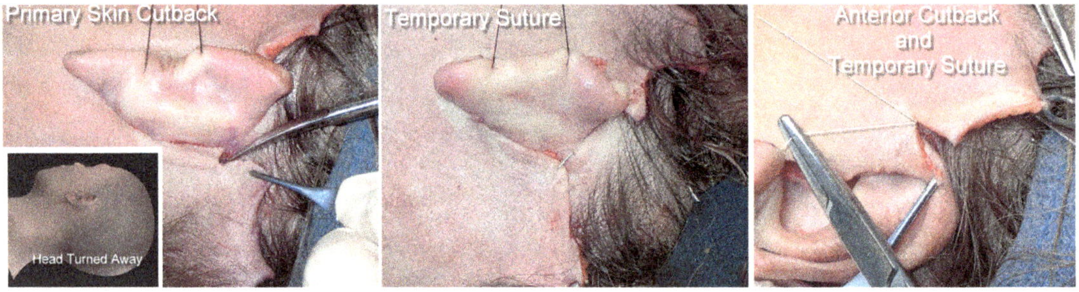

Fig. 6.139. Step 1. The head is turned away from the surgeon and the initial skin cut back is made. A temporary key suture or staple is placed and the postauricular skin is trimmed.

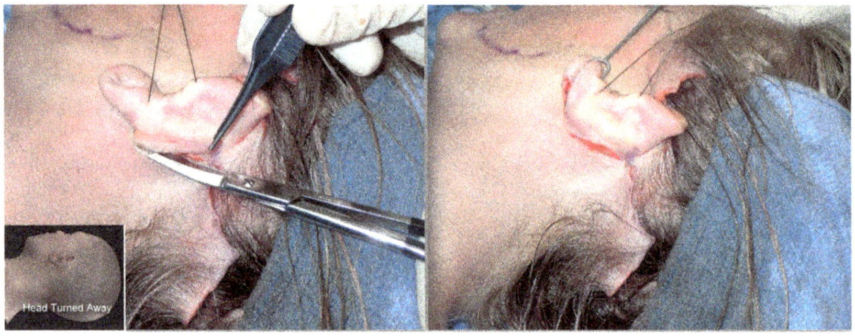

Fig. 6.140. Step 2. With the head turned away, a skin cut back (*left* image) and key suture is placed (*right* image). The skin tension vector is superolateral with more vertical direction that the posterior auricular flap.

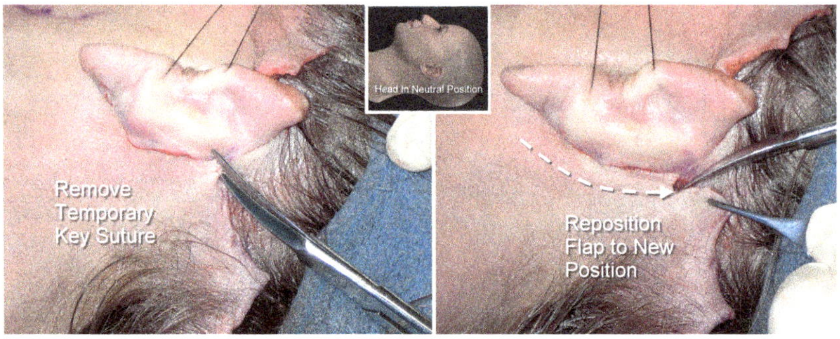

Fig. 6.141. Step 3. The head is repositioned into neutral position and the temporary key suture is removed. Due to the positional change, there is more available skin, and the flap is reset with new cutback and position.

in the proper vector. This is usually in a superolateral vector but has more vertical tension than the postauricular flap. A skin cutback is made and the flap is secured with a 4-0 Vicryl suture (we call this the anterior temporary key suture) (Fig. 6.139).

Step 2. Excess skin in the postauricular sulcus is grossly trimmed at this point (Fig. 6.140). (A new cutback and key suture will be completed later when the head is repositioned in the neutral position and which produces additional skin excess in the postauricular sulcus region).

Step 3. The head is now moved to the neutral position (face towards ceiling), and the posterior key suture or staple is removed. The surgeon will find that when the head is repositioned to the neutral position that there will now be more skin now available in the postauricular and sulcular regions and frequently laxity at the temporary key suture. A secondary skin excision is performed at the sulcus and the flap is repositioned with a new key suture position (due to the increased laxity in the neutral head position) if necessary (Fig. 6.141). It is also important to position this flap in a manner to produce a contiguous hairline as shown.

Step 4. After the final 4-0 Vicryl key suture is completed, there is usually more posterior skin excess at the sulcus region, and the final trimming is performed at this point (Fig. 6.142). Remember, the residual skin excess is a result of turning the head into the neutral position. If the surgeon were to neglect head position and perform all the steps with the head turned away from the surgeon, there would most frequently be unrecognized residual skin excess that would translate into postoperative laxity in the submental and/or neck region and an unhappy patient.

The next step in my protocol is to place a second posterior key suture with moderate tension in the sulcus region (Fig. 6.143). I have not seen this described elsewhere, but it is a very simple and demonstrable step. To best understand this simple and secondary posterior key suture, the surgeon should perform the following on themselves while reading this text. Place your finger at the angle of the mandible on your own face and pull your skin superiorly in a superiolateral direction. You will see that with very little tension, there is noticeable tightening at the mandibular border and submental region. On your

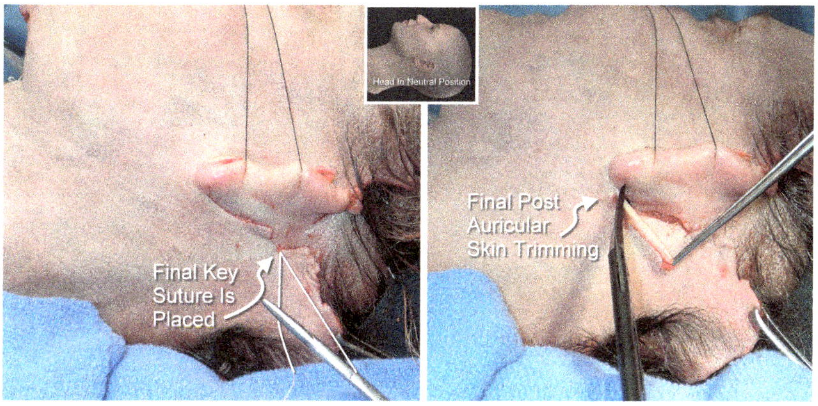

Fig. 6.142. Step 4. The *left* image shows the head in the neutral position and the flap repositioned. A new cutback is usually required due to skin excess from the head repositioning. The *right* image shows the final postauricular (sulcular) skin trimming.

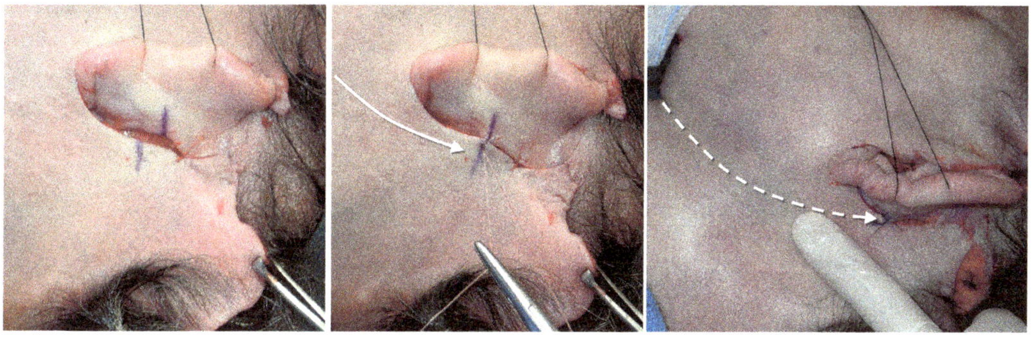

Fig. 6.143. The third key suture ("steal stich") is placed. The proximal flap is elevated superiorly as shown by the hash marks. This is a small but effective tightening maneuver when performed bilaterally. The *arrows* demonstrate the area of definition enhanced by this small suspension.

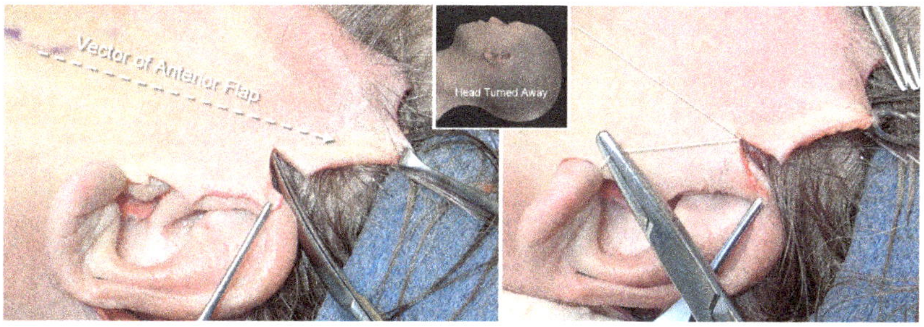

Fig. 6.144. When incising hair-bearing skin excess, it is important to match the angle of the transfollicular bevel as well as the irregularity if the incision on both surfaces. The *left* image shows the initial skin incision, and the *right* image shows the incision trimming the skin excess. The scalpel angle should be an extreme bevel and match on both surfaces to allow hair regrowth through the scar.

next facelift, perform the same procedure on the patient (with the head in the neutral position) and you will see that elevating the posterior sulcular skin margin incision will tighten the mandibular border and the submental region with very little tension. When you multiply this by both sides of the procedure you are enhancing the skin tightening and jaw definition with very little effort I also call this secondary posterior key suture the "steal stitch" because it "steals" extra skin and tightens the mandibular border and submental region.

Step 5. The final step is to readdress the anterior flap (Fig. 6.144). I have not found it necessary to reposition the head in the neutral position to treat the anterior flap. The temporary key suture or staple is removed and the surgeon will see that there is usually adjustment required in terms of vector change or new skin cutback. The anterior flap is adjusted and the final key suture is placed.

Although this stepwise treatment of skin excess may seem complicated, it is actually simple.

Step 1. Place anterior and posterior key sutures with head turned away.

Step 2. Trim posterior sulcus skin excess with head turned away.

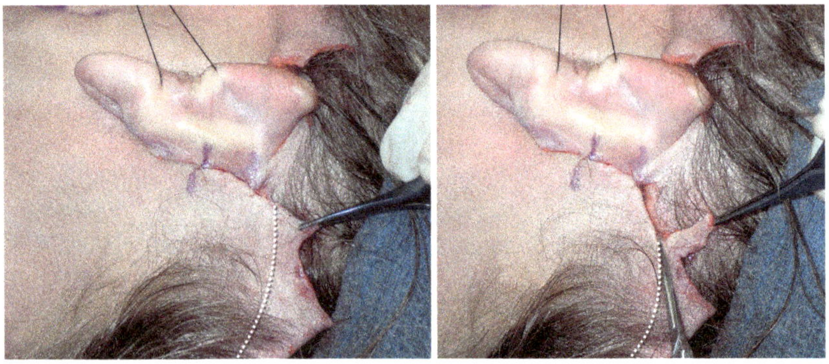

Fig. 6.145. The *dotted line* in the *left* image shows the approximate amount of skin excess. The scalpel is then used to refine the excision to match the bevel and geometry of the original incision (*right* image). For novice surgeons, it may be more accurate to excise smaller amounts of skin to avoid overcutting.

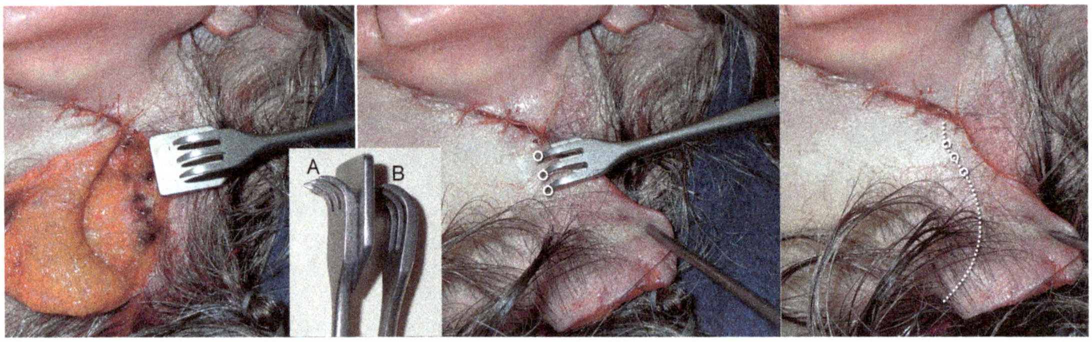

Fig. 6.146. A Pitanguy flap is shown (*left* image). The device has teeth under the square platform that are lined up with the margin of the original (distal) incision. The device is then clamped (*center* image), which makes micropunctures along the border of the original (distal) incision. This step is repeated along the entire incision, which leaves a "dotted line" (*right* image). The dotted line is then followed by scissor or scalpel excision for an exact matching pattern and configuration.

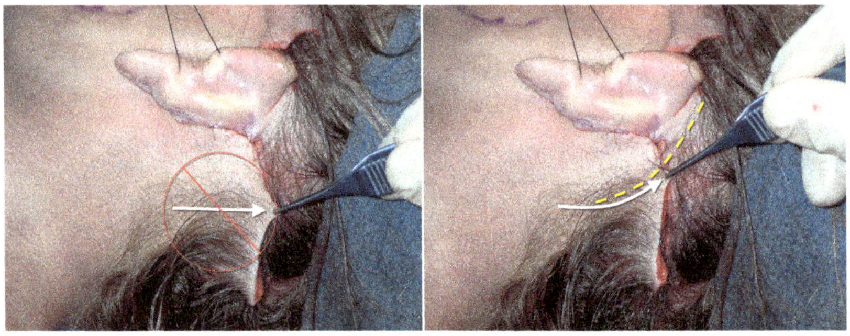

Fig. 6.147. The *left* image shows a "stepped" hairline that can result from vertical approximation of the proximal flap border. The *right* image shows the flap being advanced anteriorly to preserve the natural "S" curve of the posterior hairline (*yellow dashed line*).

Step 3. Turn head to neutral position, reposition the flap to accommodate positional skin excess on posterior sulcus and flap.

Step 4. Retrim posterior sulcus skin excess and posterior hairline excess

Step 5. Reposition the anterior flap with new vector and key suture if necessary and perform final anterior skin trimming.

The next step is to deal with the skin excess of the flaps. The gross excess is first approximated and reduced with an incision that follows the outline of the original incision (Fig. 6.145). Generally, this is done in several steps for accuracy. A gross cut is made to approximate the incision curvature. Then the precision cuts are made to exactly line up the skin edges. The surgeon should use the hyperbeveled transfollicular incision in the hairline, and the scalpel should remain at the same bevel angle as the original incision.

Experienced surgeons can freehand or "eye" the degree of bevel, irregularity, and geometry of the original incision. This is a skill that takes some time to develop. For novice surgeons it is not uncommon to use some type of flap marking device such as an Allis clamp or Pitanguy flap markers (Fig. 6.146).

In the final positioning of the posterior flap, the next step is extremely important and can save the patient and surgeon from another stigma of facelift surgery, the "stepped" hairline. If the flap is simply elevated in a vertical direction (Fig. 6.147, *left*), the hairline may have a significant discontinuity or "step." The more skin excess present, the greater the chance of "stepping" the posterior hairline when repositioning the posterior flap. To prevent this step, the

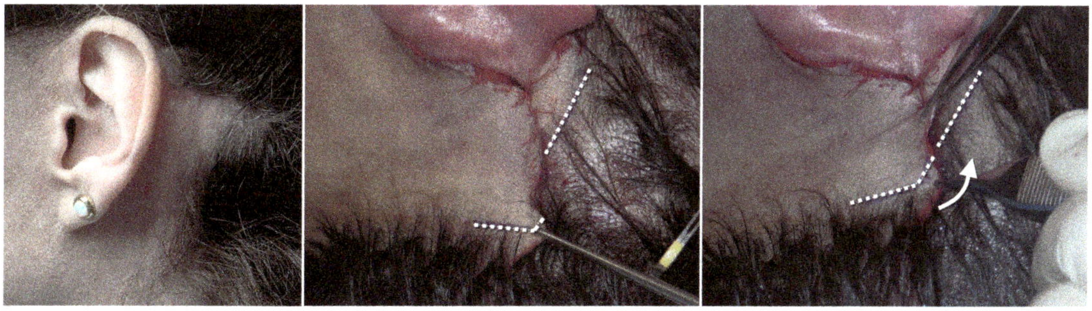

Fig. 6.148. The *left* image shows a postoperative stepped hairline. The *center* and *right* images illustrate how advancing the proximal flap medially prevents an irregular step in the hairline.

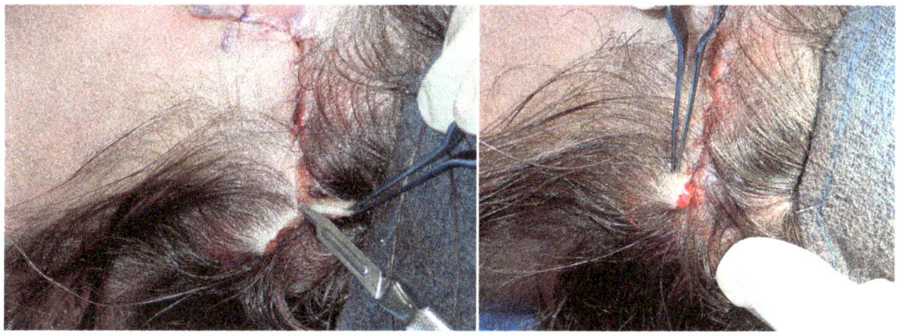

Fig. 6.149. The *left* image shows final skin excess being trimmed, and the *right* image shows tissue bunching (dog-ear) at the incision terminus.

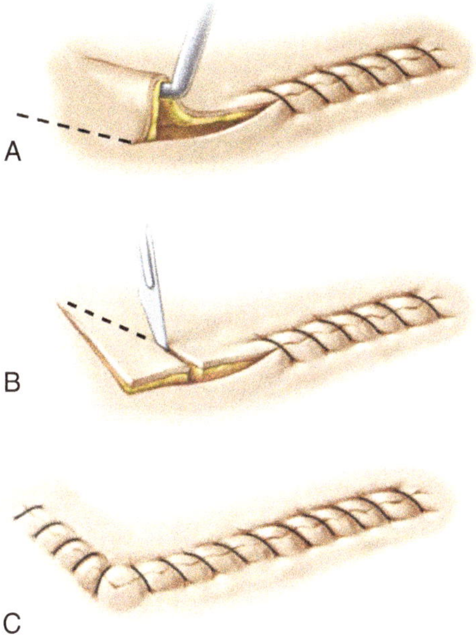

Fig. 6.150. This illustration shows a simple means of tissue release for the dog-ear bunching at the base of the incision. (A) shows elevation of the skin bunching and the *dashed lined* at the base is incised. (B) shows the overlapping excess trimmed on the *dashed line*, and (C) shows the final closure.

surgeon must advance the proximal flap border in a medial direction during closure (Fig. 6.147, *right*). Advancing the posterior flap to match the existing hairline may leave small puckers between the suture, but these resolve with wound contracture during healing.

Fig. 6.148 (*left*) shows a patient with an undesirable "stepped" hairline. The center and right images show how to advance the flap medially to avoid this stigma of facelift surgery.

As the final flap trimming progresses, it is not uncommon, especially on larger lifts, to end up with a dog-ear at the most distal portion of the postauricular incision (Fig. 6.149). Although there are numerous ways of dealing with this, the simplest method is to remove a wedge of skin at the region of the dog-ear. I prefer a simple hockey stick release where an accessory releasing incision is made at approximately a 30-degree angle from the long axis of the posterior incision (Figs. 6.149–6.151).

At this point the continuity of the natural hair line is confirmed and the surgeon verifies that no significant skin excess or bunching remains. The final postauricular incision can be closed with staples or 4-0 suture. I do not use any subcutaneous or nonresorbable sutures in my facelift cases.

If a drain is contemplated, the last centimeter of the terminus of the incision may be left open to accommodate the drain.

The order of skin trimming and closure is up to the preference of the surgeon. I personally prefer to close and trim the postauricular incision first, then transition to the preauricular incision, the sideburn, and finish with the earlobe. Some surgeons leave all incisions open after trimming and suture both sides of the facelift at the end of the case. This technique was described in the previous edition of this text.

Attention is now focused to the preauricular incision and skin excess. Trimming of the preauricular excess is different for pretragal and retrotragal approaches, and both methods are illustrated beginning with the pretragal incision.

The first step in the anterior skin tailoring is making cutbacks above and below the tragus and securing the skin edges with 5-0 gut sutures (Fig. 6.152).

With pretragal incisions, then next step is to trim the skin excess on the tragal arc. The basic technique of trimming the skin access for this approach is to simply excise three arcs of skin at the lobe, the tragus, and the helical attachment (Figs. 6.153

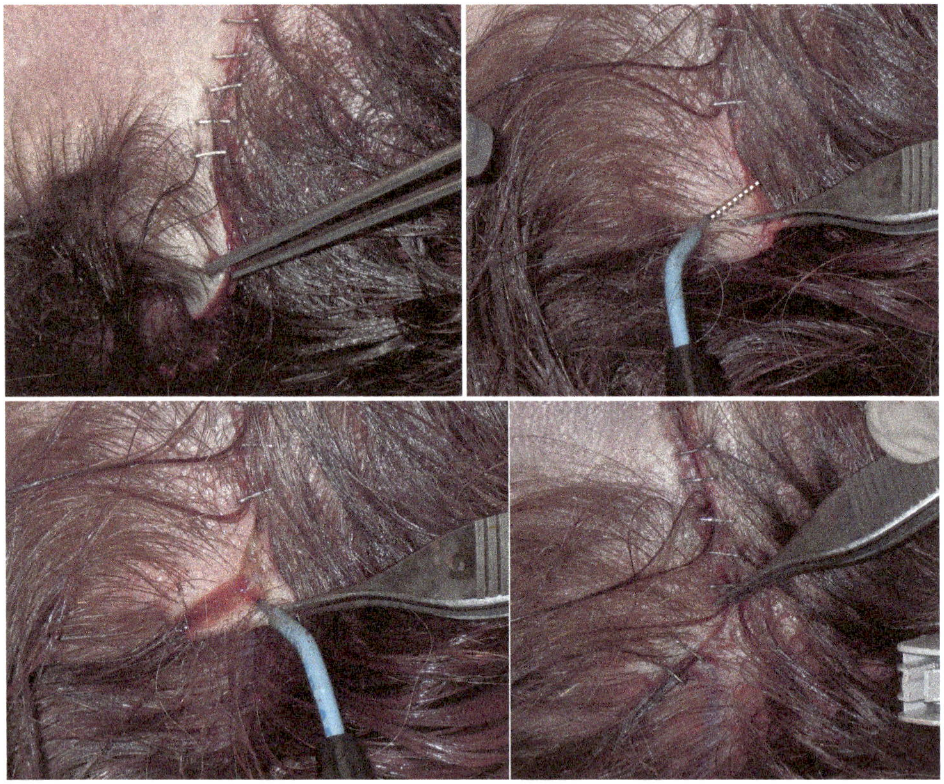

Fig. 6.151. A residual dog-ear at the flap terminus is not uncommon and requires some type of releasing incision (*top left*). The *top right* image illustrates a hockey stick releasing incision. This accessory cut is approximately a 30-degree angle incision. After the releasing incision is made, the skin excess is overlapped and removed. *Lower left* image shows the incision after trimming skin excess, and the *lower right* image shows the skin excess removed and ready for closing.

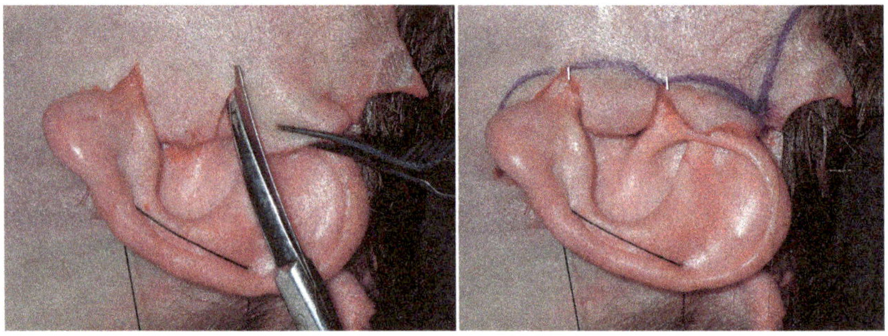

Fig. 6.152. The *left* image shows the pretragal cutbacks, and the *right* image shows the cutbacks secured with 5-0 gut sutures. The skin markings show the "triarcuate" incision pattern to be trimmed.

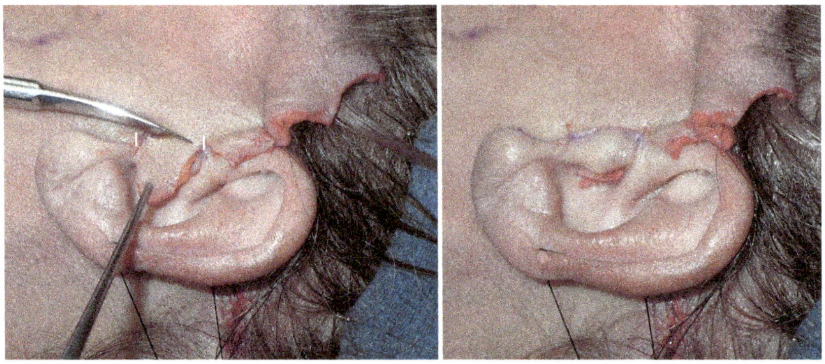

Fig. 6.153. The curved facelift scissors are used to negotiate the gentle arcs of the preauricular incision (*left* image). The *right* image shows the finished pretragal trim.

and 6.154). Facelift scissors are curved for a reason and by gently adjusting the angle of the cut as it progresses produces a very accurate curvilinear pattern (Fig. 6.155). This will be highlighted in the accompanying videos.

With practice this can be performed with great accuracy and almost perfectly abutted skin margins (Fig. 6.154).

To address the posttragal skin tailoring, the first step is to perform skin cutbacks superior and inferior tragal region and secure them with 5-0 sutures (Fig. 6.156). This not only creates the cutback, but also stabilizes the mobile tragal skin, which allows easier trimming. Some surgeons advocate thinning the subcutaneous fat on the tragal skin (Fig. 6.157). I, too, frequently trim the fat in a conservative manner. Care must be used to not overthin and skeletonize the final tragus. It is also very important when using a posttragal incision to protect the delicate cartilage in all steps.

The 5-0 gut sutures stabilize the otherwise mobile tragal skin to allow more precise contouring. I personally am more accurate using a radiowave fine wire microneedle then I am using scissors or scalpel when performing this step (Figs. 6.158 and 6.159).

After trimming the posterior and anterior auricular incisions, I proceed to the temporal tuft. As with all the hair-bearing incisions, the excess skin is removed in the same angle of bevel and contour as the original incision in a transfollicular (trichophytic) manner (Fig. 6.160). If a dog-ear is produced when closing, it is addressed in the same manner as discussed with the posterior incision (Fig. 6.150). It is imperative that whatever method is

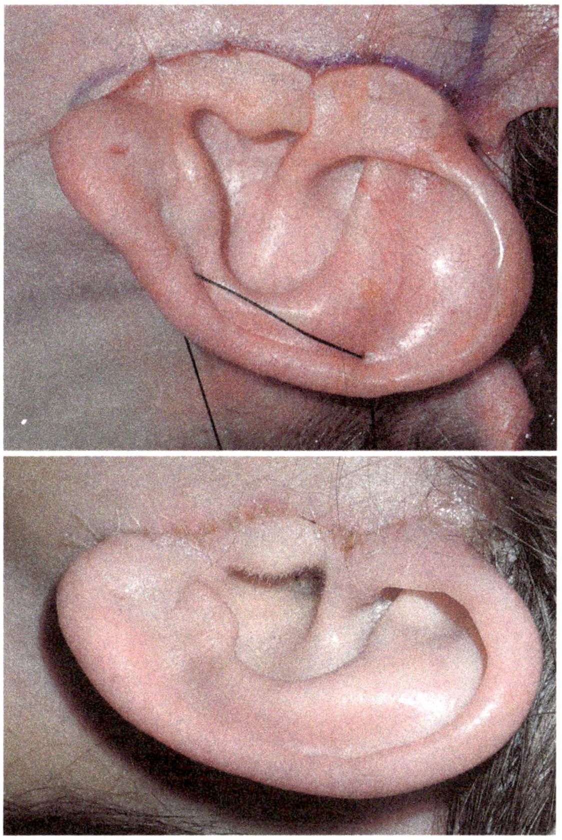

Fig. 6.155. Utilizing the natural curve of the Pagett facelift scissors can craft very accurate skin margins that heal exceptionally. The *top* image is intraoperatively, and the *bottom* image is 7 days postoperatively.

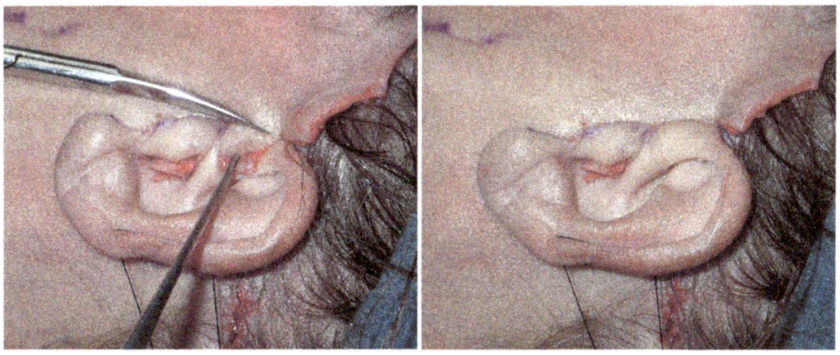

Fig. 6.154. The helical attachment region is trimmed.

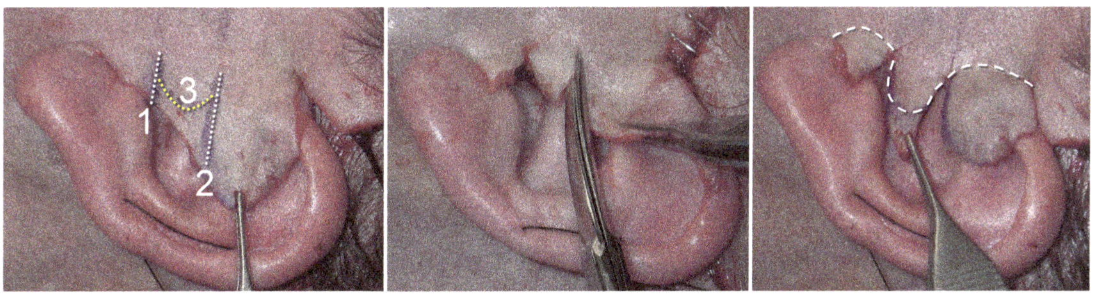

Fig. 6.156. The *left* image shows the two cutback incisions (*1* and *2*) and the planned tragal skin excision (*3*). The *center* image shows the cutbacks being fabricated. The *right* image shows the required tragal contour (*yellow dotted line shown in the left image*) and the *white dotted* lines (*right* image) show the excision pattern of the remainder of the preauricular skin excess.

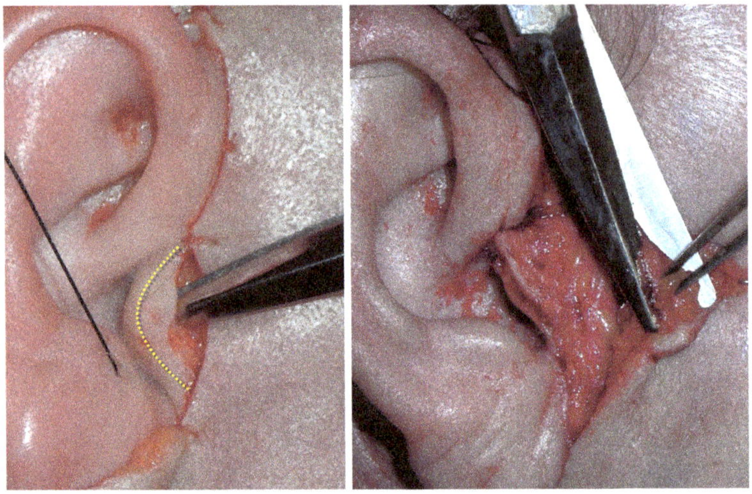

Fig. 6.157. The *left* image shows tragal undermining with the pretragal approach. This ensures there is less tension on the tissue. The *right* image shows the dermal fat being reduced on the underside of the tragal flap when using a posttragal approach. These are both ancillary techniques and not performed by all surgeons.

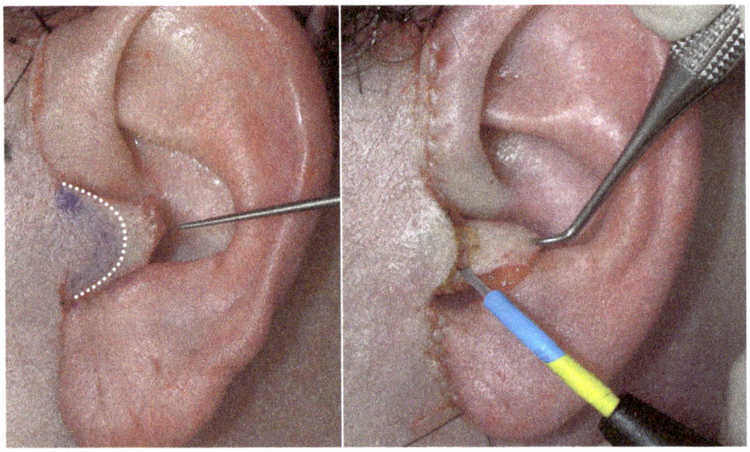

Fig. 6.158. The *left* image shows the anticipated pattern of skin excision (*dotted line*). The *right* image shows a radiowave fine wire incising the excess tragal skin with precise recontouring.

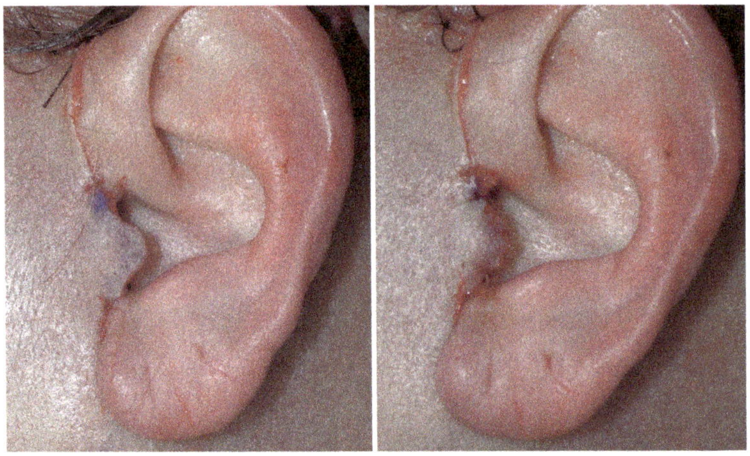

Fig. 6.159. The *left* image shows the reconstructed and delicate tragal skin after trimming. The *right* image shows the final closure using 5-0 or 6-0 gut suture.

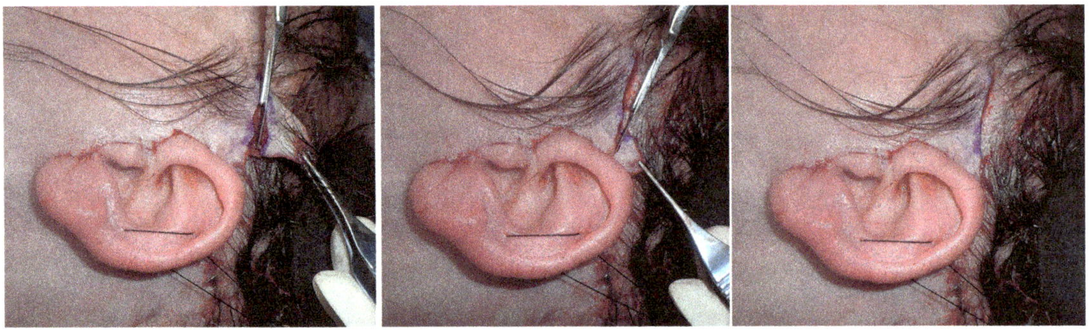

Fig. 6.160. The *left* image shows the temporal tuft excess being grossly excised. The *middle* image shows further and more precise excision. The *right* image shows the finalized temporal tuft trimming. Note that the incision will remain within the hairline, which is my goal on all hair-bearing skin incisions.

used to trim this tissue that the temporal tuft is not elevated to an unnatural position. In some cases, especially larger ones, several millimeters of sideburn elevation may occur and still be acceptable and natural looking. Significant elevation in this area stands out like a sore thumb and again screams poor surgery, poor surgeon. As a side bar, hairdressers see many scars and when you start getting referrals for salons, you are on the right track!

On occasion, the surgeon will find a bulge of fat at the sideburn area because of repositioning the SMAS and skin. This can be reduced with a small-bore liposuction cannula (Fig. 6.161). Failure to appreciate this excess can bother the patient postoperatively when they look in the mirror and notice bilateral temporal bulges.

The next step involves trimming the extra skin at the base of the earlobe. As stated earlier, it is one of the most important facets of natural-appearing facelift surgery. It has been illustrated and discussed numerous times how distorting the earlobe can produce an unnatural result and a very unhappy patient. We always must remember that we may take a patient's face apart and put it back together and do a lot of work on the inside, but the only thing that the patient and the people around them ever see is the incision, so it is so important to have all the areas of incision appear natural. The incision is the signature of the surgeon.

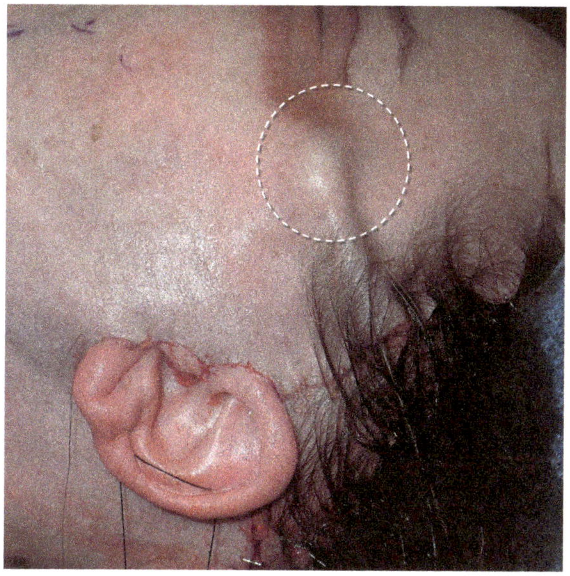
Fig. 6.161. On occasion, the surgeon may notice a bulge in the temporal region from repositioning the SMAS and the skin. This is generally adipose tissue and can be reduced with a small-bore liposuction cannula.

Most patients have more pendulous lobes that are rounded and separate from the cheek, while some patients have "fixed" earlobes that blend into the cheek and are attached (Fig. 6.162). On occasion, a patient may want fixed lobes converted to unattached lobes (Fig. 6.163).

It is important to have documented and discussed the patient's earlobe anatomy preoperatively. There are instances when somebody wants to change the way their lobe looks or is positioned and this warrants preoperative discussion. I've had numerous patients that had fixed earlobes and were unhappy because they could never wear earrings and asked me to provide more of an actually rounded lobe at the time of surgery. Having the preoperative pictures in the operating suite assists this part of the operation.

I address the earlobe as the final step in skin tailoring. The excess skin on the sulcular incision has been previously trimmed (Fig. 6.142). Precision trimming of the flap at the base of the earlobe is now performed (Fig. 6.164).

When attempting to quantify a natural earlobe position, it is often discussed that the earlobe sits about 15 degrees from the long axis of the ear. I think that this is a measurement that is difficult to quantify, especially when the patient is lying down, as the tissues are separated and distorted with tumescent anesthesia and edema. I feel that the easiest way to set the earlobe is to simply observe how it looks when the first positioning suture is placed (Fig. 6.165). When I secure the ear lobe with the first suture, I closely examine for natural placement and contour. Experienced surgeons can make accurate observations concerning lobe position in the same manner that they

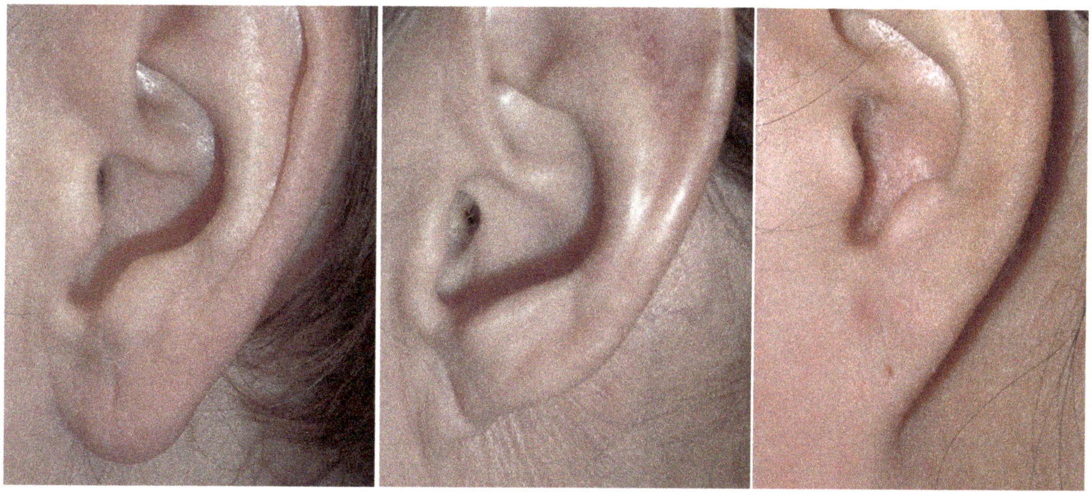
Fig. 6.162. These images illustrate the variability of earlobe shapes, sizes, and attachment. Proper reconstruction requires preoperative discussion regarding the patient's wishes for how their "new" earlobe will look.

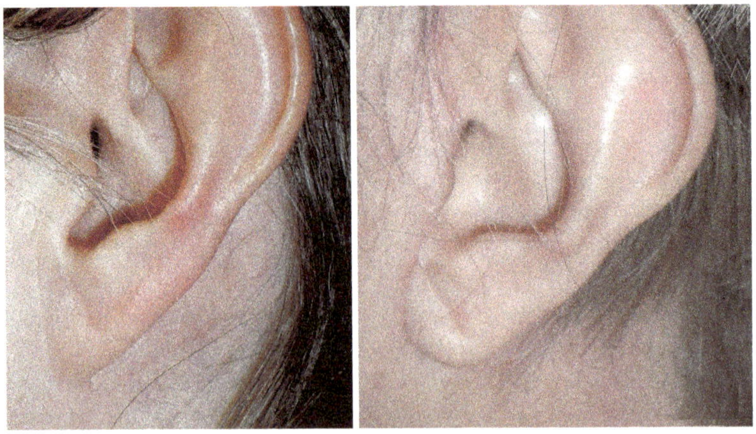

Fig. 6.163. The *left* image shows the preoperative earlobe of a patient who desired a more rounded and unattached lobe after surgery. Rounding the lobe with position adjustment and elevating it to a more superior position during the surgery allowed that change (*right*).

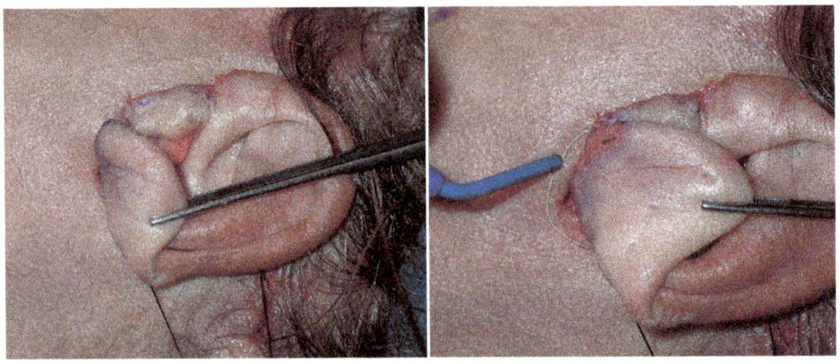

Fig. 6.164. Precise and conservative trimming of the skin excess at the base of the earlobe is performed. The *right* image shows tissue trimming with a Soniquence radiowave fine wire tip.

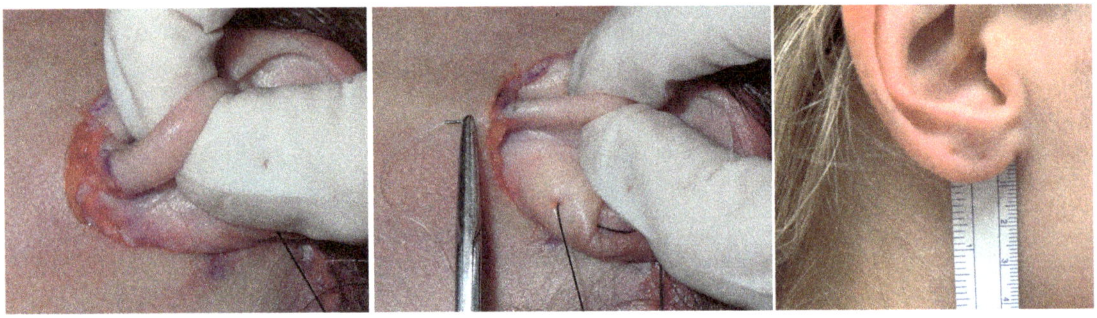

Fig. 6.165. The *left* image shows the excised flap, and the *middle* image shows the lobe being properly positioned. This can be facilitated by pinching the lobe and placing the suture in the center of the base between the pinched skin. The *right* image shows a correctly positioned earlobe where the fixation suture is superior to the base of the lobe.

treat the other tissues without measuring. Setting the lobe with the first suture is a very important step, and if it is not in a natural position, the stitch is removed and replaced until the earlobe is properly positioned. Understanding and being able to create normal position and contour is the art of facelift surgery. All the above is not possible if an excessive skin cutback is made on the flap earlier in the case when delivering the earlobe (Fig. 6.135). A sturdy 4-0 Vicryl suture is used here as patients can more easily tear the lobe sutures when smaller sutures are used. Patients need to be continually reminded pre- and postoperatively that placing or removing collared clothing over the head or sleeping on the earlobe can tear the repair and separate the lobe.

It is important not to close these incisions under tension. The only areas that will be under moderate tension are the three key sutures (preauricular, postauricular, and the sulcus steal stitch) (Fig. 6.166).

In some cases, placing the suture line superior to the lobe base may pucker or "accordion," the lobe but with return to the upright position and wound contraction, it will most commonly lie passive.

At the completion of the skin closure, I prefer to have all my suture lines hidden in the hair (Fig. 6.167).

At this point, the entire first side of the lift is completed, and the same procedures are performed on the contralateral side. During this time where, when the patient is repositioned,

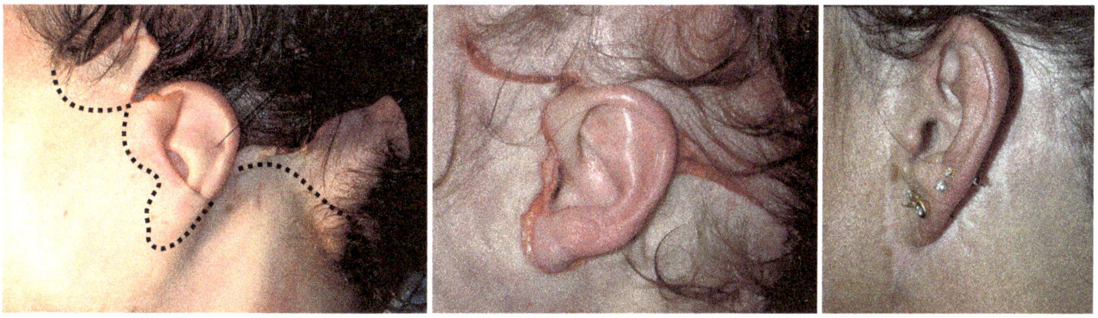

Fig. 6.166. The *left* image shows typical skin excess in a moderate-sized facelift, and the *right* image shows the incision before closure. It is tension free and the only areas of this closure that will have any tension are the three key sutures. Closing facelift incisions under tension can produce serious scarring and contracture as shown in the patient from another surgeon (*right* image).

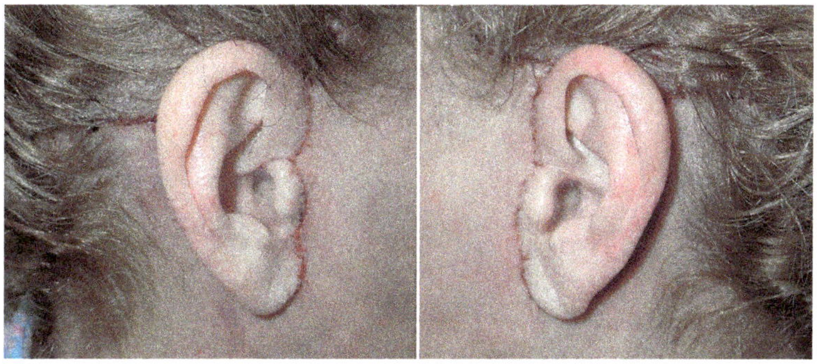

Fig. 6.167. These images show the final closure of the facelift procedure. The postauricular sutures are 4-0 gut, and the preauricular sutures are 5-0 gut and can be alternated with 6-0 gut. I prefer to keep all my incisions hidden in the hairline whenever possible.

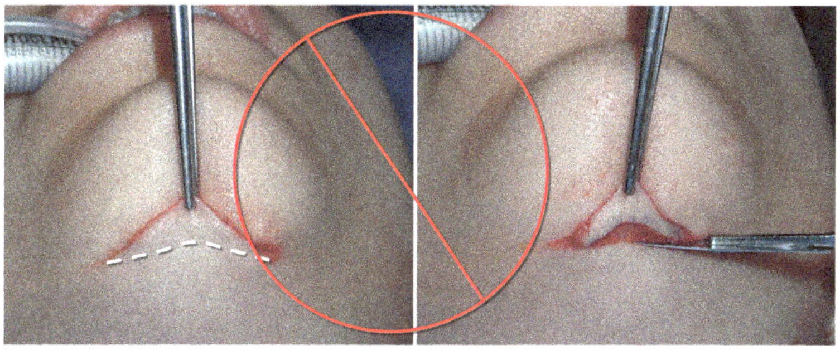

Fig. 6.168. In previous texts, I advocated removing some extra skin in the submental area; however, I no longer perform this procedure, as the extra skin is needed to fill the submental region after deep neck lift. In addition, removing this skin can produce a hollow in the submental region with a raised area on each side of the excision.

the team usually reorganizes the instruments and surgical tray and performs their preliminary sponge count. Physically turning the head on an intubated patient can be very stimulating, causing the patient to react with coughing and gagging. This is frequently accompanied by a spike in blood pressure, which may cause bleeding on the completed side of the facelift. I have seen this happen where the blood pressure spike and stimulus from coughing caused an intraoperative hematoma that required stopping the case and reopening the completed side. To maintain a smooth anesthetic and to prevent unwanted changes in blood pressure, the operative team informs the anesthetist 5 minutes in advance of turning the head or significantly repositioning the patient. This allows the anesthesia provider time to deepen the level of the anesthetic and have better control over the patient and the vital signs.

In pervious texts I recommended excising overlapping submental skin (Fig. 6.168). *I have abandoned this procedure* as my neck treatment has become more aggressive. When resecting significant soft tissue (fat, platysma, deep fat, submandibular gland tissue), the extra skin is needed to fill in the void left by deep neck treatment.

I have added a step before closing the submental incision. I routinely perform very conservative liposuction on each side of the incision (Fig. 6.169). This is mostly on patients with heavier necks. I began doing this because I noticed that after closing the submental incision, I sometimes noticed residual fullness despite my aggressive release of the mandibular ligament and submentoplasty. This is the only time I ever do "reverse liposuction" (turn the liposuction cannula orifice toward the dermis). I do very brief and conservative liposuction on that area, which has helped produce a flatter submental region.

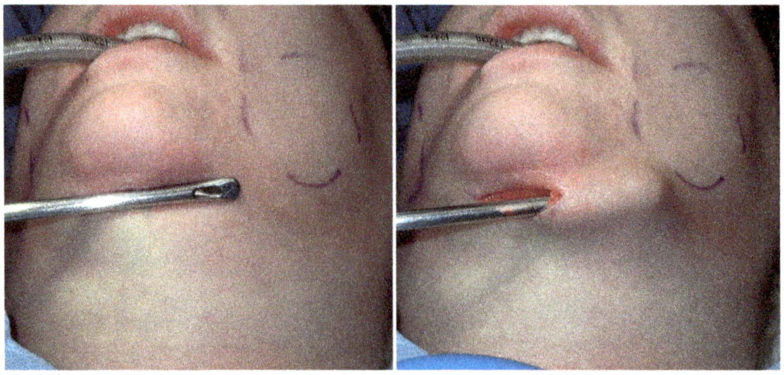

Fig. 6.169. Before closing the submental incision, I perform what I refer to as "reverse liposuction" where the orifice of the cannula is facing the dermis. I perform a very conservative and brief, several stroke liposuction in this region, especially on patients with heavier necks. Doing this has provided a flatter submental region on my patients.

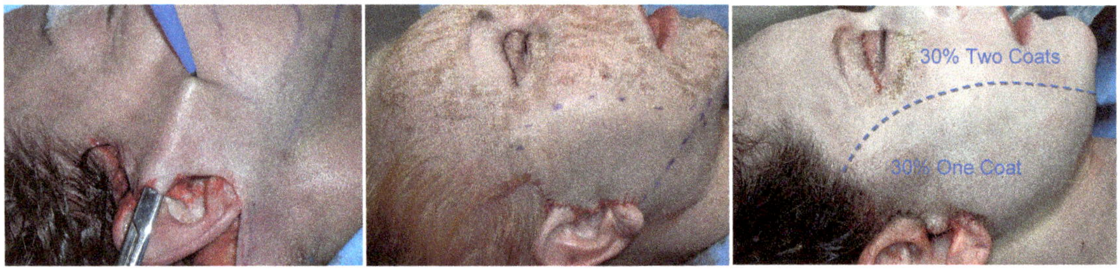

Fig. 6.170. When performing simultaneous facelift and laser resurfacing, the extent of the undermined flap is marked (*left* image). The central oval of the face can be treated with high fluence and multiple passes, but the undermined flaps are treated with lower energy and a single pass (*middle* image). Similarly, when performing medium-depth chemical peel with a facelift, the central oval can be treated with a higher acid concentration and more coats than the undermine flap (*right* image).

Simultaneous Facelift and Skin Resurfacing

I have performed almost 500 facelifts with simultaneous full-face CO_2 laser resurfacing in my career (Fig. 6.170). At one time this was a very common combination of procedures in my practice. In the last several years, I have discouraged patients from having aggressive laser resurfacing at the same time as facelift surgery. The main reason for doing this is that adding a full-face laser treatment to a facelift significantly increases the recovery and makes postoperative care significantly more complex. The other reason I perform far fewer of these simultaneous procedures is the difference in treatment depth. Although the central oval of the face can be aggressively lasered during facelift surgery, the undermined flaps are treated at a lower energy so as not to compromise flap viability. Lasering the central oval of the face aggressively and the undermined flaps at a lower setting can produce texture and color changes between the two areas that sometimes requires a revision laser procedure. It is now my preference to perform aggressive laser skin resurfacing several months before or after the facelift. This has simplified the postoperative care for me, my patients, and my staff.

I do perform light laser treatment where the entire face and flaps are treated at a lighter setting, which is much easier to care for and has less complications. I will also perform medium-depth chemical peeling with facelift but treat the undermined flaps with less concentrated acid or fewer coats.

The subject of postoperative drains is controversial, and some surgeons use two drains on every case, some use a single drain on every case, and many surgeons never use drains. I performed approximately my first 800 facelifts without ever using a drain. I did experiment with placing two 14-gauge angiocatheter "vents" to allow drainage for several days. This was a simple solution for the surgeon desiring some component of passive drainage without cumbersome Jackson-Pratt drains. After watching many of my friends use them and swear that their postoperative course was better, I began using #15 Jackson-Pratt drains for several years. My personal drainage technique consisted of a single drain that ran from the posterior auricular area on one side, at the most inferior part of the midline cervical, and exited the distal postauricular incision on the contralateral side. The drain was placed at the very end of the case and was held in place with several 4-0 got sutures that encircled the drain as it exited the incision (Fig. 6.171). Drains were left in place anywhere from 24 hours to 5 days (Fig. 6.172).

My experience was not overwhelming, and the main problems I had with drains were that the patients hated them, and if I left them in place longer than several days, a visible tunnel or drain tract was present and sometimes took weeks to resolve. Finally, and most importantly, I did not see any significant advantages of using the drains compared with my experience of not using them. I do not routinely use drains in any of my facelift procedures unless I have a patient with significant intraoperative oozing. Using drains probably does decrease seroma formation, but it does not prevent hematoma formation. Some advocates of drain placement say that it also decreases postoperative bruising, but again that was not my observation. The use of drains is a personal operator preference. I performed 109 facelifts the year of this writing and probably used drains on six patients. I will admit that I had several patients with seromas but I am not sure that a drain would have prevented these or not. The decision on whether to use or not to use drains is a personal decision based on practitioner experience. I do use drains more often on patients with heavy necks and deep neck lifts where I am removing extensive soft tissue and/or submandibular glands. I will generally use a #10 Jackson-Pratt drain in these cases for 24–72 hours.

When all procedures are finished, any blood in the hair is rinsed with hydrogen peroxide and the entire hair is washed with sterile water and hydrogen peroxide. A curl detangler is used to facilitate combing the hair (Fig. 6.173).

At the end of the case the anesthesia emergence is begun, and the patient is slowly awakened. As the patient returns to a normotensive state, it is important to closely monitor any oozing, bleeding, or hematoma formation on the operating room table. Intubated patients can become stimulated and "fight" the endotracheal tube with severe coughing and bucking. This can cause an increase in blood pressure and hematoma formation, which can make an otherwise successful case problematic. The art of anesthesia is integral for successful facelift and neck lift surgery. Accomplished and busy facelift surgeons have very capable anesthetic support, and the continual communication with anesthetist and the surgical team is imperative. Besides the obvious skills of maintaining vital signs on an anesthetized patient, avoiding hypertension throughout and especially at the end of the case is critical. Hypertension is the most common cause of postoperative hematoma. There are few things more frustrating for a facelift surgeon than having to return to the operating room after a long surgical case to drain a hematoma.

After hair is washed and the patient is cleansed of all blood and debris, a postoperative facelift dressing is applied. The type of dressing is operator preference, and facelift dressings vary from complex football helmet–sized dressings to no postoperative dressing at all. Most facelift surgeons prefer light compression after surgery, but it is critical not to have a dressing so tight

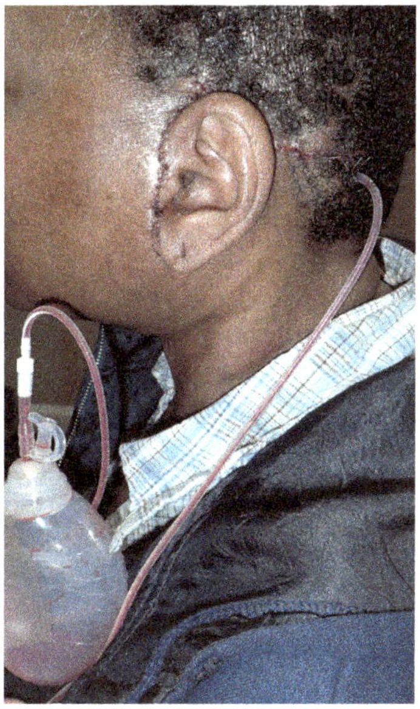

Fig. 6.172. A typical Jackson-Pratt drain is shown on a patient 48 hours after surgery.

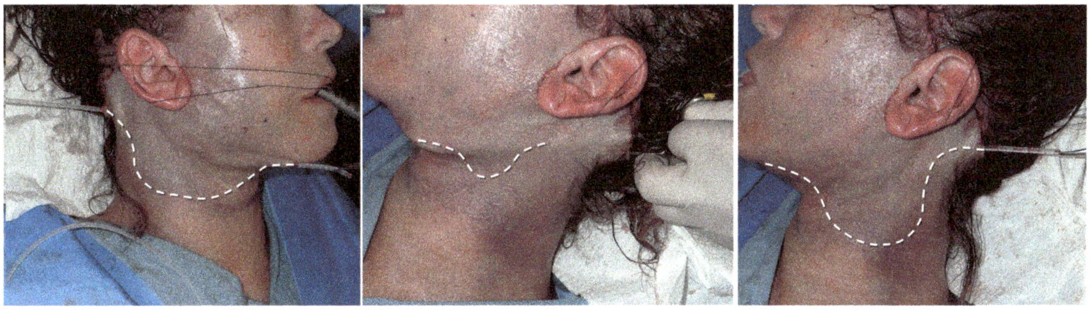

Fig. 6.171. A Jackson-Pratt drain is placed through the posterior incision on one side (*left* image), traverses the lowest portion of the dissection across the midline (*center* images shows tonsil clamp fetching the free end of the drain), and exits at the terminus of the contralateral incision (*right* image).

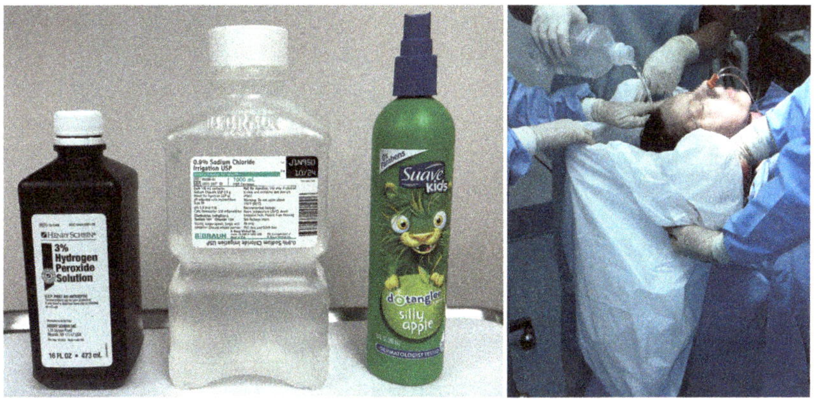

Fig. 6.173. At the very end of the procedure the hair is washed with hydrogen peroxide to remove blood with sterile water and an over-the-counter hair detangler.

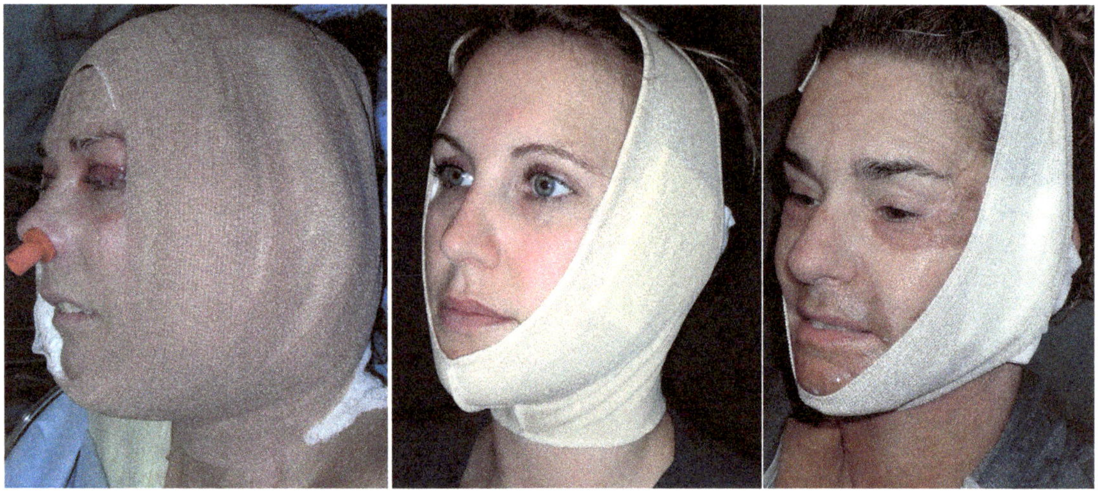

Fig. 6.174. These images show my evolution of postfacelift dressings from large bulky dressings (*left*) to commercial "jaw bra"-type dressings over several layers of gauze (*center* image) to a simple elastic bandage over several layers of gauze (*right* image).

that it compromises vascularity. It is also important for the operator to understand that a pressure dressing in itself does not prevent hematoma formation. In earlier years I too used a large, bulky, multilayer dressing (Fig. 6.174, *left*); as I progressed, I downsized to a simple "jaw bra"–type facial compression dressing (Facial Support, Medicointernational.com) with Velcro closures on the top of the head and behind the neck. After this dressing is placed, several layers of gauze pads are inserted over all incision lines (Fig. 6.174, *center*). With supply chain issues during the COVID-19 pandemic and the inability to procure previous dressings, I switched to a simple ACE-type elastic bandage, which has worked equally as well and is much more economic (Fig. 6.174, *right*). This bandage is simply tied in a bow on the top of the head and can be removed and replaced by the office or patient. I have not found any difference when using any type of dressing in terms of hematoma prevention or healing. When I perform simultaneous CO_2 laser resurfacing with a facelift, I don't use any dressing because it abrades the lasered skin. In the cases where I don't use any dressing, I have not seen any problems, which makes me wonder if I need them at all. Some surgeons feel that if suction drainage is used, then the vacuum will keep the skin in close approximation to the deeper tissues and will therefore negate the need for a drain.

Some surgeons employ a complex "net" of sutures to limit bleeding or hematoma. These surgeons say that it is effective, but I have never used it and personally find it a lot to go through (Fig. 6.175). The sutures are removed 48 hours after surgery.

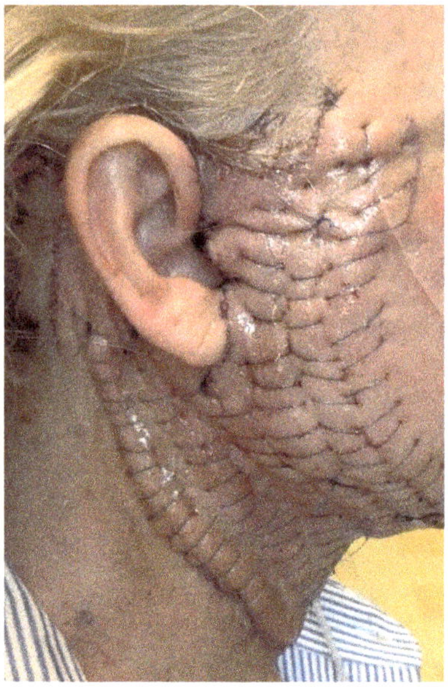

Fig. 6.175. A suture netting (described by Dr. Andre Aursvald) used by some surgeons to prevent hematoma.

After all the previous steps are complete, the patient is dressed in their postoperative clothing in the operating room and taken to the postanesthesia recovery room. Over the years, I have used several systems to move and recover patients. At one time I had two hospital beds in my recovery room and moved the patients in and out of this suite with wheelchairs. I found the beds to be bulky and they took up needed space. Also, when a patient is in a bed, they want to sleep, and this can slow down the discharge process. I now use Stryker recovery chairs (www.stryker.com) (Fig. 6.176). These have wheels that allow easy transfer from the operating suite to the recovery room, and the patient can recover in this chair until they are discharged. The chair has many different positions for comfort including Trendelenburg position in case of emergency. There are also trays to place personal effects or postoperative beverages and medications. In the recovery suite the patient is kept warm with Bair Hugger system (www.bairhugger.com), and all vital signs are monitored until discharge (Fig. 6.177).

The initial time in the recovery suite can be vulnerable. The staff is busy turning over the operating room, cleaning instruments, and preparing for other patients while the anesthesia personnel are finishing their paperwork. In my office, a dedicated person is assigned to recovery and sits with the patient, tending to their postoperative care, comforting them, and monitoring vital signs until discharge.

During this time, the patient's caregiver is watching our postoperative videos and discussing postsurgical care with our staff. The caregiver is not brought back to the recovery suite until the

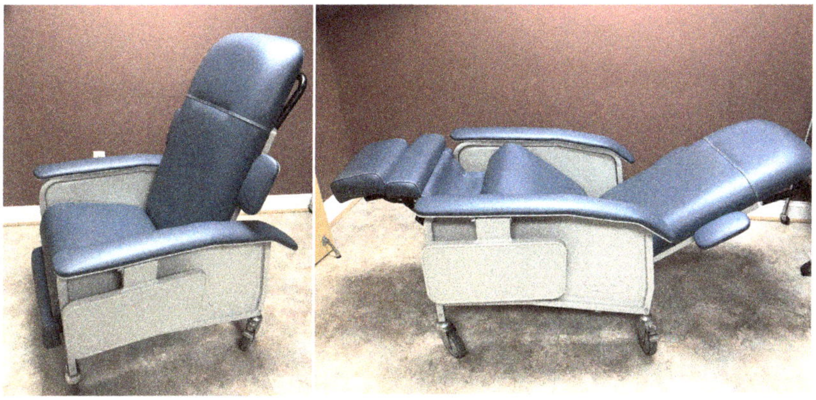

Fig. 6.176. The Stryker recovery chair is an affordable and convenient method of transport and recovery in the ambulatory outpatient office surgery center.

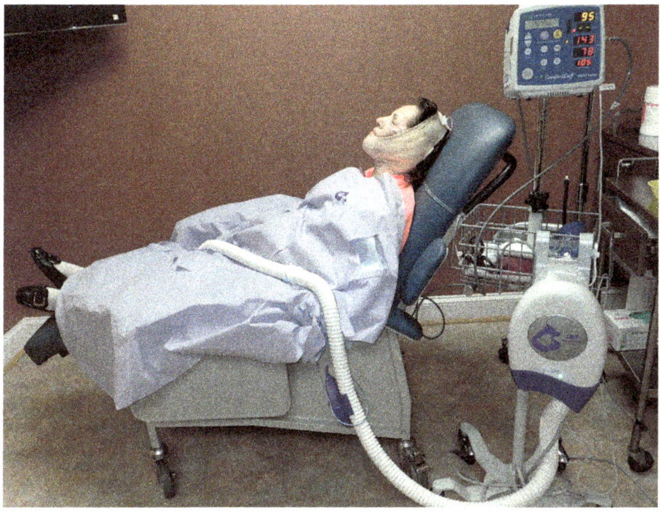

Fig. 6.177. The patient is kept warm and reclined in the recovery suite with continual monitoring of vital signs.

patient is comfortable and lucid. Pain and nausea can be common situations after facelift anesthesia. The conundrum with pain is not to administer narcotics in the recovery room as it will delay the patient's discharge as well as possibly contribute to nausea. I prefer to give the patient 200–400 mg of Celebrex (celecoxib) (www.pfizer.com) as soon as they are able to swallow a pill. The patients are asked to bring their postoperative medications with them in the case their pain is significant. Postoperative nausea is treated with Zofran 4 mg (www.gsk.com) IV or orally. The intravenous line is left in place until the patient is discharged. It is very important to document as many things as possible at the time of discharge. This discharge criteria would include vital signs, level of consciousness, pain level, ambulation, ability to understand instructions, and having a capable caregiver and a safe place to recover. Premature or unsafe discharge can result in lawsuits, serious injury, and death. I personally explain to the caregiver that respiratory distress, bleeding, or hematoma may be emergent and to notify me immediately. All patients have my cell number and that of my nurse. One of the staff will check on the patient the night of surgery, and this is recorded in the chart. The patient is scheduled to be seen in the office the next morning. Having written postoperative instructions as well as postoperative videos on my website prevents any confusion on what to do and not to do the night of surgery.

It is important to have a clean instrument setup as well as availability of anesthetic medications if the patient must return to the office for hematoma treatment. It is also important to have a plan in place with assigned staff and anesthesia personnel to report to the office in case of emergency. Seeing a patient by oneself and not having access to instruments, drugs, and assistants can be a nightmare. All competent surgeons will plan ahead for a workable situation in case of emergency or return to the operating room.

I personally never have the patient apply ice or heat to undermined facelift flaps. Although some surgeons do, my goal is to not vasoconstrict the delicate flaps with ice, and I have seen numerous patients sustain severe full-thickness burns over flaps from various heat sources. Since they are numb over the flaps, they can cause serious burns due to the lack of pain perception.

The patient is seen in the office the following morning, and the dressings are removed and the surgical sites are inspected for hematoma, seroma, or compromise of tissue viability. Motor nerve function is also documented. All incisions are cleansed with peroxide and saline and a triple antibiotic ointment is applied to all suture lines (Fig. 6.178). Any fluid collections are aspirated at this time. The postoperative elastic dressing is then replaced, and the patient is asked to wear this as much as possible for the next 7 days on a 24-7 basis. In-town patients are asked to return at 1 week, 2 weeks, 1 month, and 3 months. At the 2-week appointment any remaining staples or Vicryl sutures are removed. Obviously, any patients with problems are seen on an as-needed basis. Almost 60% of my facelift patients are from out of town and leave after a week. If they have any issues, I usually know a colleague close to them, but this is one of the big problems of a fly-in practice. Patients that have seromas are followed more closely as multiple aspirations may be necessary. Patients with induration or firmness (which is usually the submental or anterior neck regions) are seen several times a week for complimentary ultrasound treatments. Dilute steroid (triamcinolone 10 mg/mL) is also injected into indurated areas. Fig. 6.179 shows patients at various postoperative stages. It is important to understand that the average surgeon can explain many things to patients with great predictability in detail

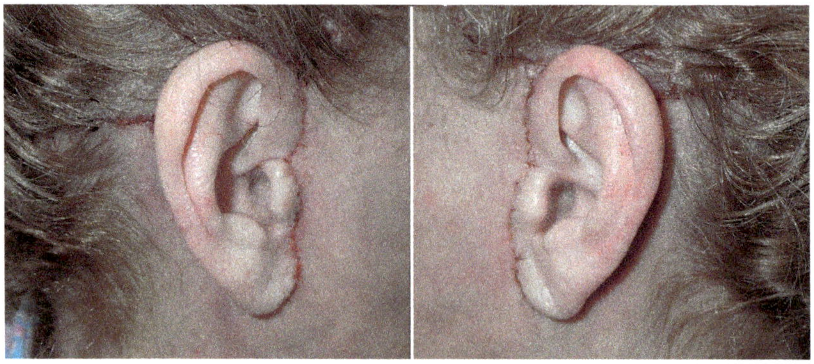

Fig. 6.178. The incision line of a typical patient is shown 24 hours after surgery.

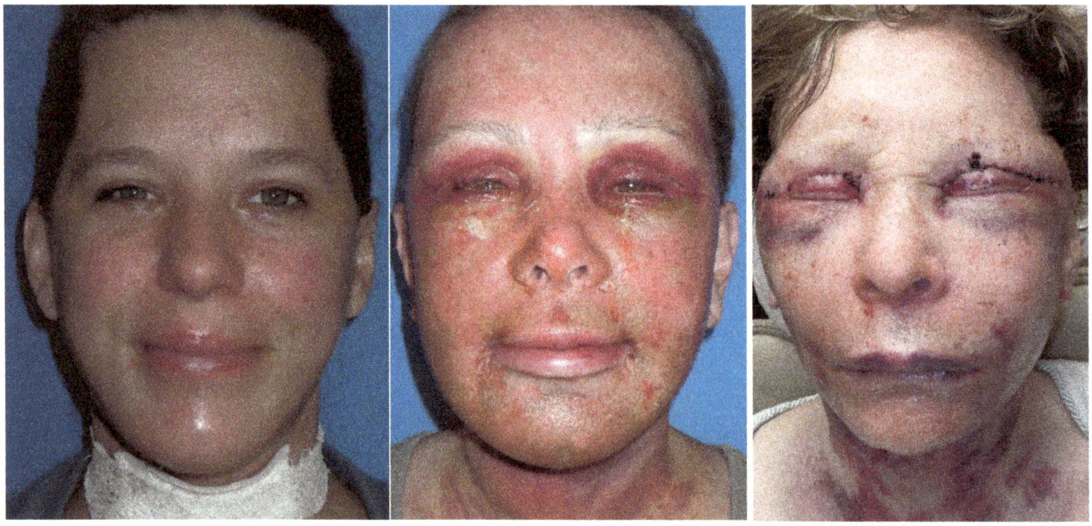

Fig. 6.179. All three of these patients are shown 24 hours after comprehensive facelift and neck lift. Postoperative healing, swelling, and bruising can be extremely variable based on many factors, including but not limited to, the number of procedures performed at same operation, the age of the patient, and their state of health. The young patient on the *left* had a small facelift only. The patient in the *center* had four quadrant blepharoplasty, facelift, and full-face laser resurfacing. The older patient on the *right* had four quadrant blepharoplasty and facelift.

including incisions, the operative procedures, prescriptions, and anesthesia. Trying to attach predictability to swelling and bruising can be much more difficult as there are so many intrinsic (heredity and clotting) and extrinsic (age, health status, meds that affect coagulation, etc.) variables in play.

This must be explained to patients preoperatively. I've had many older patients that tell me that they bruise at the slightest touch and they did not have any postoperative bruising, and I had other young healthy patients that say they never bruise, and they had significant ecchymosis. The variability of healing is a significant factor!

Further information about follow-up will be discussed in the facelift complications chapter.

Advanced Ancillary Procedures

As stated earlier in this text, I am trying to produce information that is useful for not only the novice surgeon but the expert surgeon as well. The following procedures are performed by experienced surgeons to enhance neck and profile of selected patients. As stated earlier, deep plane facelift has become extremely popular for several reasons. Number one, it is an effective procedure, and number two, social media has propelled this procedure into extreme popularity. Experienced surgeons will, on occasion, reduce the submandibular glands and digastric muscle and some surgeons advocate hyoid suspension, parotid gland reduction, and posterior laryngeal positioning. It has become common to hear from the podium who can remove the most tissue from the neck. I humorously say that it is a race to the spine! Although many of these cases look extremely aesthetic, I feel that some of them look very skeletal, and this will only amplify as the patient ages. Although this may work in their hands, trying to perform these advanced procedures as a novice surgeon can be a prescription for disaster. As I have said many times in this book, and I'll probably say it many more times, don't worry about what other people are doing—progress at your own speed until you become proficient at adapting new techniques. I will outline a brief overview of how I perform these procedures, and these same procedures will be covered in greater depth later in this book.

Treating heavy-necked patients and patients with little fat is approached differently. While aggressive soft tissue reduction may be performed in heavy-necked patients, overtreatment must be avoided in patients without significant submental fullness or fat. The submandibular glands are frequently approached by undermining the medial platysmal border and retracting the muscle laterally to reveal the gland. I perform an aggressive submental dissection on heavy-necked patients, which has really improved my cervicomental aesthetics. I remove two to three fingerbreaths of soft tissue in the midline, which includes subcutaneous fat, platysma, and subplatysmal fat. At the inferior portion of the excision, the dissection may extend the the pretracheal fascia. The lateral extent of this excision will often uncover the submandibular glands. If they are bulging or ptotic below the mandibular border, I will reduce the glands. Some surgeons reduce the gland from the submental incision, and others approach the gland from the preauricular incision (Fig. 6.180).

Generally, platysmaplasty involves removing a midline segment of muscle. This allows access to the medial platysmal borders. They can be undermined with electrosurgery or scissors and retracted laterally to a point where the submandibular gland is visible or palpable lateral to the junction of the anterior belly of the digastric muscle and the hyoid bone (Fig. 6.181). Some surgeons further retract the platysma (and marginal mandibular nerve) by placing a suture through the underside of the undermined platysma, then upward through the skin. The suture is then clamped, and pulling the suture retracts the platysma and allows better vision and access to the region. On occasion, I resect the ptotic platysma lateral to the submandibular glands and this allows direct visualization.

I have also used a tonsil snare to assist in retraction and hemostasis during gland reduction (Fig. 6.182 *left*). After the capsule is incised and the superior lobe of the gland is freed by dissection, the loop of the snare is secured around the portion of the gland to be reduced. This is generally the portion of that gland that is ptotic below the mandibular border (Fig. 6.182 *right*). The freed portion of the gland is then elevated, and the tonsil snare loop is placed around the

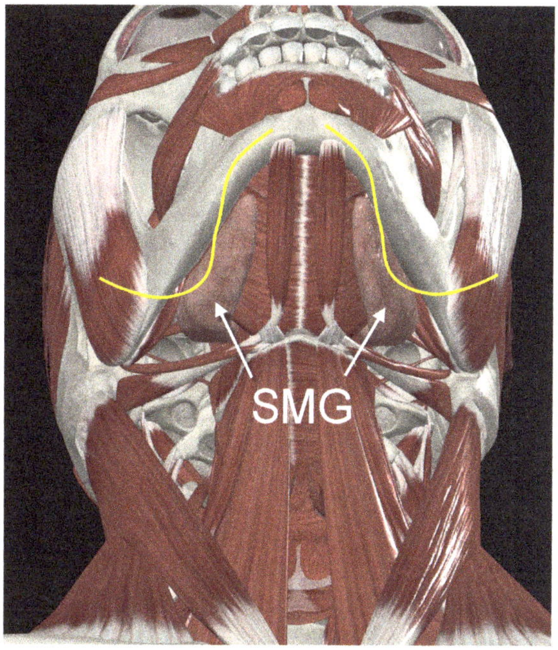

Fig. 6.181. This image shows the submandibular glands and their relationship to the digastric and hyoid structures. *SMG* points to the glands, and the *yellow lines* represent the approximate position of the marginal mandibular nerves. (Base image, courtesy *Complete Anatomy*, Elsevier.)

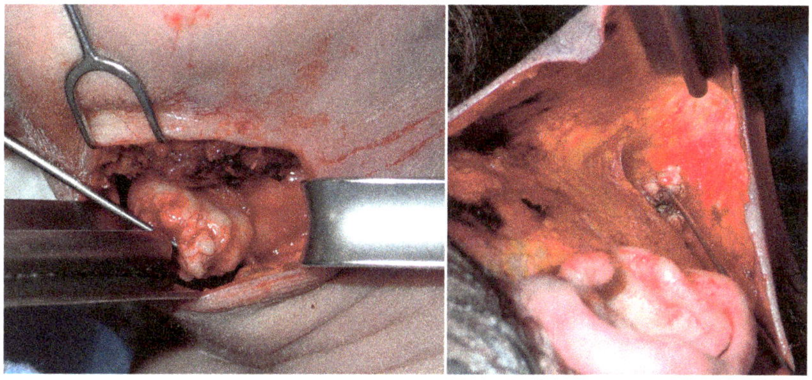

Fig. 6.180. The *left* image shows a submental approach and the *right* images illustrates a lateral approach to the submandibular gland during facelift surgery.

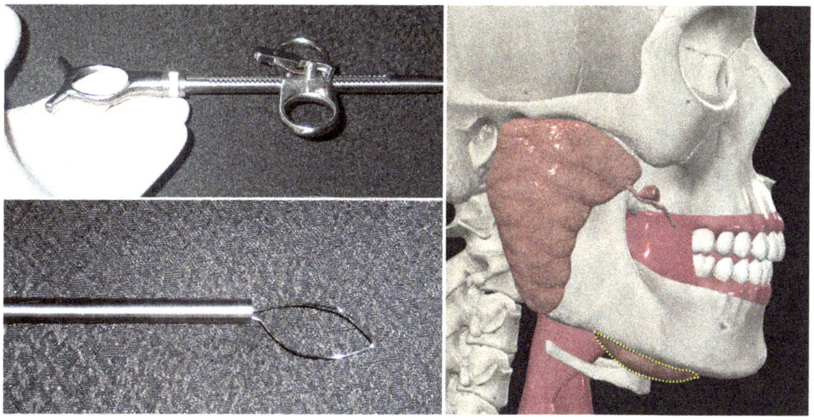

Fig. 6.182. The *left upper* and *lower* images show a tonsil snare instrument that can be used to ligate the submandibular gland for control and hemostasis. The *right* image shows the area of ptotic submandibular gland which lies inferior to the mandibular border. The *dotted line* shows the amount of ptotic gland to be removed.

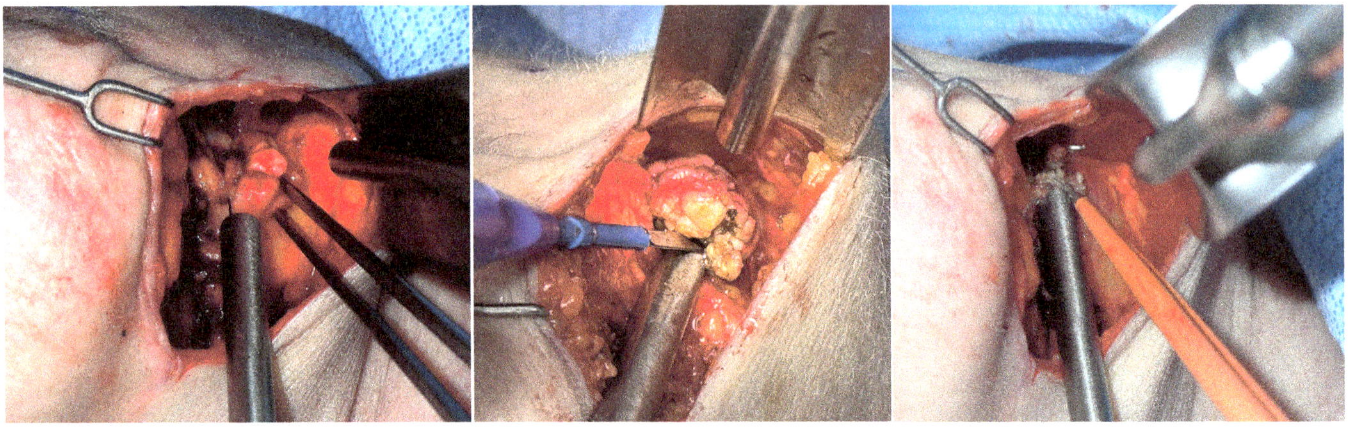

Fig. 6.183. The *left* images shows the tonsil snare loop placed over the gland that has been freed from the capsule. The *center* image shows the snare retracted which ligates the gland which is in turn sectioned at the base with a Bovie or radiowave electrode. The *right* image shows the sectioned base which is then cauterized further, in this case with a bipolar forceps.

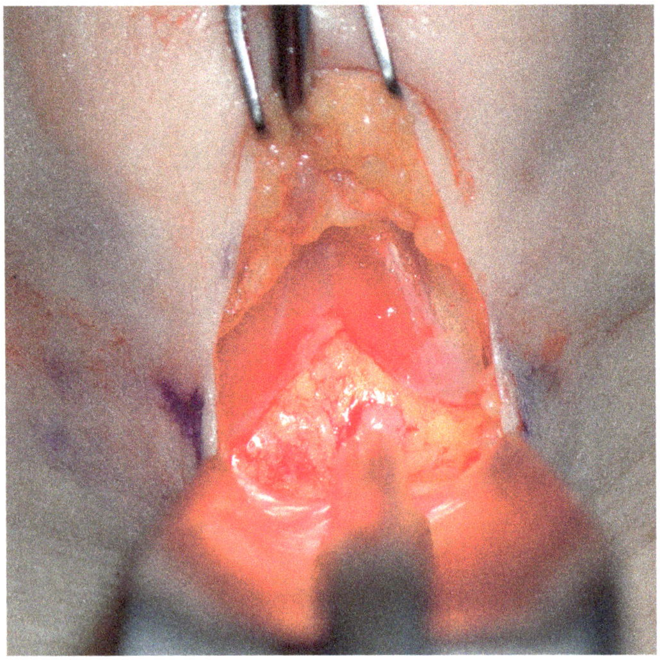

Fig. 6.184. This image shows full digastric muscles that I would consider reducing during surgery. Notice the subcutaneous fat at the top of the picture and the subplatysmal fat below and between the anterior bellies of the digastric muscle.

gland and the loop is retracted (Fig. 6.183 *left*). This places a tight temporary ligature around the base of the ptotic gland. The glandular excess is then transected using a Bovie or radiowave cutting tip for hemostasis (Fig. 6.183 *center*). After resection and before the snare is released, the base of the gland is cauterized to insure complete hemostasis (Fig. 6.183 *right*). I close the gland capsule with 4-0 Vicryl suture after the gland is reduced. Although some surgeons advocate drains in the area or neurotoxin injection of the remnant gland, I don't perform either of these steps.

Complications with this procedure include nerve damage, severe bleeding, hematoma, and sialocele.

Digastric Muscle Reduction

Thinning the anterior belly of the digastric muscle is an additional means of debulking the heavy neck. I perform this procedure on selected patients when I notice thick muscle when working in that area of the neck (Fig. 6.184). I have not found it to make a huge difference by itself, but the cumulative effects of other debulking procedures can add up to make a difference.

Reducing the digastric muscles is relatively simple and involves filleting a longitudinal section to thin the muscle. A hemostatic modality such as electrosurgery or radiowave surgery is used to prevent muscle bleeding (Fig. 6.185).

Reinforcing previous points, minimally invasive or aggressive procedures will come and go in facelift operative technique. Just because something is new does not mean it's better, and novice surgeons should not rush to adopt these techniques until their skill level justifies so.

Aggressive neck and jawline procedures became popular in the 1990s and led to some very skeletonized results (Fig. 6.186).

Facelift Case Presentations

My goal in this section is not to show only my best cases, but to provide a representative reference of various patients in various shapes, sizes, and forms. I will begin by showing some early results in the first week of surgery.

Figs. 6.187–6.190 show various patients in the first 24 hours to 7 days after surgery. Watching patients transform from the "caterpillar to the butterfly" stage is one of the great joys of our profession.

Figs. 6.187–6.239 show before-and-after pictures of facelifts and neck lifts performed by the author. Some of these patients have also had concomitant cosmetic facial procedures as well. All of the after pictures were taken at least 90 days after surgery. Cases are shown in increasing order of skin excess with smaller cases shown first progressing to larger lifts, and all pictures show before on the left and after on the right.

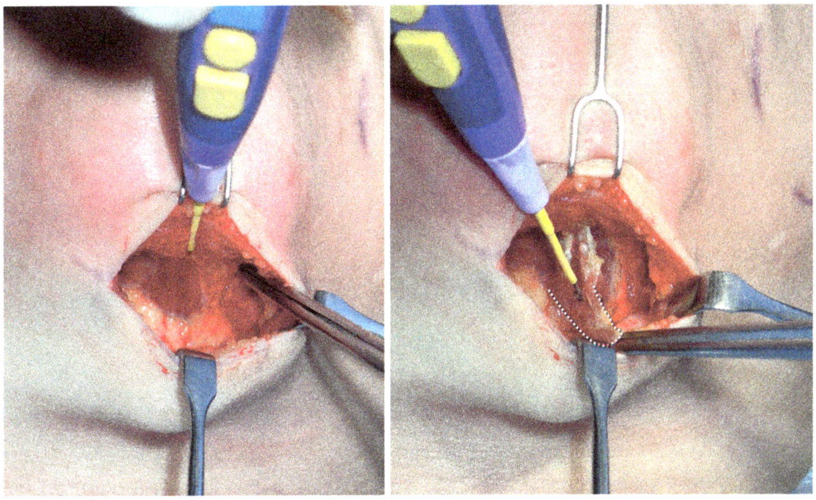

Fig. 6.185. The *left* image shows the left anterior digastric belly, and the *right* image shows a horizontal reduction using the Soniquence radiowave microneedle.

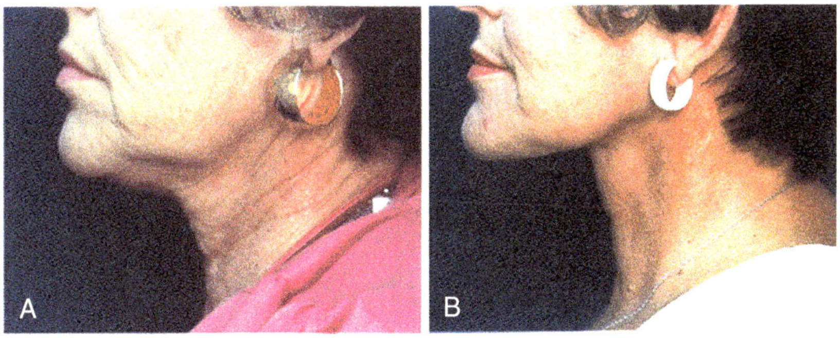

Fig. 6.186. These images show overtreatment of the deep neck structures resulting in an unnatural skeletonized appearance. (Baker DM. Face lift with submandibular gland and digastric muscle resection: radical neck rhytidectomy. *Aesthetic Surg J* 2006;26(1):85–92.)

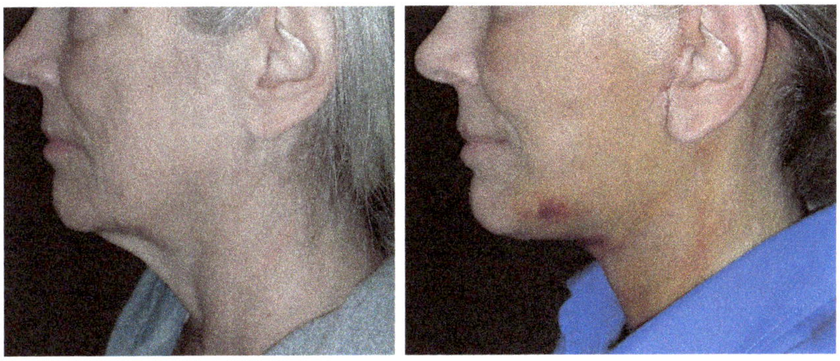

Fig. 6.187. This 62-year-old female is shown before and 24 hours after deep plane facelift and neck lift.

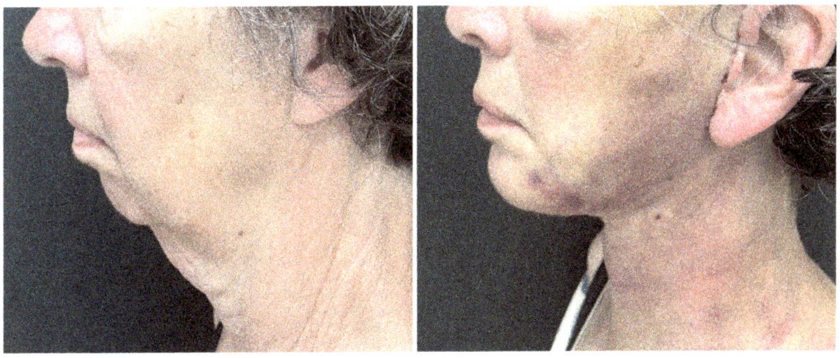

Fig. 6.188. This 63-year-old female is shown before and 24 hours after deep plane facelift and neck lift with chin implant.

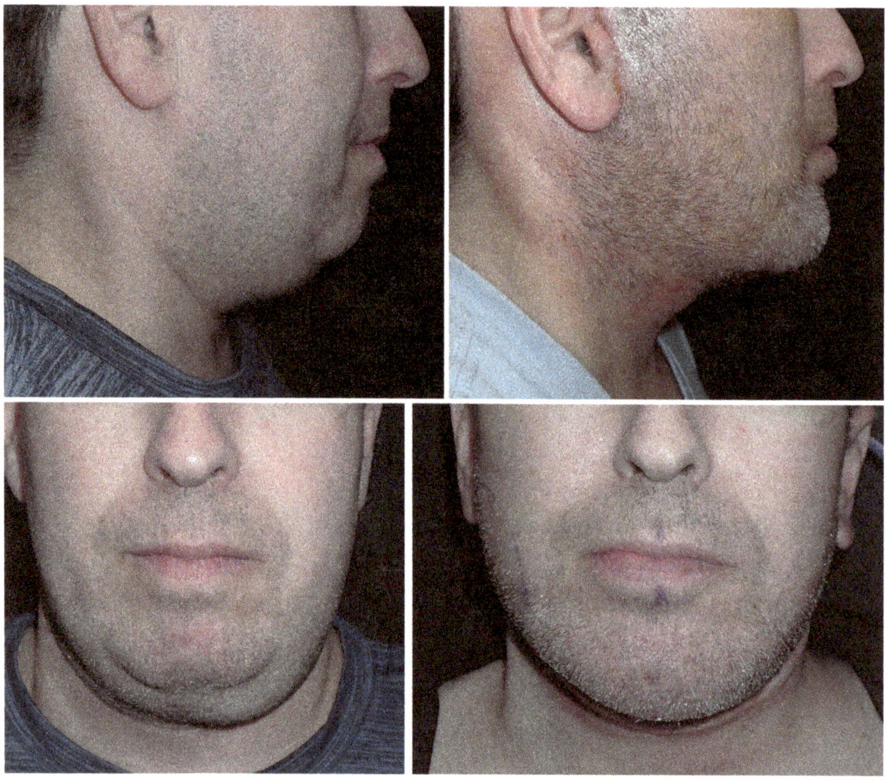

Fig. 6.189. This 50-year-old male is shown before and 5 days after deep plane facelift and neck lift and chin implant.

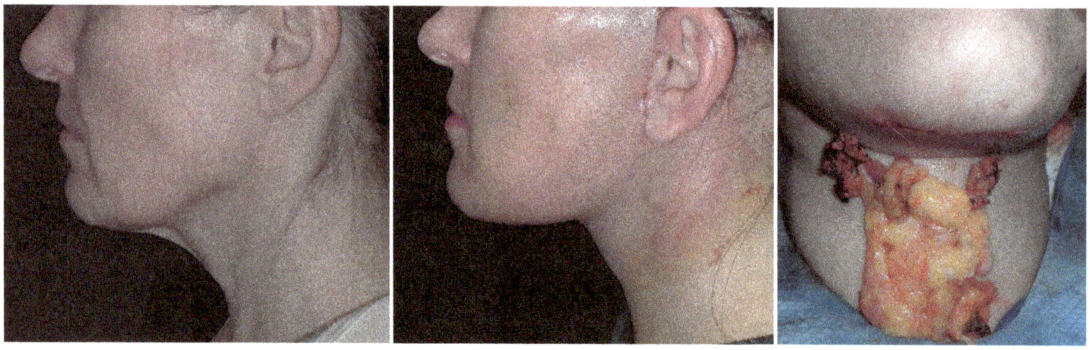

Fig. 6.190. This 56 year old female is shown 1 week after deep plane facelift with deep neck lift and submandibular gland reduction. The *right* image shows excised tissues.

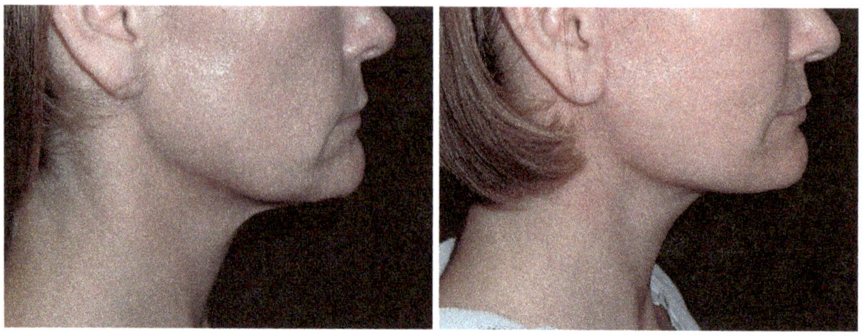

Fig. 6.191. This 47-year-old female is shown before and after facelift with SMASectomy.

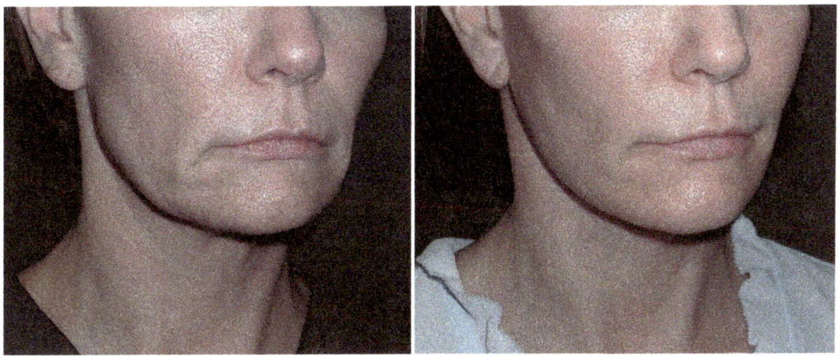

Fig. 6.192. The patient shown in Fig. 6.191 is shown in the right three-quarter view.

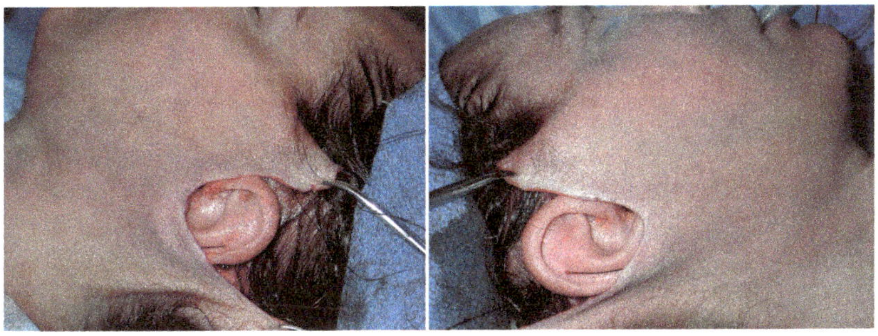

Fig. 6.193. These images is the same patient shown in Fig. 6.191 showing the intraoperative skin excess.

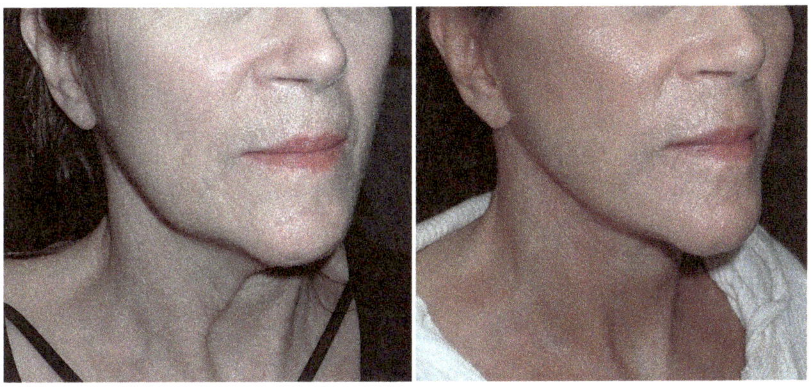

Fig. 6.194. This 72-year-old female is shown in the three-quarter view before and after deep plane facelift with deep neck lift.

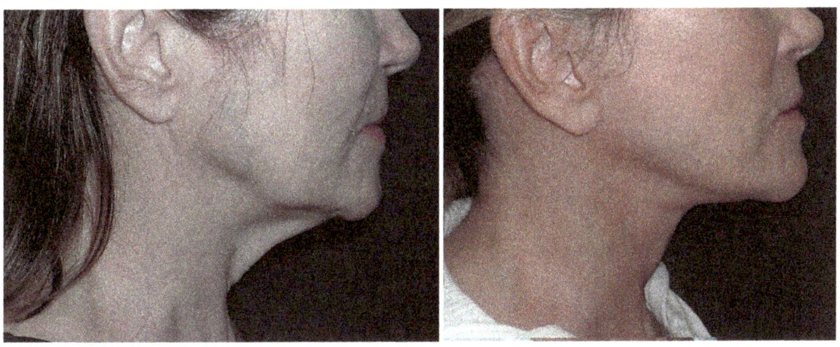

Fig. 6.195. This 72-year-old female shown in Fig. 6.194 is shown in the right lateral view before and after deep plane facelift with deep neck lift.

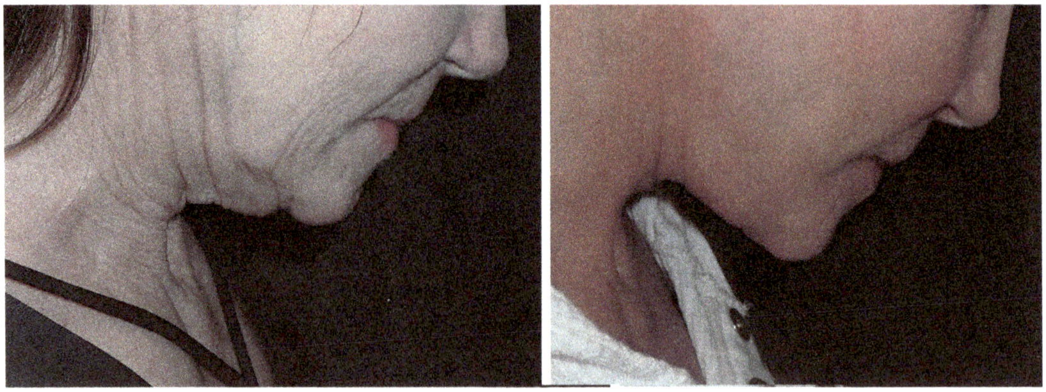

Fig. 6.196. This 72-year-old female shown in Fig. 6.194 is shown in the right downward view before and after deep plane facelift with deep neck lift.

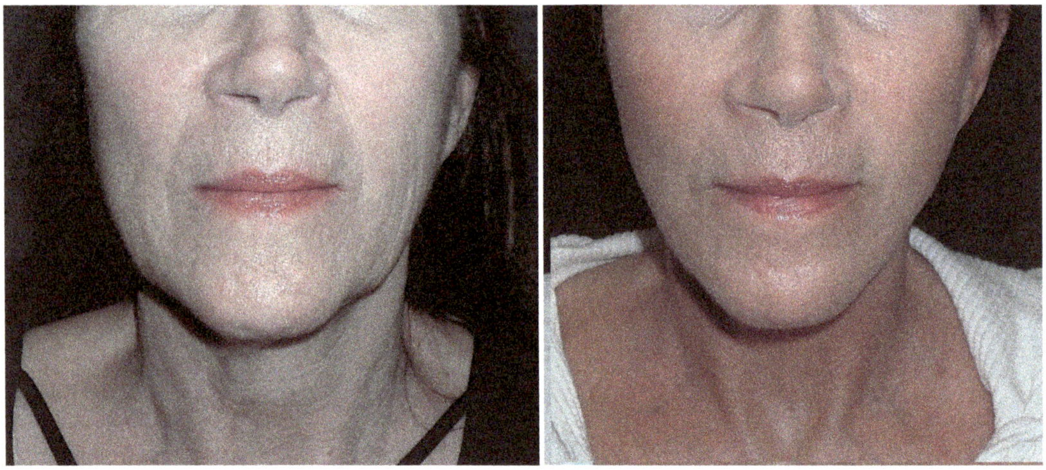

Fig. 6.197. This 72-year-old female shown in Fig. 6.194 is shown in the right frontal view before and after deep plane facelift with deep neck lift.

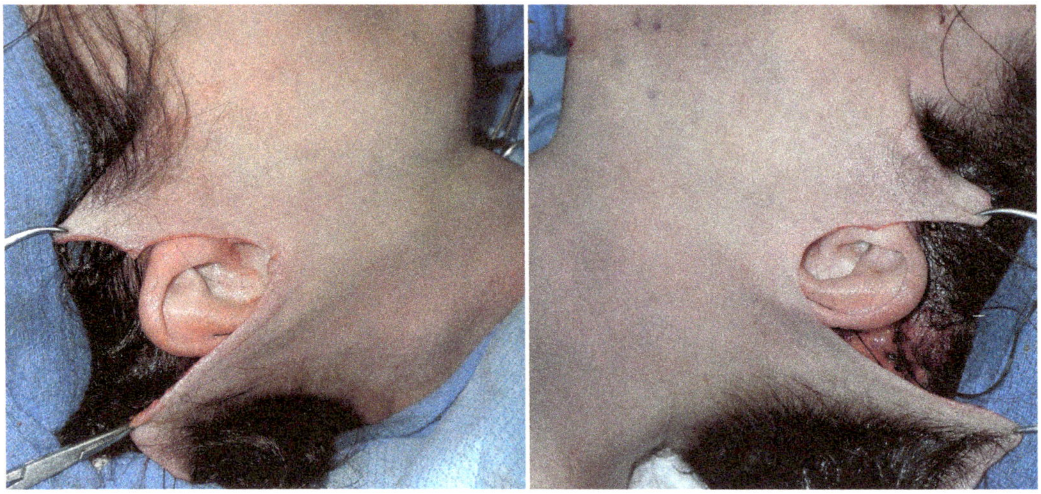

Fig. 6.198. This 72-year-old female shown in Fig. 6.194 is shown with the amount of intraoperative skin excess.

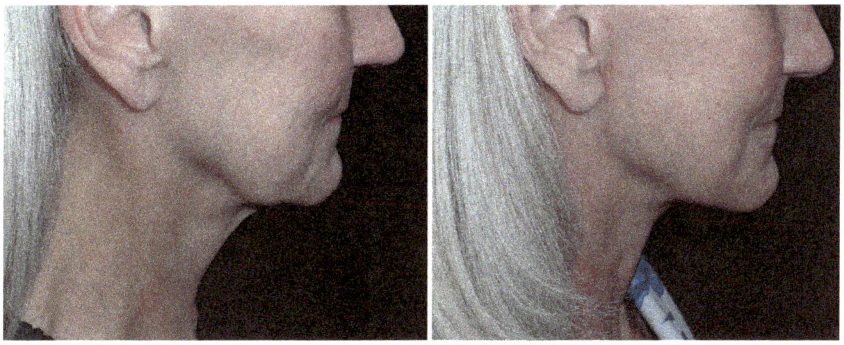

Fig. 6.199. This 69 year old female is shown before and after deep plane face and neck lift with submandibular gland reduction.

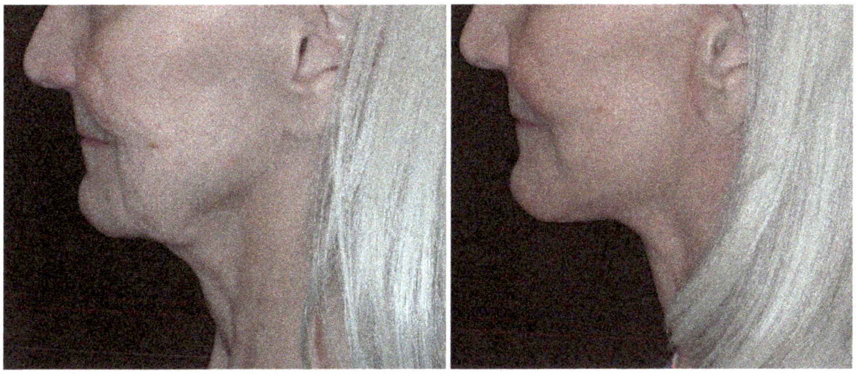

Fig. 6.200. The same patient shown in Fig. 6.199 is shown in the left lateral view.

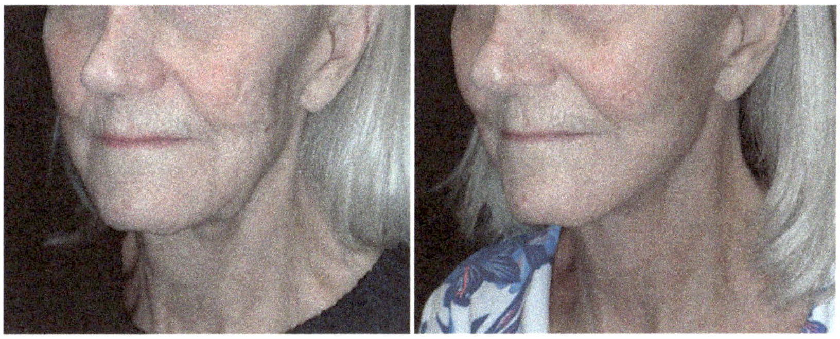

Fig. 6.201. The same patient shown in Fig. 6.199 is shown in the left ¾ view.

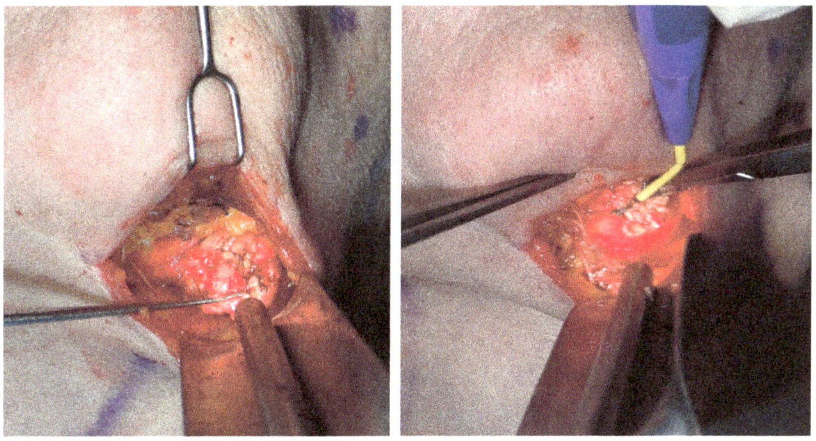

Fig. 6.202. These intraoperative images are from patient shown in Fig. 6.199. The *left* image shows her left submandibular gland exposed and the *right* image shows the gland being reduced with a Soniquence radiowave micro needle.

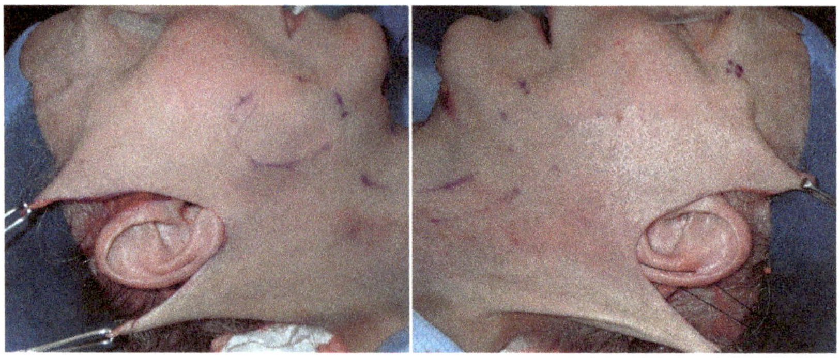

Fig. 6.203. This image shows the skin excess during surgery on the patient shown in Fig. 6.199.

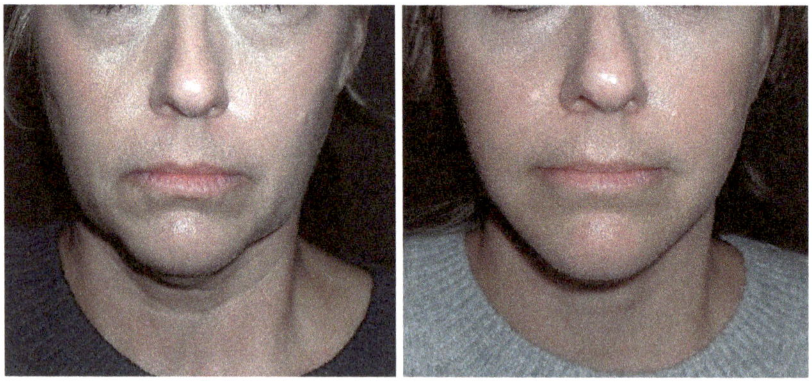

Fig. 6.204. This 57-year-old female is shown in the frontal view before and after deep plane facelift with deep neck lift.

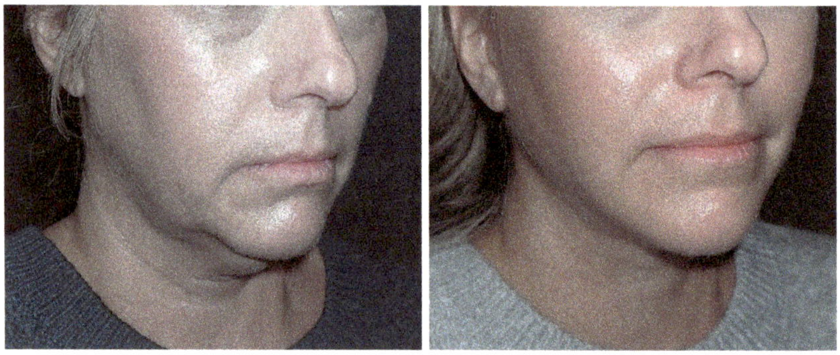

Fig. 6.205. The same patient shown in Fig. 6.204 in the right three-quarter view.

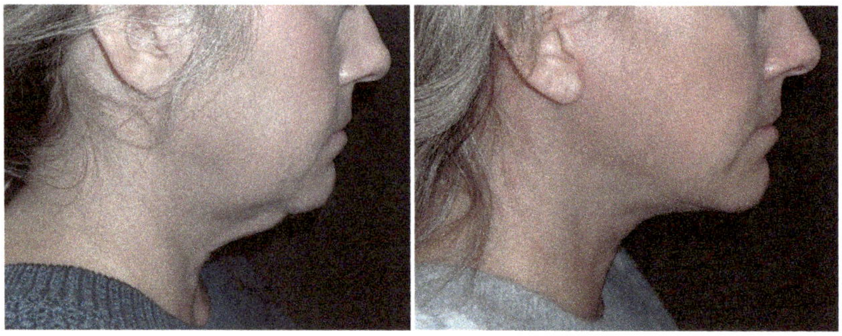

Fig. 6.206. The same patient shown in Fig. 6.204 is shown in the right lateral view.

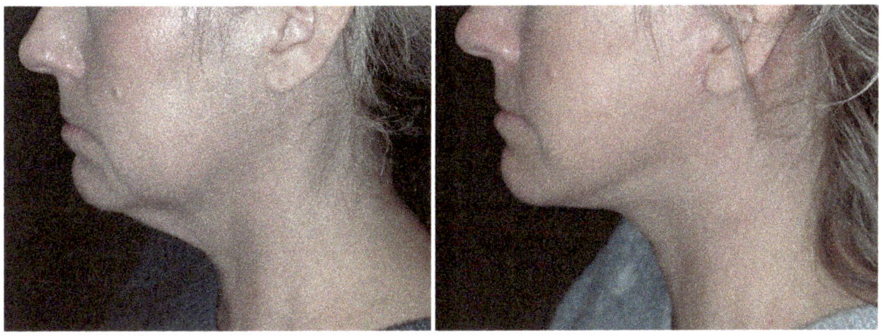

Fig. 6.207. The same patient shown in Fig. 6.204 is shown in the left lateral view.

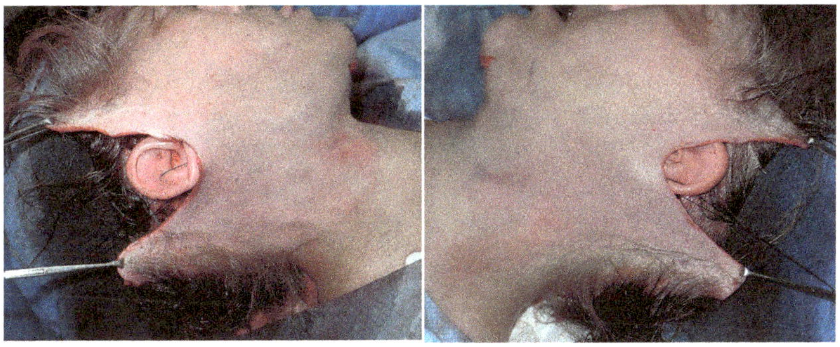

Fig. 6.208. The same patient shown in Fig. 6.204 is shown with the intraoperative skin excess.

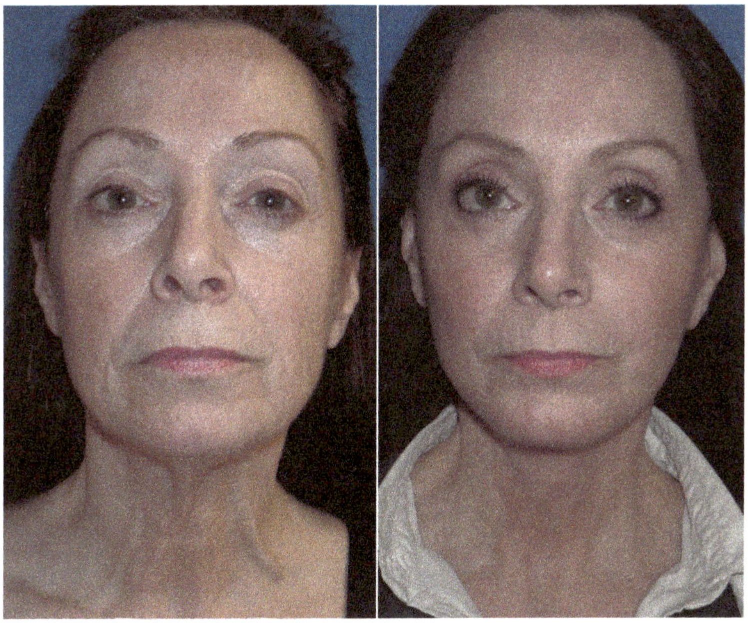

Fig. 6.209. This 52-year-old female underwent facelift and neck lift with SMASectomy and cheek and chin implants.

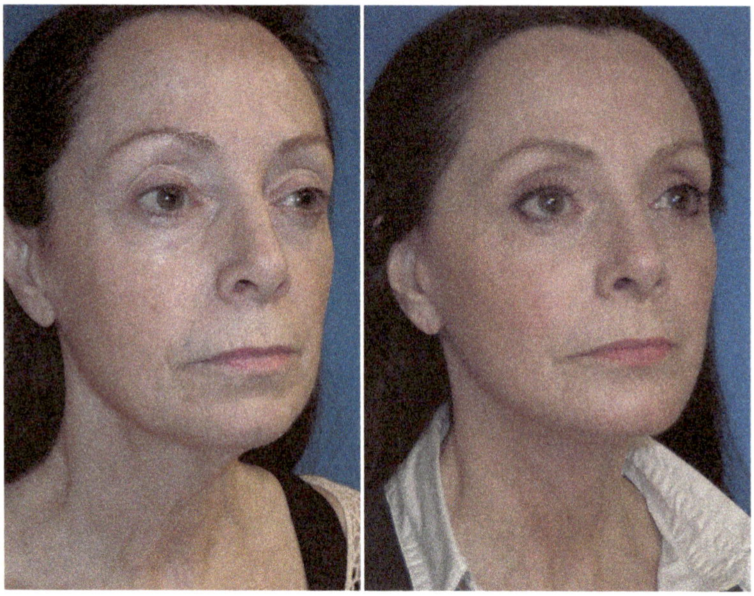

Fig. 6.210. The same patient shown in Fig. 6.209 is shown in right three-quarter view.

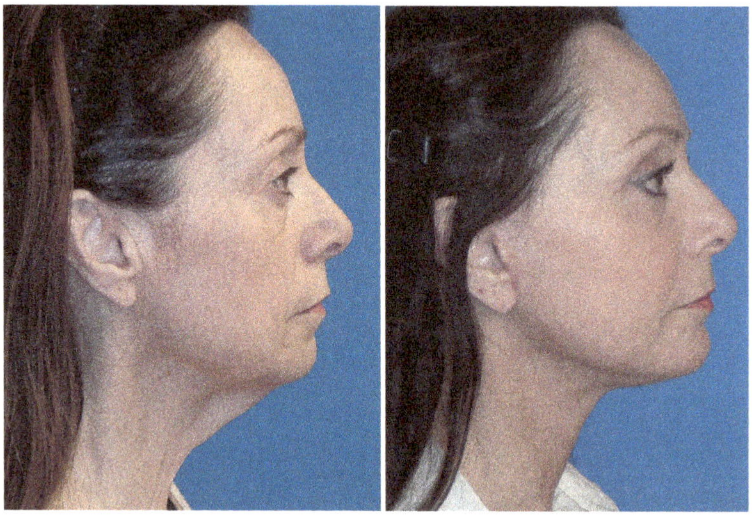

Fig. 6.211. The same patient shown in Fig. 6.209 is shown in right lateral view.

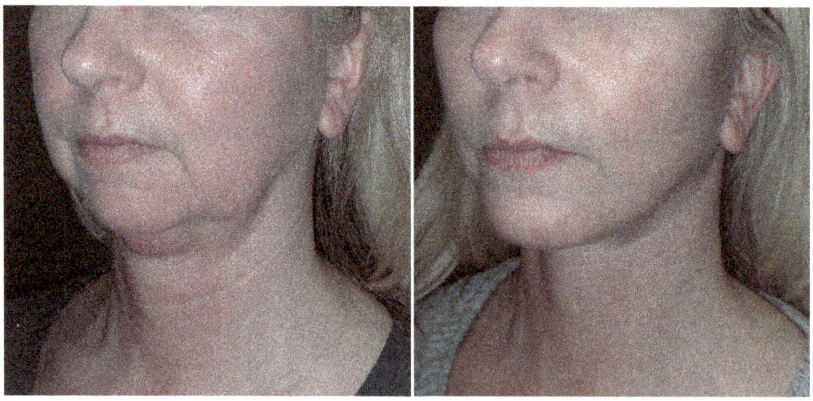

Fig. 6.212. This patient is shown in the left lateral view and underwent facelift and neck lift with SMASectomy and chin implant.

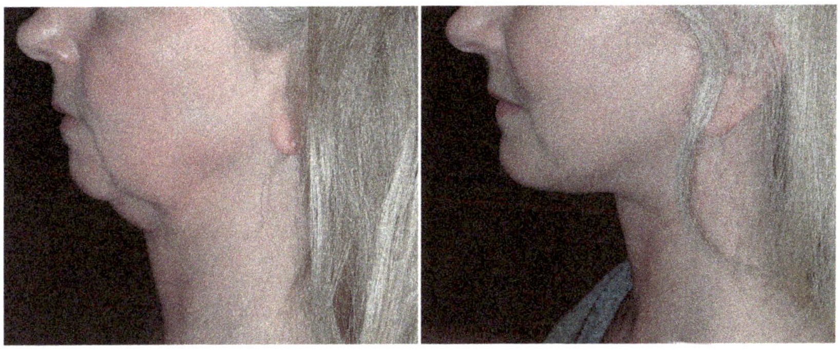

Fig. 6.213. The same patient shown in Fig. 6.212 is shown in the left three-quarter view.

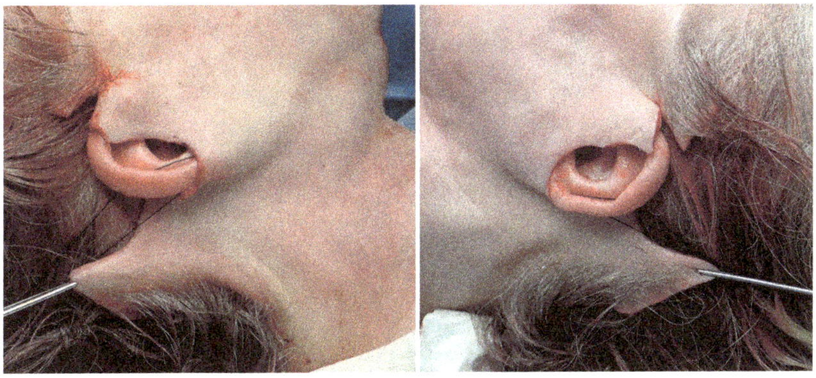

Fig. 6.214. The same patient shown in Fig. 6.212 is shown with the amount of intraoperative skin excess.

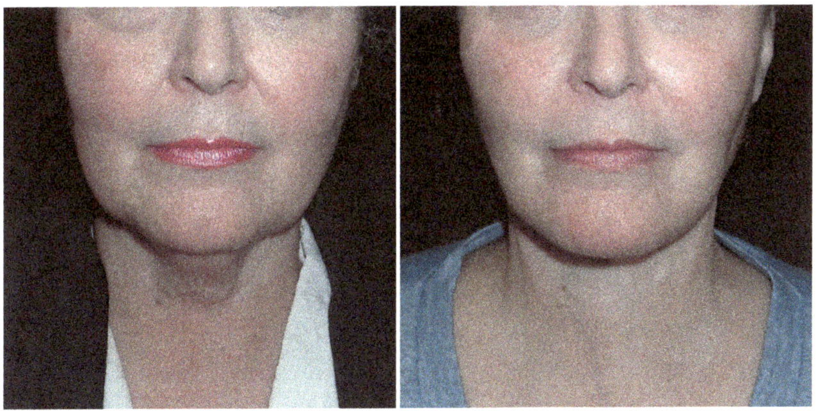

Fig. 6.215. This 64 year old female is shown before and after deep plane face and neck lift and buccal fat reduction.

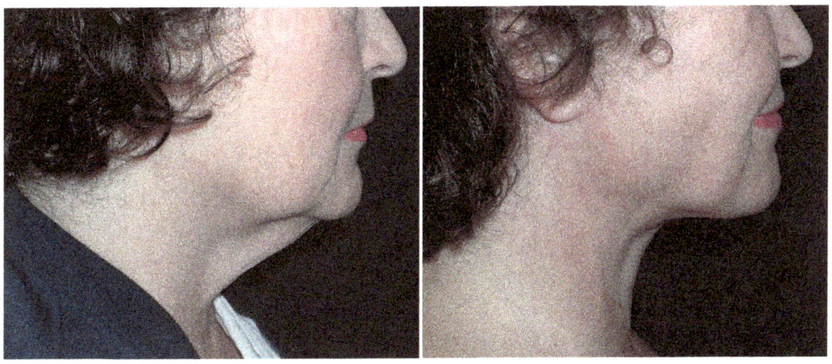

Fig. 6.216. The same patient shown in Fig. 6.215 is shown in the right lateral view.

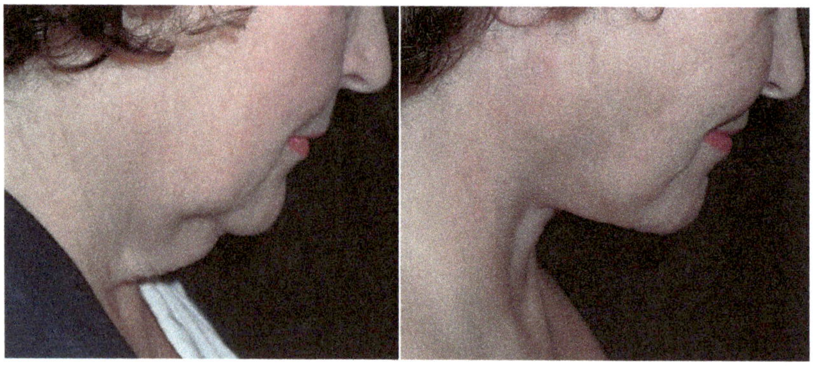

Fig. 6.217. The same patient shown in Fig. 6.215 is shown in the right lateral flexion view.

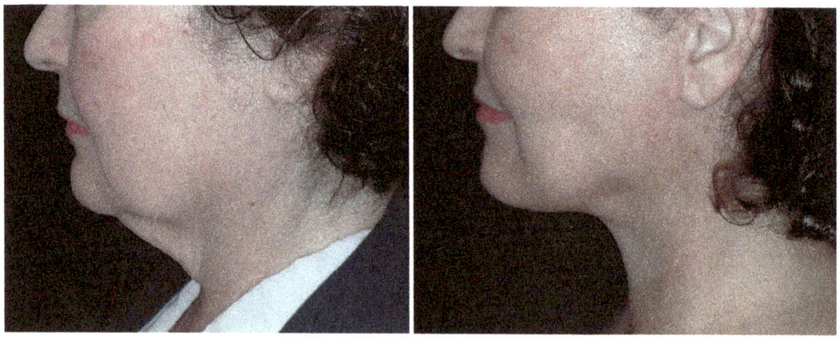

Fig. 6.218. The same patient shown in Fig. 6.215 is shown in the left lateral view.

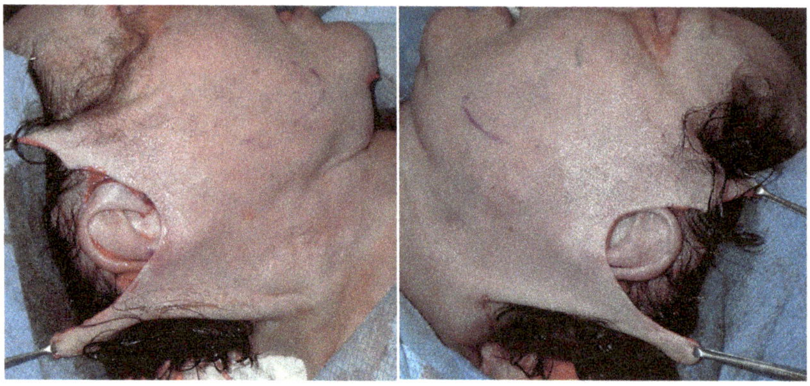

Fig. 6.219. The intraoperative skin excess of the patient shown in Fig. 6.215 is shown.

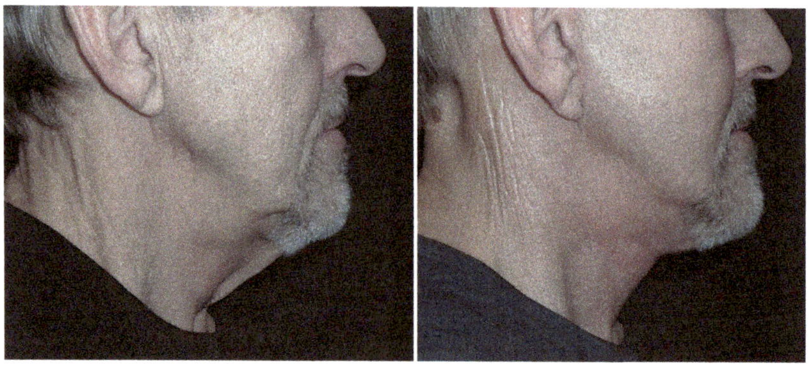

Fig. 6.220. This 69 year old male is shown before and after deep plane face and neck lift in the right lateral view.

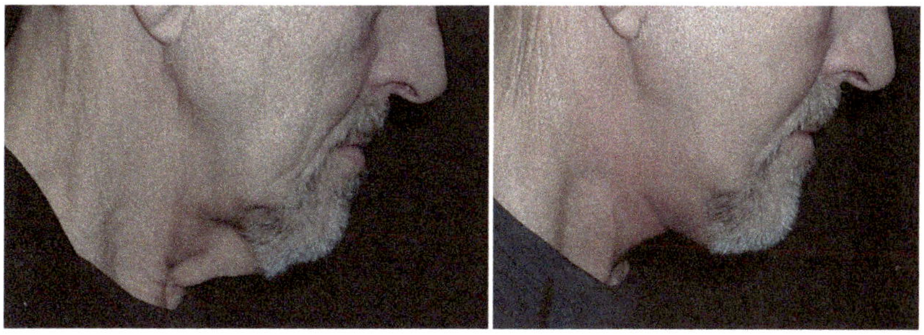

Fig. 6.221. The same patient shown in Fig. 6.220 is shown in the right flexion view.

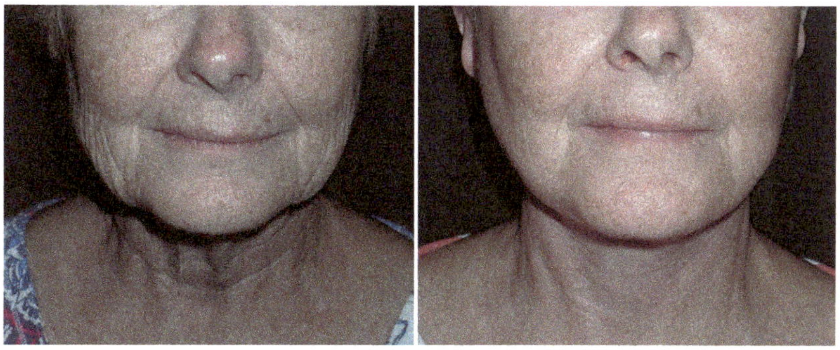

Fig. 6.222. This 72-year-old female underwent deep plane facelift with deep neck lift, buccal fat reduction, and perioral CO_2 laser resurfacing.

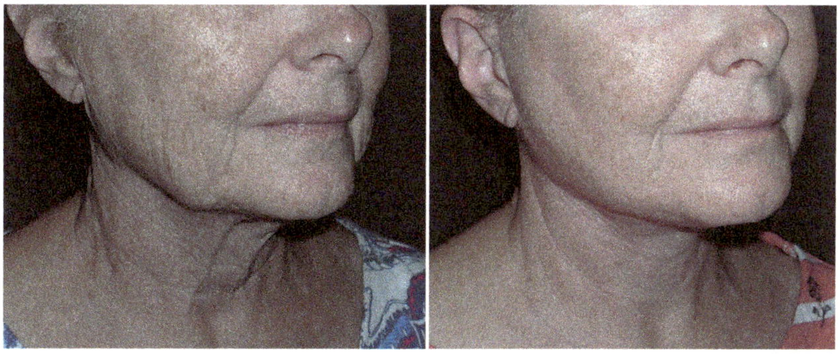

Fig. 6.223. The same patient shown in Fig. 6.222 is shown in the right three-quarter view.

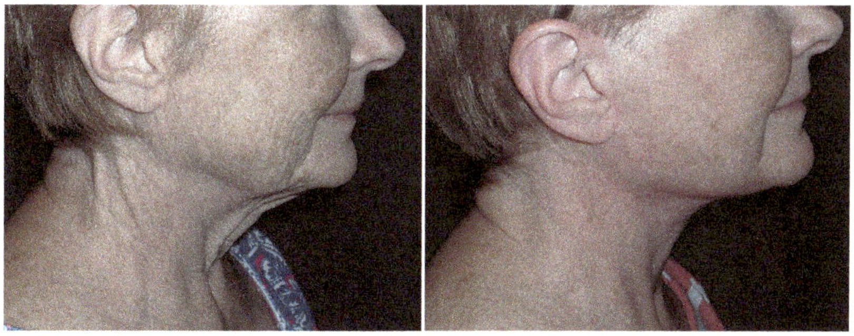

Fig. 6.224. The same patient shown in Fig. 6.222 is shown in the right lateral view.

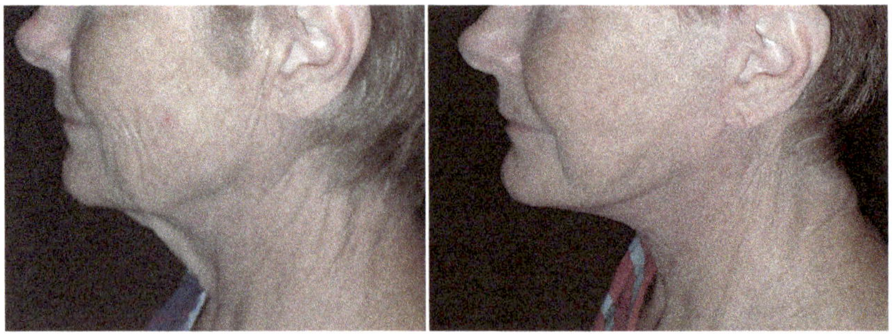

Fig. 6.225. The same patient shown in Fig. 6.222 is shown in the left lateral view.

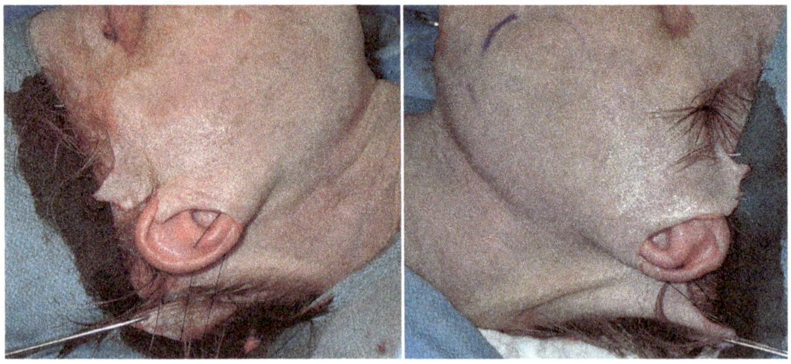

Fig. 6.226. The same patient shown in Fig. 6.222 is shown with the intraoperative skin excess.

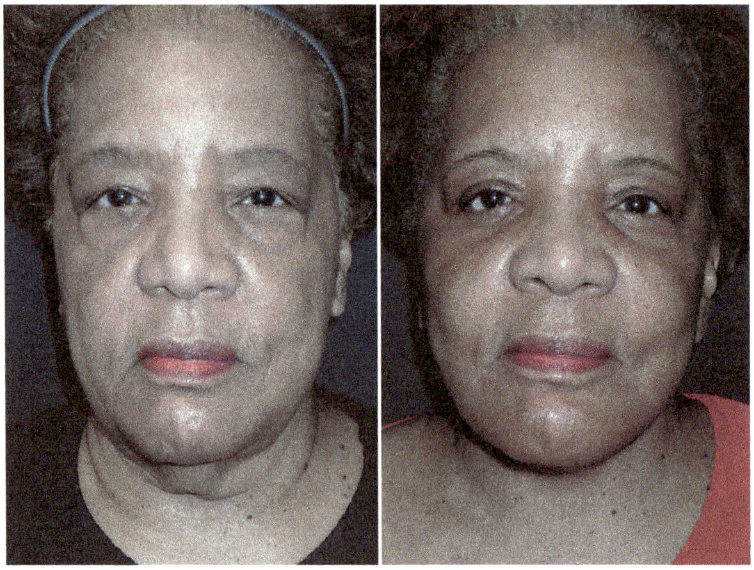

Fig. 6.227. This 68-year-old female underwent deep plane facelift and neck lift.

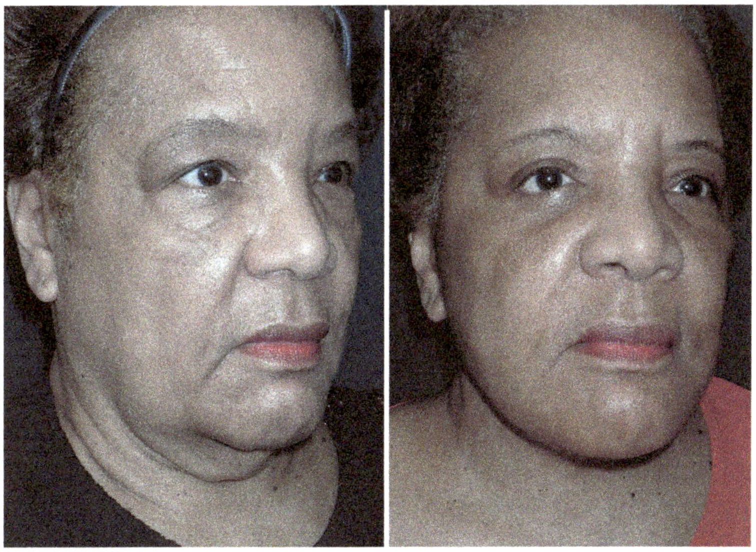

Fig. 6.228. The same patient shown in Fig. 6.227 is shown in the right three-quarter view.

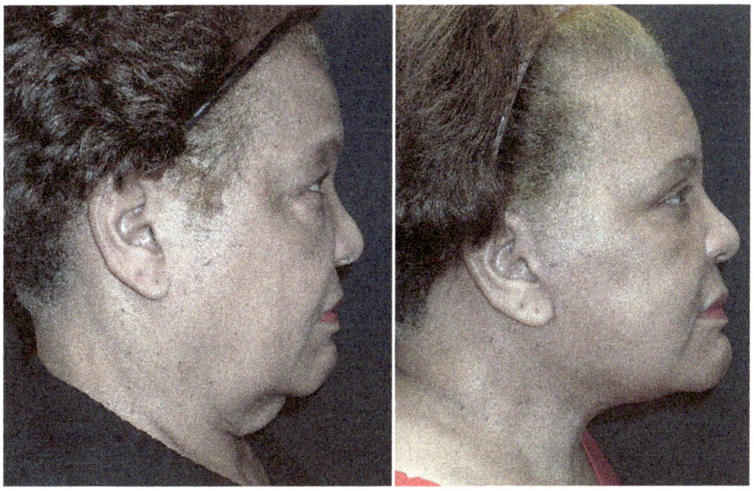

Fig. 6.229. The same patient shown in Fig. 6.227 is shown in the right lateral view.

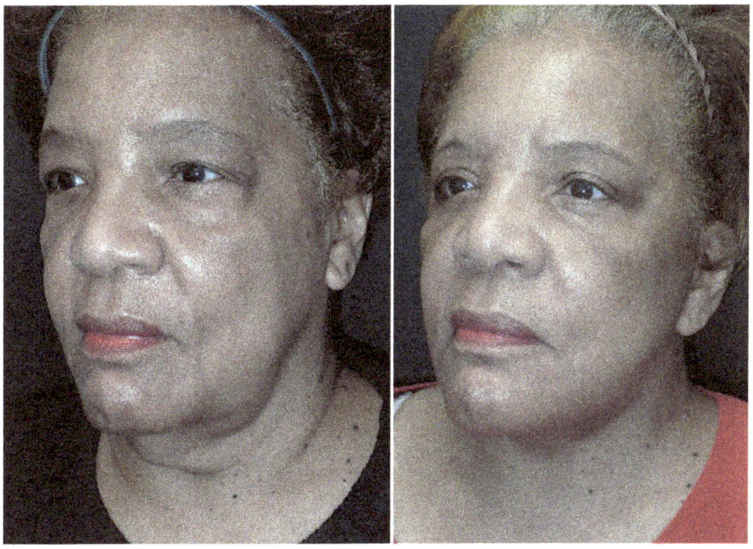

Fig. 6.230. The same patient shown in Fig. 6.227 is shown in the left three-quarter view.

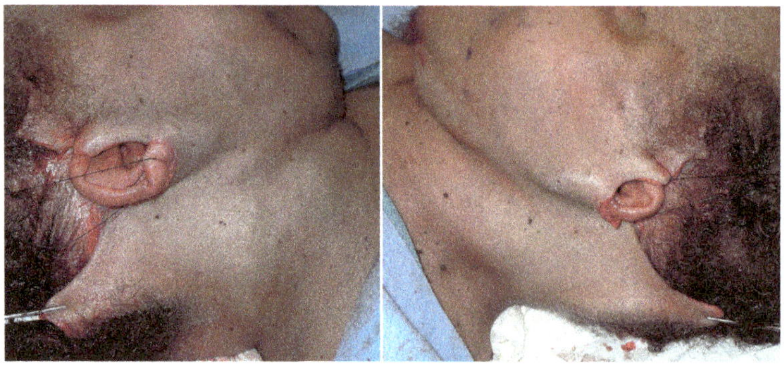

Fig. 6.231. The same patient shown in Fig. 6.227 is shown with the intraoperative skin excess.

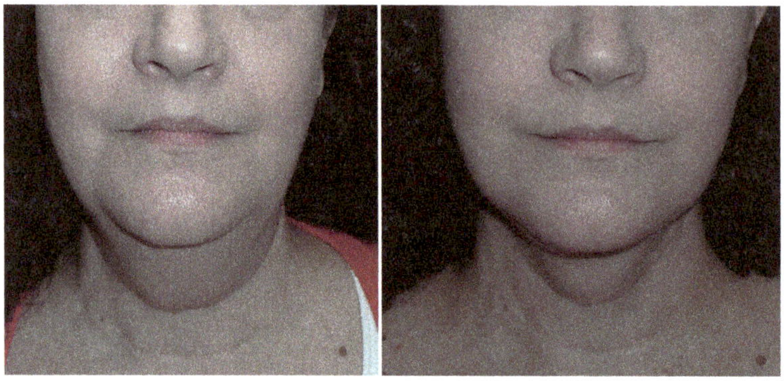

Fig. 6.232. This patient underwent facelift and neck lift with SMASectomy.

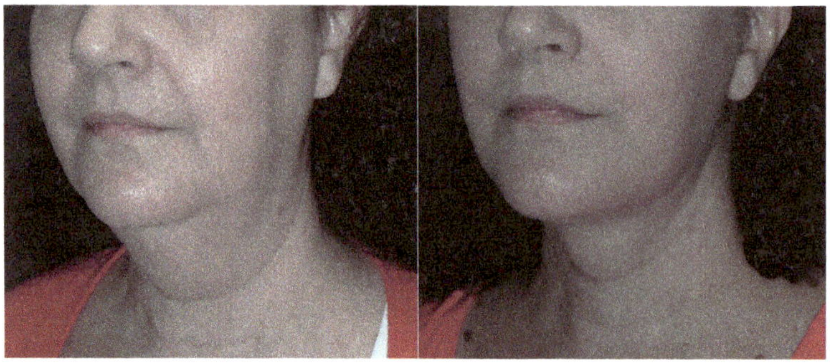

Fig. 6.233. The same patient shown in Fig. 6.232 is shown in the left three-quarter view.

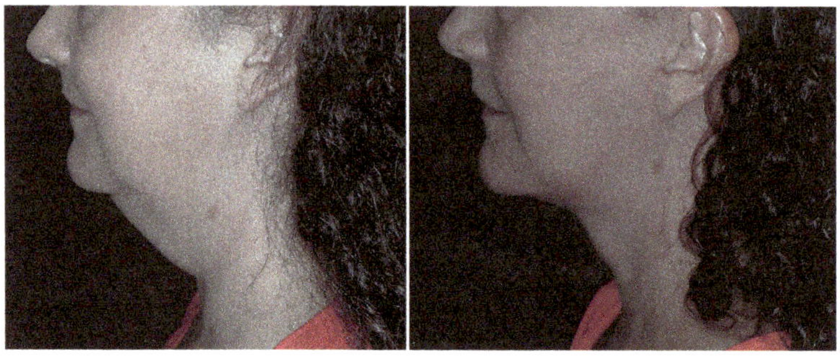

Fig. 6.234. The same patient shown in Fig. 6.232 is shown in the left lateral view.

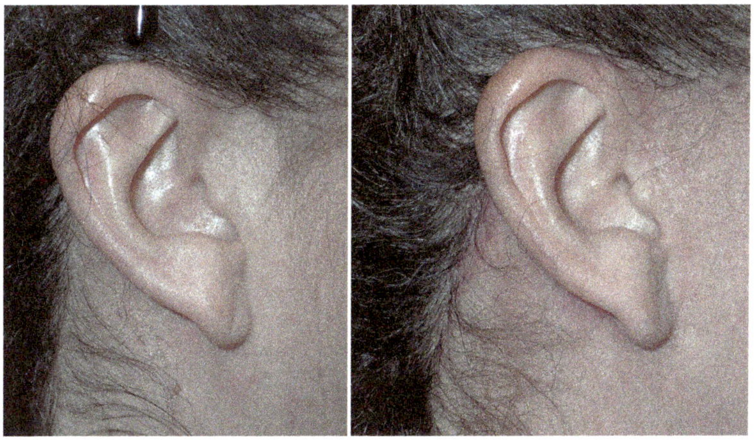

Fig. 6.235. This patient is shown with right side before (*left*) and after (*right*) incision scars.

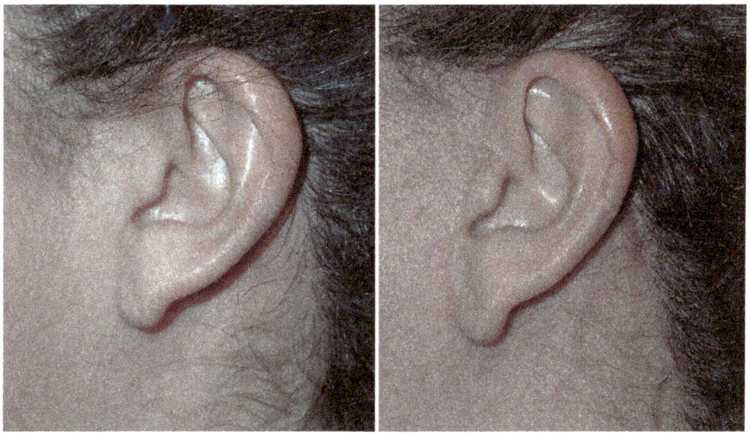

Fig. 6.236. This patient is shown with left side before (*left*) and after (*right*) incision scars.

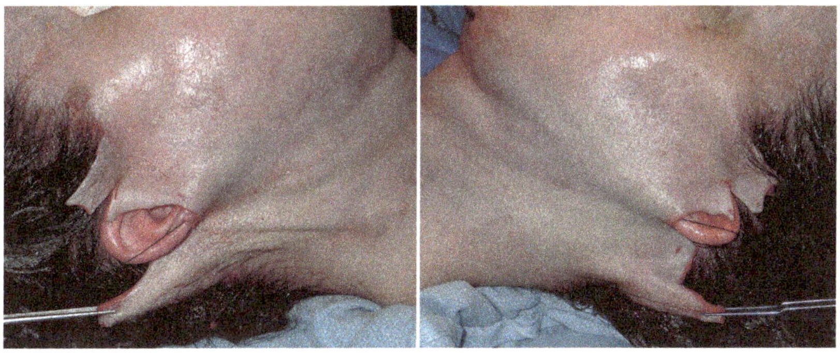

Fig. 6.237. The same patient shown in Fig. 6.232 is shown with the intraoperative skin excess.

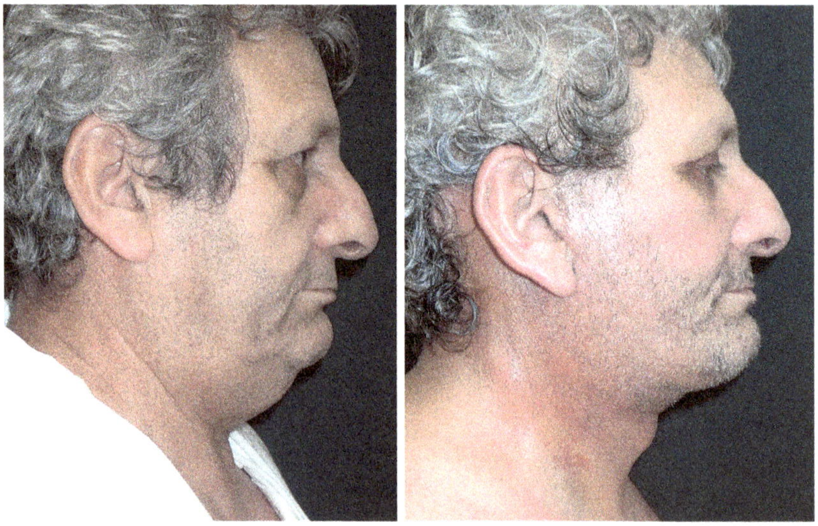

Fig. 6.238. This 63-year-old male is shown before and after deep plane facelift with deep neck lift.

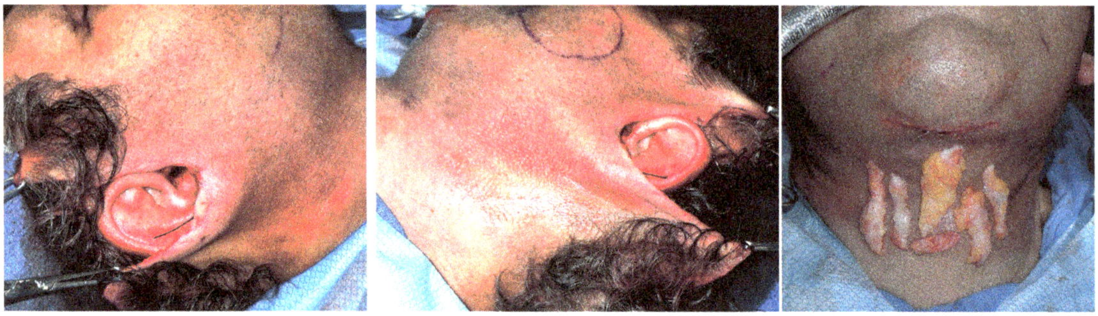

Fig. 6.239. This figure shows the introaperative skin excess on the patient shown in Fig. 6.238.

CHAPTER 7

Deep Plane Facelift and Deep Neck Lift

Laxmeesh Mike Nayak, Joe Niamtu, III

Chapter Outline

The goal of all facelift surgery is to powerfully, durably, and tastefully reposition the sagging tissues of the middle and lower thirds of the face. At its best, a facelift should eliminate jowls, improve midface ptosis, and improve the contours of the neck.

Various approaches to facelifting exist and are discussed in detail elsewhere in this book. All of them demonstrate meaningful jowl improvement; indeed, the jowls are a subcutaneous feature and seem to be the easiest aging face feature to improve. The lateral and anterior midface, however, is typically resistant to treatment with techniques that do not release the dense ligamentous attachments that resist repositioning of those areas (Fig. 7.1). Specifically, the zygomatic and upper masseteric ligaments tether the upper midface in place, making it resistant to improvement with superficial musculoaponeurotic system (SMAS) plication, imbrication, and limited sub-SMAS dissection lifts. Anteriorly extended sub-SMAS approaches, however, directly release these ligaments and allow for passive, natural, powerful midface repositioning.

Even the lower portion of the face can be lifted more naturally and more durably if the lifting is performed in the sub-SMAS plane, releasing the lower masseteric and platysma-auricular ligaments that inhibit repositioning of the lower facial

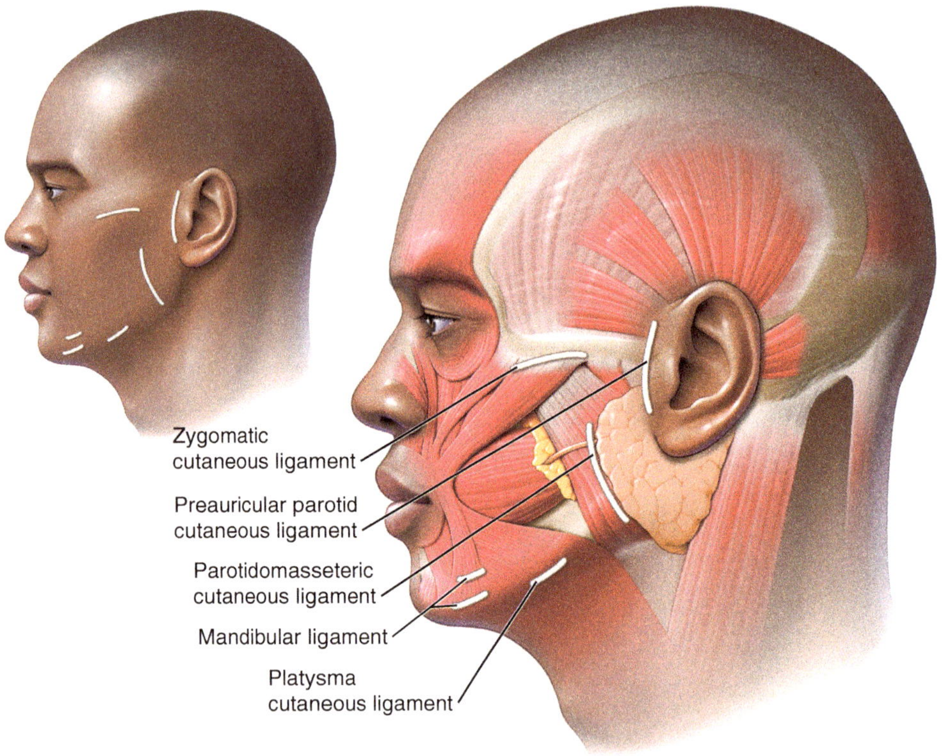

Fig. 7.1. The deep plane facelift addresses the zygomatic and masseteric ligaments in subsuperficial musculoaponeurotic system plane and the mandibular ligament in the subcutaneous plane.

tissues. The final major ligament that must be released for excellent results is the mandibular ligament. Unlike the others, it must be released in the subcutaneous plane, which may be done from the submental incision, if present, or from the lateral approach after deep plane dissection has been performed.

Although subtleties exist, it is practical to consider the SMAS plane as a single, contiguous sheet of fibromuscular tissue that invests the head and neck. The sheet comprises the platysma, lower-face SMAS, orbicularis, temporoparietal fascia, and frontooccipitalis. Many anatomists refer to all of these structures as "layer 3," and the potential space beneath them is described as "layer 4." Sub-SMAS lifting is performed in layer 4 (Fig. 7.2).

In the lateral face and neck, the platysma, lower facial SMAS (including remnants of the platysma along and over the jawline), and orbicularis components of the SMAS are best defined and easiest to identify. The lower-face SMAS, in particular, is relatively easy to raise in layer 4, with the parotidomasseteric fascia serving as an easily identified floor. Many so-called "deep plane" or "SMAS flap" lifts are performed in the sub-SMAS plane in the lower part of the face, but transition to supra-SMAS/supraorbicularis in the midface, leaving the midface SMAS and orbicularis down. These lifts are most effective in the jawline and jowl but offer minimal mechanical advantage in the midface region.

The "high SMAS" technique remains in layer 4 and incorporates the SMAS of the midface as well, up to the level of the midpoint of the zygoma. The advantage is by lifting from that high in the face, lifting power is extended to the anterior malar region. A relative disadvantage of this technique is that a large skin flap is raised first, and the SMAS is raised as a second, independent flap starting just anterior to the ear. The SMAS in this region is thin, delicate, and densely adherent to the parotid. Dissection of this posterior/superior SMAS is tedious and does nothing in particular to contribute to enhanced mobility of the anterior/inferior facial tissues, where ptosis is most clinically important. Finally, this elevation of the high/posterior SMAS, although safe in expert hands, is performed in close proximity to the temporal branch of the facial nerve. This adds risk but no particular cosmetic benefit over the lift described below.

The suborbicularis deep plane (SO-deep) lift provides the high vector and midface control of the high SMAS lift, plus the full mobility from anteriorly extended sub-SMAS ligament release, all while being safer due to the design of the SMAS entry. It is also technically easier to execute because the deep SMAS flap is left attached to the skin while it is being raised (although it may optionally be delaminated afterward if desired). When the entire skin flap is raised first, as with a high SMAS lift, there is often minimal SMAS integrity left down to elevate a robust SMAS flap, especially in the superior/posterior section of the flap. Leaving the SMAS attached to the overlying skin during dissection allows even thin-SMAS faces to be safely and easily dissected in the sub-SMAS plane. Unlike with a basic deep plane lift, the lateral portion of the orbicularis oculi muscle is raised and repositioned by the SO-deep lift, which provides a fascial-layer lift of the anterior malar region. The orbicularis myopexy also enhances lower eyelid support. This effect is so powerful that the authors recommend that if transconjunctival

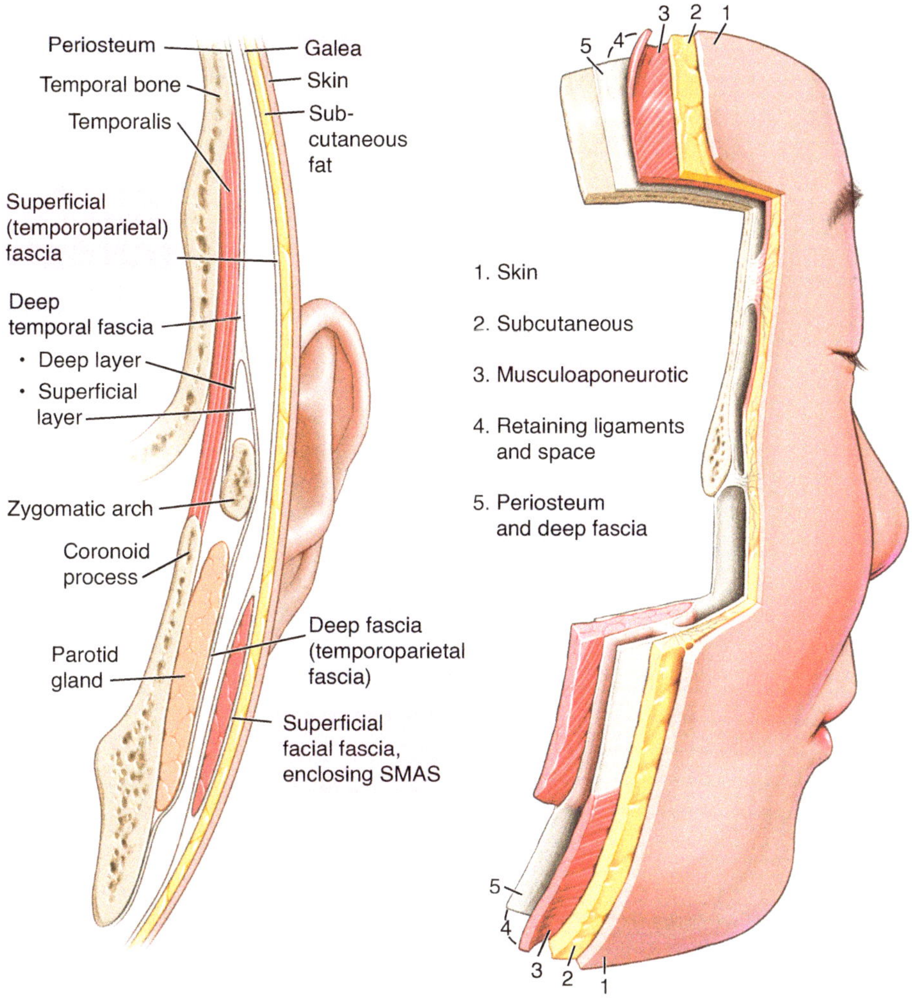

Fig. 7.2. The so-called "layer 4" is best shown as "Number 4" on the *upper right* image. This is the where potential space and retaining ligaments lie in the subSMAS layer.

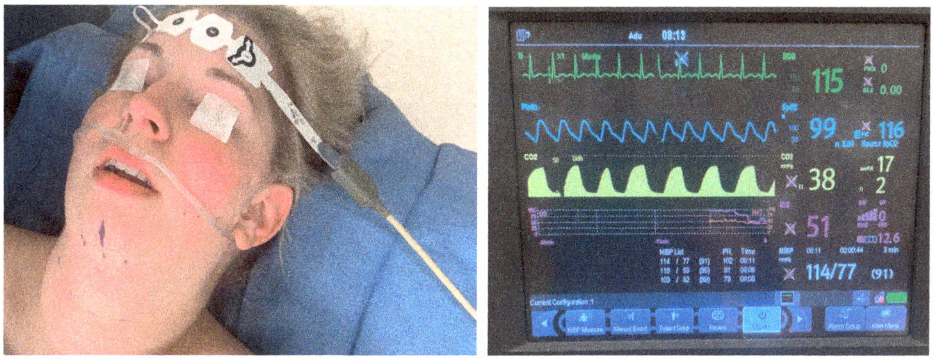

Fig. 7.3. The Bispectral Index monitoring defines the anesthetic plane of the patient throughout the case.

blepharoplasty is planned, it should be done before the SO-deep facelift, while the lid is easily distracted. Anesthesia for this procedure, as performed by the author (MN) is, propofol/ketamine sedation with Bispectral Index monitoring (Fig. 7.3).

Anesthesia

The patient is taken to the operating room, positioned supine, with pressure points padded and pneumatic boots placed, and anesthesia is induced. Deep sedation or general anesthesia without paralysis (to allow for monitoring of electrocautery facial nerve stimulation) are both acceptable options, in each case with a Foley catheter to monitor fluid status and prevent hypertension from bladder fullness. Due to the time-consuming nature of the procedure and the extreme sensitivity of the submandibular glands, local anesthesia alone or with light sedation is unlikely to be adequate for safe, comfortable surgery.

The senior author (MN) prefers a modified Friedberg PK-BIS deep sedation technique. Due to the length of the surgery, in a deviation from Friedberg's protocol, propofol/ketamine sedation with Bispectral Index monitoring is complemented with 2 mg of midazolam at the case outset. Long infusions of propofol eventually fill muscle stores, prolonging the typically short time to emergence from propofol sedation. The addition of midazolam at the beginning of the case decreases the total propofol requirement, and midazolam may also be reversed in recovery if needed with flumazenil. In addition to routine intravenous antibiotics, additional routine premedications are administered prior to the ketamine bolus aiming to decrease the tendency for laryngeal hyperreactivity common in the first 20 minutes after a ketamine bolus. They include 50 mg of intravenous lidocaine to decrease laryngeal reactivity and 0.2 mg glycopyrrolate to help dry secretions.

Once the premedications have been given and the midazolam bolus with propofol infusion have achieved a steady-state BIS reading of 45–60, a Foley catheter is placed. The patient is then dissociated with a 50 mg ketamine bolus. Propofol is titrated to maintain the BIS in the 50s. In the 3 minutes necessary for full N-methyl-D-aspartate blockade ketamine dissociation, the patient is sterilely prepped with betadine on the skin and benzalkonium chloride (BAK) in the hair, and sterilely draped. The operative field is then tumesced with 0.075% lidocaine, 1:500,000 epinephrine, and 0.1% tranexamic acid (TXA) solution (750 mg lidocaine, 1000 mg TXA, 2 cc 1:1000 epinephrine added to 1 L of normal saline). Usually 350–500 mL of solution is required to adequately tumesce the face and neck, with additional solution being appropriate for tumescing the brow or fat donor sites if indicated. If local anesthesia infiltration requires more than about 20 minutes, it may be necessary to administer a second, 25 mg bolus of ketamine to complete infiltration.

The tumescent anesthetic is an important part of this procedure, as the infused volume makes planes more obvious, and the fluid serves as a heat sink to protect motor nerves from thermal injury. Cautery should be low during this portion of the case, on the order of 15–18 watts.

Incision design is largely surgeon preference. The SO-deep lift can be performed with any of the common periauricular facelift incision patterns. Due to the powerful midface lifting effect, this lift can generate significant temporal skin excess. Temporal hairline trichophytic incision designs are generally preferred to prevent lifting of the sideburn (Fig. 7.4). Similarly, a browlift may need to be considered to prevent "crowding" in the temple soft tissue that can occur when a ptotic brow tail is not addressed.

The deep plane entry incision is planned from the lateral orbital rim (which is well anterior to course of temporal branch of the facial nerve over the zygoma) to the angle of mandible (which is posterior to the eventual parotid exit of marginal mandibular branch of the facial nerve) (Fig. 7.4). The deep plane incision then turns inferiorly along the anterior border of the sternocleidomastoid (SCM) at least 4–6 cm to release platysma/auricular ligament to provide maximum passive facial lifting.

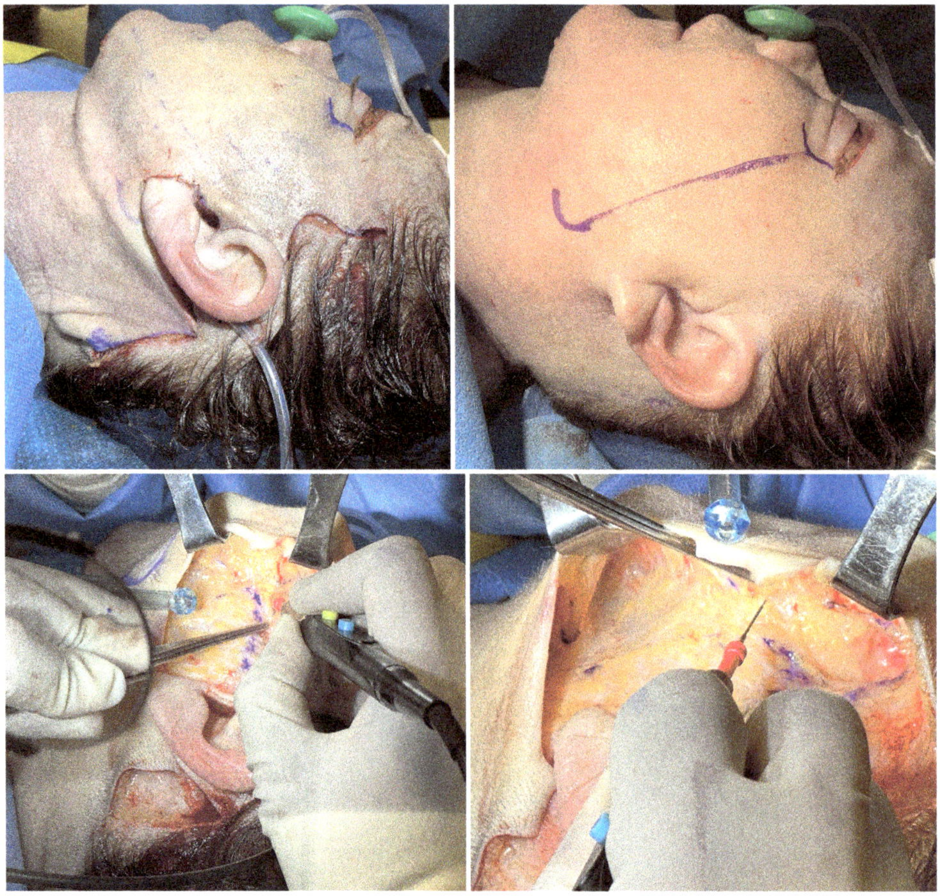

Fig. 7.4. The *top* images show the skin incision used with this technique (*top left*), and the *top right* image shows a marking where the SMAS entry point will be. The *lower* images show the SMAS entry and electrocautery dissection.

The SO-deep lift begins by elevating a skin flap raised to just beyond the deep plane entry line. The skin is left attached to SMAS from there forward, as well as along jawline, so that radial (outward) traction on the flap also pulls on the SMAS, which helps demonstrate and emphasize the sub-SMAS plane.

Deep plane entry begins by incising the SMAS over the angle of the mandible, where platysma is most robust and easily identified. The surgical assistant uses two Army Navy retractors, toeing in and strongly lifting the skin flap away from parotid. Low-current cautery is used to broadly incise the flap over the lower third of the face while the assistant and scrub tech watch for nerve stimulation. The tumescent lidocaine does not seem to inhibit twitching, though higher concentrations and systemic muscle relaxation may. As the incision is developed, one can usually identify the pink/gray/purple fibers of platysma as they are incised to enter the loose areolar plane between SMAS/platysma and parotidomasseteric fascial floor of the dissection. Once this area has been opened broadly, gentle vertical spreading with scissors or a Trepsat dissector easily opens the potential space (Fig. 7.5).

It is imperative that the parotidomasseteric fascia is not violated and left down, covering (the often visible) buccal and marginal branches of the facial nerve. The spreading dissection end point is just anterior to the masseter, which completes disruption of the lower masseteric ligaments. There is no benefit to dissect further but doing so does put the terminal branches of the facial nerve at risk.

Attention is then turned to creating the upper extent of the SMAS incision, over the malar eminence. As that incision is made, one can usually see the pink/purple fibers of lateral orbicularis muscle being incised, then the opening potential space between orbicularis and malar periosteum. Again, the surgical team aids the dissection with strong radial/outward tension and careful surveillance for nerve stimulation. Once the plane has been entered, blunt spreads of the Trepsat open it anteriorly to the lateral nose. The surgeon will feel the tight, restrictive zygomatic ligaments inferior to this tunnel, especially the main ligament at the origin of zygomaticus major.

To complete the sub-SMAS dissection and ligamentous release, one Army Navy retractor is placed into each of the two previously created sub-SMAS pockets, and the flap is retracted. The SMAS incision is continued to connect upper and lower pockets, and dissection is carried forward in the sub-SMAS plane. A loose areolar tissue plane is definitely present and visible, though not as apparent as in the upper and lower pockets. The zygomaticus major can often be palpated and/or seen in the floor of the dissection. There is no need to skeletonize the muscle or carry the dissection more than 1.5 cm forward over the muscle. Doing either risks creating at least temporary smile dysfunction. The plane of dissection *must* remain superficial to zygomaticus major to protect the all-important zygomatic branch of the facial nerve. The surgeon should utilize the superior and inferior pocket planes as a guide and work from known to unknown. The final step of release is the zygomatic ligament itself, which should be performed immediately under the SMAS flap, rather than deep, near the zygomaticus major and the zygomatic branch of the facial nerve.

Next, the SMAS is undermined under the bare platysma along the anterior border of the SCM, which is both superficial to the deep cervical fascia and posterior to marginal mandibular nerve's exit from the parotid. The platysma is then released from the anterior border of the SCM for 4–6 cm with scissors or cautery, little by little, under direct vision, to protect the external jugular vein. This step completely releases the platysma-auricular ligament (Fig. 7.6, *left*).

Attention is turned back to the lateral face, and the skin is freed from the edge of the SMAS flap as needed just enough to create a 1 cm cuff (Fig. 7.6, *right*). The skin for about 3 cm over the mandible border is also released from the SMAS flap to connect to subcutaneous neck dissection. At this point, one may also ensure that the mandibular ligament has been completely released in the subcutaneous plane. If this skin and ligament are not free, it will be nearly impossible to access the submental neck at the end of the case, after both SMAS flaps have been secured.

The SMAS is now draped under moderate tension in a 60- to 75-degree superior/posterior vector. The redundant portion of SMAS overlapping the parotid anterior to the lobule and tragus may be designed into an inferiorly based SMAS transposition flap. Inset begins at the angle of the mandible, securing the SMAS flap edge to the SMAS overlying the parotid. SMAS repositioning and lifting is continued toward the malar eminence with a running 2-0 Vicryl progressive tension suture (Fig. 7.7, *left*). As the superior end of the incision is reached, one may need to change

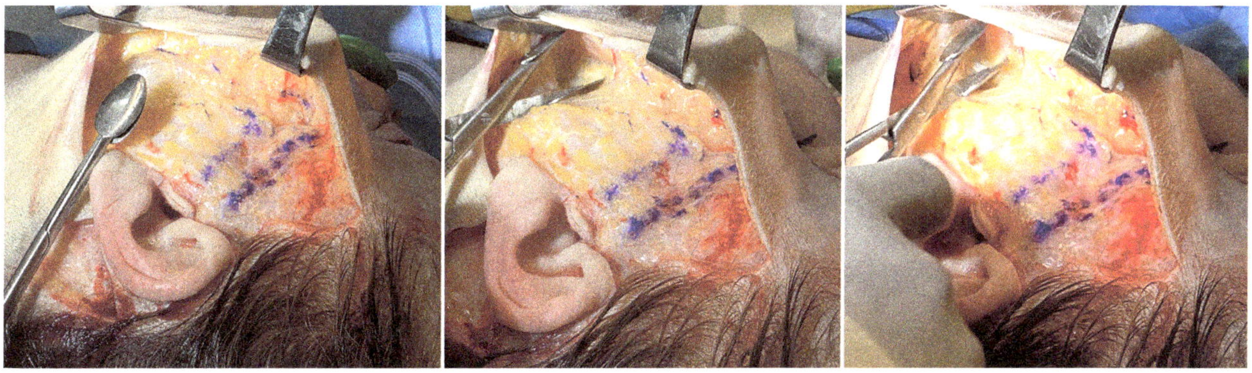

Fig. 7.5. These images show the Trepsat dissector spreading the loose areolar plane between the SMAS and parotidomasseteric fascia.

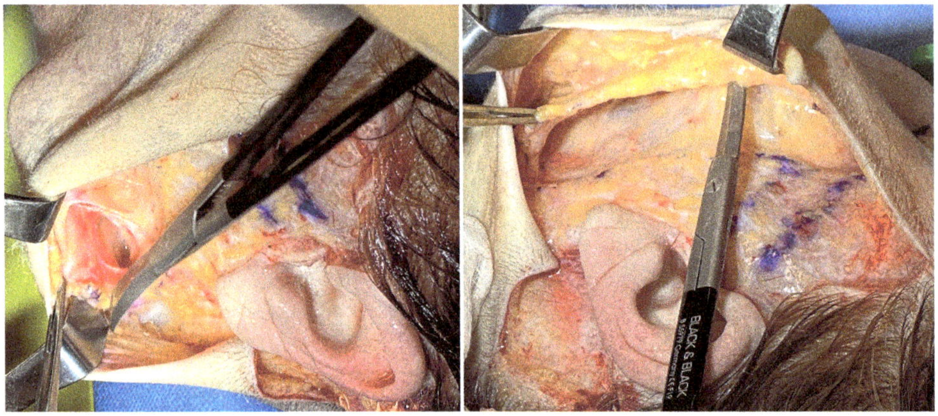

Fig. 7.6. The *left* image shows the undermined platysma along the border of the sternocleidomastoid muscle, and the *right* image illustrates the SMAS cuff.

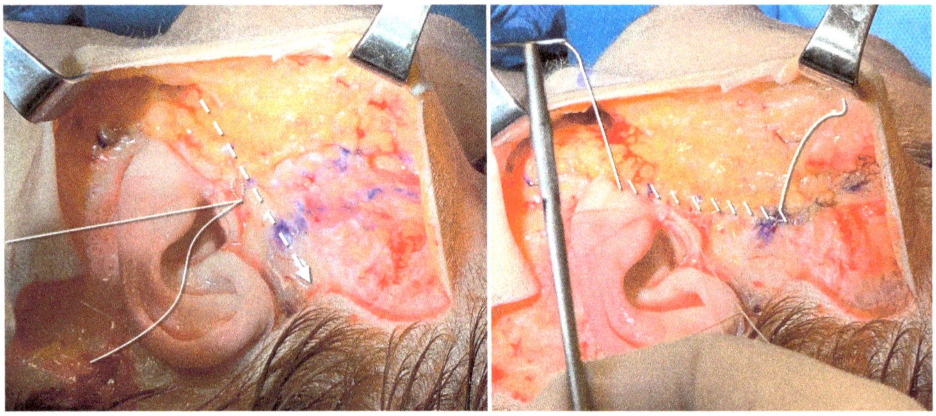

Fig. 7.7. The SMAS is draped in a superior posterior vector. The *dashed arrow* indicates posterior/lateral vector of pull. The *right* image shows a second layer of closure.

the angle of SMAS tension to 45 or 30 degrees (more posteriorly) to prevent lower lid bunching. The same suture is then used to run a second layer of strength back to starting point at angle of mandible, where the suture is tied (Fig. 7.7, *right*).

This second layer of closure does not create additional lifting, but is useful in settling down any small bumps and creates a second layer of support to prevent the SMAS from being torn with mouth opening, facial expression, and similar stresses. The SMAS transposition flap, if created, is transposed behind the lobule and secured to the mastoid. No additional tension is placed on this flap, as doing so will make closure of the infrahyoid platysma impossible. The purpose of the flap is not to create additional tension at rest. Instead, it creates dynamic tension in the chin down head position. The mastoid rises relative to the hyoid as the head pivots on the atlantoaxial angle, and the SMAS flap auto-tensions the hyoid angle at that position only.

The procedure concludes by a final hemostasis check of both sides of the face and of the neck. If a deep neck lift (see later in this chapter) has been performed, a drain is placed from a left postauricular stab and run subcutaneously into the submental neck. There, it is transitioned to the subplatysmal plane by introducing a hemostat or right angle from under the anterior belly of the platysma and pushing the tips out through the plasma laterally to pull the drain tip into the submental, subplatysmal space (Fig. 7.8).

The platysma is closed with 2-0 Vicryl simple inverting sutures from symphysis down to at least cricoid, taking care not to ensnare the deep drain. If low platysma cannot be approximated, the closure may stop at hyoid angle, but the risk of the submental platysma becoming dehiscent increases because that closure is not "protected" by muscle closure of the vertical neck.

A second drain is introduced from the right side and kept entirely in the subcutaneous plane traversing low in the neck all the way across to the left SCM region.

A final check for hemostasis and skin drape is performed, and the skin flaps are tailored and closed without tension (Fig. 7.8). No dressings are used, as they prevent early detection of hematomas and can cause pressure wounds or skin bunching.

Postoperatively, standard hematoma precautions are followed, including blood pressure management and strict avoidance of exercise and nonsteroidal antiinflammatory drugs (NSAIDs) for 2 weeks. The patient is encouraged to rest supine rather than elevated, to drive edema toward the undisturbed posterior column of lymphatics. Patients are instructed to ice through a cloth barrier for 20 minutes on, 20 minutes off cycles while awake. Diet is restricted to soft foods and small bites, and sialagogues are avoided for 5 days if submandibular gland surgery was performed.

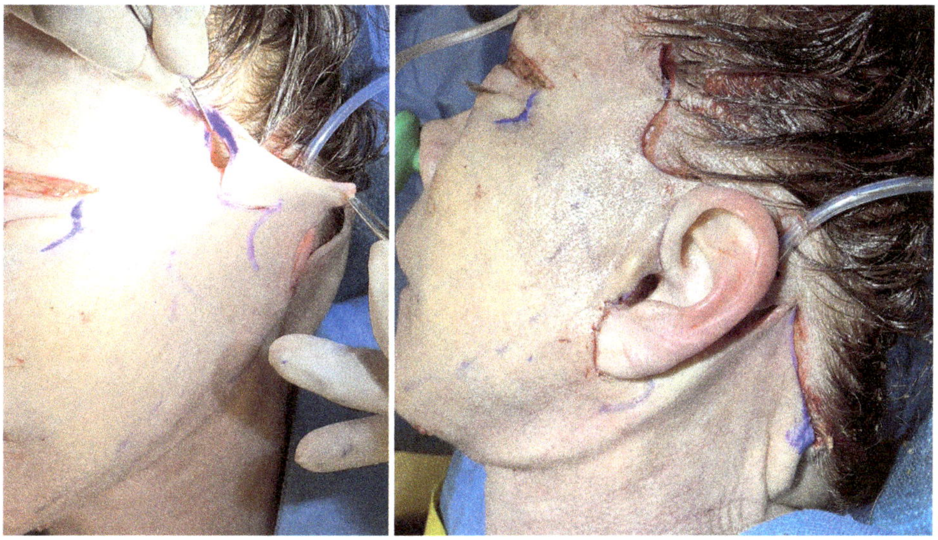

Fig. 7.8. The *left* image shows the skin excess before trimming. The *right* image shows the trimmed skin and the drain under the neck skin and exiting behind the ear.

Although drain output may seem minimal on day 1 or 2, it is not uncommon for output to pick up on day 3 or 4 as the patient becomes more ambulatory and active. If output remains robust, the drains may be required for longer periods of time.

Walking is encouraged as soon as the patient feels well, usually the evening of surgery or the morning after. Mild to moderate aerobic exercise is acceptable at 2 weeks. Weightlifting and other endeavors that put muscular strain on the neck must be avoided for 6 weeks, when fraying of the SMAS and platysma closures is no longer a risk.

The previous description is specific for the deep plane facelift. The cervical region can be managed in numerous ways including the typical midline platysmaplasty (as previously described) or via the deep plane neck lift technique described later in this chapter.

Complications are commensurate with the other types of lifts and described in the complication section of this chapter.

Drains are removed when output has decreased sufficiently, usually on day 5. The patient shown in the operative figures above is shown 1 week after the procedure (Fig. 7.9). Figs. 7.10 to 7.17 (all Dr. Nayak's patients) show before-and-after cases of deep plane facelift with deep neck lift (some patients had concomitant procedures such as rhinoplasty, eyelids, facial implants).

Deep Plane Neck Lift and Isolated Deep Plane Neck Rejuvenation

Laxmeesh Mike Nayak

Acknowledgment

Although I am a board-certified, fellowship-trained head and neck and facial plastic surgeon, I did not fully comprehend the power of deep neck surgery until I learned its value from Dr. Timothy Marten. Most of the techniques below are modifications of Dr. Marten's (which, in turn, originated with Dr. Bruce Connell).

Introduction

Many patients who present with complaints of facial aging, laxity, volume malposition, and excess skin also have similar concerns regarding their neck. In fact, in many patients, unfavorable neck contours may be congenital or may occur earlier in the aging process than corresponding changes of the face.

In traditional neck lift surgery, most surgeons aggressively liposuction or otherwise defat the subcutaneous plane of the neck and treat platysmal laxity/malposition via anterior excision and plication with or without lateral traction from a facelift. Although these interventions can improve the contour of the neck to some degree, they rob the skin of its vital backing of subcutaneous fat and neglect treatment of the subplatysmal foundation of the neck altogether. Initial results are suboptimal compared with the deep neck lift, and long-term results are "surgical" appearing, with accelerated aging of the fat-depleted skin, fibrosis of the dermis to the platysma, and accentuation of platysmal banding.

Liposuction and nonsurgical approaches to treatment of the full or loose neck (injection lipolysis, cryolipolysis, radiofrequency lipolysis, etc.) suffer from these same shortcomings while also being less effective than traditional neck lift surgery.

The deep neck lift is a procedure that can be done independently or in combination with other procedures, most commonly a deep plane facelift. The deep neck lift addresses submental and submandibular *subplatysmal* fat, platysma muscle laxity, submandibular gland hypertrophy, and floor of mouth muscle excess and/or malposition. Through changing the internal topology of the neck, pseudo-excess neck skin is also treated (Fig. 7.18). Subcutaneous fat sculpting, when performed, is a final step of the operation. Its extent is minimized and is often totally unnecessary to achieve dramatic contour improvement.

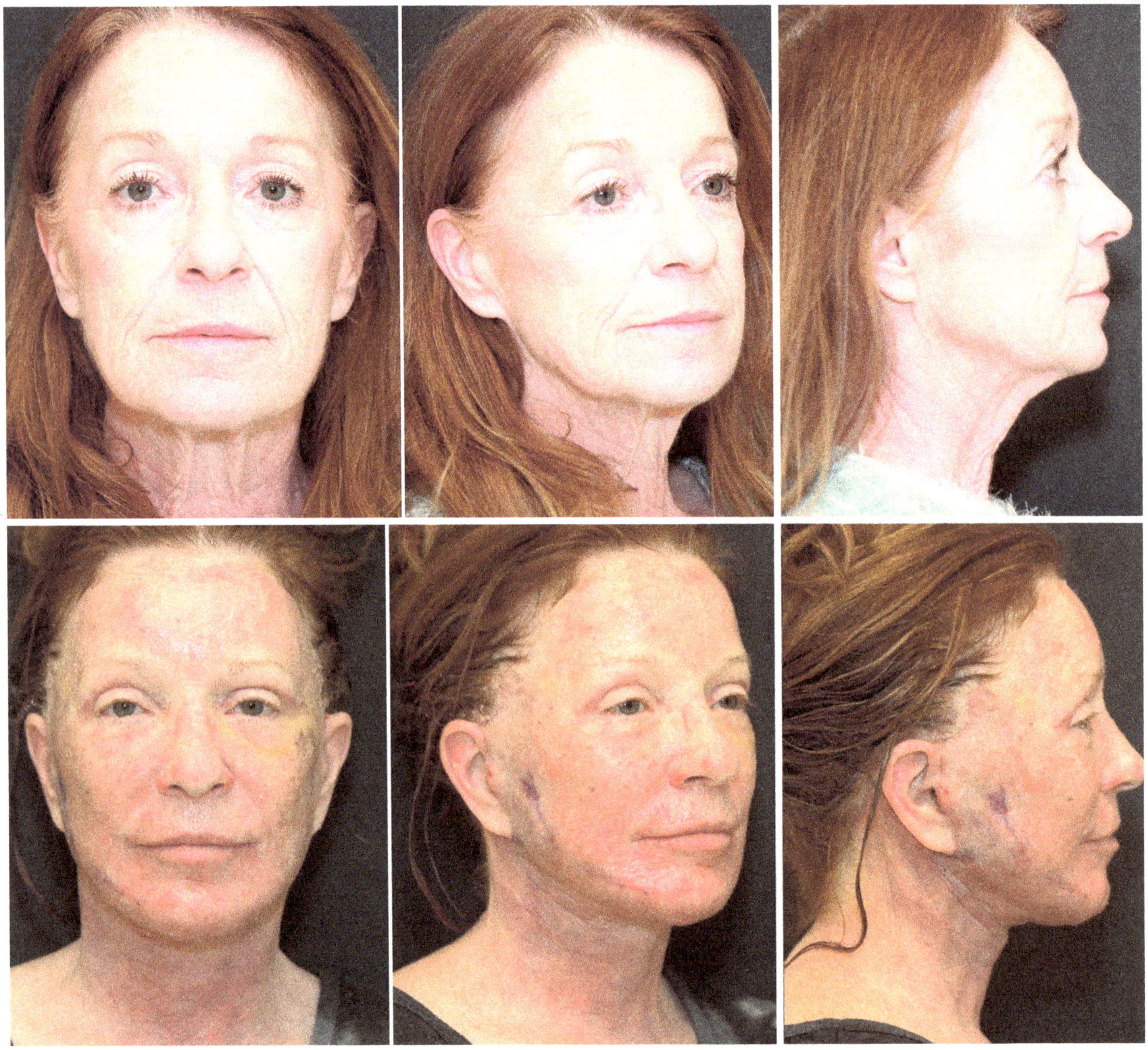

Fig. 7.9. The *top* images show a patient before surgery and the *bottom* images show the patient 1 week after the deep plane facelift and deep neck lift.

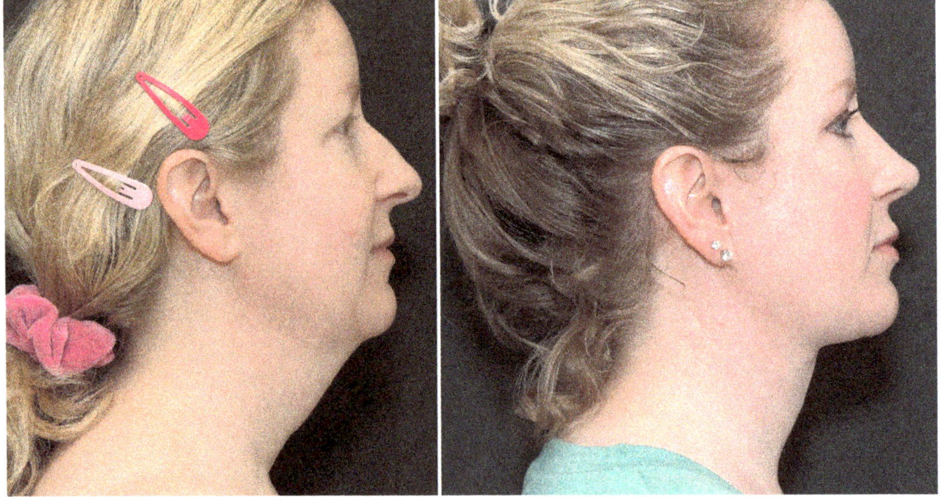

Fig. 7.10. This patient is shown before and 10 months after deep plane facelift with deep neck lift.

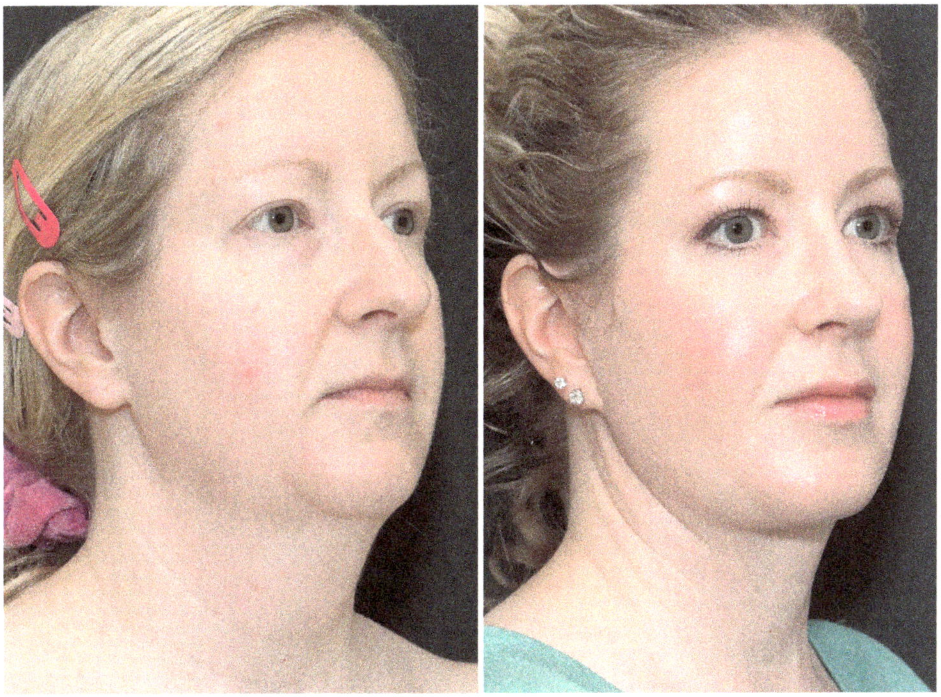

Fig. 7.11. The same patient shown in Fig. 7.10 is shown in the right lateral view.

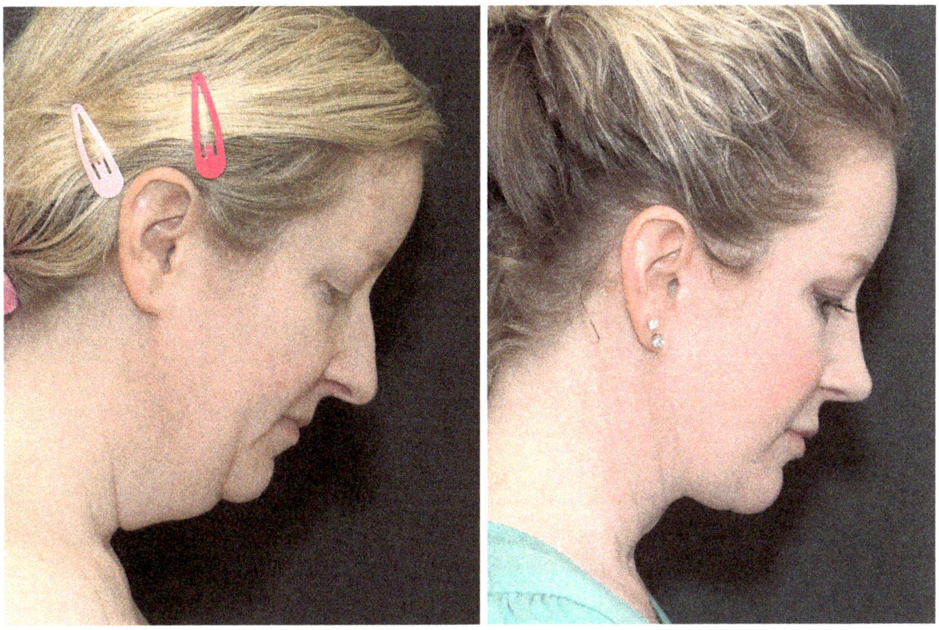

Fig. 7.12. The same patient shown in Fig. 7.10 is shown in the left lateral view.

This chapter will address the relevant anatomy of the deep neck, including indications for submandibular gland reduction as a part of the deep neck lift. The detailed surgical procedure, postoperative considerations, and possible complications will also be discussed, and cases will be presented.

Deep Neck Anatomy

The ideal neck shape includes a sharp cervicomental angle, flat submental plane, defined mandibular border, smooth skin drape without platysmal banding (Fig. 7.19). The goal of the deep neck lift is to create these features in a natural appearing, long-lasting way.

As with rhinoplasty, external shapes and contours of the neck are reflections of internal anatomy, and it is better to correct these contours on a structural level than attempt to camouflage them on a superficial level. Although SMAS/platysma system looseness can be a major contributor to unflattering shapes in thin, "empty" necks, more "full" aging necks are reflections of excess subplatysmal bulk. Tightening the skin and platysma in these patients creates a fraction of the improvement available by addressing the root cause of the problem: the excess subplatysmal bulk.

Offending subplatysmal structures can be diagnosed by an experienced hand. Subcutaneous fat usually feels soft and is

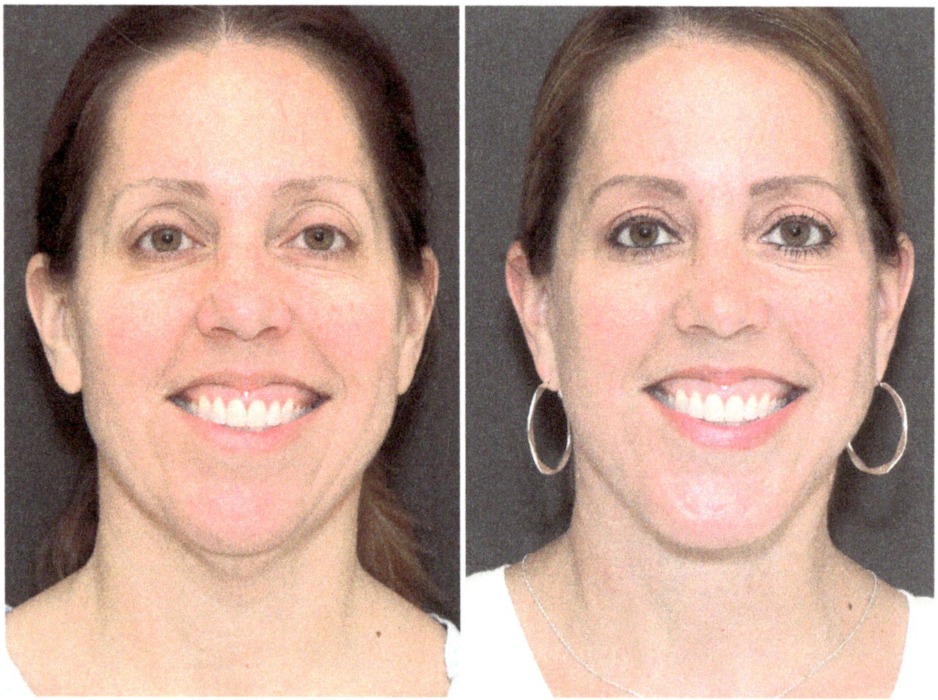

Fig. 7.13. This patient underwent deep plane facelift, deep neck lift, and rhinoplasty is shown in the right lateral view 10 months after her procedure.

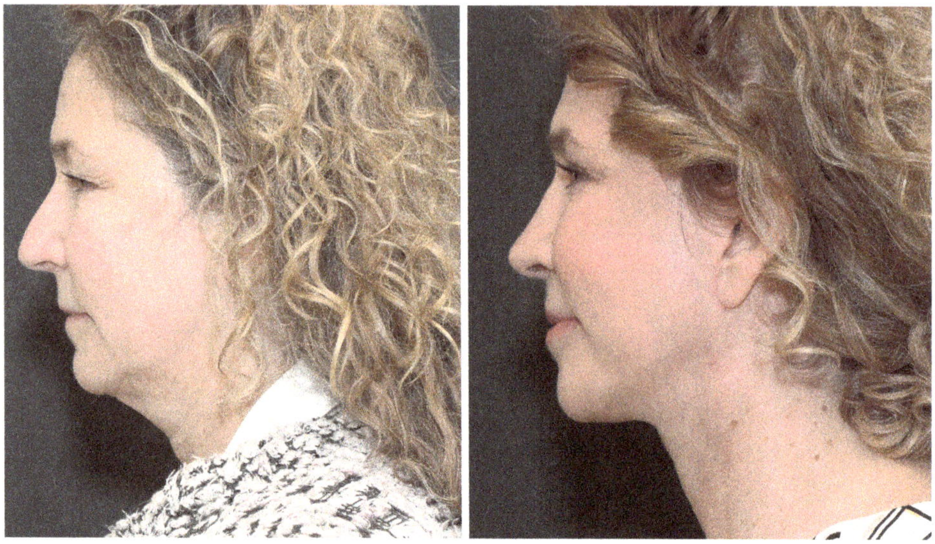

Fig. 7.14. The same patient shown in Fig. 7.13 is shown in the left flexion view.

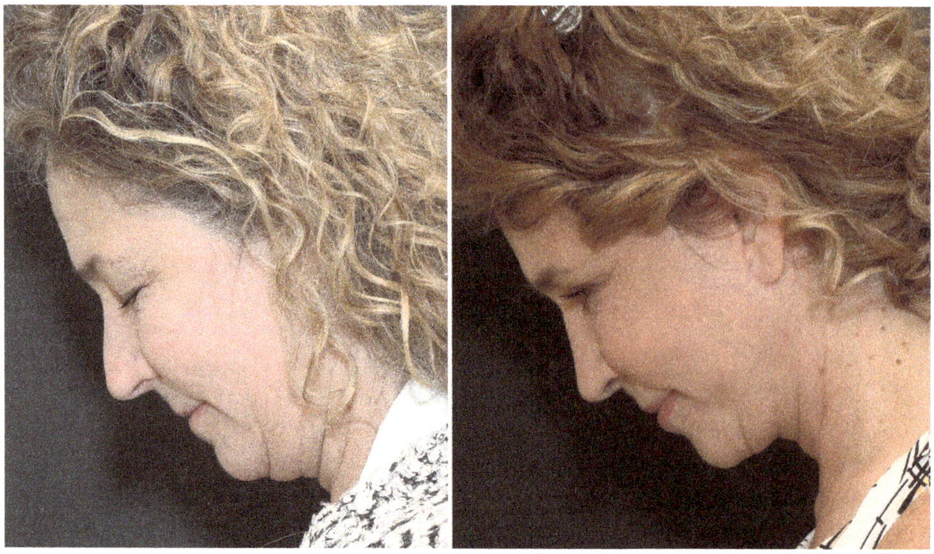

Fig. 7.15. This patient is shown 10 months after deep plane neck lift, deep neck lift, and rhinoplasty.

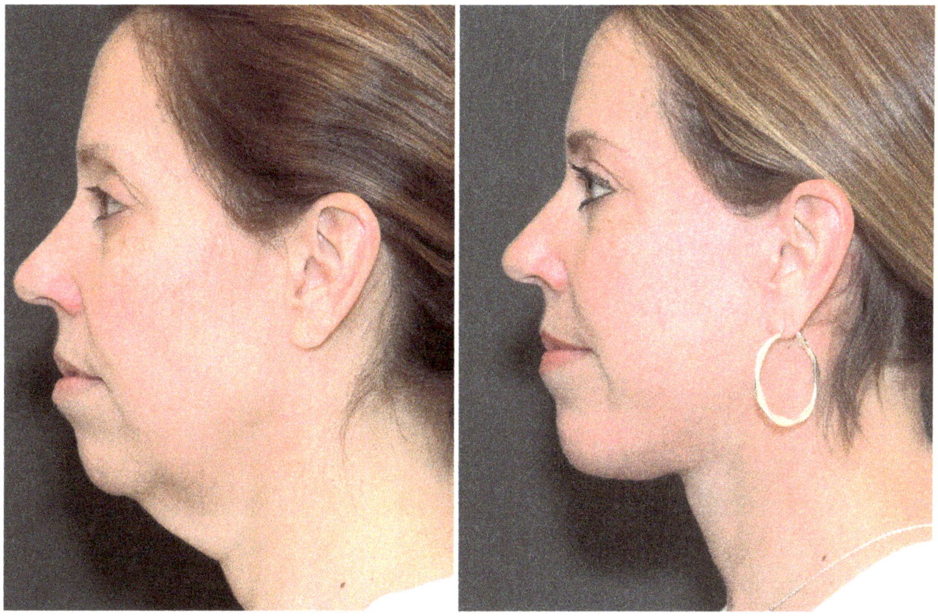

Fig. 7.16. The same patient shown in Fig. 7.15 is shown in the right lateral view.

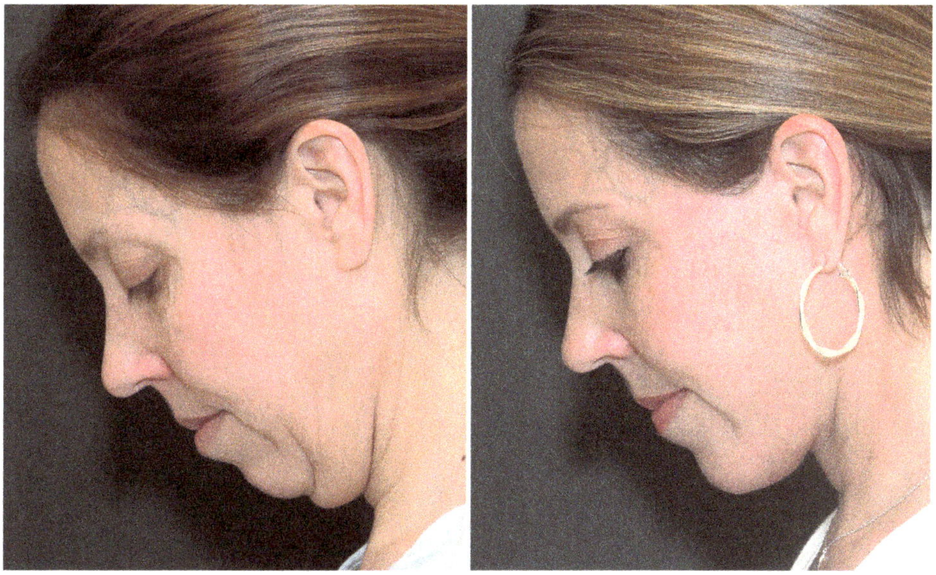

Fig. 7.17. The same patient shown in Fig. 7.14 is shown in the flexion view.

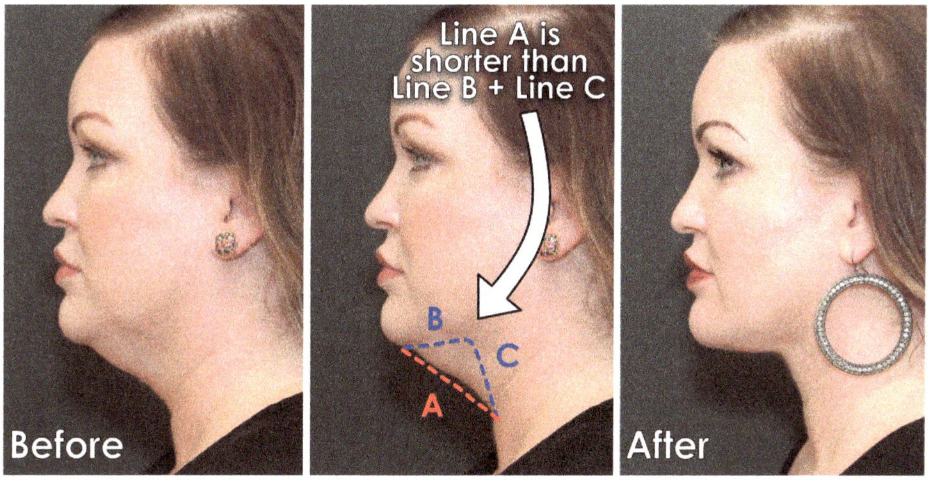

Fig. 7.18. This series of images illustrates the geometry associated with changing the convex neck to the concave neck.

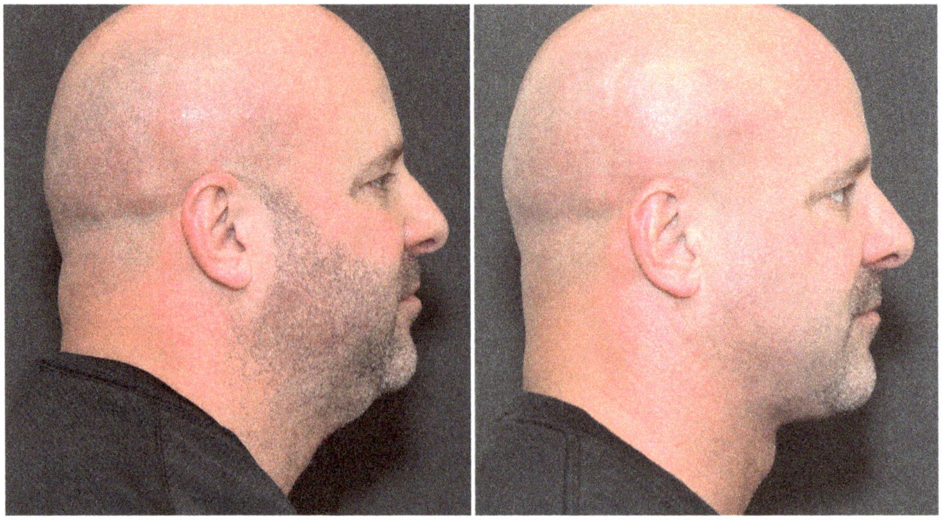

Fig. 7.19. The *left* image shows the described cervical aging changes and the *right* image shows a rejuvenated neck using the deep plane neck lift technique described.

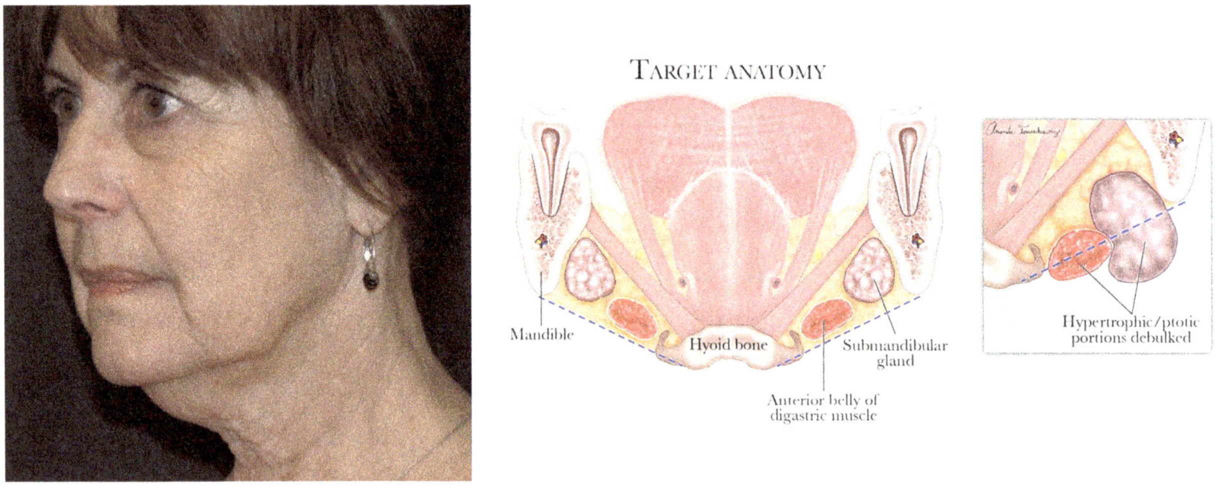

Fig. 7.20. The *left* image show ptotic submandibular glands preoperatively. The *right* image illustrates some of the deep neck anatomy addressed with this technique.

most prevalent in patients in their 20s and 30s. Subplatysmal fibrofatty tissue is usually dense and firm and is more prevalent in patients in their 40s and older but may also plague certain younger patients with a hereditarily obtuse, firm, "woody" neck.

Hypertrophic submandibular gland contours are also palpable as ovoid, mobile, firm masses in the submandibular triangle (Fig. 7.20). Externally, these contours (medial and inferior to the mandibular border) are distinct from the jowl fullness (lateral and largely superior). Hypertrophic gland contours are almost universally absent in patients under 35 and become increasingly prevalent with age, even in lean necks. Although treating submandibular gland hypertrophy is stressful to do and tempting to omit, doing so is important. Extensive defatting the submental region of the neck without sculpting excess submandibular gland bulk results in a "cobra" or "gunshot" deformity.

The most important anatomical considerations for safe deep neck surgery are the course of the marginal mandibular nerve, lingual nerve, and hypoglossal nerve, as well as the facial and retromandibular vein and the intraglandular arterial perforators. The marginal mandibular nerve lies on the lateral surface of the submandibular gland capsule, whereas the lingual and hypoglossal nerves lie deep to the digastric tendon/submandibular gland fossa. The facial and retromandibular vein also lie extracapsular, lateral, and posterior to the gland respectively (Fig. 7.21). These relationships together are the basis for the anterior-inferior approach to intracapsular gland debulking described later.

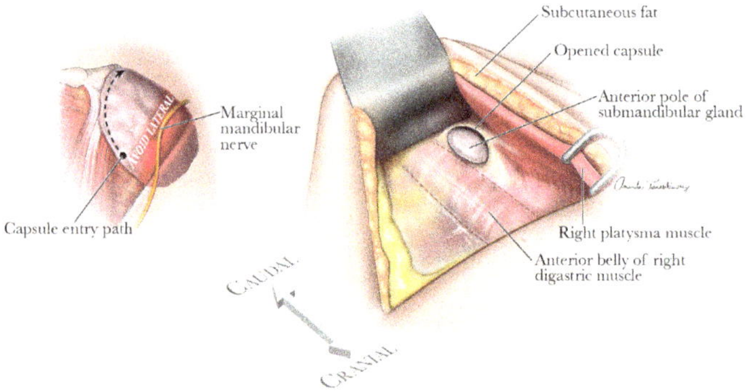

Fig. 7.21. This image shows some of the relevant neuroanatomy associated with the submandibular glands and deep neck.

Planning

An in-depth discussion and physical exam are the two best ways to determine if a deep neck lift is the best procedure for the patient. Considerations include recovery time, physical limitations after surgery, risks involved, and how dramatic of a result the patient is looking to achieve. Although extensive sub-SMAS and subplatysmal surgery is capable of creating the most dramatic results, it is also the most invasive approach and comes with greater risk than traditional facelift or neck lift surgery.

It is critically important to diagnose and discuss microgenia at this stage. Correction of microgenia via sliding genioplasty or chin implant at the time of deep neck lift can be the difference between an acceptable result and an amazing one (Fig. 7.22).

A full preoperative visit to review instructions, review routine lab work and electrocardiogram as per American Surgical Association criteria, obtain consent, and collect prescriptions is performed 2 weeks preoperatively. Patients are advised to strictly avoid NSAIDs and other blood thinners beginning at this point.

SURGICAL PROCEDURE

Marking

Prior to the procedure, standardized photography is performed, and informed consent is obtained. Preoperative inspection and palpation are once again performed, and skin markings are made. The facial midline as well as the submental skin crease are marked. Although many surgeons advocate placing the submental incision posterior to the crease, we find the placement of the incision in the crease to be most favorable in terms of imperceptible healing. Such placement does not deepen the crease, and, if the mandibular ligaments are released, allows for the incision to be adequately mobile to access the deep neck structures including the submandibular glands. Jowl fullness and pre-jowl sulcus emptiness are marked.

Anesthesia

The patient is taken to the operating room and positioned supine, pressure points are padded and pneumatic boots are placed, and anesthesia is induced. Deep sedation or general anesthesia without paralysis (to allow for monitoring of electrocautery facial nerve stimulation) are both acceptable options, in each case with a Foley catheter to monitor fluid status and prevent hypertension from bladder fullness. Due to the time-consuming nature of the procedure and the extreme sensitivity of the submandibular glands, local anesthesia alone or with light sedation is unlikely to be adequate for safe, comfortable surgery.

I prefer a modified Friedberg PK-BIS deep sedation technique. Due to the length of the surgery, in a deviation from Friedberg's protocol, propofol infusion is complemented with 2 mg of midazolam at the case outset. Long infusions of propofol eventually fill muscle stores, prolonging the typically short time to emergence from propofol sedation. The addition of midazolam at the beginning of the case decreases the total propofol requirement, and midazolam may also be reversed in recovery if needed with flumazenil. In addition to routine intravenous antibiotics, additional routine premedications are administered prior to the ketamine bolus aiming to decrease the tendency for laryngeal hyperreactivity common in the first 20 minutes after a ketamine bolus. They include 50 mg of intravenous lidocaine to decrease laryngeal reactivity and 0.2 mg glycopyrrolate to help dry secretions.

Once the premedications have been given and the midazolam bolus with propofol infusion have achieved a steady-state BIS reading of 45–60, a Foley catheter is placed. The patient is then dissociated with a 50 mg ketamine bolus. Propofol is titrated

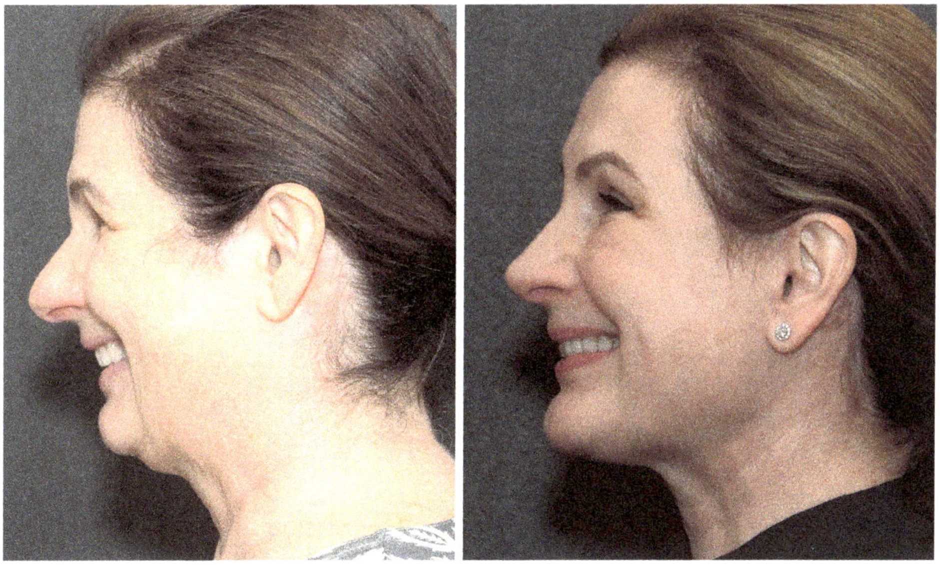

Fig. 7.22. This image shows a patient before and after deep plane facelift with a simultaneous chin implant, rhinoplasty, and periorbital rejuvenation.

to maintain the BIS in the 50s. In the three minutes necessary for full NMDA blockade ketamine dissociation, the patient is sterilely prepped with betadine on the skin and BAK in the hair, and sterilely draped. The operative field is then tumesced with 0.075% lidocaine, 1:500,000 epinephrine, and 0.1% TXA solution (750 mg lidocaine, 1000 mg TXA, 2 cc 1:1000 epinephrine added to 1 L of normal saline). Usually 350–500 mL of solution is required to adequately tumesce the face and neck, with additional solution being appropriate for tumescing the brow or fat donor sites if indicated. If local anesthesia infiltration requires more than about 20 minutes, it may be necessary to administer a second, 25 mg bolus of ketamine to complete infiltration.

If chin augmentation, blepharoplasty, or buccal fat reduction are being performed, those sites are infiltrated with smaller nontumescent volumes. V1/V2/V3 nerve blocks are also performed with this same anesthetic mix as appropriate.

In the first 20 minutes after ketamine administration, airway irritability and tendency toward laryngospasm are possible. At the first sign of any airway irritability (cough, sneeze, stridor), a rescue bolus of 100 mg of lidocaine plain is administered to desensitize the larynx. Jaw thrust with inward finger pressure at the "laryngospasm point" is also helpful. Muscle relaxation and intubation capabilities are important to have as fail safes. Intubation, however, is truly a very remote possibility, and I have never had to resort to those steps.

Once the local anesthesia has been infiltrated, the remainder of the sedation is carried out with propofol titration alone, aiming to maintain a BIS of 45–70 to prevent both over sedation/delayed recovery and awareness/recollection. No narcotics are administered whatsoever, and management of pulse and blood pressure is carried out with cardioactive/vasoactive drugs as per routine. Further details regarding this anesthesia technique may be found at goldilocksfoundation.org.

Procedure Details

The procedure begins by making the submental skin crease incision with a #15 blade. The incision is usually about 4 cm long and must be kept within the confines of the inner tables of the mandible to avoid lateral visibility. On males, it is important to bevel with the hair follicles and keep the incision superficial. The deep dermis is then pried apart with the tips of a small, sharp scissor to minimize transection of the hair follicles bulbs with the blade.

If genioplasty or augmentation mentoplasty are indicated, they are performed at this stage, and the mentalis/platysma muscle coat is closed over the implant.

Next, via the ends of the submental incision, microcannular liposuction of the jowl (usually 1–2 cc per side) is carried out with a 1.8 mm spiral cannula, and the fat harvested may be transferred to the prejowl sulci with a 0.9 mm cannula. This step is especially important in the borderline candidate who is on the verge of needing a facelift and has early to moderate jowls.

Next, a lipocutaneous flap is elevated in the submental and submandibular regions using a combination of cutting and spreading with facelift scissors. Broad undermining is necessary to allow passive skin redistribution and drape. Typical undermining is from one anterior border of the SCM to the other, with the inferior extent beyond the cricoid level (Fig. 7.23, *left*). Flap thickness is checked frequently during this dissection to ensure maintenance of an even 3–4 mm of fat on the flap. The flap is also undermined in the subcutaneous plane for 2–3 cm over the mandible border, and the mandibular ligaments are released to allow the incision to be moved freely left, right, superior, and inferior to maximize visibility without having to make a larger skin incision. If the plane is kept subcutaneous over the mandible, and the lip depressors are not violated, the marginal mandibular nerve is not at risk of transection. Low current (15–18 watts) insulated needlepoint electrocautery is used to control the perforating vessels that commonly accompany the mandibular ligaments, as well as perform broad hemostasis of the entire undermined area.

All of the subcutaneous, preplatysmal fat that was not elevated with the flap is left intact on the platysma at this point. It may be tempting to debulk or suction some of it at this stage, but doing so makes the next step, raising subplatysmal flaps, much more difficult. The platysma is stronger and more easily handled and raised with its "backing" of subcutaneous fat completely intact. The subcutaneous fat will be sculpted at the conclusion of the submentoplasty, and it is often surprising how

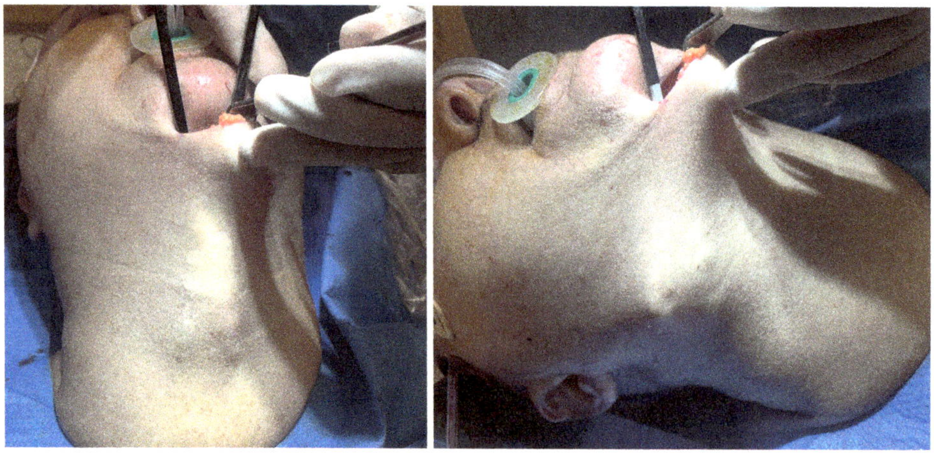

Fig. 7.23. These images show undermining of the submental and submandibular regions.

little needs to be removed. Leaving the maximal amount possible in situ minimizes contour irregularities and premature aging of the submental skin seen with aggressive defatting.

A vertical mark is made from symphysis menton to cricoid on the platysma's overlying fat. The platysma is entered at the midline using scissors or electrocautery and opened inferiorly to the cricoid, exposing the subplatysmal fat at the midline. Electrocautery energy is increased at this stage to 30–35 watts in preparation for subplatysmal surgery. The platysma is then undermined bilaterally in the submandibular and submental triangles immediately under its posterior surface, trying to leave all of the subplatysmal fat down (Fig. 7.24). The surgical assistant team keeps a constant vigil for marginal mandibular nerve stimulation.

The pyramidal-shaped subplatysmal fat is then sculpted out (Fig. 7.25). Surgical boundaries are the digastrics at the deep surface, the hyoid inferiorly, body of mandible superiorly, and anterior pole of the submandibular gland laterally. Any portions of the anterior belly of the digastric or other floor of mouth muscle that are vertically malpositioned or present caudally to the ideal, flat submandibular plane are also debulked with electrocautery.

If debulking of the submandibular gland is indicated, it is performed at this stage. A minimum of two assistants, together with suction and appropriate lighting, are necessary to safely perform this portion of the procedure. The gland capsule is entered with electrocautery via its anterior pole and spreading intracapsular dissection is carried out to mobilize the gland within its capsule (Fig. 7.26). The capsulotomy may be extended along the inferior/caudal edge of the gland as needed. Manipulation of the gland is extremely stimulating to even deeply sedated patients.

Therefore, once the gland is mobilized, 0.5% lidocaine, 0.25% Marcaine, 1:100,000 epinephrine (half-and-half mix of 1% lidocaine 1:100,000 epinephrine with 0.5% Marcaine 1:100,000 epinephrine) is injected into the parenchyma, and attention is turned to identifying, mobilizing, and anesthetizing the contralateral gland while the local anesthetic takes effect.

Attention is returned to the first gland. The portion of the gland positioned inferior to the body of the mandible is removed using coagulative current electrocautery while the assistants monitor for marginal mandibular nerve stimulation (Fig. 7.27). During this portion of the procedure, the surgeon must seek out and control intraglandular perforators of the facial artery with cautery, clips, or suture ligation. Failure to do so will result in brisk arterial bleeding either intraoperatively or on a delayed basis up to 2 weeks later.

After the completion of the contralateral gland debulking, the subplatysmal submental plane should be flat, even with the axial level of the body of the mandible. Twenty units of onabotulinum toxin A are injected into the stump of each gland to help minimize the chance of excess saliva production requiring the drains to remain in place for a prolonged amount of time. Two 10-French closed suction drains are placed via stabs posterior to each lobule. One is brought through the platysma with a hemostat and left in the subplatysmal plane to drain both gland fossae, and the other is left in the subcutaneous plane at the lowest extent of flap undermining to drain the subcutaneous space and allow the redraped skin to take shape immediately. 3-0 PDS or 2-0 Vicryl sutures are used to close the platysma down to the cricoid level.

At this stage, the cautery current is returned to 15 to 18, and cautery, scissors, or a 2- to 3-mm spatulated cannula is used for any subcutaneous defatting that is needed to optimize the submental, submandibular, and gonial angle contours. In most cases, almost no fat is removed in the submental region, but more is removed inferior and posterior to the posterior portion of the

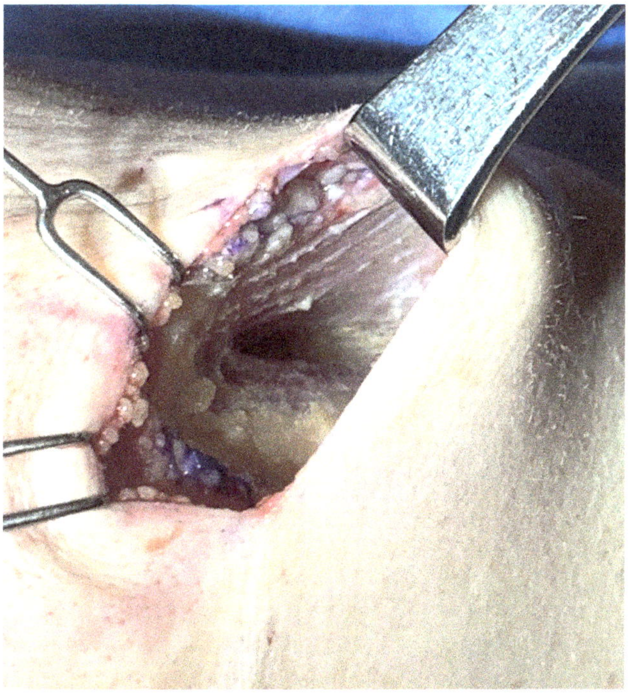

Fig. 7.24. This image shows subplatysmal dissection.

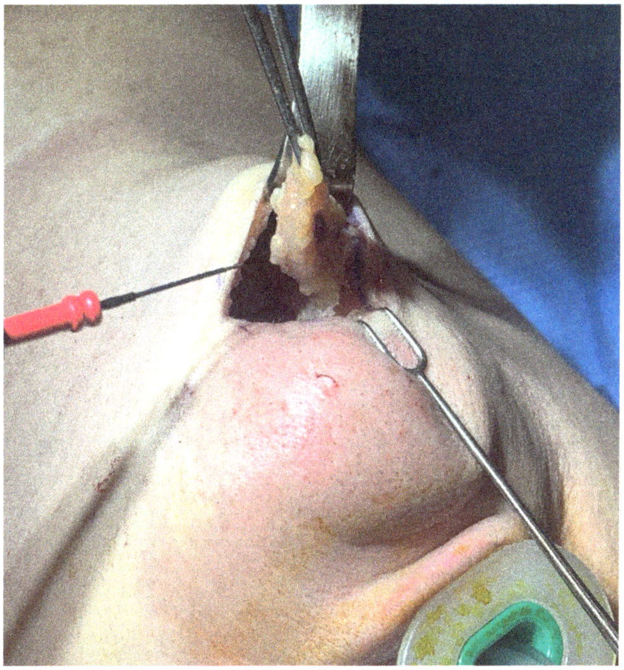

Fig. 7.25. This image shows the subplatysmal fat, which will be sculpted to in part debulk the submental region.

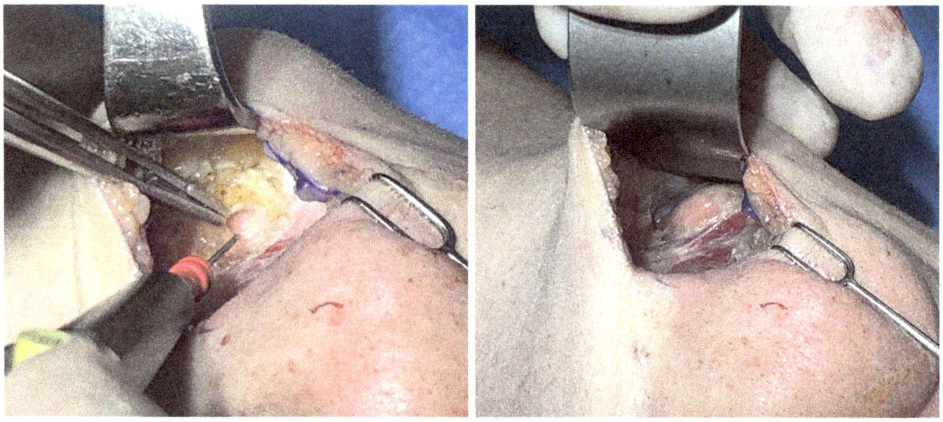

Fig. 7.26. The submandibular gland capsule is incised with the electrosurgery electrode.

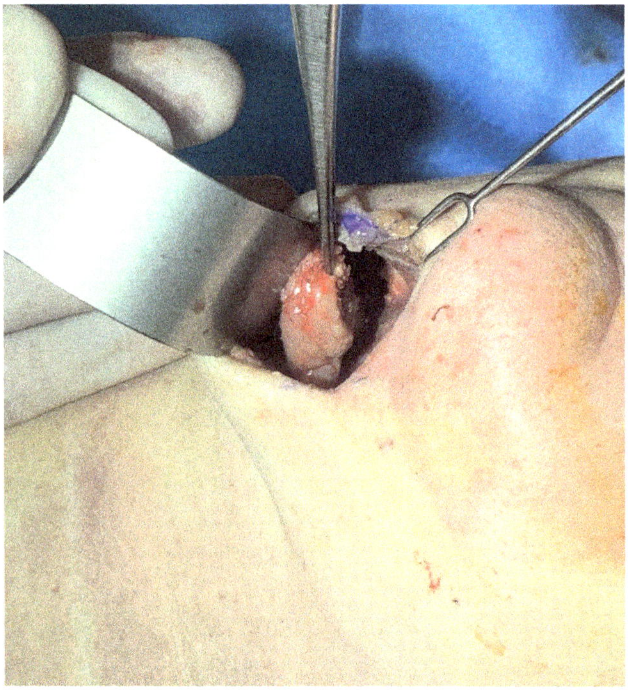

Fig. 7.27. The portion of the submandibular gland that lies below the inferior border of the mandible is resected.

body of the mandible and gonial angle. Hemostasis is confirmed one last time, the wound is irrigated thoroughly, and the skin incision is then closed.

Postoperative Care Considerations

Patients are discharged home with an adult caregiver after reaching an Aldrete discharge score of 8 or above. For two weeks, they are advised to avoid NSAIDs, sleep on their backs, and avoid exercise, sex, or masturbation to prevent pulse and blood pressure extremes that might lead to hematoma. They are also advised to avoid spicy, sour, salty, or dry foods that promote salivary flow, as well as alcohol, for the first 5 days.

The first routine follow-up visit is on postoperative day 1. The skin flap is inspected, fluid collections are ruled out or treated if present, and nerve function is documented. Postoperative instructions are reviewed and reinforced, and wound care is performed. Drains are typically removed on postoperative day 5, presuming drain output is minimal.

Sutures are removed at 1 week, and men are allowed to shave. Light aerobic exercise without straining or extremes of neck motion that might jeopardize the platysma repair are allowable at 2 weeks, and all restrictions are lifted at 6 weeks.

Complications

Complications for this procedure are similar to facelift complications. Possible complications include hematoma (both immediate and delayed), sialocele, nerve injury, skin drape irregularities, contour irregularities, and infection. Transient telogen effluvium of the beard in the submental region may also be seen.

It should be noted that this is not a beginner's procedure. Access is limited, and vital structures are encountered.

Case Presentations

Figs. 7.28–7.31 show before-and-after cases utilizing the described deep plane neck lift techniques.

Conclusion

Overall, the deep neck lift is a safe and very effective procedure in the right hands and for the right patient. It does not come without risks, so long discussions must take place between the surgeon and the patient to decide what outcome they want to achieve. Downtime after surgery, complications, and limitations must all be discussed prior to surgery to determine if invasive surgery is the best option. The same surgery cannot be performed on every patient, as every patient's anatomy and expected outcome is different. It is important to tailor each procedure to each individual patient. Remember, external shape and structure is dictated by internal anatomy. Understanding the anatomy is essential and knowing major anatomic structures to avoid is key to a successful surgical procedure and a happy patient.

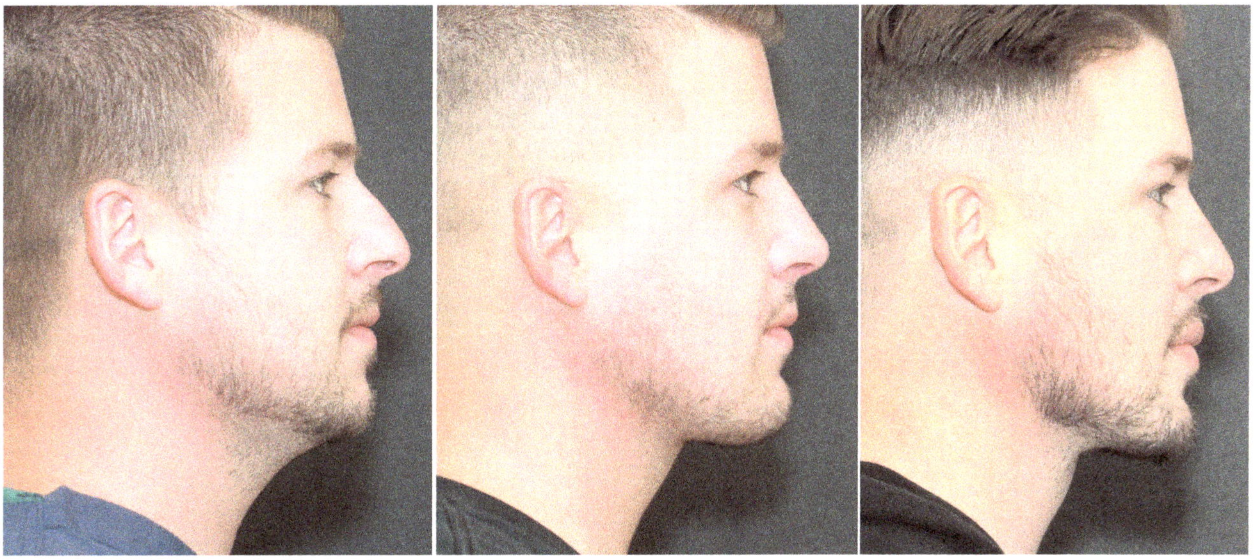

Fig. 7.28. This is a 33-year-old male with oblique neck, microgenia, poor jawline definition, and buccal fat fullness. He wanted a more masculine-appearing face with a stronger jawline and chin. Surgery performed: chin implant, deep neck lift, transoral buccal fat reduction, and simultaneous rhinoplasty. After photos are 3 months (*center*) and 3 years (*right*) postoperatively.

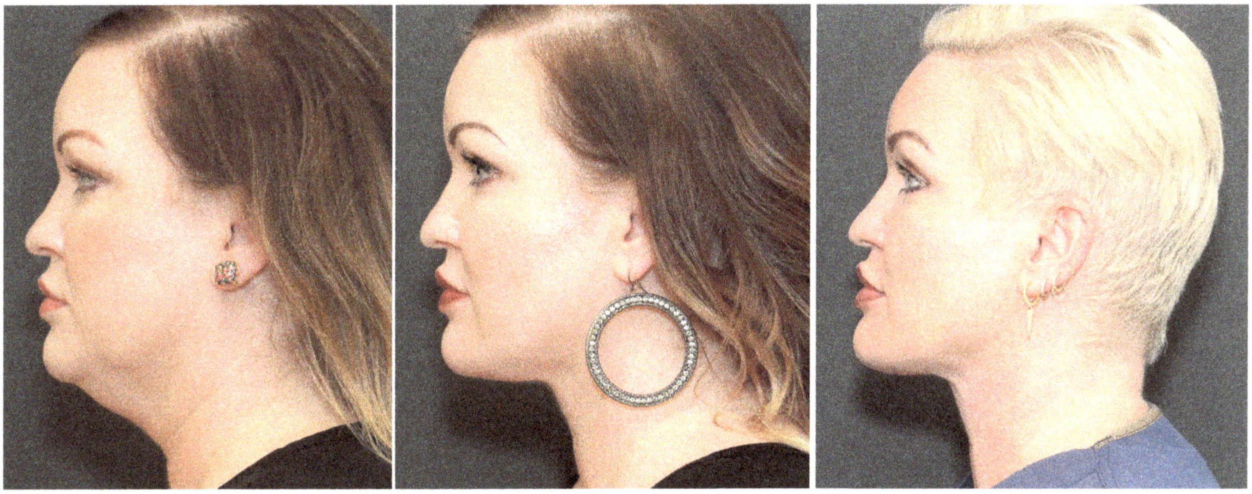

Fig. 7.29. This patient is shown before and after deep neck lift *without* a chin implant. After photos are 3 months (*center*) and 3 years (*right*) postop.

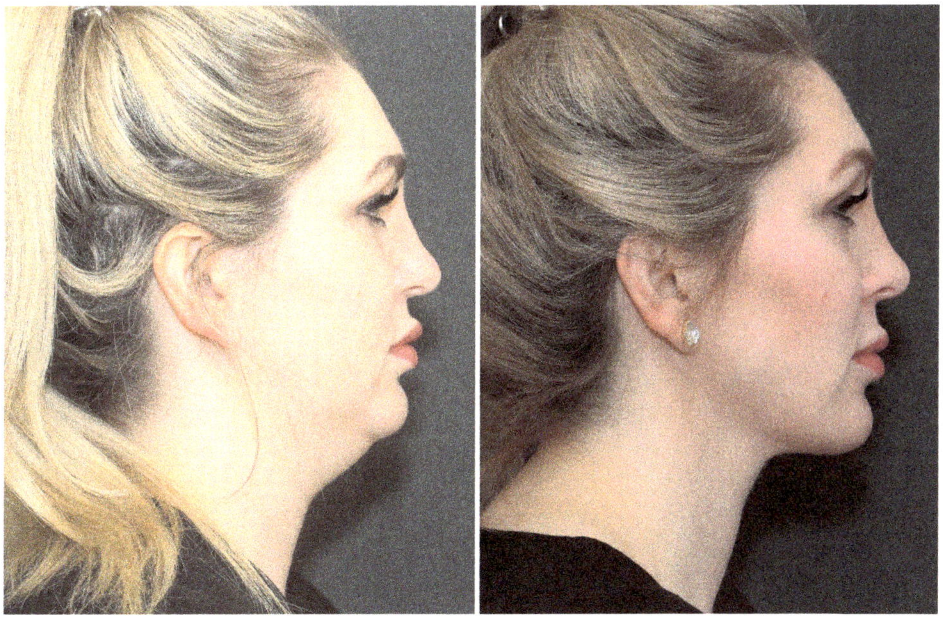

Fig. 7.30. This patient is shown before 1 year after deep neck lift, and 7 months pregnant.

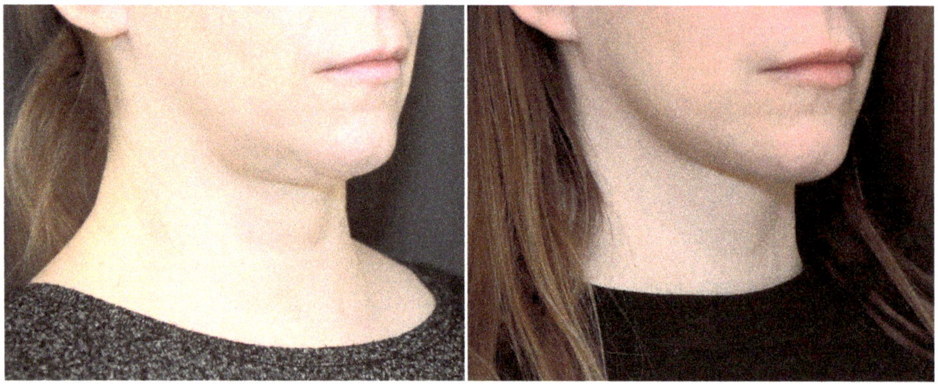

Fig. 7.31. This patient is shown before and 6 months after isolated deep neck lift.

Isolated Submentoplasty

Joe Niamtu, III
Angelo Cuzalina

Doctor Nayak is truly an innovator and a giant in our profession and in face and neck lift surgery. I am honored to once again have his contributions in my textbook. Doctor Nayak speaks from decades of experience as well as his exceptional talent and experience in deep structures of the face and neck. The previous discussion on the deep plane neck lift is certainly about advanced techniques. I think it is important for an author to understand that although there will be experts reading this text, many of the people that purchased this textbook will be reading their first ever chapter on these techniques and have little or no experience. For that reason, I feel it is always important to balance chapters to suit all reading from novice to expert. Not every neck procedure requires deep plane techniques such as reduction of digastric muscle and submandibular glands. Many surgeons do not perform these deep procedures with their facelifts or neck lifts. Aggressive deep plane procedures have certainly become more popular in recent years, which I believe is partially attributed to social media. I predict that there will be significant injury and litigation arising from inexperienced surgeons attempting to perform these techniques. For that reason, I have added an array of procedures that vary in technical difficulty and will do that in this chapter as well.

Isolated submentoplasty (neck lift without traditional upper facelift) can be a very effective in selected patients without the need to remove deep structures.

Introduction

The demand for various aesthetic procedures that improve the neck has increased steadily along with public savvy for cosmetic surgery options. Patients often request a more defined jawline and preferably without undergoing a formal lower facelift. Various procedures exist but when a diagnosis of both submental fatty excess and platysmal banding both exist, then a submentoplasty is typically necessary to obtain maximal results. The question then becomes whether a submentoplasty can be performed as an isolated procedure or in combination with a facelift.

Patients who complain of poor neck contour may be entirely willing to undergo a full lower facelift and neck lift in combination with a submentoplasty to maximize the improvement to their jowls and neck. However, many patients prefer not to undergo a more invasive procedure but still desire improvement in their neck or submentum. As the name suggests, submentoplasty is a procedure that addresses the neck in the submental. Patients who have submental aesthetic issues such as fatty excess, platysmal laxity, or even submandibular gland excess may be good candidates for a "submentoplasty," classically performed through an isolated incision under the chin adjacent the submental crease.

Limitations of an isolated submentoplasty are that there is minimal or no improvement to sagging jowls and fair to good skin elasticity must be present, since no skin is removed in the classic submentoplasty. It is important for the surgeon to recognize the limitations and counsel patients appropriately. If a patient desires improvement of their sagging jowls or if their neck skin is poor quality and reveals major laxity, then a formal facelift will likely be required. However, even a very poor chin-neck angle that is obtuse in nature may potentially be treated with an isolated submentoplasty and no ear incision or skin excision in the appropriate candidate.

Neck Evaluation

After obtaining a thorough medical and family history, it is important to rule out any pathologic process that may be contributing to the patient's unattractive neck aesthetics such as thyroid hyperplasia or salivary gland pathology. Low hyoid position or hypertrophic digastric muscles may also contribute to a poor submental shape in addition to the usual complaints of submental fatty excess and platysmal bands.

The patient's skin tone and laxity are also evaluated. Younger patients (<40) with great skin tone and no muscle laxity are likely candidates for isolated liposuction. This is most ideal if most of the fat is in the preplatysmal area (superficial to the platysma) compared with fat below the platysma (subplatysmal). Gently pinching the submental skin with your fingers can give one a good idea of how much superficial fat is present. If much more thickness is present below the average pinch by fingers, deeper subplatysmal fat is likely in the majority. That cannot be adequately improved by liposuction alone and a submentoplasty may be required. The "heavy" neck patient with a 180-degree or obtuse "ski slope" neck classically has the majority of their submental fat below the platysma muscle and requires open submentoplasty to adequately remove this fat that does not extract well via liposuction.

A finding of a low hyoid bone, as noted by palpation, is an example of a difficult neck to treat. A low and anterior positioned hyoid bone is characteristically associated with an obtuse cervicomental angle that creates limitations in aesthetic improvement despite excellent surgical technique. Mandibular hypoplasia, isolated microgenia, or a combination of the two are often seen with poor neck aesthetics and should be recognized and discussed with the patient. Proper diagnosis will allow the surgeon to discuss the limitations of the procedure or alternatives such as orthognathic surgery, geniotomy, or chin implant.

Platysmal banding from aged, thin, or weak platysmal muscle often causes classic neck bands on each side of dehiscence of the fibers in the neck midline. Platysmal banding may be dramatically improved with a well-performed isolated submentoplasty provided the skin is healthy enough to shrink and redrape adequately. However, severe platysmal banding or laxity is often seen in combination with sagging jowls and skin laxity, which is a rationale for performing a standard lower facelift and neck lift plus submentoplasty. Platysmal banding is extremely variable as is the amount of midline dehiscence seen in each patient (Fig. 7.32). The thin nature of the platysma and the variable nature of missing areas of muscle make treatment decisions challenging. Options besides simple midline plication are needed to be able to treat the wide variety of platysmal problems.

Submandibular gland ptosis or general gland enlargement with obvious visibility in the submandibular triangle region is another important variable to note on preoperative exam and was addressed earlier in this chapter. If unrecognized, the cosmetic result will potentially be less than acceptable following traditional liposuction, submentoplasty, or a facelift. Aggressive liposuction may cause the patient to recognize submandibular gland fullness that they did not notice before their surgery. Therefore, the patient must be informed of the limitations if the redundant submandibular gland will not be addressed or treatment can be performed to reduce, resect, or suspend the gland. If the enlarged or ptotic gland is not addressed, the patient will have a residual bulge in the submandibular triangle that may be more obvious following fat reduction or skin tightening around the gland.

Liposuction Technique (Alone vs. Combined With Submentoplasty)

The ideal candidate for liposuction alone is generally a patient less than 40 years old that has good skin tone with a favorable hyoid position and localized submental and submandibular fat deposits mostly superficial to the platysmal muscle. If there are minor platysmal bands, botulinum toxin A injections can be used to treat the minor bands. Severe platysmal banding or laxity will need to be treated with submentoplasty since liposuction alone may make the banding look visibly worse.

The technique for neck liposuction has advanced subtly over the past decades. Formerly, surgeons used large (8–10 mm) spatulated cannulas to extract as much fat as possible from the neck. The preliminary results were often good, but with time patients developed a skeletonized appearance of the neck and irregularities from fibrous adhesions for the dermis to the platysma. Areas devoid of fat can cause the dermis to effectively "stick down" to the underlying muscle. This creates an uneven or even lumpy appearance that is unnatural compared with a neck with a smoothly moving freely movable plane. Contemporary treatment employs small microcannulas 1–2 mm in diameter to sculpt the neck by removing selective fat but not all the fat. Three small punctures can be made for microcannula liposuction via a submental crease region and behind each ear.

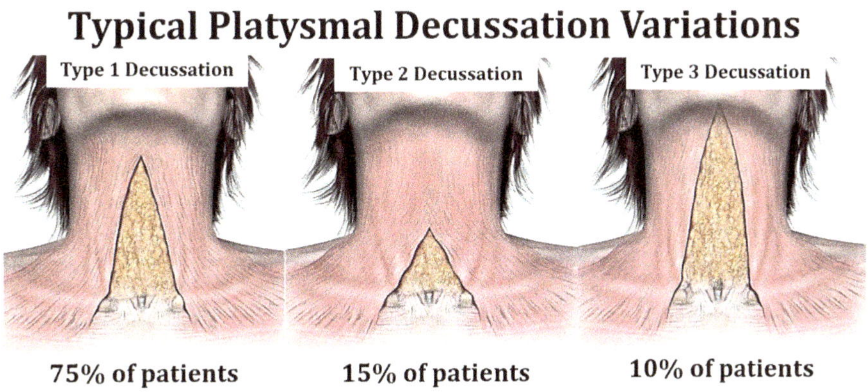

Fig. 7.32. Decussation, which means a crossing of fibers, typically in an X fashion, happens in the midline of the neck from bilateral platysmal muscle fibers in extremely variable patterns. Simplistically demonstrated above, the open portion or window is the dehiscence of the platysma. Patients with a larger dehiscence can have more fat or soft tissue protruding in the same manner as an abdominal hernia where abdominal contents protrude through dehisced rectus muscle.

The cannula should be moved in a smooth in-and-out motion each time, trying to enter a new location and avoid repeating in the same area, which can lead to sunken areas of irregularities that can be difficult to correct. The opposite or nondominant hand should always be held carefully over the skin to feel the depth of the cannula tip. Additionally, the surgeon should frequently stop to feel the skin below the cannula tip to ensure even removal of fat and proper plane of fat removal. The cannula tip should typically be superficial to the platysma with the port facing toward muscle and not dermis to help prevent fibrosis from exposed dermis to muscle adhesion.

Subplatysmal fat is difficult to adequately remove via closed microliposuction, and open submentoplasty is generally needed to properly address excess fat deep to muscle. When a submentoplasty is planned to reduce deep subplatysmal fat, then liposuction is performed much differently than liposuction alone. A submentoplasty elevates all the skin in the submentum sharply in the subcutaneous plane. Although microcannula liposuction prior to skin elevation can make the skin flap a bit easier to elevate, it also can produce a more irregular skin flap. Therefore, elevating the skin flap sharply in the submentum is performed prior to any liposuction to achieve a smooth skin flap with an even 5–8 mm of thickness and fat immediately below dermis (Fig. 7.33).

Next, open liposuction with a large 5- to 10-mm cannula can very safely and smoothly "clean off" fat via an "open" liposuction technique. The remaining fat still attached immediately above platysma is removed easily via open liposuction across the neck to clearly see the platysma remaining below while leaving a healthy and smooth layer of fat attached to the skin above in the elevated flap.

Regardless, if liposuction is performed alone or combined with an isolated submentoplasty, it is important to select patients that have quality skin tone to allow for nice shrinkage. The ability of skin to shrink adequately is the difference between choosing a submentoplasty alone or combined with a facelift to remove the excess skin.

Patient Selection for an Isolated Submentoplasty

As discussed in the chapter on neck evaluation, the patient that has platysmal banding and significant subplatysmal fat deposits is likely a candidate for submentoplasty. If there is major submental skin laxity or jowling that is a complaint, then the submentoplasty needs to be performed in conjunction with a rhytidectomy (facelift). But if there is no significant jowling and the patient has fair to moderate skin elasticity, then an isolated submentoplasty may be considered.

The ideal patient for an isolated submentoplasty is a patient with reasonable skin tone, moderate, deep (subplatysmal) fat, minimal to moderate muscle laxity, normal mandibular bone structure, and a family history of an obtuse shaped neck. Patients that are candidates for a submentoplasty without a facelift often say something like, "I just want my neck improved and preferably without a facelift or any incisions around my ears." The ideal patient must still be cautioned that it is riskier than liposuction alone and if the skin does not shrink adequately, a facelift may be necessary to correct.

The hyoid bone serves as great landmark for location of the deepest portion of the ideal cervicomental angle. The position of the hyoid bone influences the result that can be achieved in a submentoplasty particularly if it is a low and anterior positioned hyoid, which makes it difficult to obtain a well-defined or near 90-degree cervicomental angle. Hyoid position can also be used to guide where potential back-cutting of the platysma is performed. Horizontal cutting of the platysma immediately below the level of the hyoid allows for the cervicomental angle to fall in a more ideal position when trying to deepen an obtuse chin-neck angle with the deepest portion near the hyoid level. A low hyoid is often associated with microgenia, and in that case a chin implant can be used to help camouflage the poor hyoid position and thereby also improve the resulting chin neck angle following a submentoplasty. A less common anatomical concern is when the paired anterior digastric muscles are obviously enlarged and are aesthetically not pleasing. The surgeon should inform the

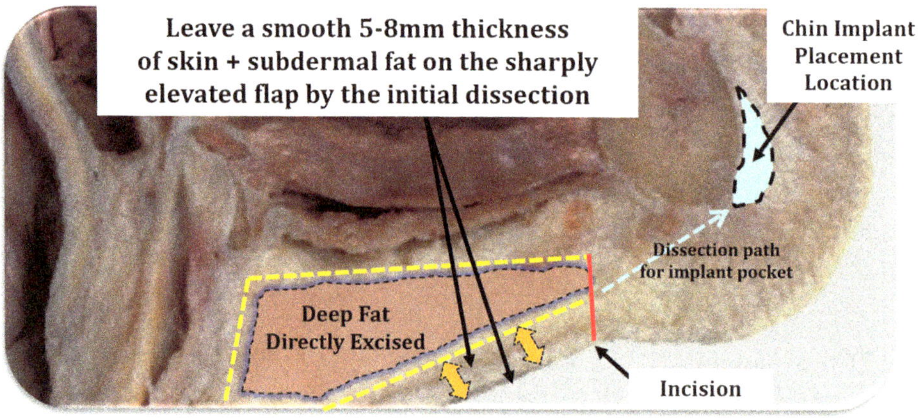

Fig. 7.33. This diagram shows a key component to a successful submentoplasty by maintaining an even, healthy layer of fat on the skin surface when planning direct excision of deep fat. Therefore, a smooth thin layer of fat remains both superficially and above the deep musculature.

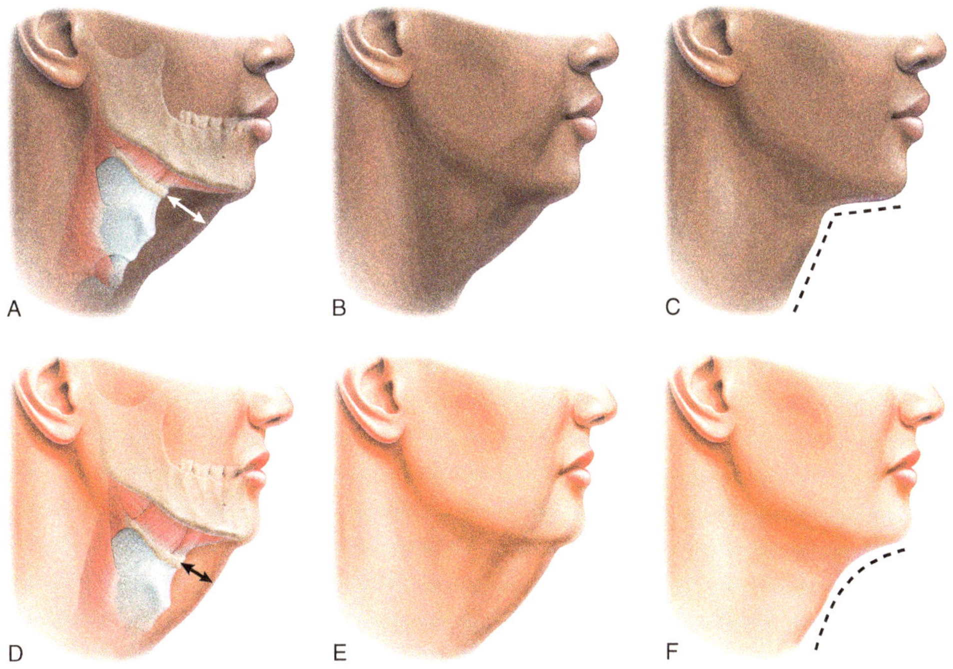

Fig. 7.34. The *top* images show a representation of a patient with normal (superior and posterior) hyoid, laryngeal and floor of the mouth anatomy. Figure A shows the anatomic position, Figure B shows a representation of the preoperative appearance and Figure C shows a representation of the possible angular result after face and neck lift surgery in the "high/posterior" neck. Figure D shows a representation of the anatomy of a patient with low and anterior hyoid, laryngeal and floor of the mouth. Figure E shows a representative preoperative appearance (similar to Figure B). Figure F shows a representation the lack of angular result after face and neck lift as a result of the "low/anterior" anatomic relationship.

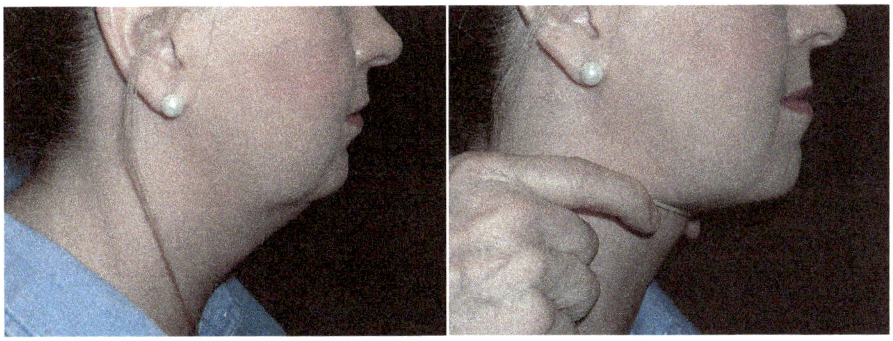

Fig. 7.35. Retracting the soft tissues in the submental region can be useful to estimate a result by exposing the submental anatomic outlines.

patient of the limitation and not treat or consider an anterior muscle belly reduction or shave in this isolated group of patients with this less common but occasional problem.

Like many of these truncated procedures, submentoplasty represents a compromise in that it is only applicable to very select patient populations. This procedure generally works best on younger patients with significant submental excess by without significant skin excess (see before-and-after images). As discussed earlier in the diagnostic section, this procedure is also more dramatic on patients that have an acute cervicomental angle and is less effective on patients with an obtuse cervicomental angle (Fig. 7.34). In addition, this procedure is less effective on patients that have significant jowling. To recap, any patient with significant submental fullness, skin excess, and jowling is a candidate for facelift surgery and not submentoplasty. As I have said numerous times in this textbook, if a surgeon attempts to perform a smaller procedure on a patient that needs a bigger procedure, both parties will be disappointed. An estimation of result can be made by retracting the submental soft tissues posteriorly (Fig. 7.35).

Some patients (and surgeons) do not understand how a concavity can be made from a convexity. Basically, when considering surface area and contour, it takes the same amount of tissue for a concavity or convexity in the submental region (Fig. 7.18).

Surgical Technique

The submentoplasty procedure is basically the same as the submental treatment described in the submental part of the facelift chapter. It concerns:

- Submental incision
- Submental liposuction
- Possible deep platysmal lipectomy
- Platysmal plication (or platysectomy)
- Chin implant if indicated
- Buccal fat reduction (if indicated)

The goal of the procedure is to debulk the region and redrape the skin, thus creating a more youthful neck and cervicomental angle.

The first step is to inject tumescent anesthesia and all of the area to blanch. A routine submental incision is made at or below the submental crease (Fig. 7.36). The incision should be a small enough to be aesthetic and large enough to allow access without traumatizing the skin margins.

Figs. 7.37–7.46 show a stepwise surgical technique. Submental liposuction is performed in this area commensurate with the amount of preplatysmal fat present with the goal of not overthinning the skin flap. At this point the platysma is generally visualized and I prefer to excise several centimeters of muscle on each side the platysmal midline. This exposes the subplatysmal fat, which lies between the mandibular border and the anterior bellies of the digastric muscle. If this is excessive, it is reduced. Some patients may need significant reduction of the subplatysmal fat and others have very little adipose tissue here. Care is always used as not to create an overcorrection, which results in hollowing. Concomitant jowl liposuction can be performed either through this incision or through stab incisions in inferior lobe region. Many of these patients have full faces and may also benefit from simultaneous and buccal fat reduction. Figs. 7.47–7.53 show before-and-after images for surgeries I have performed.

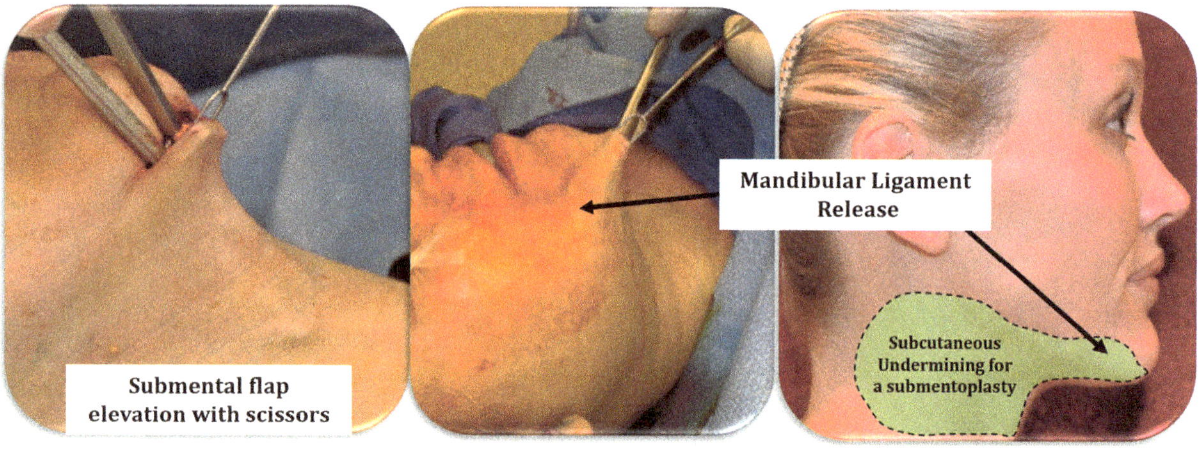

Fig. 7.36. A submental skin flap is made through the submental incision and performed sharply using facelift scissors. Cautious sharp subcutaneous release of the mandibular ligament dramatically improves redraping of the skin and the outcome of the prejowl region. Adequate subcutaneous release is required as shown with the green highlight in the *right* image.

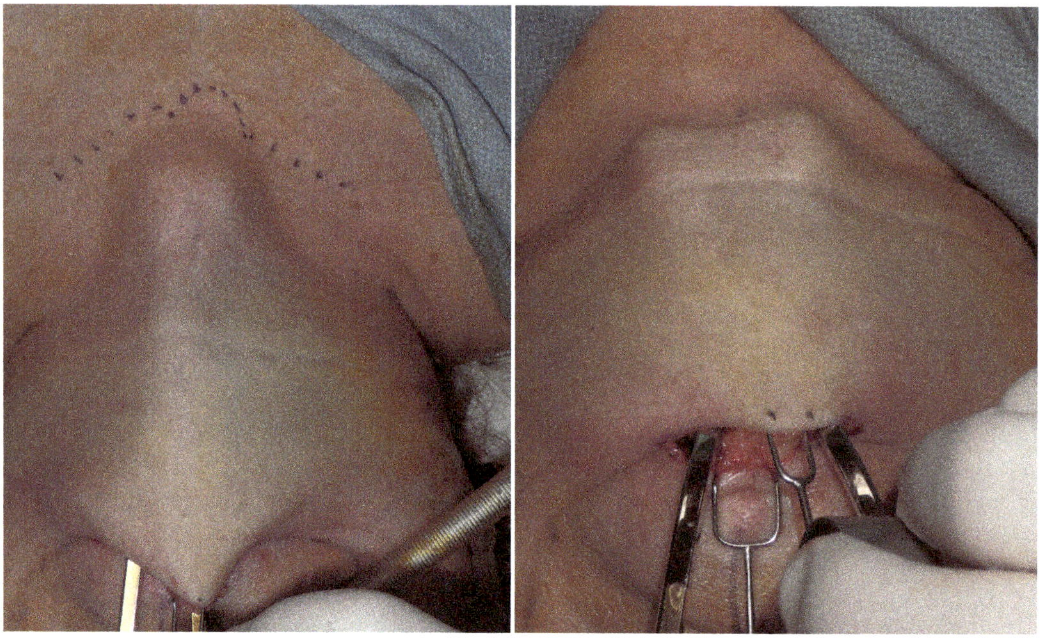

Fig. 7.37. These images show the undermining of the submental region. As stated earlier, when deep fat or tissues are to be reduced, the subcutaneous flap needs to be thicker to mitigate visible irregularities. This is analogous to putting a thick rug over a crooked floor, much of the irregularity can be hidden.

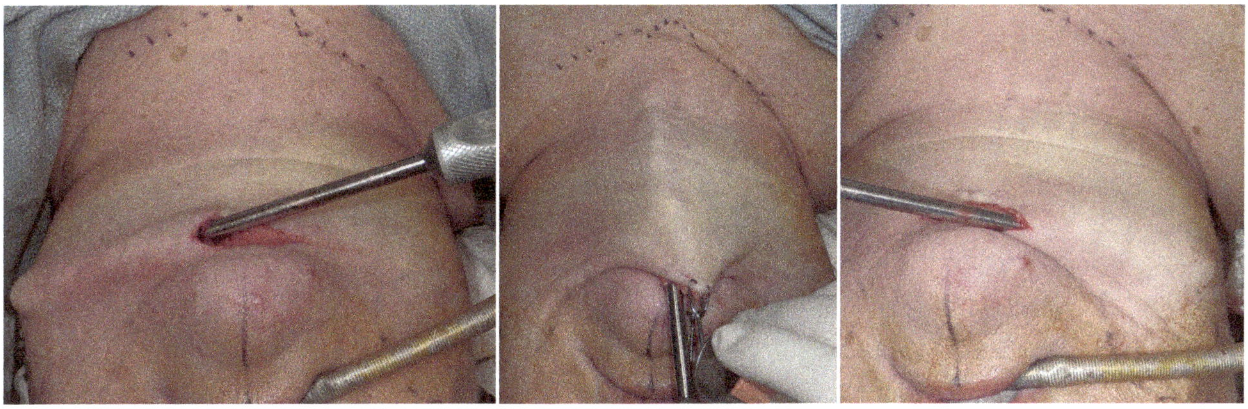

Fig. 7.38. Judicious liposuction can be performed after undermining the skin envelope. This is done under direct vision, and the surgeon has left a thicker amount of subcutaneous fat on the flap with initial dissection. More fat can be liposuctioned at the end of the case if necessary.

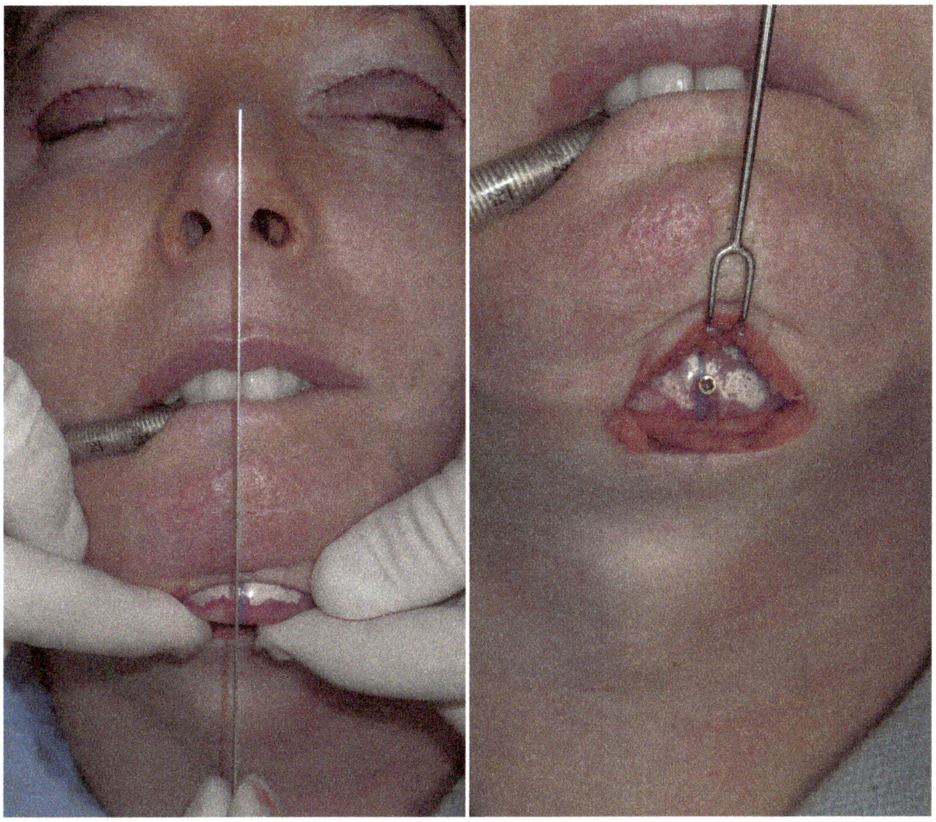

Fig. 7.39. Improving a recessive mandibular profile with a chin implant can dramatically improve the submentoplasty result, and I perform this procedure after the initial skin dissection.

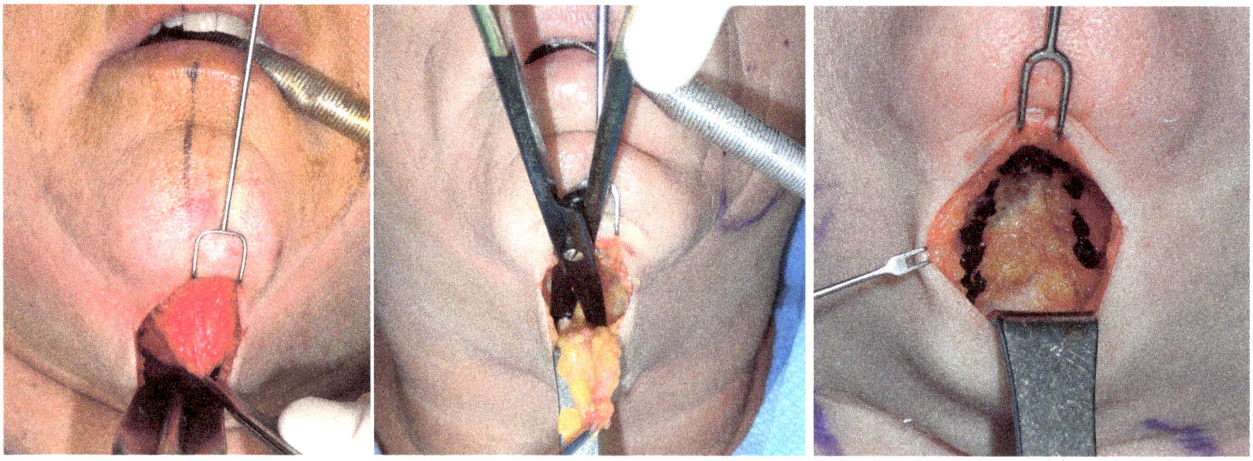

Fig. 7.40. The *left* image shows fibro-musculo-fatty tissue picked up with tension, and the *middle* image shows the midline segment of excess fat and platysma muscle being excised. The *right* image shows the operative field after excision with the lateral platysma borders marked with a pen. The deep tissue in the center of the image is the deep platysmal fat.

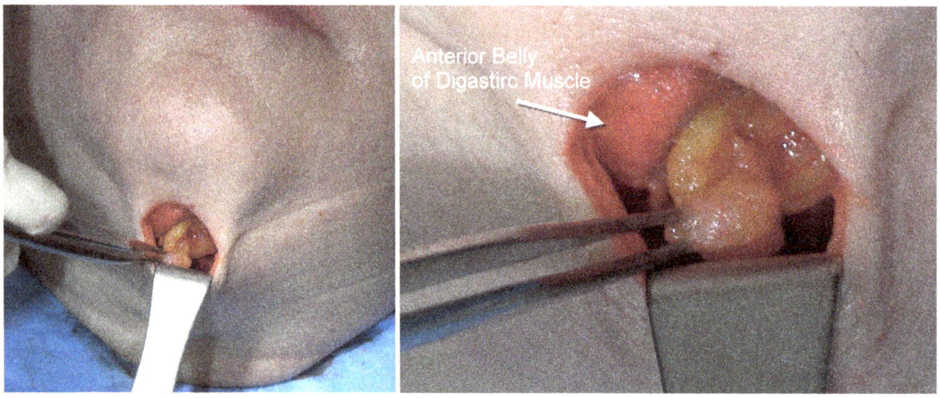

Fig. 7.41. This image shows the deep platysmal fat that sits between the anterior bellies of the digastric muscle. This deeper fat is almost always addressed with submentoplasty.

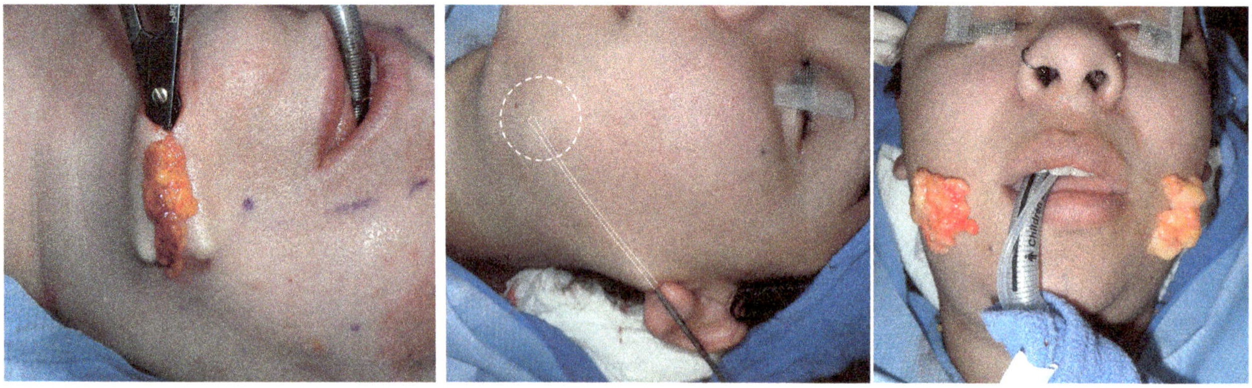

Fig. 7.42. In cases with very heavy and obtuse necks, further excision of fibrofatty tissue and or platysma may be performed to slim the region.

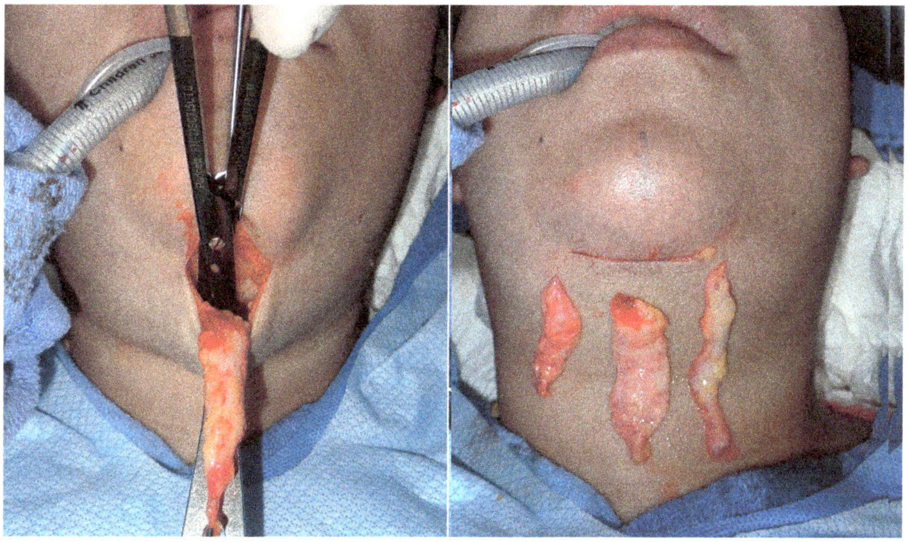

Fig. 7.43. The key to an isolated submentoplasty procedure is to sculpt areas of excess fat so the skin drape can lie on a more defined mandible, submentum, and neck. You can't make an obese person skinny, but on the right patient, results can be dramatic.

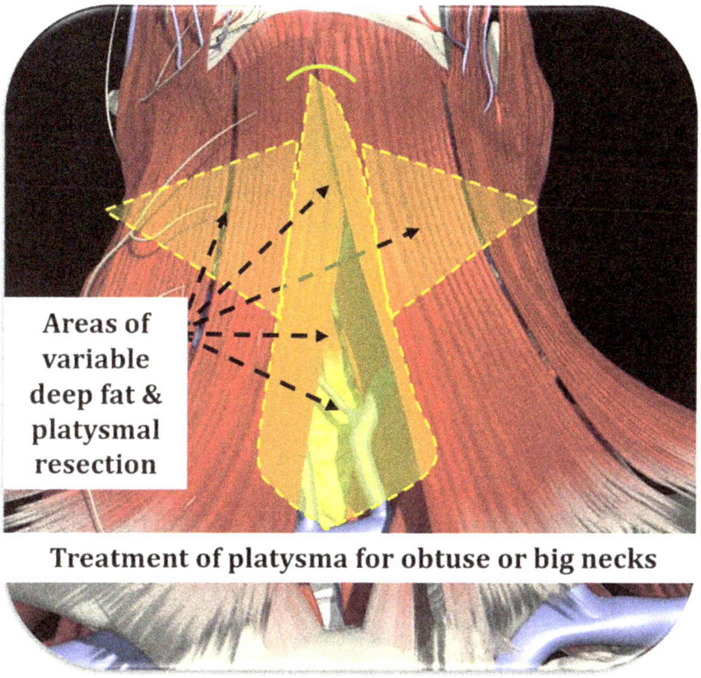

Fig. 7.44. The yellow areas between the *dotted lines* on the *left* image show platysma resection that is performed in patients with heavier necks. Instead of sewing the platysma back together, it is simply excised to debulk the neck. The patient on the *right* is shown before and after submentoplasty with platysectomy. (Surgery by Dr. Angelo Cuzalina.)

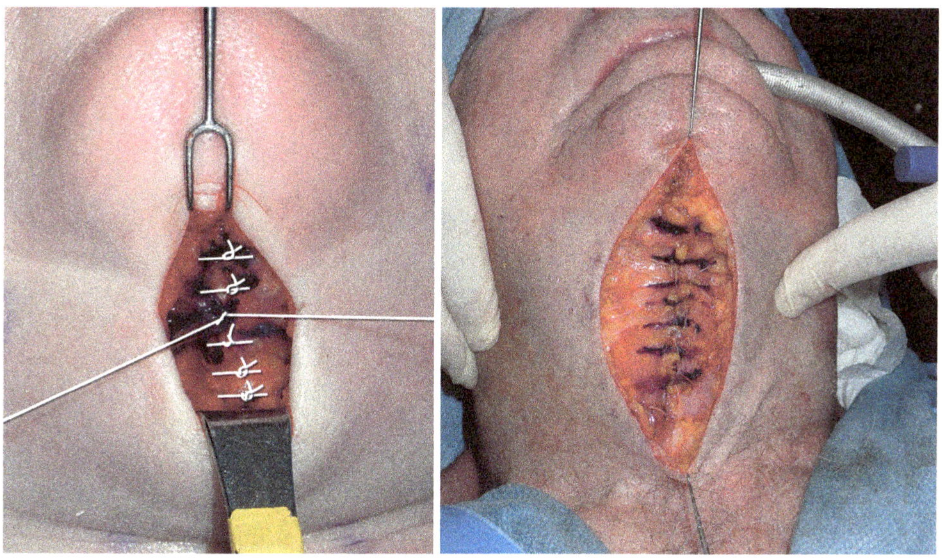

Fig. 7.45. The *left* image shows a representation of a midline platysmaplasty using 3-0 Vicryl sutures. The right image (from direct neck Z-plasty case) shows what the sutured platysma would look like under the skin.

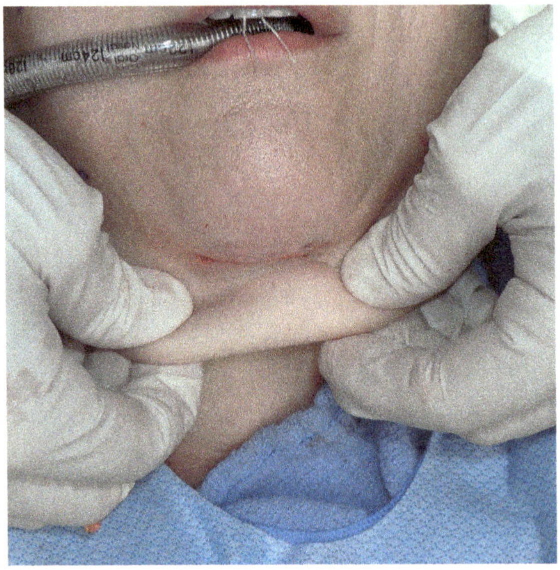

Fig. 7.46. This image shows a patient at the end of a submentoplasty procedure and illustrates the amount of excess skin that is now available to reposition on the neck. This skin was convex at the beginning of the case, and the patient's profile will be concave when repositioned.

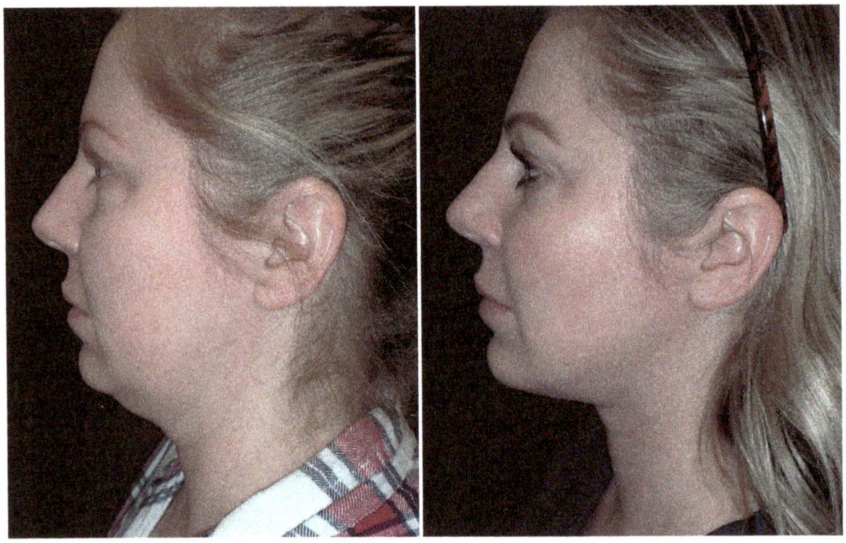

Fig. 7.47. This patient underwent submentoplasty with sumbental liposuction, subplatysmal fat reduction, digastric muscle reduction, platysma reduction with platysmaplasty, jowl liposuction, and buccal fat reduction. (Surgery by Dr. Joe Niamtu, III.)

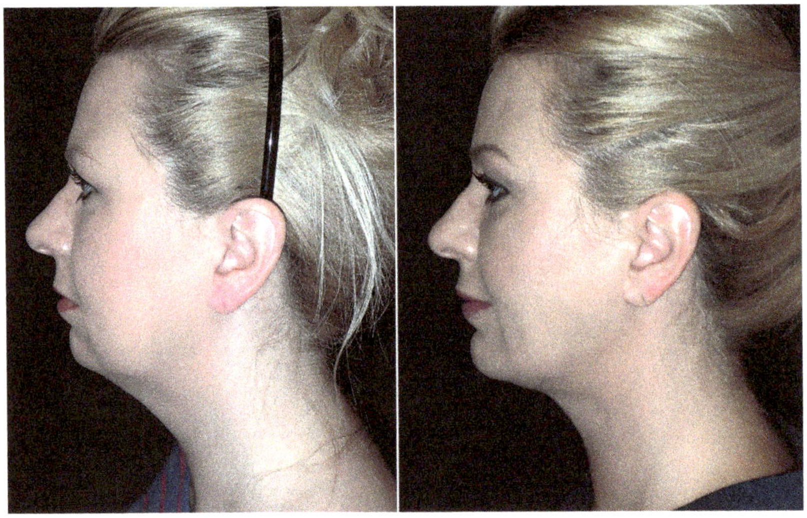

Fig. 7.48. This patient is shown 3 months after submentoplasty with submental liposuction, subplatysmal fat reduction, digastric muscle reduction, platysma reduction with platysmaplasty, jowl liposuction, buccal fat reduction, and silicone chin implant. (Surgery by Dr. Joe Niamtu, III.)

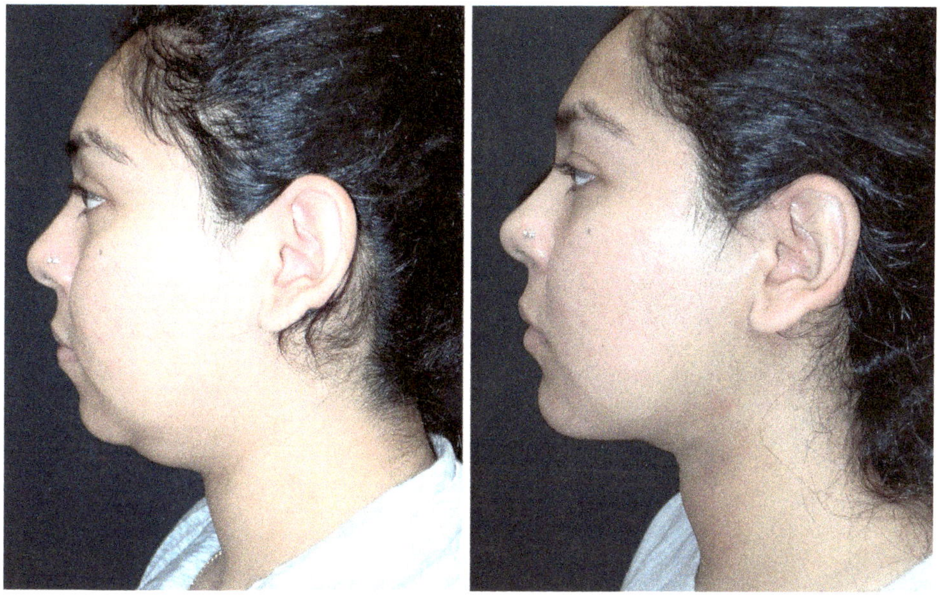

Fig. 7.49. This patient underwent submentoplasty with liposuction, jowl liposuction, midline platysma resection, deep platysmal fat reduction, buccal fat reduction, chin implant, and midline platysmaplasty. The *left* image is before and the *right* image is 24 hours postoperatively. (Surgery by Dr. Joe Niamtu, III.)

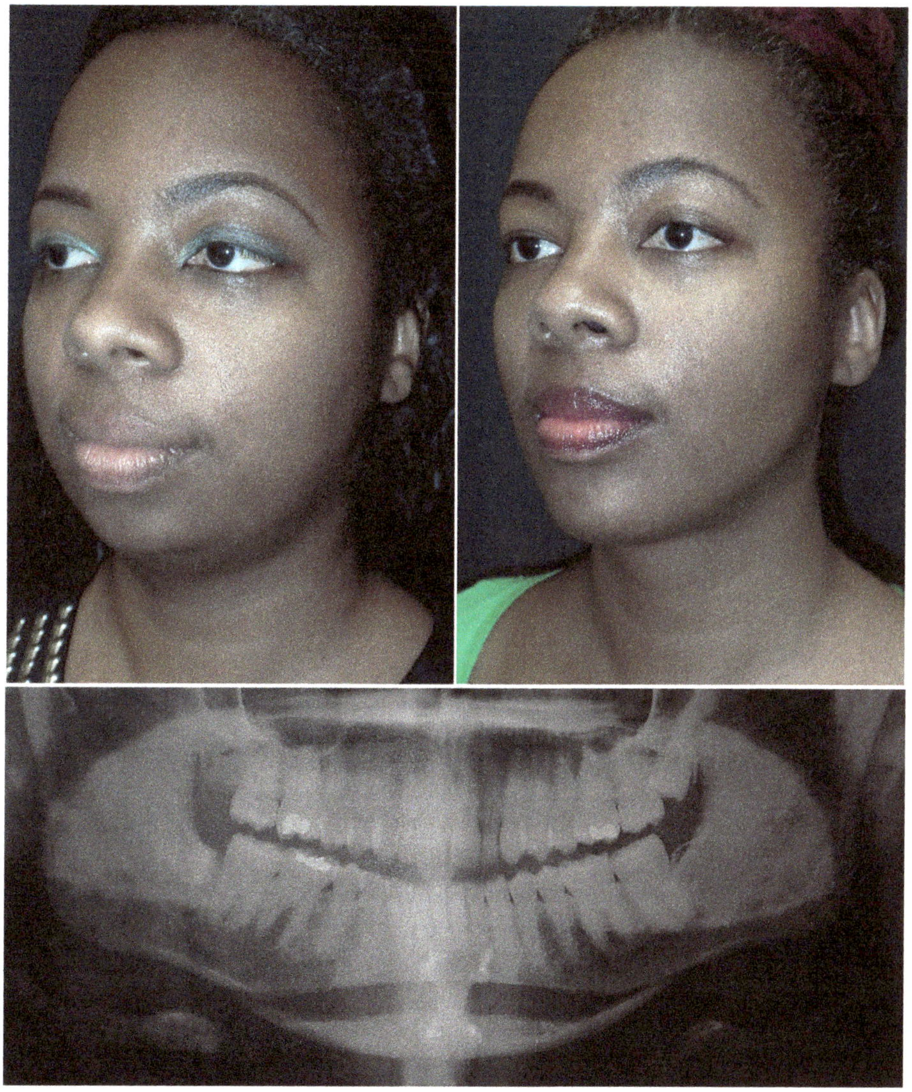

Fig. 7.50. This patient underwent submentoplasty with liposuction, jowl liposuction, midline platysma resection, deep platysmal fat reduction, buccal fat reduction, genioplasty, and midline platysmaplasty. The *left* image is before and the *right* image is 24 hours postoperatively. (Surgery by Dr. Joe Niamtu, III.)

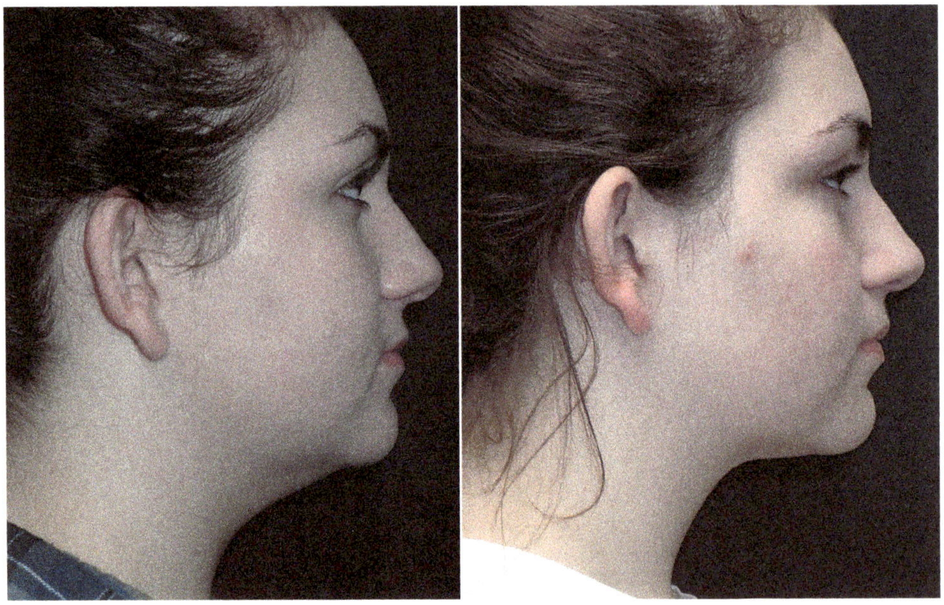

Fig. 7.51. This patient underwent submentoplasty with liposuction, jowl liposuction, midline platysma resection, deep platysmal fat reduction, buccal fat reduction, chin implant, and midline platysmaplasty. The *left* image is before and the *right* image is 90 days postoperatively. (Surgery by Dr. Joe Niamtu, III.)

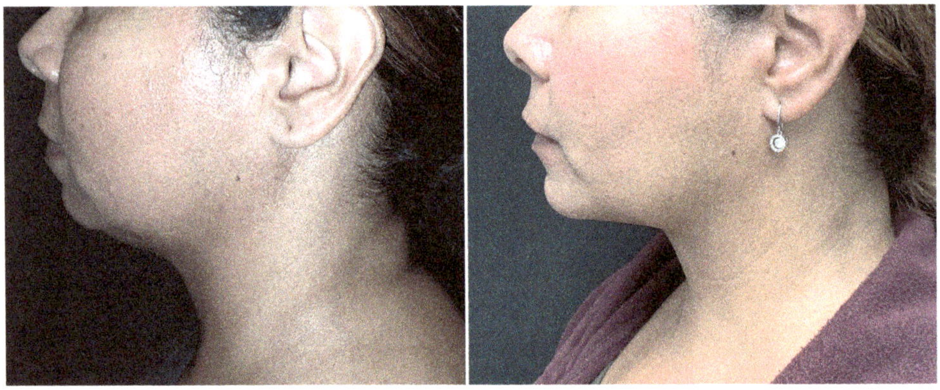

Fig. 7.52. This patient underwent submentoplasty with liposuction, jowl liposuction, midline platysma resection, deep platysmal fat reduction, buccal fat reduction, chin implant and midline platysmaplasty. The *left* image is before and the *right* image is 24 hours postoperatively. (Surgery by Dr. Joe Niamtu, III.)

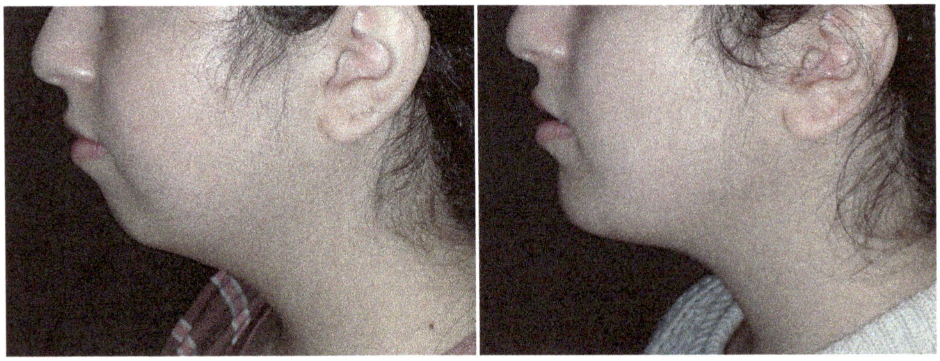

Fig. 7.53. This patient underwent submentoplasty with liposuction, jowl liposuction, midline platysma resection, deep platysmal fat reduction, buccal fat reduction, chin implant and midline platysmaplasty. The *left* image is before and the *right* image is 90 days postoperatively. (Surgery by Dr. Joe Niamtu, III.)

CHAPTER 8

Abbreviated Facelift and Neck Lift Procedures: Short Scar Facelift

Malcolm D. Paul, Joe Niamtu, III, Laxmeesh Mike Nayak

Chapter Outline

SHORT SCAR FACELIFT

Joe Niamtu, III

As with any procedure, people are always trying to find a shortcut way that produces results. Like anything else in life, if a shortcut is taken, there is usually some compromise in the result. This text has thus far shown several ways of performing facelift and neck lift surgery to suit surgeons with intermediate to expert abilities. Abbreviated procedures are more for the beginning surgeon and do have a place in cosmetic facial surgery, if performed on the proper patient. These smaller-type facelifts are often referred to collectively as "weekend facelifts," "S lifts," and "minilifts." A more accurate name is "short scar facelift" because most of these approaches utilize minimal incision techniques. Attempting to perform a short scar or minilift procedure on a patient with advanced aging is a recipe for failure. One cannot overcome large aging changes with these small types of procedures. They can be effective, however, if used on the correct patient population. These procedures frequently serve as the introductory facelift that surgeons learn and perform early in their careers. In my experience, these abbreviated facelift procedures are not common in the mainstream, busy facelift practice. But again, I do believe that they have a place.

The same preoperative scrutiny and operating room preparation is used regardless of the type of facelift performed. Numerous practitioners perform the short scar procedures with tumescent anesthesia only or tumescent anesthesia and oral sedation. Again, in my office, all procedures are performed under sterile technique with general anesthesia. One of the attractive things about short scar face lift is the fact that they can frequently be done without IV or general anesthesia.

Who Is a Short Scar Facelift Candidate?

This is a limited incision facelift and is only applicable to a very selective patient population. If a patient requests a short scar facelift in my office, I explain to them that almost every time I do this procedure, the incisions are not big enough to capture the amount of excess skin, even on younger patients. When I do perform this type of lift (once every several years), I obtain written permission and consent to extend the incision superiorly up the sulcus area and into the posterior hairline like a conventional facelift so I can adequately manage the skin. I would say that in 100% of these cases I end up extending incisions, but I have done very successful short scar lifts without these extended incisions on patients in their 30s or sometimes early 40s.

The best patients have minor jowling and minor submental skin excess and no platysmal banding. Patients with significant jowling or significant submental skin excess and significant platysmal banding are absolutely not candidates for this procedure. The crux of this procedure is to use a limited incision that is similar to the regular facelift incision anteriorly, but usually terminates in the mastoid region. The "limited incision" in this case is the fact that the incision does not extend superiorly on the postauricular sulcus region and does not extend into the posterior hairline. Eliminating the posterior auricular sulcus incision as well as the hairline incision streamlines the procedure with less surgery, dissection, and skin trimming. Reducing traditional incisions facilitates the procedure, but it also significantly decreases the control of skin tightening vectors. A submental incision can be made with platysma plication, but each additional step such as this nullifies the reasoning for performing "limited incision surgery."

Minimal procedures have great patient appeal, and patients may push for them. A problem that can exist is that a patient may beg for a "mini" procedure, even with extreme consent about what the procedure won't do. If the patient becomes unhappy with the smaller result, they will tell everyone that Dr. X performed a bad facelift. They won't mention that it was an abbreviated procedure and/or that they were adequately informed about the expected results—only that you were a poor surgeon! Due to situations like this, some surgeons avoid this type of procedure, as it can turn into negative PR.

Short scar facelift approaches are a great way for surgeons to learn facelift surgery as long as they understand the limitations of the procedure. It is absolutely important that the patients also understand the limits of the procedure and that the consent contain verbiage on not only what this small facelift will do, but what it also will *not* do.

The first step is to mark the incisions (Fig. 8.1). The preauricular incision is the same as the previously described comprehensive facelift. The posterior incision is much shorter and extends around the lobe just to the lobe attachment. The incision can be extended more superiorly along the post-irregular sulcus for patients with more excess neck skin.

The aforementioned incisions are made with a scalpel and the sideburn incision is irregular and beveled as previously described. Fig. 8.2 shows the completed incisions for the short scar facelift.

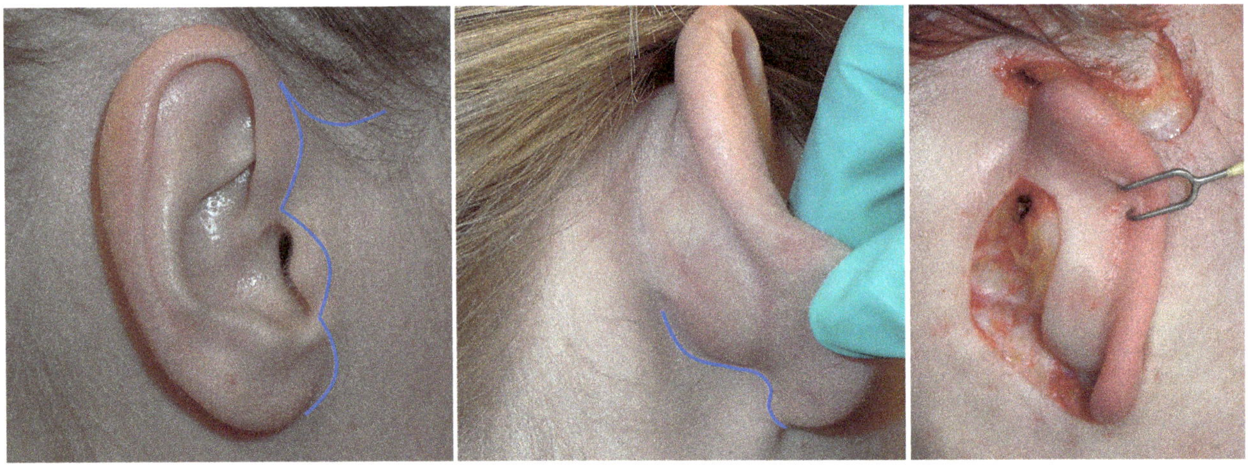

Fig. 8.1. The *left* image shows the preauricular incision, and the *right* image shows the posterior extension (the incision is continued more cephalad) frequently used in short scar facelifts.

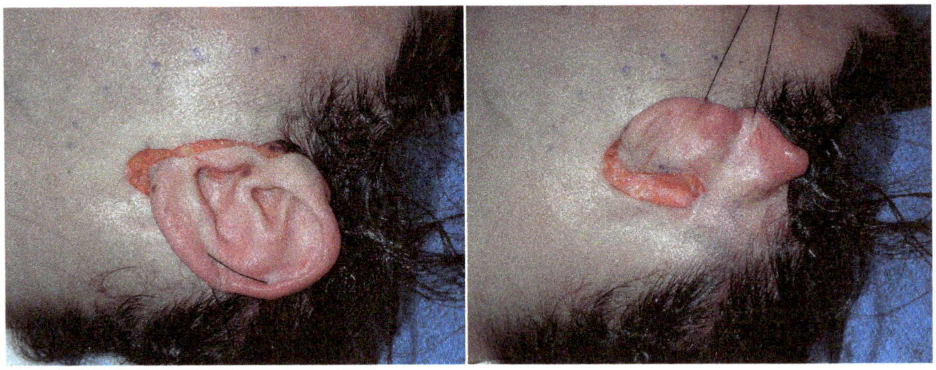

Fig. 8.2. These images show the completed incision for the short scar or "weekend facelift." A pretragal approach is shown but it can also be made behind the tragus.

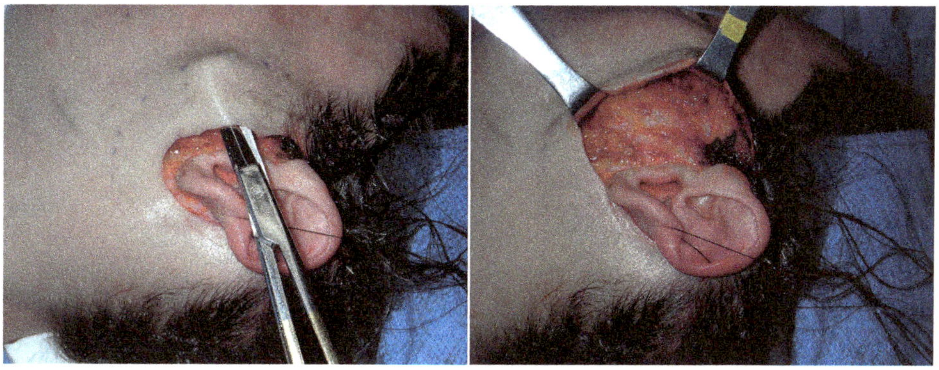

Fig. 8.3. These images illustrate the typical preauricular dissection with the short scar approach.

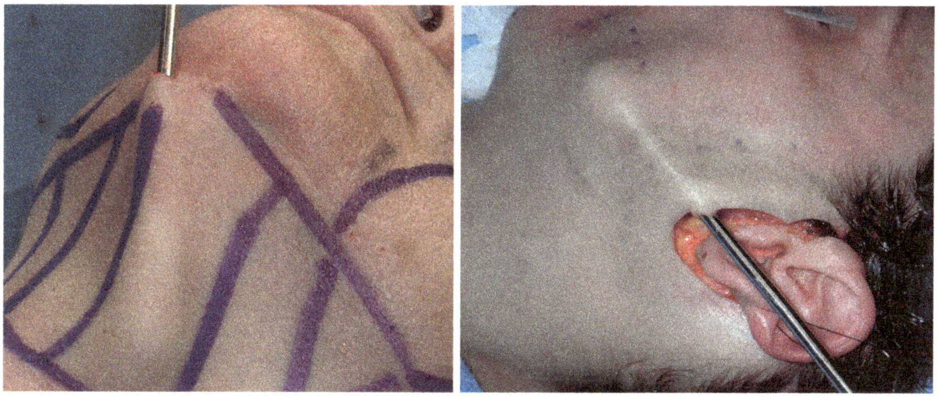

Fig. 8.4. Submental and jowl liposuction is usually performed with short scar lifts. I generally perform the submental liposuction first and the jowl liposuction after the cheek flap dissection.

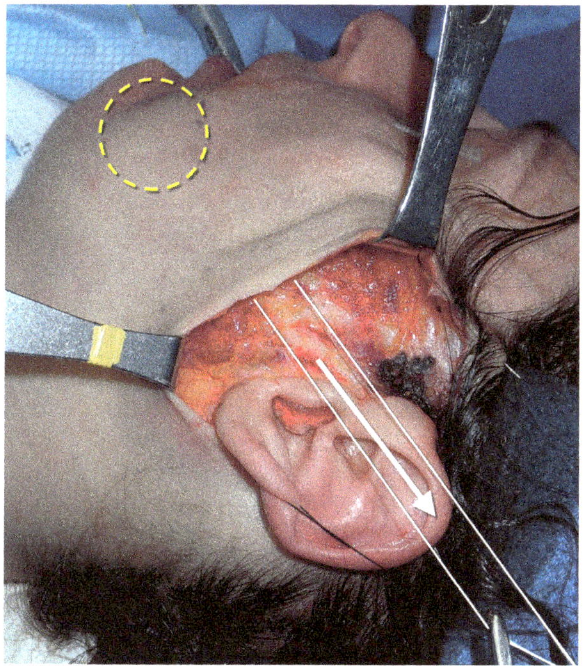

Fig. 8.5. This image shows the first SMAS placation suture, which commonly extends from the jowl region to the tragus. The *yellow circle* shows the area of the jowl that will be improved with this type of suspension.

The preauricular dissection is more conservative than the comprehensive facelift and generally extends anywhere from 2–5 cm and is commensurate with the amount of aging or jowling present (Fig. 8.3).

Meticulous attention to surgery, vital signs, and hemostasis is performed as with any other type of facelift. Liposuction is usually performed in the submental and jowl regions with short scar lifts (Fig. 8.4). The incision is extended around to the mastoid area and the superficial musculoaponeurotic system (SMAS) is addressed. The SMAS-plication is the simplest means of affectively managing the deeper tissues (Fig. 8.5).

Multiple SMAS-plication sutures are placed until the ptotic tissues are taut and repositioned. Fig. 8.6 shows several SMAS-plication sutures outlined with a marking pen. Note the most inferior suture is at or below the level of the mandibular border and assists in tightening the neck and defining the jawline.

For surgeons skilled at SMAS ectomy this can be performed in the same manner as described for the comprehensive facelift but in a smaller and more conservative manner (Fig. 8.7).

After the SMAS sutures are placed, the skin is addressed. Obviously, these small facelifts have much less detailed skin management than their bigger counterparts. An important fact with the anterior-only approach is that the vector of skin pull is much more vertical (Fig. 8.8).

When the correct vectors are verified, and the tension tightens the cheek, jowl, and upper part of the neck, the flaps are then set with anterior skin cutbacks and key sutures (Fig. 8.9).

After the key suture is placed, the excess skin is trimmed as described in the previous techniques (Fig. 8.10).

As discussed earlier, one of the main drawbacks of the short scar face lift is the inability to accommodate posterior auricular skin excess. If a patient has significant posterior auricular skin excess, they were a poor candidate for this procedure. Minor skin excess in the posterior auricular region can be managed with a small horizontal cut back at the mastoid region (Fig. 8.11). This should not extend past the pinna of the ear or it will be visible after surgery. Fig. 8.12 shows the sutured incisions at the end of the short scar procedure.

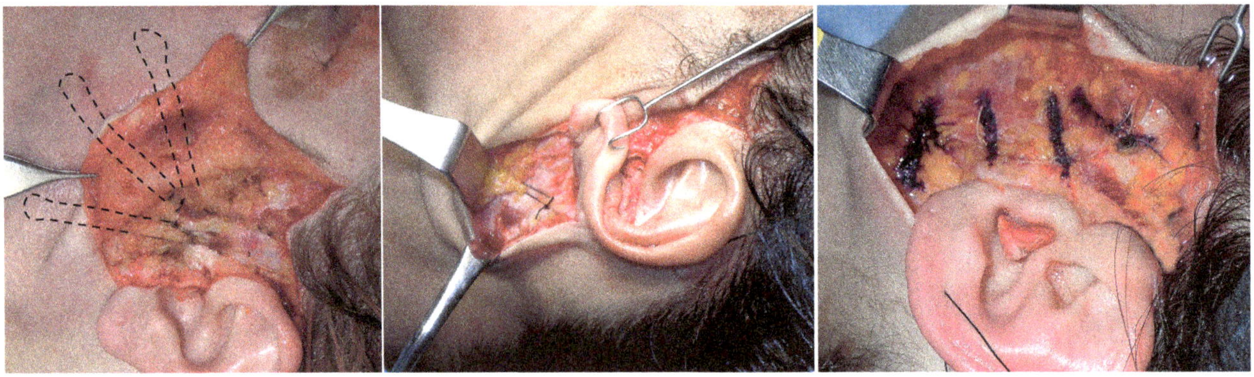

Fig. 8.6. The *left* image shows typical cheek plication sutures for the short scar lift. The *center* image shows the most inferior suture is at or below the mandibular border (preferred) and assists in tightening the neck and defining the jawline. A surgical marker outlines the SMAS-plication sutures in the *right* image.

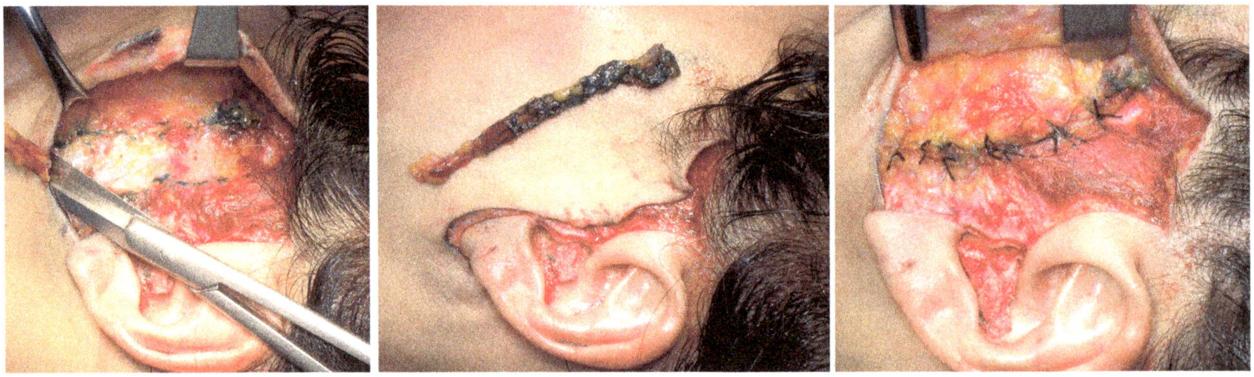

Fig. 8.7. Conservative SMAS ectomy (in experienced hands) is an optional way of SMAS management with short scar lifts.

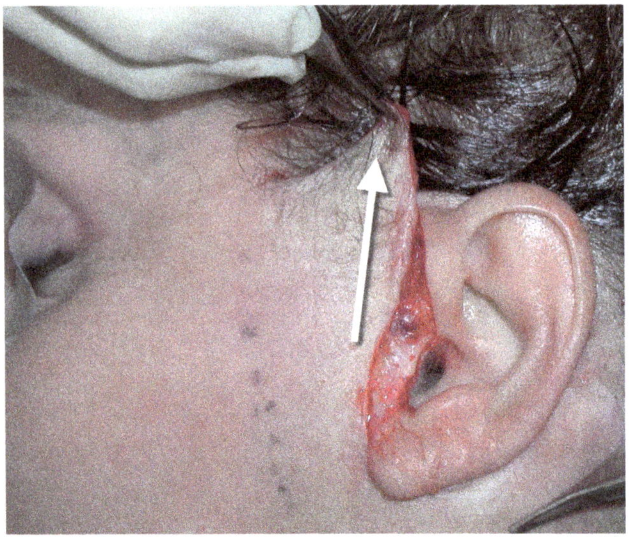

Fig. 8.8. The direction of skin pull and tension in the short scar face lift has a more of a vertical component. This image shows a pure vertical vector; however, in reality the vector is superior and lateral but more vertical than the previous lead described techniques. With short flaps, the surgeon must make sure the chosen vector will allow sufficient skin to close the incisions without tension. Only the key suture will hold tension, all other sutures must be passive so they don't scar.

Fig. 8.13 illustrates a typical case of skin excess in a short scar face lift. In the event that there is significantly more skin or a much larger dog-ear present, I personally convert the lift to a minilift as described. This would be the addition of a standard postauricular incision to manage this skin excess.

Sometimes surgeons make numerous compromises with small lifts to avoid several inches of posterior incision. Those several additional inches of posterior incision and dissection can "save" the case by making a significant impact on neck tightening and posterior auricular skin management. Chin implants in patients with profile deficiency can significantly impact the final result.

Postoperatively, no drains are used, and due to the small area of dissection, a pressure dressing may be omitted although it does not hurt to use light compression for several days.

Complications are similar to other facelift procedures but with less incidence. Hematoma is possible but rare due to limited undermining. Nerve damage, seroma, poor scarring, and undertreatment can occur. One big problem that can be encountered is attempting to perform this procedure on a patient with excessive neck skin. Since the incision does not extend up into the posterior hairline, there will be tissue bunching. This bunching will usually resolve but can last a year. Fig. 8.14 shows two cases about a month after surgery.

Figs. 8.15–8.17 show before-and-after pictures of short scar facelift performed by Dr. Niamtu. Patients must understand that a procedure for "small aging" will yield "small results." Accurate patient expectations are critical when performing abbreviated procedures.

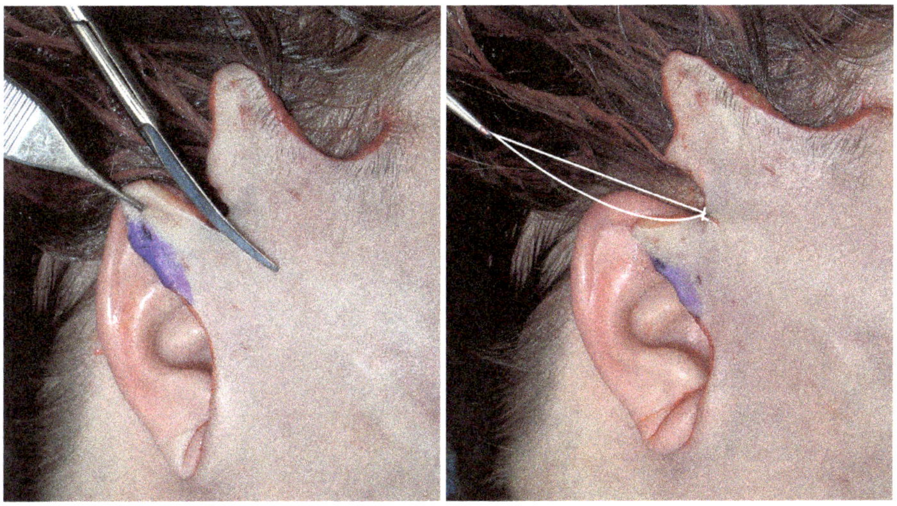

Fig. 8.9. The *left* image illustrates the skin cut back with scissors, and the *right* image illustrates the anterior 4-0 Vicryl key suture.

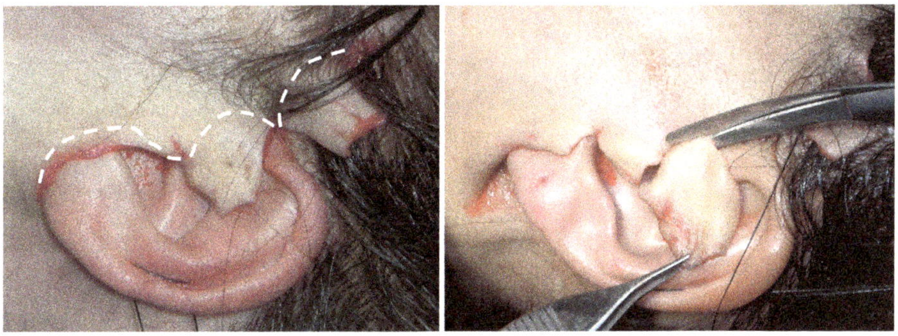

Fig. 8.10. The skin access is illustrated by the *dashed lines* on the *left* image, and the *right* image shows the excess skin being trimmed.

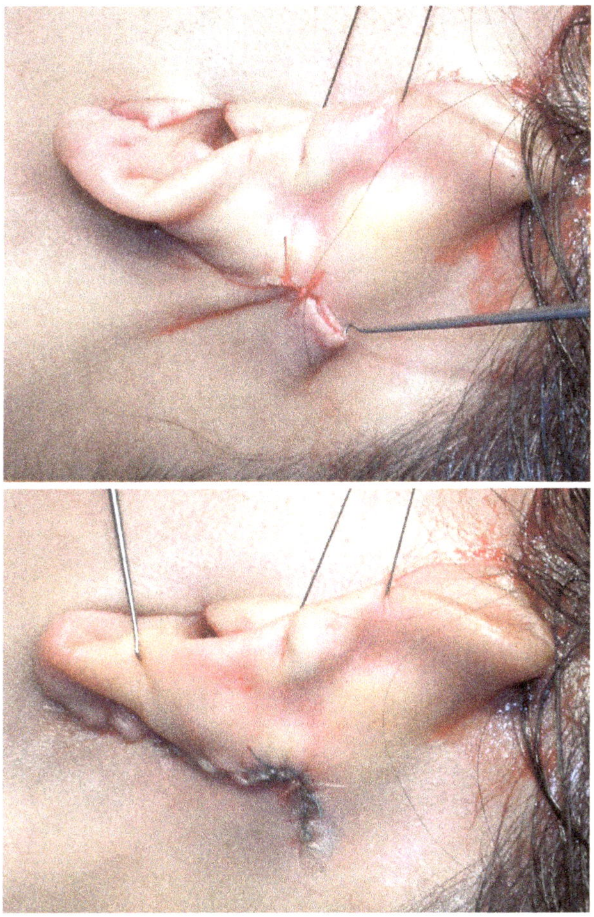

Fig. 8.11. When retracting the posterior auricular skin in an effort to tighten the neck, there is frequently excess skin or dog-ear that requires a release to prevent bunching. This release needs to be hidden behind the ear so it will not be visible after surgery.

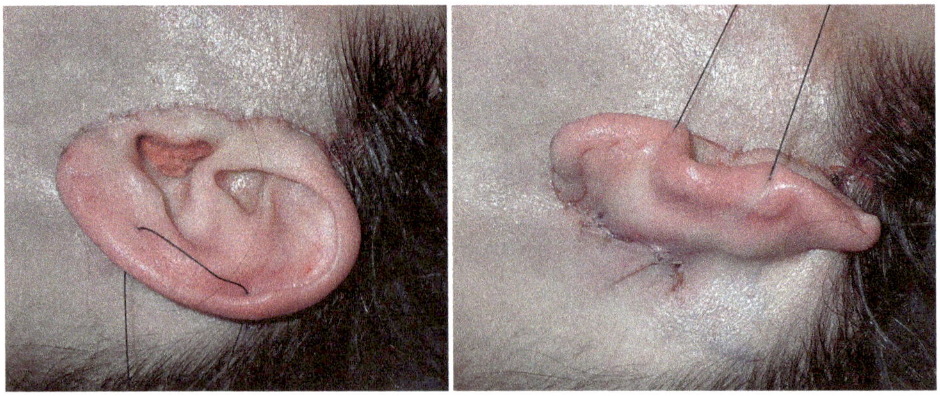

Fig. 8.12. These images show the final closure of the short scar lift. The front is closed with alternating 5-0 and 6-0 gut sutures.

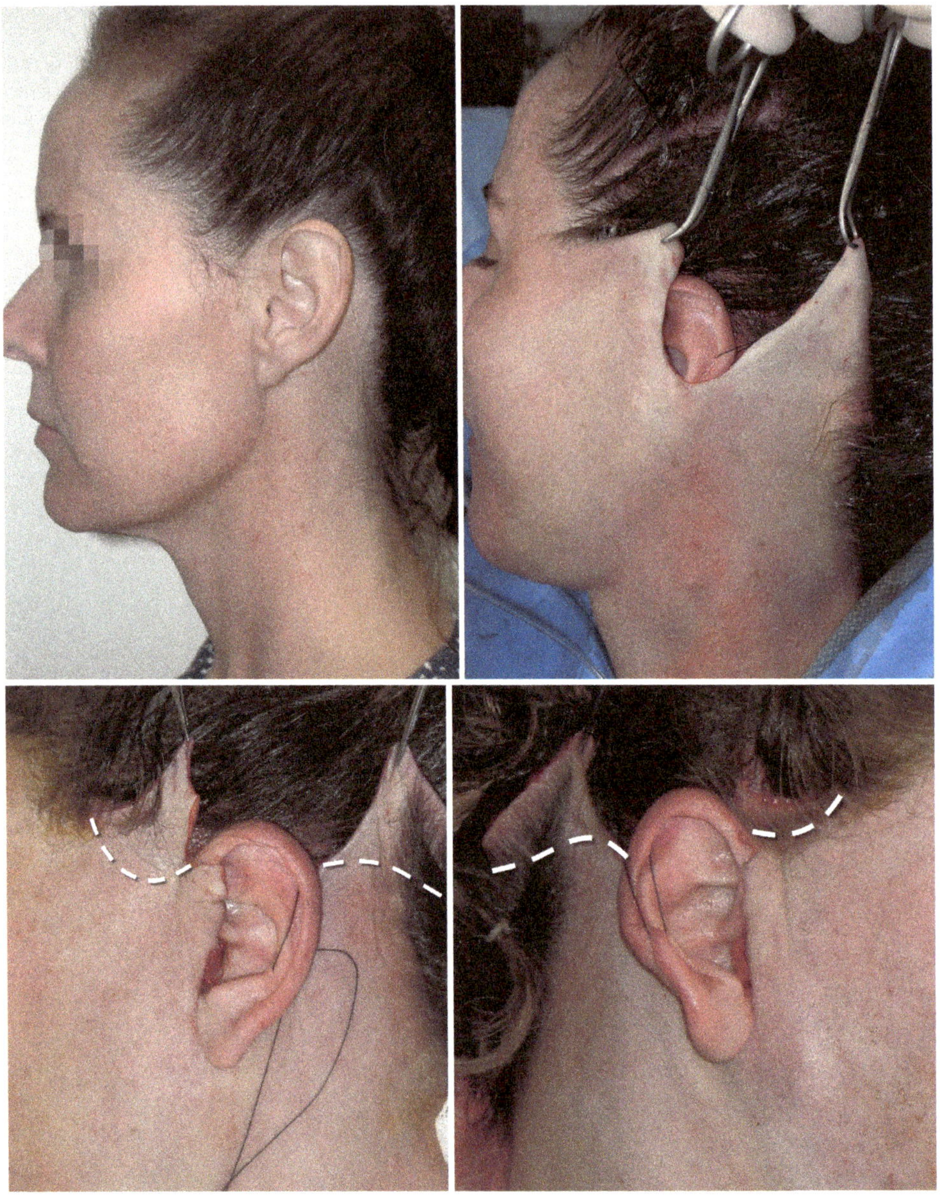

Fig. 8.13. The *upper left* picture shows a patient that appears to be suitable for a "short scar" lift, but the *upper right* picture shows the amount of actual skin excess that required conversion into a more traditional pre- and postauricular incision case. The *lower* images show the skin excess to be excised. Numerous times I have been faced with a "short scar" case that required conversion to a larger lift. Failure to do so would cause a decreased result with skin excess.

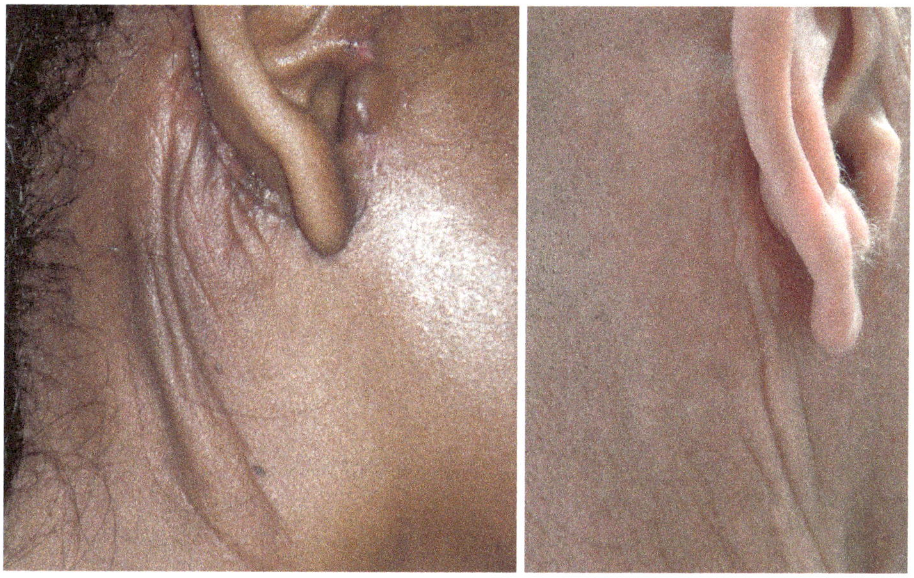

Fig. 8.14. The *left* image shows bunching on the posterior region 30 days after surgery that took a year to resolve. The *right* image shows another patient with noticeable bunching. The remedy for this would have been to perform a conventional facelift with pre- and postauricular flaps.

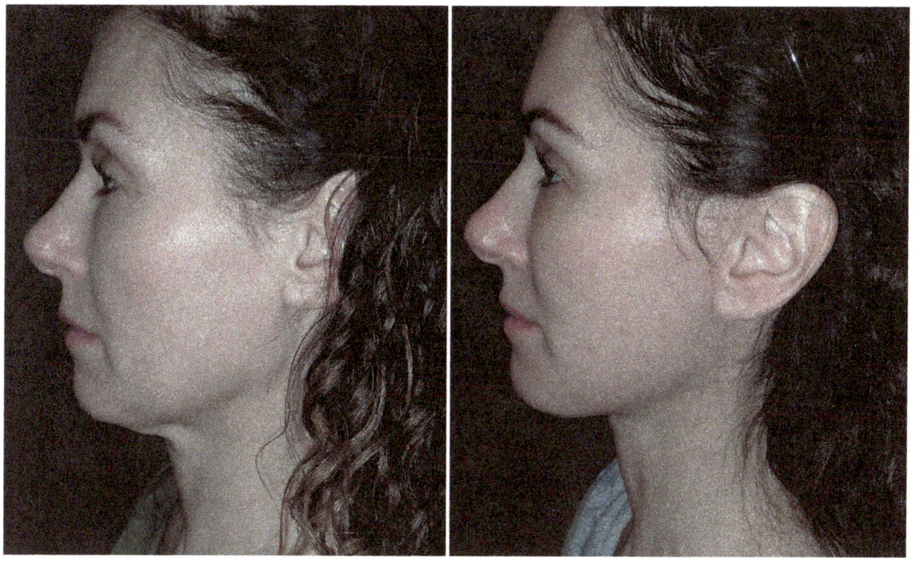

Fig. 8.15. This patient is shown before and 3 months after short scar facelift.

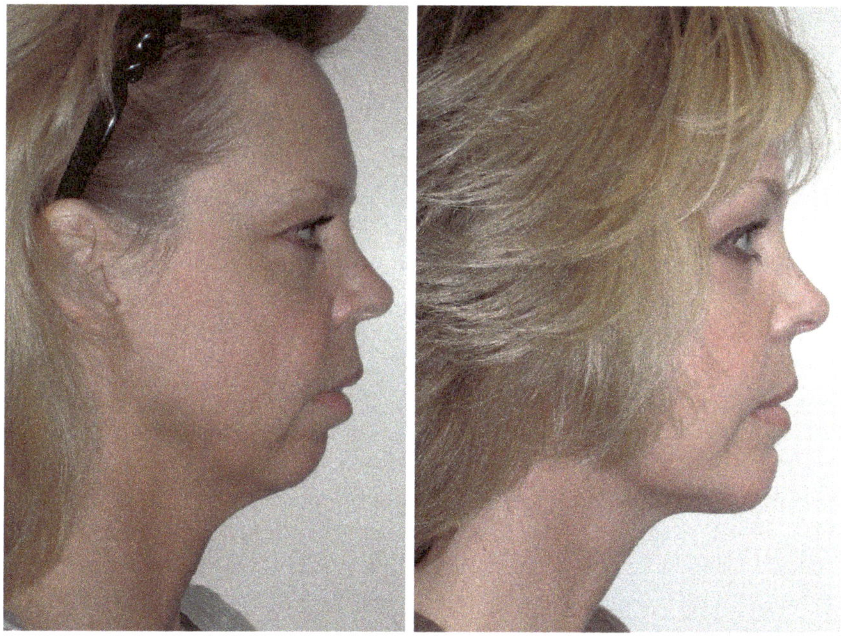

Fig. 8.16. This patient is shown before and 3 months after short scar facelift with a large silicone chin implant.

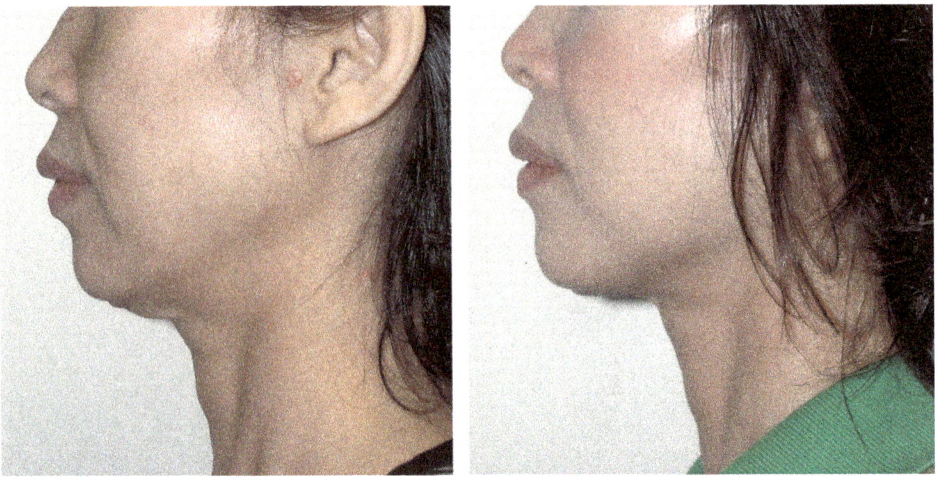

Fig. 8.17. This patient is shown before and 3 months after short scar facelift with a small silicone chin implant.

SHORT SCAR FACELIFT: MY EVOLUTION OF THOUGHT, PROCESS, AND TECHNIQUES

Malcolm D. Paul

History of Short Scar Facelifting

The concept of performing facial rejuvenation through a short scar has a long history. Beginning at the start of the 20th century, Passot used very short excisions of lateral facial skin to tighten the lateral face. Noel was also a proponent of short scar lifts. These procedures with limited dissection did not provide any correction of ptotic midface, lower face, and neck age-related shifts of soft tissue. Of course, we now appreciate the combined effect of loss of volume and gravitational changes in the aging face and neck. The goal of facelift surgery has always been to provide a safe approach with minimal scarring, minimal downtime, and effective long-lasting improvement in the maintenance of elevated and repositioned soft tissue along with autologous and nonautologous fillers as needed for volume enhancement. I have performed a variety of procedures with various incisions, SMAS manipulation, vectors, and soft tissue auto-augmentation by shifting midface ptotic tissues to a more elevated, youthful position including the shortening of the lid-cheek junction.

Problems Encountered With the Short Scar Facelift

The popularity of short scar facelifts occurred as a response to the request from our patients for shorter, less noticeable incisions; a faster recovery time; and longevity of the result obtained. Original proponents of short scar facelifting included the Saylan (S lift), Baker (lateral SMAS ectomy), and Tonnard and Verpaele (minimal access cranial suspension [MACS] lift). Limiting the incision to the temporal sideburn and the preauricular area, ending at the ear lobule, was the pattern published by these surgeons. Unfortunately, for the short scar facelift, some of these requests were not met with these most popular short scar techniques. That is not to say that there are not patients who will benefit from the short scar approach. On the contrary, many younger patients with minimal skin laxity, thin facial soft tissue, minimal neck laxity, short platysma bands, and so on can undergo this procedure with success. However, patients need to be properly informed as to the expected result to be achieved with a short scar facelift. It is best to underpromise and overdeliver. Before surgery, what we tell patients is an explanation. After surgery, when patients' expectations are not met, it is perceived by our patients as an excuse!

The drawback to the short scar facelift is the vertical vector that is required to avoid a postauricular incision needed to redrape skin excess, which in conventional facelifts is in a superolateral pull (Marchac and Nasr au lieu de Nask 2008). This brings me to the next and even more important concept: Why avoid a postauricular incision when this incision can be hidden if placed properly and closed without excessive skin tension? So, I believe that one should never compromise on the incision placement to allow the facelift to be performed through short incisions. Moreover, the vertical pull required the excess skin to be redraped at the temporal sideburn with an extension from the horizontal to the vertical. Incisions placed in the horizontal sideburn area can be covered by the downward direction of the hair. However, extending the incision to the vertical sideburn/temporal hairline creates a scar that is visible because the hair grows up and back, revealing a permanent scar, which can be hypopigmented and/or hypertrophic. Tonnard and Verpaele worked with a zigzag pattern to incorporate the excess skin. Vertical extensions should be avoided. (When I have had to tailor the excess skin in this area, I performed a backcut in the temporal hair to avoid a visible scar, but this can advance the temporal hairline posteriorly with a greater than 6–7 cm distance from the tail of the eyebrow, which is undesirable.)

Another negative effect of the short scar facelift is the frequent occurrence of a pleat of skin behind the ear lobule. Often this incision, despite our best intentions and reassurance to the patient, does not flatten and become a nonissue. So the correct solution is to extend the incision along the retroauricular sulcus to allow the excess skin to be tailored for better approximation. At that point, one is nearly at a standard facelift pattern except for the extension into the scalp, which, again, can be invisible when properly planned and performed. My preference is to start the backcut of the postauricular incision at the touch point of the helix and the postauricular skin and be certain to realign the hairline when the flap is inset. This becomes a traditional facelift and neck lift pattern and is no longer a short scar approach. Again, this illustrates the desire for a "short scar" but the need for a longer scar.

The neck cannot be adequately addressed in the short scar approach without additional maneuvers. A 2 to 3 cm extension of the short scar in the retroauricular sulcus with additional undermining followed with lateral platysma myotomies and suspension to the mastoid fascia has been published (Jacono 2020) and allows precision contouring of the neck from the lateral approach without extending the incision into the hair-baring scalp. Certainly, the central neck can most directly be approached through a standard submental incision (my preference).

Evolution of My Technique in Short Scar Facelifting

For many years, I have attempted to limit the postauricular incision to the postauricular crease without crossing into the hair-bearing scalp. For 90+% of my facelifts, I have not had to add the horizontal component behind the ear. Several technical modifications have allowed me to avoid extending the incision into the hair-bearing scalp. My protocol for over 90% of my facelifts is as follows:

1. Use of tumescent anesthesia has significantly improved the ease of soft tissue dissection (Fig. 8.18).
   500 mL of lactated Ringer's solution
   1 mg epinephrine
   500 mg of tranexamic acid to diminish bleeding and ecchymoses
2. I use standard facelift incisions mostly along the tragal edge and the temporal sideburn horizontally (Fig. 8.19). I avoid adding vertical incisions in the temporal hairline area, preferring a backcut into the temporal scalp to blend in the excess skin. The trade-off is a modest posterior movement of the temporal hairline.
   The postauricular incision stays within the postauricular crease including an inverted V where the contour changes.
3. The submental incision for liposuction of the neck, management of the interplatysmal and the subplatysmal fat, platysma undermining, platysmaplasty including the digastric fascia, and a backcut in the inferior platysma muscles for long, thick bands (Fig. 8.20, *left*).
4. The use of sequential dilators to release the skin and subcutaneous tissue from the underlying superficial cervical fascia in the neck and from the anterior SMAS in the cheek.
5. The SMAS is infiltrated with saline approximately 10 mm per side (I use 1% lidocaine with epinephrine in cases performed under oral sedation and analgesia to avoid the

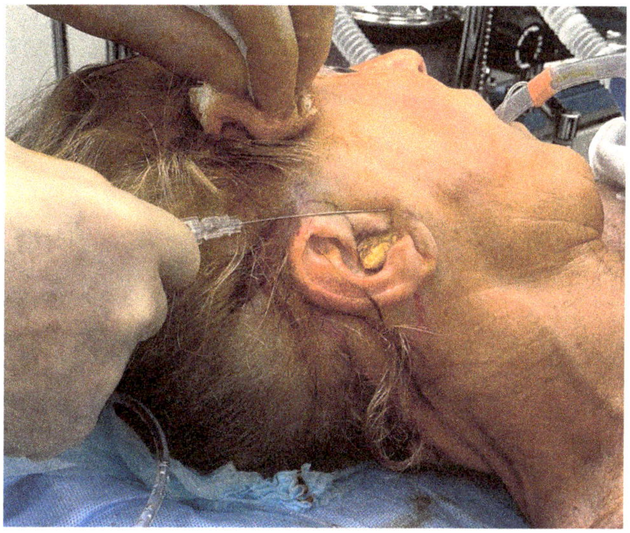

Fig. 8.18. This image shows the tumescent infiltration.

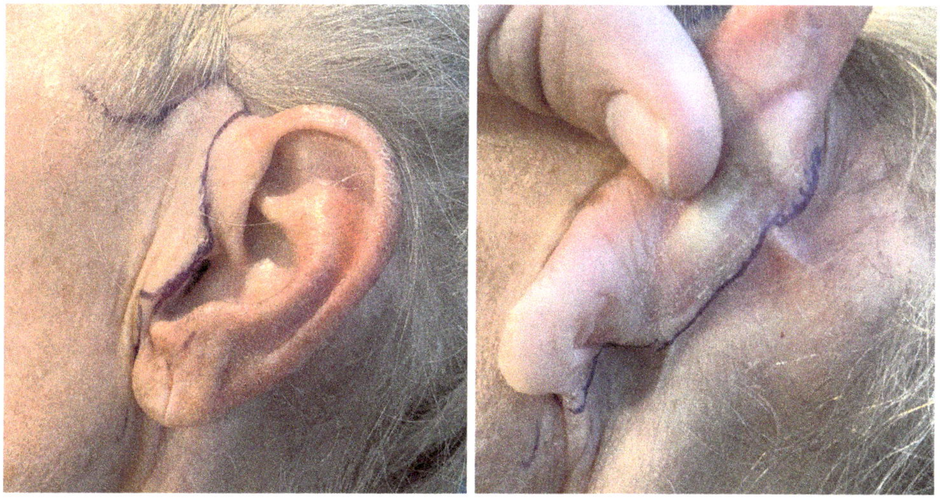

Fig. 8.19. This image shows the pre- and postauricular incisions utilized in 90% of my facelifts.

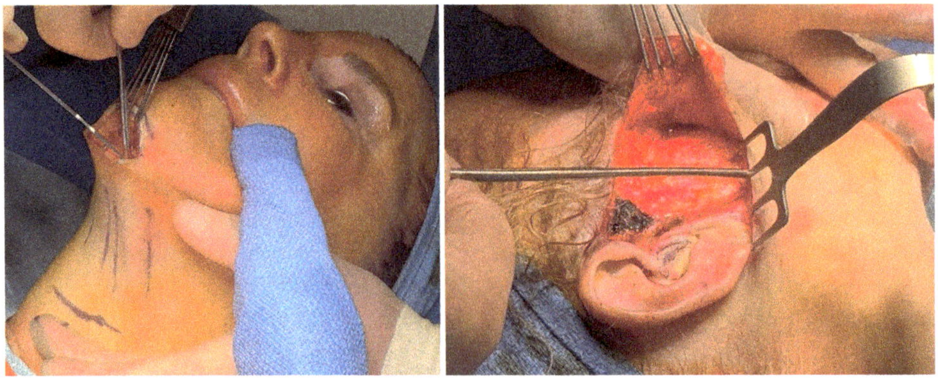

Fig. 8.20. The *left* image shows both the submental incision and the use of a dilator to "pretunnel" the dissection. The *right* image shows a dilator being used to pretunnel the anterior portion of the area to be undermined. The Hegar uterine dilators are available online and for less than $20 and come in a kit from 3 to 20 mm. When used sequentially, the entire flap can be undermined and raised with literally no sharp dissection.

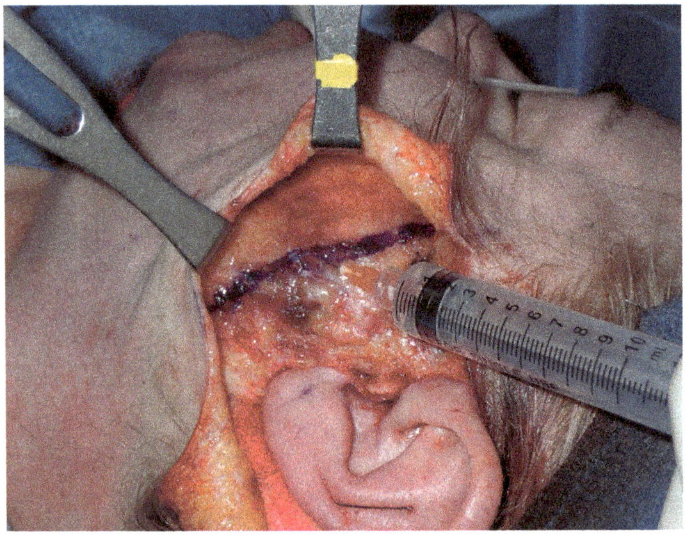

Fig. 8.21. This image shows local anesthetic injection to SMAS before surgical entry of this plane.

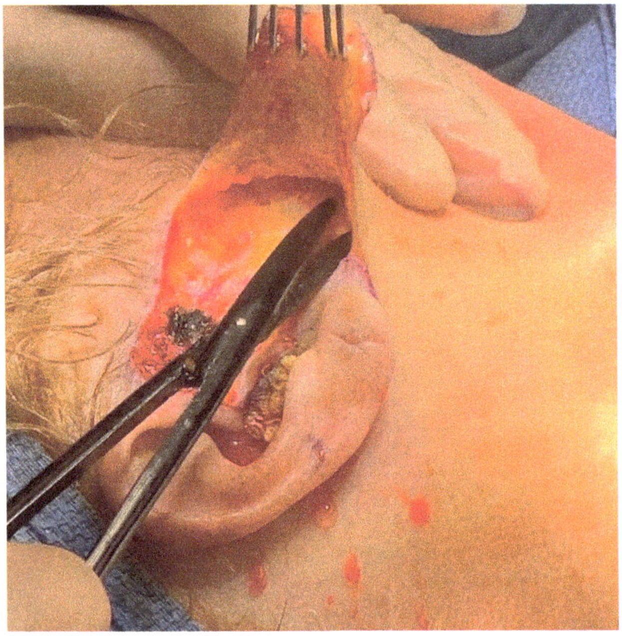

Fig. 8.22. The SMAS incision and dissection are carried to the anterior cheek.

discomfort of the sub-SMAS dissection) prior to incision and undermining (Fig. 8.21). The anterior SMAS incision and dissection is carried to the anterior cheek (Fig. 8.22) to advance the SMAS including the repositioning of ptotic midface fat superiorly after ligamentous release, thereby shortening the lid-cheek junction. This maneuver has allowed me to avoid adding fat grafting except in overly deflated cases.

6. Superolateral SMAS suspension is performed beginning at Lore's (platysma auricular) fascia, ending over the malar region. Irrigation of the wound with hydrogen peroxide has a remarkable effect on reducing troubling oozing before closure.
7. Redraping the skin with proper vector correction of ptotic soft tissues (Fig. 8.23).
8. Skin incisions are closed without tension to avoid hypertrophic scars, and drain placement is optional depending on the requirement in each case (Fig. 8.24).

This technique is, in effect, a short scar facelift and neck lift performed without compromising the result. The bidirectional lift is anatomically correct, addressing all components of the aging face and neck without visible scars, skin pleating, or incorrect vectors of correction. Patients experience an average recovery time of 7–10 days.

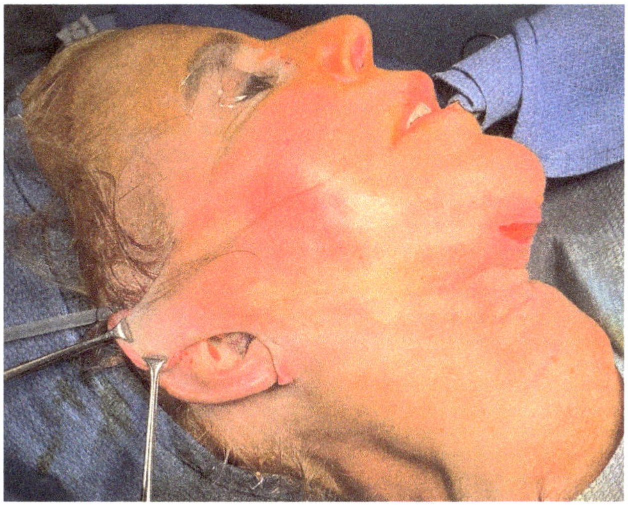

Fig. 8.23. The skin is redraped in the proper vector to correct the ptotic tissues and skin excess. This vector may be different from traditional facelift traction due to the lack of a posterior hairline incision.

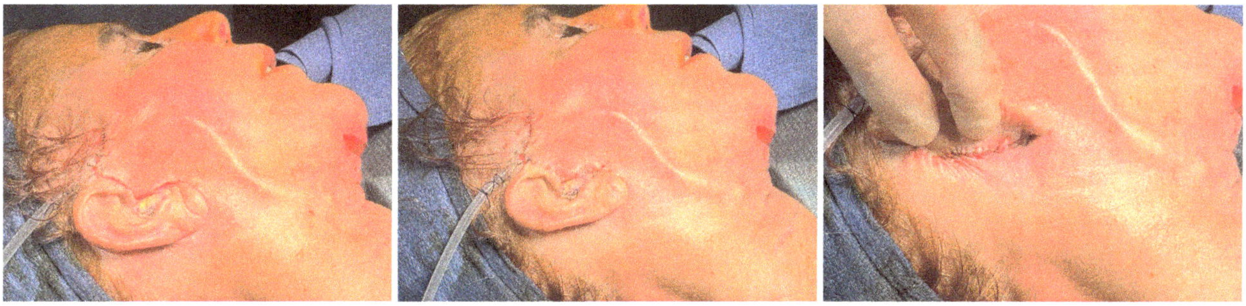

Fig. 8.24. The preauricular incision is shown after trimming and before closure (*left* image), and the *center* image shows the preauricular incision closed and an optional drain placed. The *right* image shows the postauricular incision closed passively without bunching.

Further Reading

Baker DC. Commentary on: short scar face lift. *Aesthet Surg J*. 2008;28:209–210.

Fulton JE, Saylan Z, Helton P, Rahimi AD, Golshani M. The S-lift facelift featuring the U-suture and O-suture combined with skin resurfacing. *Dermatol Surg*. 2001;27:18–22.

Jacono AA. Face-lift surgical techniques. *Facial Plast Surg Clin North Am*. 2020;28.

Labbé D, Kaluzinski E. Les innovations françaises en chirurgie esthétique de la face [French innovations in aesthetic surgery of the face]. *Ann Chir Plast Esthet*. 2010;55:384–396.

Marchac D, Nasr au lieu de Nask M. Avoiding the operated on look in multiple face lifts. *J Plast Reconstr Aesthet Surg*. 2008;61:1449–1458.

Tonnard P, Verpaele A. The MACS-lift short scar rhytidectomy. *Aesthet Surg J*. 2007;27:188–198.

Direct Neck Excision Z-Plasty

Laxmeesh Mike Nayak, Joe Niamtu, III

Editor's note

As stated many times throughout this book, my goal is to present new information. There are times, however, when historic information is useful, and to that end I have copied Doctor Nayak's awesome chapter on direct neck lift and included it in this text. It is largely the same as it appeared in my previous texts; however, sometimes things are so well done they don't need to be changed. Although this is not a commonly performed procedure, there is a place for it, and some people are interested, hence I am including it in this edition.

Introduction

The previous section detailed comprehensive treatment of lower facial aging with facelift surgery and this chapter discusses alternative lifting techniques. Comprehensive facelift and neck lift remains the gold standard for treatment of jowls and excess neck skin. Not all patients are candidates for comprehensive facelifts for medical reasons, inability to take time off, finances, or simply wanting a more conservative procedure. It is imperative for the surgeon and the patient to realize that any procedure that is more conservative will yield less of a treatment result. In cases of excess neck skin and submental aging without significant jowling, the direct excision Z-plasty neck lift may be appropriate. The positives include a small surgical procedure with minimal recovery and a dramatic change in submental aesthetics. Negatives include a visible scar and the fact that only the anterior neck is improved.

A sharp cervicomental angle is central an overall appearance of youth and strength. Defined by the intersection of the facial plane with a line from the cervical point to the menton, the cervicomental angle is acute in youth and becomes obtuse with age or even effaced. Restoration of the obtuse cervicomental angle is a key aim of surgery of the lower third of the aging face.

Widening of the cervicomental angle with age is due to the combined effects of loss of skin elasticity, increase in submental fat, and soft tissue ptosis, including the platysma muscle and submandibular glands. Abnormally low and anterior hyoid bone position and/or microgenia can accentuate these features.

Traditionally, the cervicomental angle has been addressed together with a tightening of the jawline and jowls via cervicofacial rhytidectomy and submentoplasty. Correcting these interrelated areas simultaneously contributes to a natural-appearing rejuvenation of the lower third of the face.

For selected patients, however, direct rejuvenation of the aging neck is an appropriate option. These patients may evidence primary aging changes of the neck out of proportion to adjacent facial units or may present with persistent skin laxity after facelift surgery. Other patients seek isolated correction of the lax neck or wish to avoid the stigmata of traditional periauricular facelift incisions. These groups of patients can benefit from more targeted neck rejuvenation.

Traditional approaches to direct treatment of the aging neck include liposuction, open submentoplasty, and suture suspension techniques. Although these procedures address the fat and sometimes the platysma, they can be inadequate for patients with inelastic or excessive cervical skin and will often lead to unsatisfactory rejuvenation and early recidivism. Direct excision and simple primary closure of the redundant skin in either a transverse or vertical fashion creates an unfavorable scar, prone to contracture and webbing. To address this problem, direct excision of neck skin with Z-plasty closure is a viable alternative for isolated treatment of the male neck. This chapter presents experience with direct excision of redundant neck skin with submentoplasty and Z-plasty closure in both male and female patients.

In previous articles, the application of direct neck excision has been limited mainly to male patients, especially those who are balding or have heavy beards. This has been expanded to include any patient who is uncomfortable with undergoing a traditional facelift and is willing to accept isolated rejuvenation of the neck in exchange for a fine Z-plasty incision line. Certain male patients, in particular, fear the social stigma of periauricular incisions, no matter how well executed, and are more comfortable with the more "functional-appearing" Z-plasty incision. This technique has also been adapted as a planned second-stage revision for after facelift or concomitantly with a facelift for patients with either thick, excessive, heavy skin or fine, crepey, inelastic skin.

Surgical Technique

The patient is marked sitting in the upright position, with head held in the Frankfort horizontal plane. A midline vertical, elliptiform incision is marked on the anterior neck, with its apex in the submental triangle and its inferior extent as low as necessary to encompass the redundant neck excess. In most individuals, the inferior extent of the incision is at the level of the thyroid notch; however, with extreme cases, it may be carried down as low as the suprasternal notch. The width of the ellipse is marked conservatively to avoid excessive tension in the final closure. The intended level of the new cervical point/neck crease is also marked (Fig. 8.25). In many cases the actual incision is directly on the midline, especially in patients with a symmetric "turkey gobbler" skin excess. In patients with solitary isolated lateral excess, the incision can be made off center to better address the precise excess.

A single dose of intravenous antibiotic is given for skin flora coverage. Once an adequate plane of intravenous sedation and analgesia is achieved, the anterior neck is infiltrated with 0.5% lidocaine/0.25% bupivacaine and 1:150,000 epinephrine, and sufficient time is allowed for the epinephrine to exert maximum hemostatic effect. During this time, markings are reconfirmed and the patient is sterilely prepped and draped. The procedure begins with a full-thickness skin incision using a #10 Bard-Parker blade. Dissection is then carried down through the subcutaneous fat with needle-tipped electrocautery hemostasis (Fig. 8.26). The excessive skin and midline submental/preplatysmal fat are removed en bloc (Figs. 8.26 and 8.27).

The medial platysmal borders are identified and treated in a similar manner to conventional facelift/submentoplasty.

Bilateral neck flaps are then created by elevating thin subcutaneous flaps off of the preplatysmal flaps on each side of the neck to the anterior borders of the sternocleidomastoid muscles. Most of the dissection is accomplished with sequential spreads of a medium or large facelift scissor. Bridging vessels are identified and cauterized with bipolar cautery as needed. While elevating the flaps, several millimeters of subcutaneous fat are preserved to prevent dermal adhesion to the underlying muscle as well as to protect the dermal plexus. A headlight or lighted facelift retractor can be helpful with the lateral-most extents of this dissection. Liposculpting is performed in a similar manner to conventional facelift to address any focal areas of fat. Subplatysmal lipodystrophy and/or submandibular gland ptosis may also be addressed, if needed, by elevating the platysma off of the deep cervical fascia from medial to lateral. Care is taken during debulking of ptotic submandibular glands to preserve the marginal mandibular nerve and avoid the facial vessels. If indicated, maneuvers such as debulking and plication of the anterior bellies of the digastric muscles or placement of a chin implant may also be accomplished at this time. After the fat contours have been addressed, a median platysmaplasty is performed.

A 3-0 PDS suture is used to approximate the medial edges of the platysma. The initial suture is placed at the level of the desired cervical point marked preoperatively, and a running simple stitch is used to approximate the medial edges of the platysma up to the mandibular symphysis. Care is taken not to recruit excessive amounts of platysma and fat into this suture, so as to avoid excessive bulk in the central neck. Upon reaching the mandibular symphysis, the suture is run back down to the cervical point for an additional layer of strength and is then tied. Next, a 1 cm notch is cut from the medial edges of the platysma bilaterally, inferior to the cervical point. This prevents postoperative banding of the

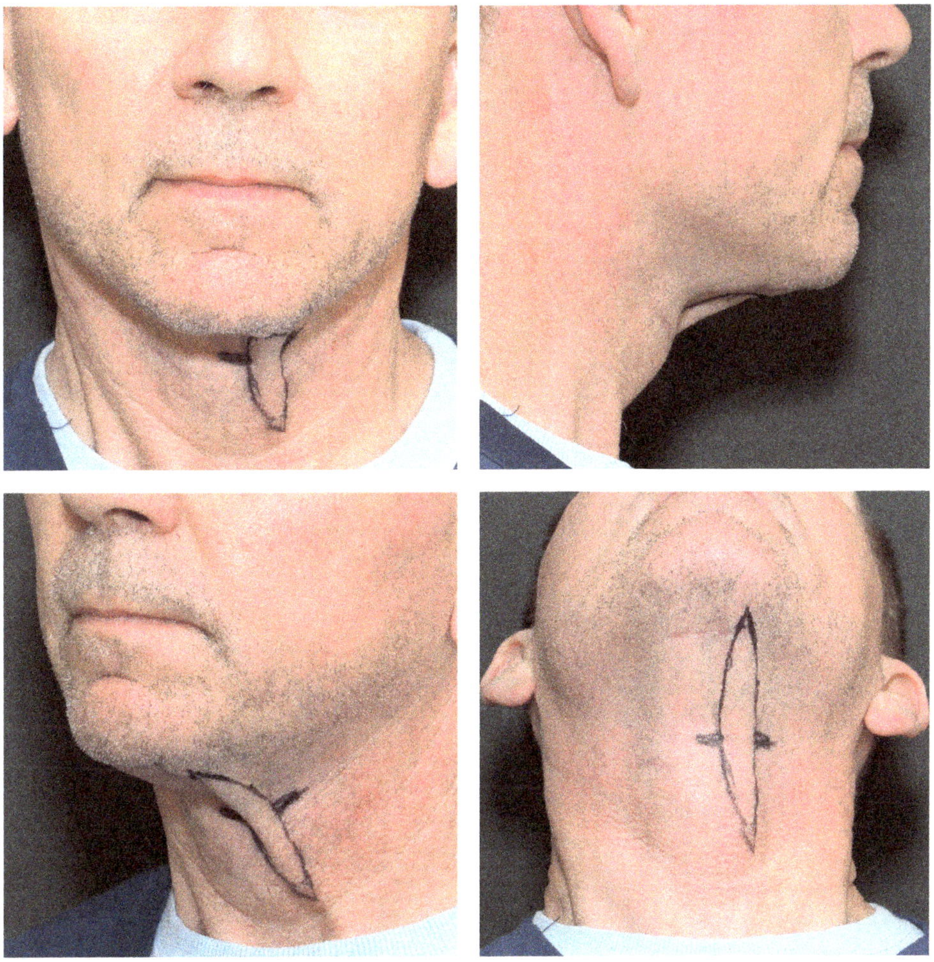

Fig. 8.25. This series of markings shows the typical incision outline. Since this patient had increased skin/muscle excess on the left medial platysmal band, the incision in this case is made lateral to the midline.

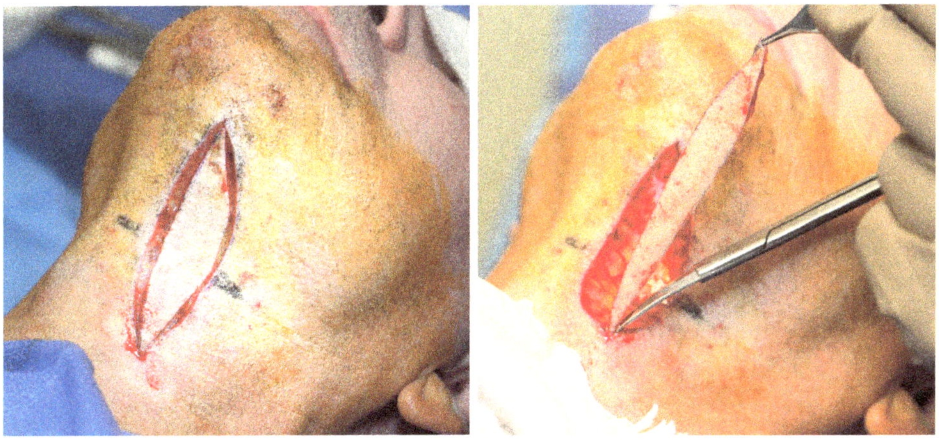

Fig. 8.26. The *left* image shows the skin incision, and the *right* image shows the en bloc resection of at the preplatysmal level.

free edges of the inferior aspect of the platysma. This process is the same as conventional midline platysmaplasty described earlier in this chapter.

With the shaping of the preplatysmal fat, platysma, and, if necessary, subplatysmal fat complete, attention is turned to the Z-plasty closure of the neck incision. The wound is temporarily closed in a simple vertical line with simple interrupted sutures (Fig. 8.27). The mark at the cervical point is once again verified, and used as the central limb for Z-plasty. An incision is made diagonally, at 30 degrees to the cervical point line, on each neck flap, creating the triangular flaps to be transposed (Figs. 8.28 and 8.29).

The temporary sutures are then removed, and the wound is closed in layers, with 4-0 and 5-0 Monocryl in the deep layer and tension-free 6-0 running, locking Prolene in the skin (Fig. 8.30). Care and time should be given to the ends of the incision. Despite the primary Z-plasty, some degree of standing

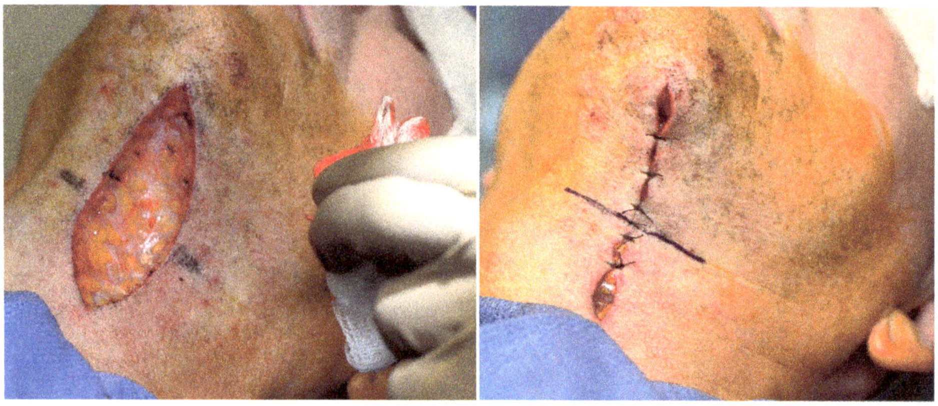

Fig. 8.27. The *left* image shows the surgical defect after resection, and the *right* image shows the temporary sutures used to determine the cervicomental angle, which is shown by the *black line*.

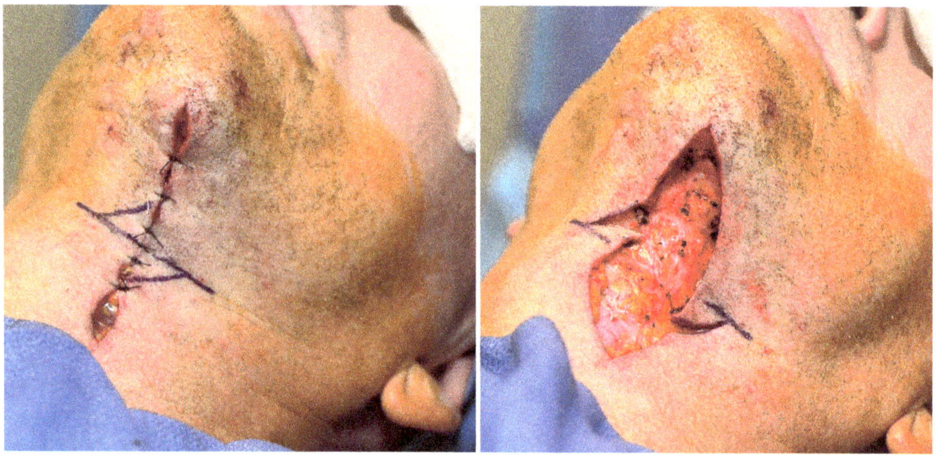

Fig. 8.28. The *left* images shows the Z-plasty markings 30 degrees to the cervical line one each flap, and the *right* image shows the Z-plasty incisions after release of the temporary sutures.

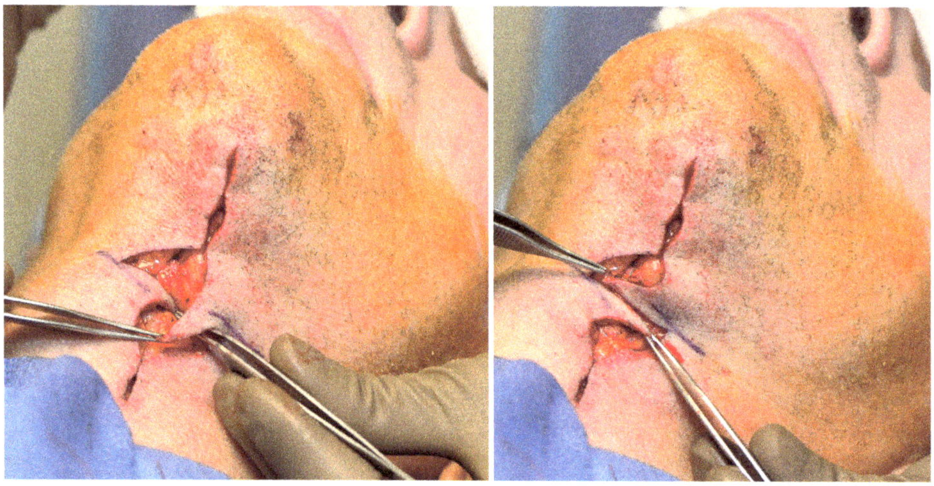

Fig. 8.29. The *left* image shows the Z-plasty incisions in position, and the *right* image shows them transposed.

cone deformity may occur at the superior and inferior extents of the incision, requiring additional careful tailoring of the skin of these areas, with possible Burow's triangle excisions.

With meticulous attention to hemostasis throughout the procedure and prior to closing, no drain is necessary. The wound is dressed with bacitracin and a nonadherent dressing, and a fluffy, facelift-type fluffy pressure dressing is applied, concluding the procedure.

The patient is examined in office on postoperative day 1, the dressing is discontinued, and sutures are removed on postoperative day 7. The patient is allowed to shower and pat the wound dry beginning on postoperative day 1.

Case Presentations

Figs. 8.31–8.35 show before-and-after cases of direct neck excision Z-plasty.

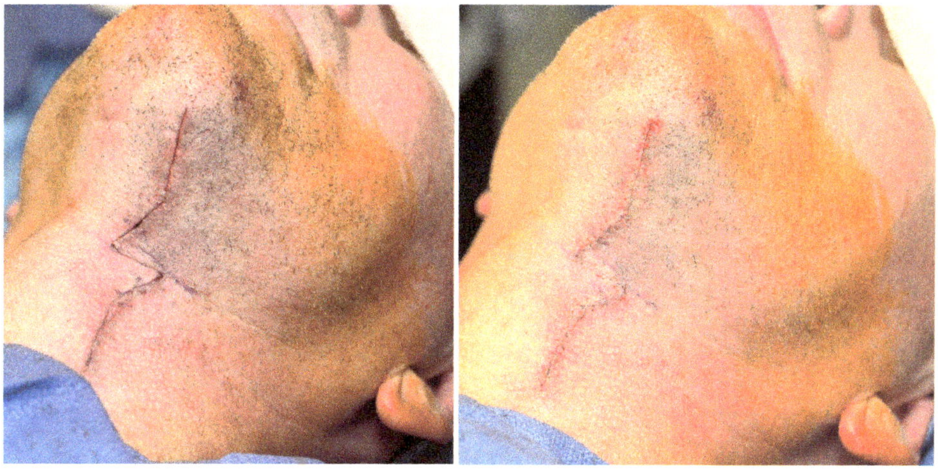

Fig. 8.30. The *left* image shows closure of the subcutaneous layer, and the *right* image shows final suture closure.

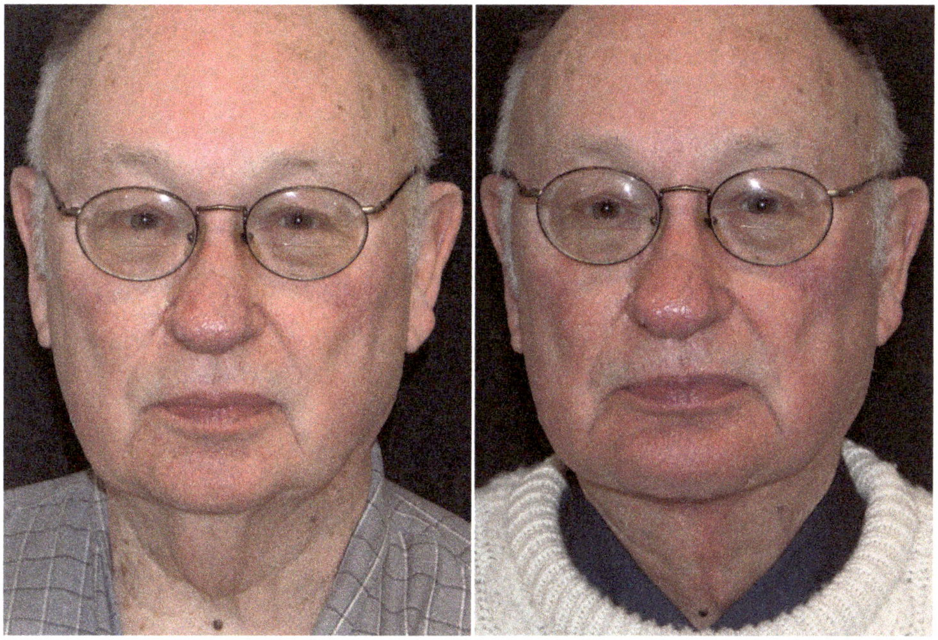

Fig. 8.31. This male patient is shown 60 days after direct excision Z-plasty. The patient also had open sculpting of the jowls and a chin placed through the main incision.

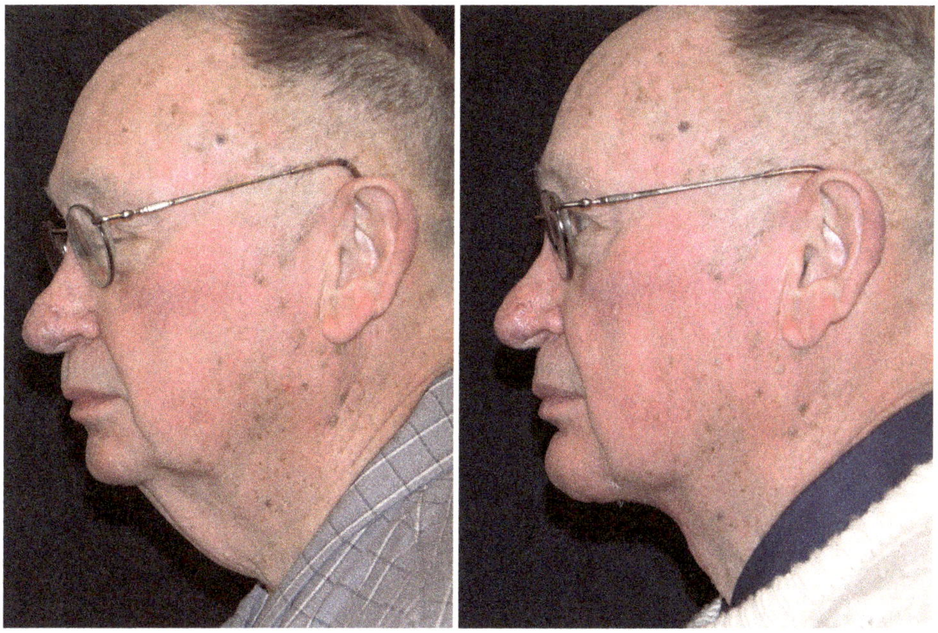

Fig. 8.32. The same patient shown in Fig. 8.31 shown in the left lateral view.

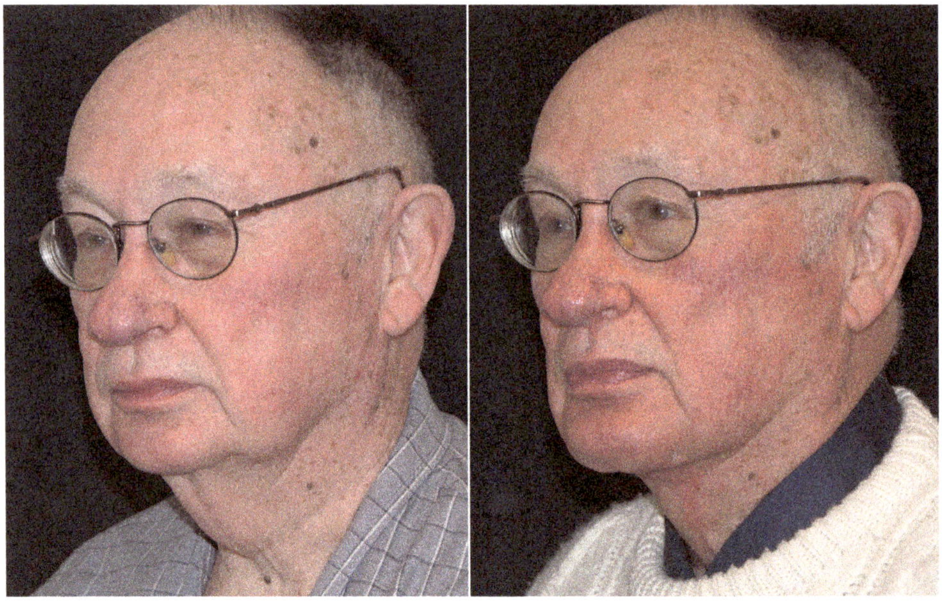

Fig. 8.33. The same patient shown in Fig. 8.31 is shown in the left three-quarter view.

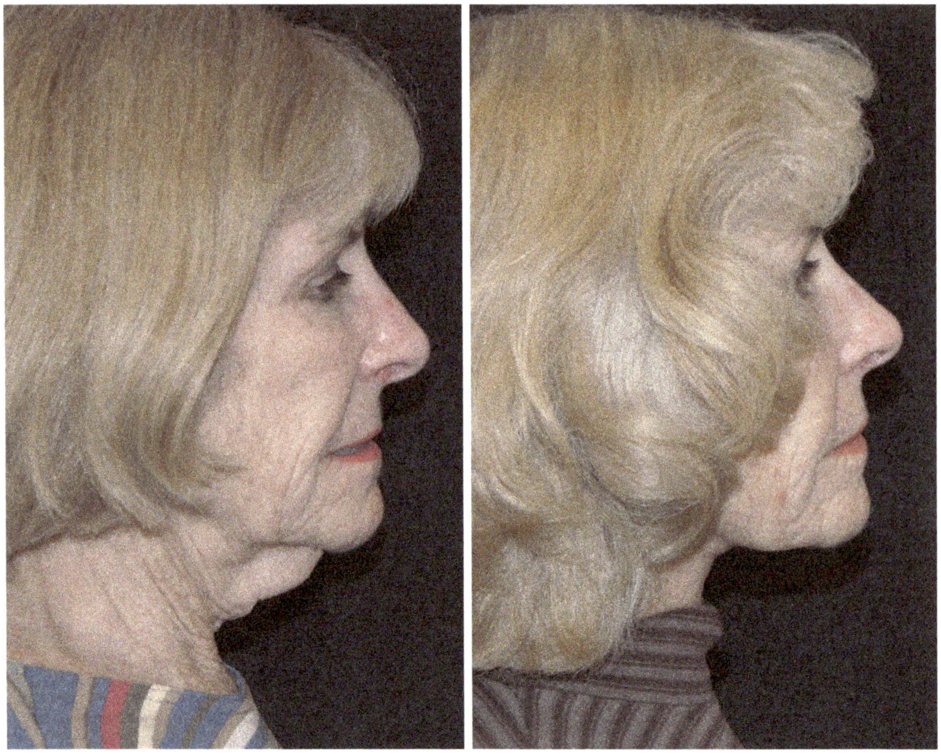

Fig. 8.34. This female patient is shown 6 months after direct neck excision Z-plasty and open jowl sculpting.

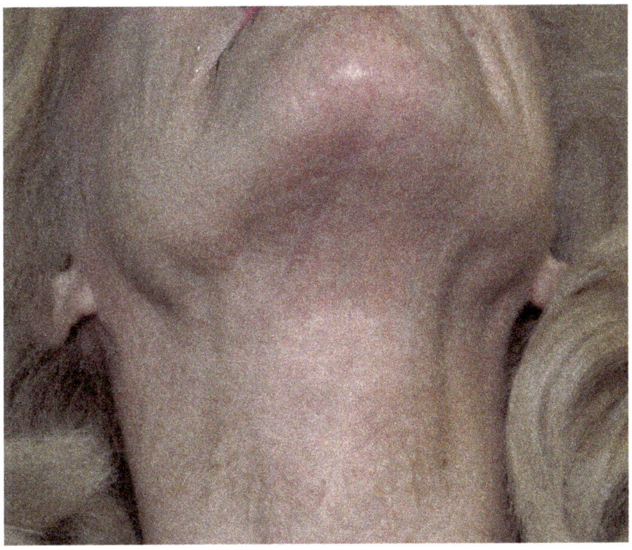

Fig. 8.35. The same patient shown in Fig. 8.34 is shown here. The aesthetic scar is a trade-off for avoiding traditional facelift.

Complications

Complications for this procedure are similar to facelift incisions and it is not uncommon for patients to undergo steroid injection for scar improvement, laser or light therapy for incision erythema, and scar revision for cone deformities at the incision edges. Major complications are rare.

Conclusion

Direct excision of the neck is a targeted procedure that specifically addresses the multifactorial issues that together created cervical ptosis and laxity. It is not a substitute for a conventional facelift, but rather an alternative. The curved and concave surface of the neck is notorious for poor scarring and banding with total vertical or horizontal incisions but when the wound tension is shifted via Z-plasty, extremely aesthetic incisions can be crafted in cervicomental region. All the patients treated were happy with their outcomes and valued the procedure and results over those of a conventional facelift.

In summary, direct neck excision is an effective technique that yields high rates of patient satisfaction when performed on patients with specific aging changes and desires. Although not as comprehensive as conventional facelift, the surgery, anesthesia, recovery, and cost are markedly less than that of a facelift. This procedure can be a viable alternative to conventional facelift for:

- Patients with cervicomental aging and minimal jowling
- Patients who desire improvement only of their neck
- Patients without the finances, recovery window, or medical clearance for conventional facelift
- Patients wanting to avoid the stigma of facelift incisions or hairline changes associated with facelift surgery

Like any surgical procedure, this technique is not applicable to all patients but rather a more select group. If the patient has the aging changes compatible with this procedure and a thorough understanding of the benefits and drawbacks, this surgery has merit for both the patient and surgeon.

CHAPTER 9

My Theory of Facelift Surgery

Robert James Troell

Chapter Outline

If you are reading this chapter, you may already be an expert on facial cosmetic surgery or just beginning your journey. Your personal training and experience will guide your decisions on treating individual patients. I have compiled information from 25 years of experience that may assist you in making a comprehensive facial aesthetic plan highlighting facelift surgery.

My most important concepts in facelift surgery are:

1. Volume replacement.
2. Osteocutaneous retaining ligament release.

Facial Rejuvenation Philosophy

Understanding your patient's target facial appearance or their aesthetic goal guides the recommendations. Confirmation of realistic expectations and comprehension of the cosmetic limitations are paramount. Although more complex than the sum of its parts, humans seek balance and harmony of proportions, near symmetry, highlighting of sexual gender identity, youthful features, and other "attractive attributes."

Defining Goals of Facial Rejuvenation Treatment

To achieve the ultimate facial beauty image, each of the "Ten Commandments of Beauty" should be addressed (Box 9.1).

Collectively, a facelift and simultaneous cosmetic procedures can address facial proportions, temporal brow ptosis, malar prominence, submalar fullness, upper and lower lip drooping, excess jowl fatty tissue; establish a straight mandibular line; may remove excess cervical fat; and create an acute cervical-mental angle.

Face Volumetric Enhancement

The underlying bony framework and soft tissue facial volume is essential to a youthful appearance and to optimize facial proportions, lines, and shapes. The anatomic sites for volume enhancement, specific substance for volume replacement, and timing related to facelift surgery needs to be jointly agreed upon between the surgeon and the patient.

Determining Facial Anatomical Sites to Undergo Volume Enhancement

The primary anatomic sites for volume augmentation along with facelifting are the midface (malar and submalar area) and the mandible (chin, entire inferior border mandibular, and angle of mandible). Secondary considerations are the temporal fossa,

Box 9.1. Ten Commandments of Beauty

1. Optimal aesthetic facial proportions
2. Optimal forehead height and brow shape
3. Absence of eyelid dermatochalasia
4. High cheek bones
5. Nose appropriate size and shape
6. Attractive white teeth (class I occlusion)
7. Full upper and lower lips
8. Straight mandibular line
9. Acute cervical mental angle
10. Smooth, flawless skin—no or few wrinkles

prejowl sulcus, tear trough, and lips. The face has numerous superficial and deep fat pads along with multiple retaining ligaments that may need to be addressed for an optimal aesthetic outcome (Fig. 9.1).

In my opinion, one of the keys to success in volume augmentation is preoperative *photographic morphing*. It is invaluable for both the patient and surgeon to confirm the postulated enhanced appearance of anatomic sites using morphing programs (Fig. 9.2). Its best to use the oblique facial view for the malar and submalar area and the front and side view for the anterior and posterior mandible. Panoramic video documentation or 3D software systems may also be valuable tools.

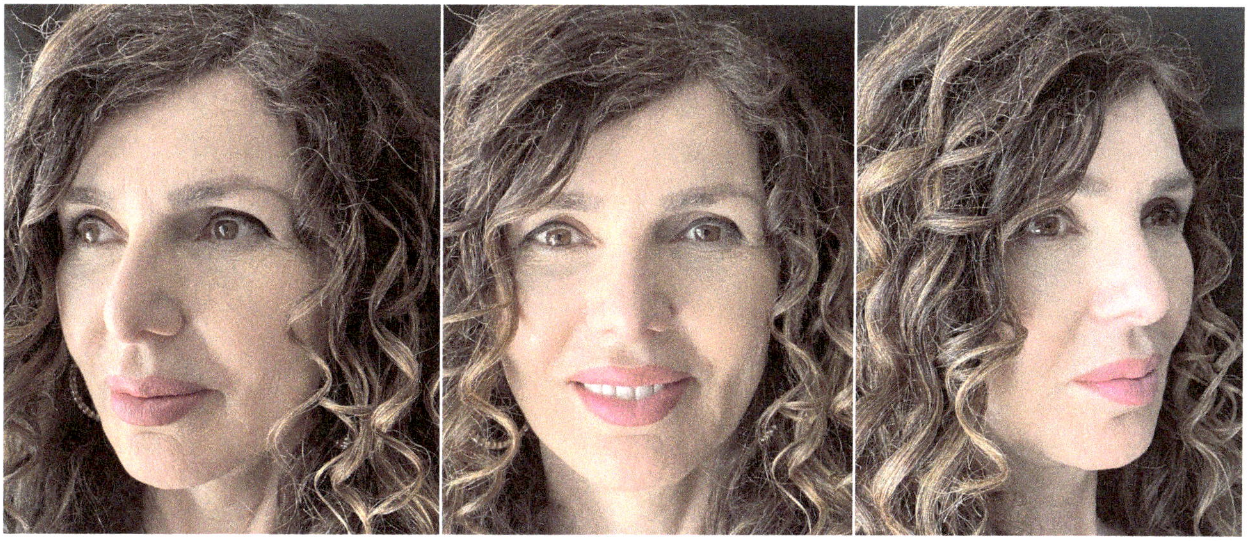

Fig. 9.1. A 56-year-old woman who displays much of the subjectivity and complexity of beauty. Implementing the "Ten Commandments of Beauty" in the preoperative facial analysis identifies the overall facial shape and anatomic sites for volume replacement, concentrating on the malar eminence, chin, and angle of the mandible. If the midface is not sufficiently wider than the lower face, either midface volume enhancement and/or lower face reduction of volume by jowl liposuction, masseter muscle hypertrophy reduction using neuromodulators, and/or face suspension should be entertained.

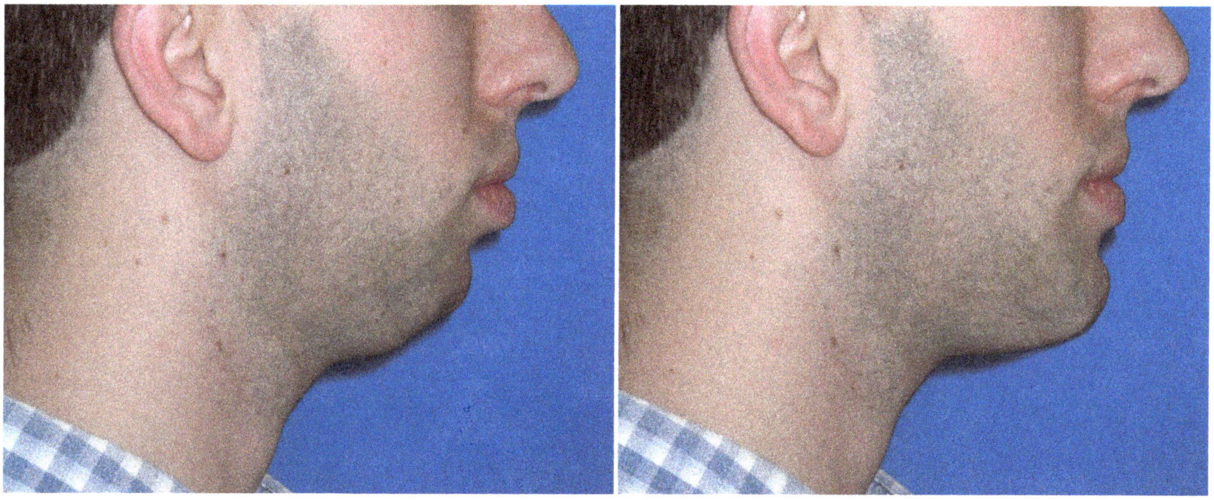

Fig. 9.2. Preoperative photographic morphing confirms volume augmentation. The lateral photograph is the best to determine the degree of anterior mandible or chin augmentation (*left* image is before, *right* image is morphed).

Methods of Permanent Facial Volume Replacement

Although temporary, dermal fillers such as hyaluronic acid are the most commonly used for volume replacement. When performing a long-term procedure such as a facelift, permanent volume replacement is often sought.

The permanent facial volume replacement options I employ are:

1. Bovine collagen gel suspended polymethylmethacrylate (Bellafill)
2. Fat grafting
3. Silicone implants

Bellafill

If small volume is necessary, such as the tear trough, prejowl sulcus, and temporal fossa, bovine collagen gel suspended polymethylmethacrylate microspheres or Bellafill (Suneva Medical, Inc., San Diego, California) is the filler I commonly use. This can be performed before surgery or as a staged procedure 1–3 months postoperatively after swelling resolution. If the deficiency in the lower eyelid area is more severe, one should consider a tear trough or extended tear trough implant.

Autologous Facial Fat Grafting

If the preoperative evaluation reveals the need for pan-facial volume replacement, I feel that facial fat grafting is the best option. Even though many expert facelift surgeons employ the fat grafting simultaneously with the facelift, I prefer staging it 1–3 sessions after swelling resolution from the facelift surgery. An alternative when only minimal pan-facial volume replacement is indicated, L-lactic acid (Sculptra, Galderma Pharmaceutic Company, Lausanne, Switzerland) can be used for injection.

There are numerous reasons to stage facial fat grafting, with the most significant being a more consistent outcome from a higher degree of adipocyte survival. In my experience, there is more intersurgeon variability of the technique of fat grafting compared with any other plastic surgery procedure. However, there are recognized best practices deemed from the cosmetic surgery literature that direct my technique with the highest fat survival rate and consistent outcomes (Box 9.2).

Purified, enriched, microaliquot fat droplets placed in the 3D extracellular matrix using 0.8–2.0 mm fat grafting cannulas is a recognized optimal technique (Figs. 9.3 and 9.4) (Videos: Fat Grafting Technique Video).

The centrifugation-filtration system (Medi-Khan Corp., Seoul, Korea) I employ yields increased cellular viability with purified, condensed fat along with stem cells and growth factors (blood and adipose source) enrichment. Centrifugation at 3000 rpm for 3 minutes has been shown to be the optimal settings for fat grafting using a weighted 60 cc syringe with a 100-μm filter. Besides improved adipocyte survival when staging facial fat grafting after a facelift, the technique yields more exactness in both the specific anatomic sites enhanced and the volume of augmentation (Fig. 9.5).

There are three types of fat grafts based on size: (1) millifat (>2.4 mm), (2) microfat (1.2–2.4 mm), and nanofat (<1.2 mm). Some suggest using millifat for deep fat compartments, microfat for superficial compartments, and nanofat for subdermal placement and the tear trough area. All surgeons must understand the specific location of the superficial and deep fat compartments. Direct enhancement of these areas that have suffered age-related atrophy is an important part of panfacial rejuvenation.

Typically, my method of purification and enrichment does not necessitate me using the microfilters to achieve superior aesthetic results.

Box 9.2. Optimal Facial Fat Grafting Technique Variables

- Harvest fat at low pressure with a 2.5–3.0 mm cannula
- Purify fat with a centrifugation-filtration system (LipoKit)
- Enrich fat with autologous stem cells and platelet-rich plasma
- Administer purified, enriched fat within 1–2 hours of harvesting
- Microaliquot injection into the 3D space of the extracellular matrix

Facial Silastic Implants: Midface

The most impactful method of facial volume replacement is using a silastic implant. A large combined malar-submalar implant equates to 4.6 mL of volume per side. The planning and marking of the deep-plane facelift with the midface implant are the first steps on the day of surgery. The midface implant is placed through a number of steps through the buccal-gingival sulcus (Videos: Midface Implant Placement). It's preferred to place the midface implant *after* the facelift surgical procedure

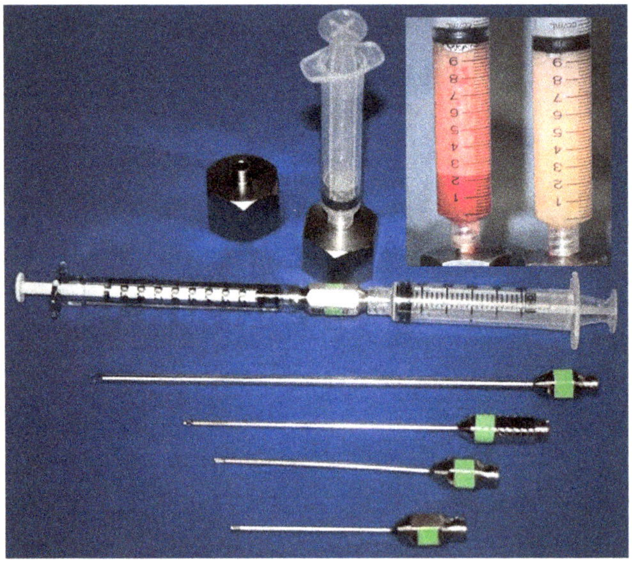

Fig. 9.3. Fat grafting instrumentation includes condensed, purified (centrifugation-filtration), enriched (stem cells and stromal vascular fraction cells with platelet rich plasma growth factors) (*inset*), and fat grafting microcannulas, syringes and female-to-female Luer-Loc adapter.

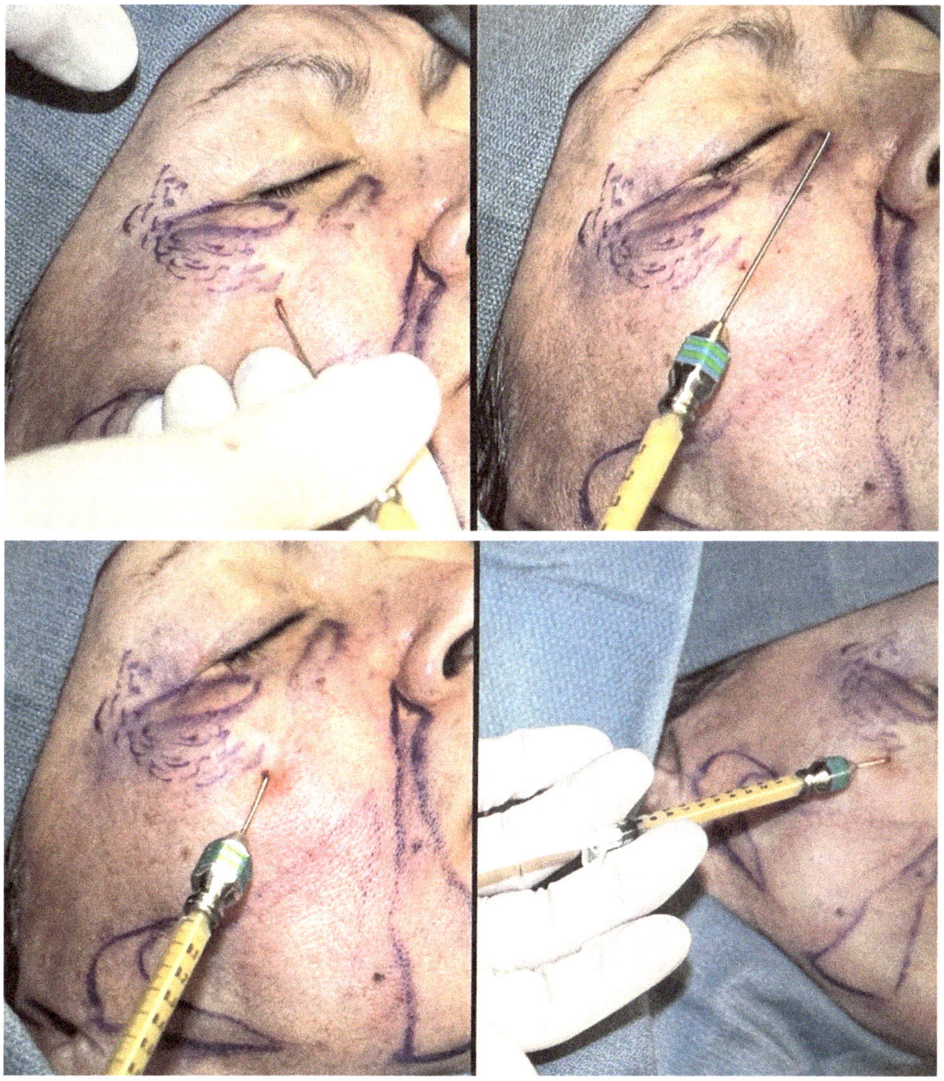

Fig. 9.4. The *top left* image shows 1.5 mm dermal punch incisions with 0.8, 1.2, and 1.8 mm microcannula placement (*top right* image). The *bottom left* and *right* images show microaliquot injections in a fanning motion placed in the 3D extracellular matrix.

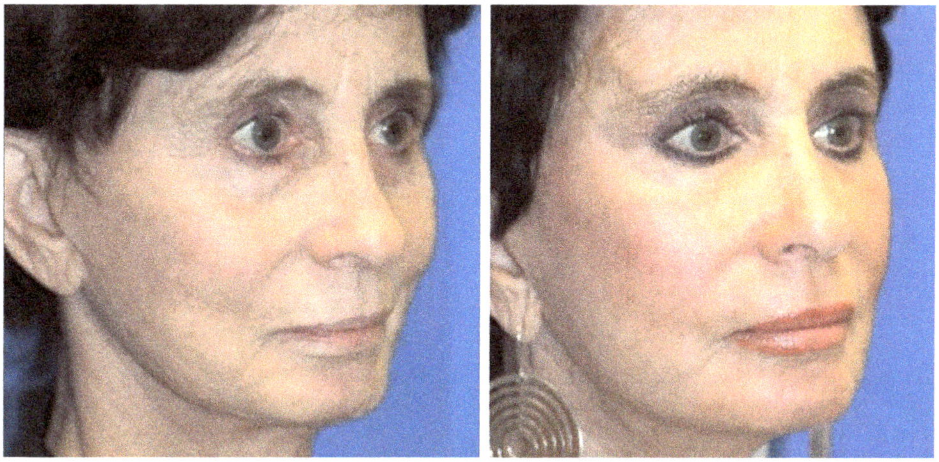

Fig. 9.5. This image shows a 74-year-old female with pan-facial volume deficiency and moderate skin photodamage treated with purified, stem cell and platelet-rich plasma growth factor enriched fat.

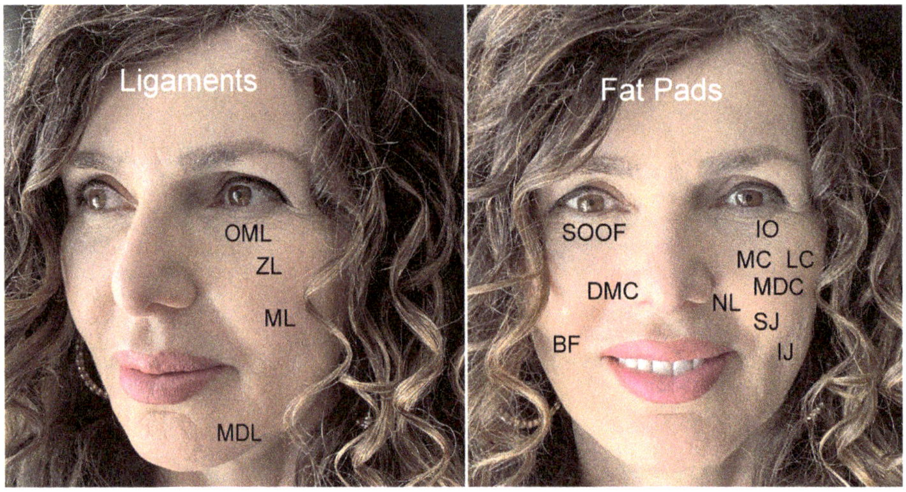

Fig. 9.6. (*Left*) Facial cheek fat compartments. (*Right*) Facial osteocutaneous ligaments. *BF*, buccal; *DMC*, deep medial cheek; *IJ*, inferior jowl; *IO*, infraorbital; *IOML*, orbitomalar; *LC*, lateral cheek; *MC*, medial cheek; *MDL*, mandibular; *MDC*, middle cheek; *ML*, masseteric; *NL*, nasolabial; *SJ*, superior jowl; *SOOF*, medial and lateral suborbicularis oculi; *ZL*, zygomatic.

is completed. This technique further suspends the face by raising the periosteum, thereby raising the osteocutaneous ligaments that typically inhibits the maximum suspension of the face. The aesthetic result is one of midface volume replacement and both midface and lower face suspension (Fig. 9.7). In patients with more extreme midface ptosis and/or ptosis more medially situated, one can add a midface lift with suborbicularis oculi fat pad suspension to optimize the aesthetic outcome (Fig. 9.7).

The style of implant is either a submalar implant (if this area of the midface is the only area of volume loss) or more commonly, a combined malar-submalar implant, which provides volume to the entire midface area. Combining implant volume enhancement with facial suspension profoundly improves the facelift aesthetic result.

In patients with facial asymmetry who may benefit from volume replacement, patient-specific or custom implants fabricated from 3D computerized scan reconstruction is the optimal method. These implants are constructed by a process known as 3D Accuscan (Implantech Associates, Inc., Ventura, California). This process uploads 1–1.5 mm cuts of axial, sagittal, and coronal computerized tomography scan views to a software program, working jointly with a technician and surgeon, to construct the desired implant size and footprint (Fig. 9.8). This image is referred to engineering for implant fabrication, a process that takes 4–6 weeks.

Chin and Complete Mandibular Border Implants

The acute cervicomental angle and the importance of a straight mandibular line in facial aesthetics is best treated by the placement of a chin (much more common in clinical practice) or a custom (patient-specific) complete mandibular implant. The anterior chin implant in women should be reduced in the paramedian area by manually carving the silastic implant. This will result in a more triangular-appearing chin than the "boxier" chin seen in men (Video: Chin Implant Carving). This augmentation typically produces a more profound cosmetic effect than the cervicoplasty itself. If a chin or mandible implant is implemented, the implant is placed *first*, followed by the deep neck lift dissection and completing the neck rejuvenation with the platysmaplasty. The augmented mandible both improves facial balance and rejuvenates the cervical area by redraping the skin (Fig. 9.9).

Deep-Plane Facelift Surgery

Even though I was taught that clinical comparison studies revealed no long-term difference with the superficial musculoaponeurotic system long-flap facelift and the deep-plane facelift, I believe the deep-plane facelift provides a better facial suspension and improved facelift longevity. The reason for the superior outcome is that disruption of the orbital, zygomatic, masseteric, and mandibular osteocutaneous retaining ligaments (Fig. 9.6, *right*) allows for the superior suspension.

The surgical steps in the deep-plane facelift are similar to surgeons' steps featured in this text with minor caveats (Videos: Deep Plane Facelift Technique). When volume replacement is performed simultaneously, either the implant or the fat grafting is performed last. Placement of the midface implant as the final step using a separate, sterile Mayo stand through a buccal-gingival incision has the advantage of lifting the periosteum attached to the osteocutaneous ligaments, further suspending the face.

Increase Successful Facelift Cosmetic Outcomes

Formatting a jointly agreed upon comprehensive aesthetic plan based on a detailed facial analysis coupled with photographic

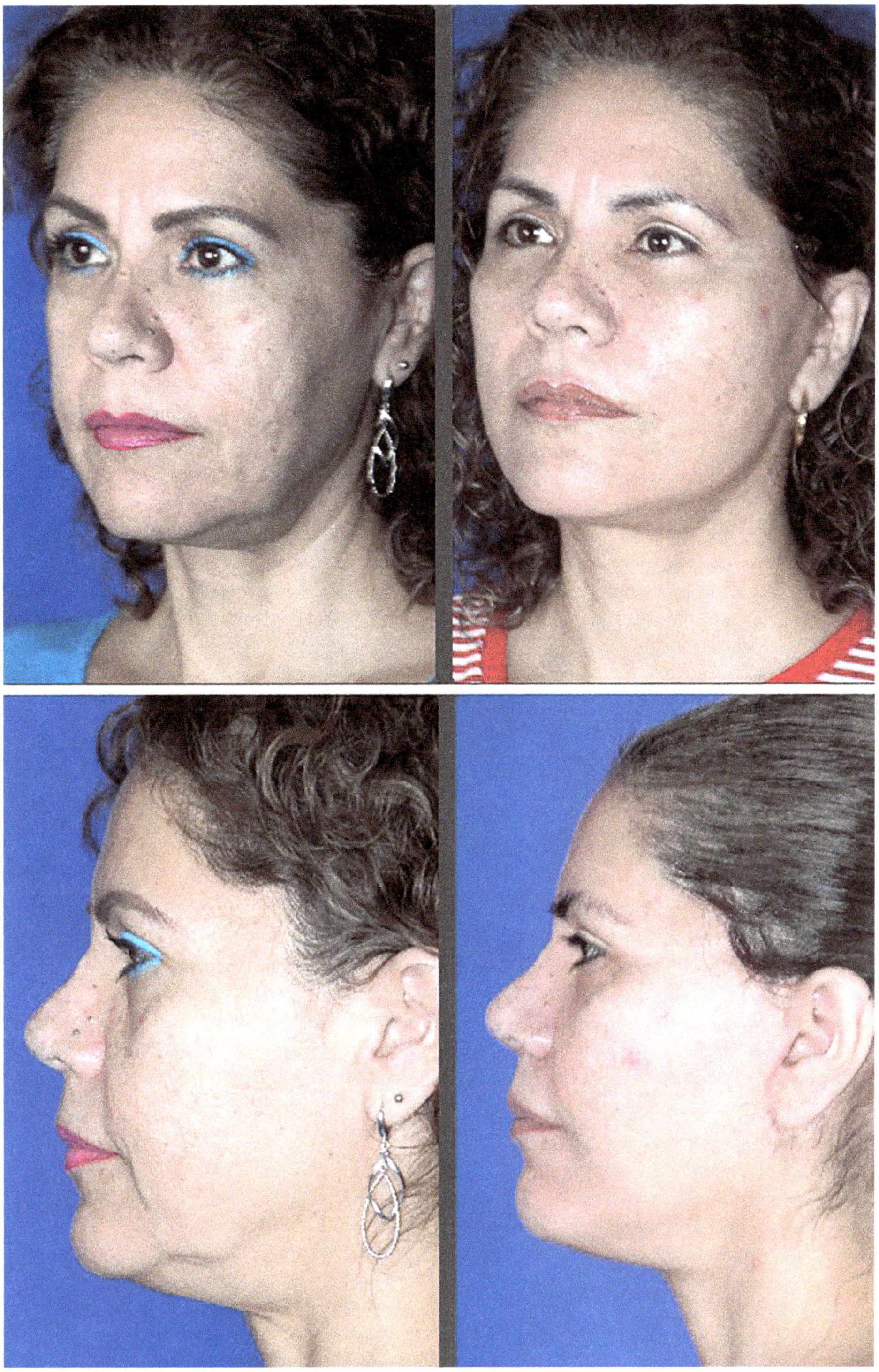

Fig. 9.7. Aesthetic result midface implant with deep-plane facelift. This 55-year-old female with moderate acne scarring, upper eyelid dermatochalasia, midface volume deficiency of the malar and submalar area, midface and lower face ptosis with excess skin, and a good neck appearance underwent upper blepharoplasty, combined submalar implant (medium size) along with deep-plane facelift.

morphing is the initial endeavor. Ensuring volume replacement perioperatively is completed and intraoperative osteocutaneous retaining ligament suspension is part of the facelift technique that will yield a superior outcome. Additionally, ancillary cosmetic procedures (laser skin resurfacing, blepharoplasty, browlift, neuromodulators, dermal fillers, lip augmentation, lip lift) will heighten the facelift result and to finalize the treatment of the "Ten Commandments of Beauty."

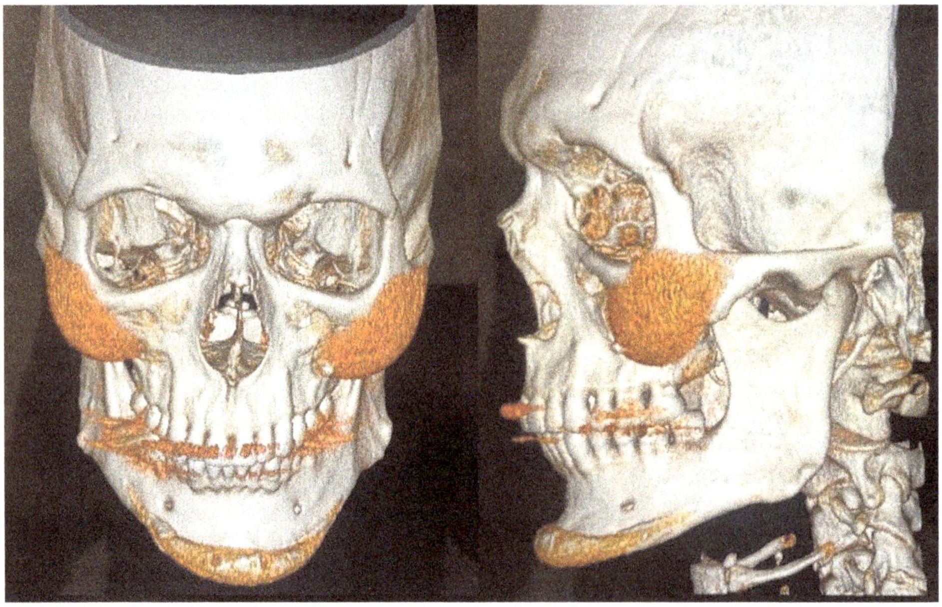

Fig. 9.8. A 3D computerized scan reconstruction. The axial, coronal, and sagittal planes can be reconstructed to evaluate the footprint and size of any facial implant. A patient-specific or custom implant is recommended in those with more than mild facial asymmetry for the optimal implant. The scan can also be used postimplant placement to determine implant symmetry.

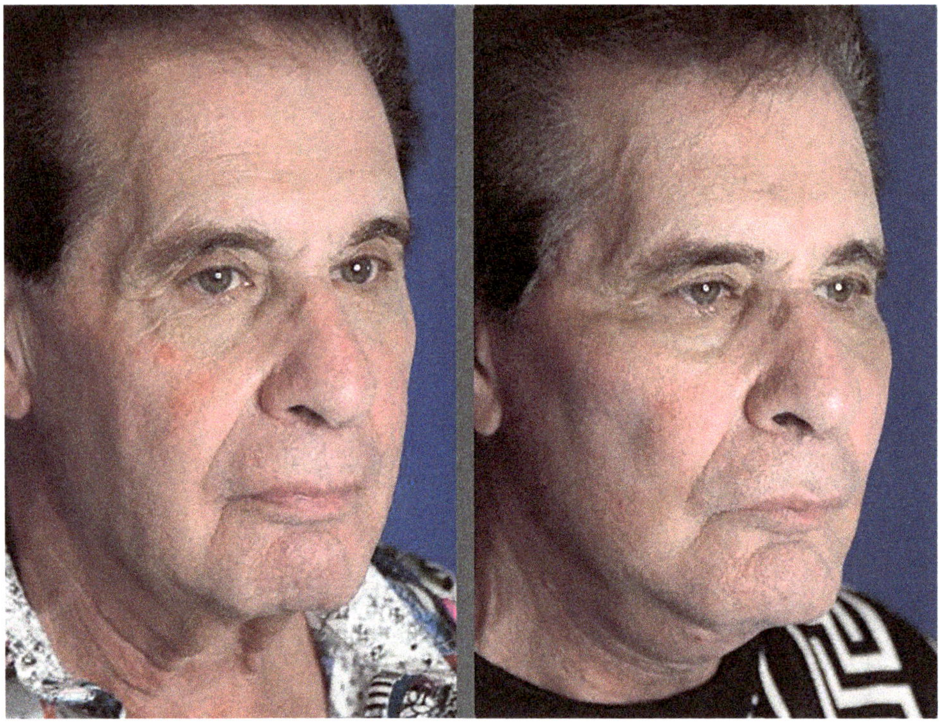

Fig. 9.9. This 73-year-old male underwent combined submalar implant (medium size), anatomic extended chin implant (large size), deep plane facelift, and anterior platysmaplasty. He refused laser skin resurfacing, tear trough volume replacement, and blepharoplasty surgery at this time.

CHAPTER 10

Facelift and Neck Lift: History and My Current Deep Plane Technique

Abdul Nassimizadeh, Michael Oca, Amit Kochhar, Kian Karimi

Chapter Outline

Introduction

The genesis of the modern facelift or "rhytidectomy" can be traced to 1907, when surgeons began performing specific and localized resections of skin along the hairline. During the first half of the 20th century rhytidectomies became increasingly popular. Early principles relied primarily on a foundation of skin excision and access to the subcutaneous layer. Despite some success, this technique did not address underlying soft tissue ptosis.

However, in the 1970s the emergence of knowledge surrounding surgical manipulation of the superficial musculoaponeurotic system (SMAS) revolutionized the modern approach to the procedure.

Two major schools of thought developed from this point. One point of view focused upon manipulation of the SMAS through imbrication or plication and a belief that this was sufficient for optimal results. The other championed a sub-SMAS or "deep plane" approach, which involved the malar fat pad, platysma, and skin. This was first described in 1986, with further advancements over the next few decades that led to improved midface control and reduced complication rates.

There are currently a myriad of styles and techniques utilized. The following discussion will categorize each rhytidectomy based upon anatomical considerations.

Incidence

Despite a century of historical progress, it is only in recent decades that rhytidectomy has become more popular, with an increase in public preference for a youthful appearance. This has been linked to a growth in common knowledge, strengthened social acceptance, and a significant increase in life span.

At the turn of the 21st century, 84% of patients seeking cosmetic rhytidectomy were Caucasian. This percentage has significantly decreased in modern times, with a rise in Hispanic and African American patients in the same period.

Although Caucasians typically have thinner skin, and therefore greater wrinkles secondary to glycation, the introduction of modern techniques that address the deep planes have attracted other ethnicities, whose principal problem lies in deep tissue drooping. Current trends within this domain have evolved toward less invasive techniques in a younger demographic.

Anatomical Considerations

Knowledge on the complex nature of facial anatomy is a fundamental prerequisite to rhytidectomy. Careful dissection through the skin, dermal plexus of blood vessels, and fat enhances viability of the facial flap, simultaneously affecting postoperative contour and shape.[1,2]

The subcutaneous layer includes fat, which interdigitates with the SMAS. There are variations to its thickness secondary to anatomical location and patient ethnicity. Subcutaneous fat is virtually nonexistent in the upper and lower eyelids, becomes thickened over the malar region, and is attached by the zygomatic ligaments to the underlying periosteum in an area known as McGregor's patch. The fibrous nature of this section must be understood when encountering resistance during dissection. Although the fat within the malar region consists of loose globules, the mentum and upper and lower lips contain densely compacted, thicker globules. There is also significant "branching" in the subcutaneous fat known as the retinacular cutis, which contributes to the formation of septa and divides the face into different compartments.

Deeper still lies the SMAS, attached to the skin above and the deep parotid-masseteric fascia below. It is contiguous with the platysma and a caudal extension of the superficial temporal fascia. It envelopes the facial musculature, as well as the corresponding motor nerves. Manipulation of this layer repositions the lateral skin in the desired vector.[3,4]

The sub-SMAS plane is a critical area and requires extensive familiarization due to the essential structures encountered. Although the facial nerve branches exit deep to the parotid-masseteric fascia laterally, they become more superficial in the anterior face as they pass over the buccal fat pad to innervate mimetic muscles. During a rhytidectomy, great care is afforded to operate superficial to parotid-masseteric fascia laterally. Loose areolar tissue extends from the parotid gland to the anterior border of the masseter. Blunt dissection of this layer can be performed; however, the facial nerve branches are intimately located, especially as they cross the masseter muscle.[2]

In addition to anatomical planes, facial retaining ligaments play a key role in optimal patient outcomes. These are condensations of connective tissue, which divide the face into compartments and connect the skin superficially with deep bone. In a vertical boundary immediately lateral to the lateral orbital rim lie the temporal ligamentous adhesion, lateral orbital thickening, zygomatic-cutaneous ligament, and mandibular-cutaneous ligament. Release of these ligaments facilitates mobilization and repositioning of soft tissue. Division of the zygomatic-cutaneous ligament allows for vertical elevation of the soft tissue complex, and release of the mandibular-cutaneous ligaments is required to adequately address the prejowl sulcus.

There are several other structures of note to be aware of during rhytidectomy procedures. The greater auricular nerve lies superficial to the SMAS layer and provides sensory innervation to the lobule of the ear. In close proximity to the great auricular nerve and the sternocleidomastoid muscle sits the external jugular vein.

Patient Approach

The key focus of all cosmetic interventions is patient evaluation and a reproducible workflow. At the initial consultation, a photographer captures a complete set of digital preoperative photos. Patients have jewelry removed and hair tied back. Photographs include full-face frontal, left and right oblique, left and right lateral, and chin tuck views (Fig. 10.1).

On certain occasions we would supplement this further with close-up visuals of submental neck tissue and the auricles.

In our experience digital videos are as powerful, if not more so, as photography to highlight dynamic movement of tissue. This acts as both a surgical and patient aid during preoperative planning and postoperative follow-up.

Within our workspace, we also utilize digital three-dimensional imaging software, namely Canfield's Vectra 3D imaging in some patients. Multiple cameras take images of the patient from numerous angles and create a three-dimensional virtual image, with the ability for manipulation on a monitor. Patients place great value in this technology, and it provides both the surgeon and patient with a tangible goal (Fig. 10.2).

Patients are reviewed with their imaging and information is garnered, which includes their primary complaint, medical history, allergies, medications, and an accurate psychological profile. Isotretinoin and vitamin E are particularly of note due to their adverse effects on healing. Smoking and alcohol also play a prominent role in affecting viability of the facial flap. In addition to surgical considerations, anesthetic pitfalls must also be considered.

Once everything is collected, patients are thoroughly examined and information is gathered related to skin laxity and other anatomical cues. The skin of the surgical site is assessed for appropriate scar maturation and quality. Documentation regarding hairline is made for surgical incision planning.[5] The senior author prefers a retrotragal incision for most of his patients but on occasion will favor a pretragal incision for some female patients and many male patients (Fig. 10.3).

Anatomical variants to give special consideration to in the submental region include retrognathia, low anterior hyoid, and a short vertical height of the neck.

Patients with a previous history of rhytidectomy require caution, due to distortion to organic tissue planes and location of the facial nerve. The combination of this workflow allows the ability to plan optimal treatment plan and potential outcomes.

Although age is not an essential factor, postoperative recovery is typically better in a demographic younger than 50. The ideal patient would be in good health, with a sound psychological profile, desiring to address skin irregularities in cheeks or jowls, prominent lines or folds in the commissure-mandibular grooves, or slack subcutaneous tissue. A thorough history of prior injectables, biostimulators, and energy-based treatments

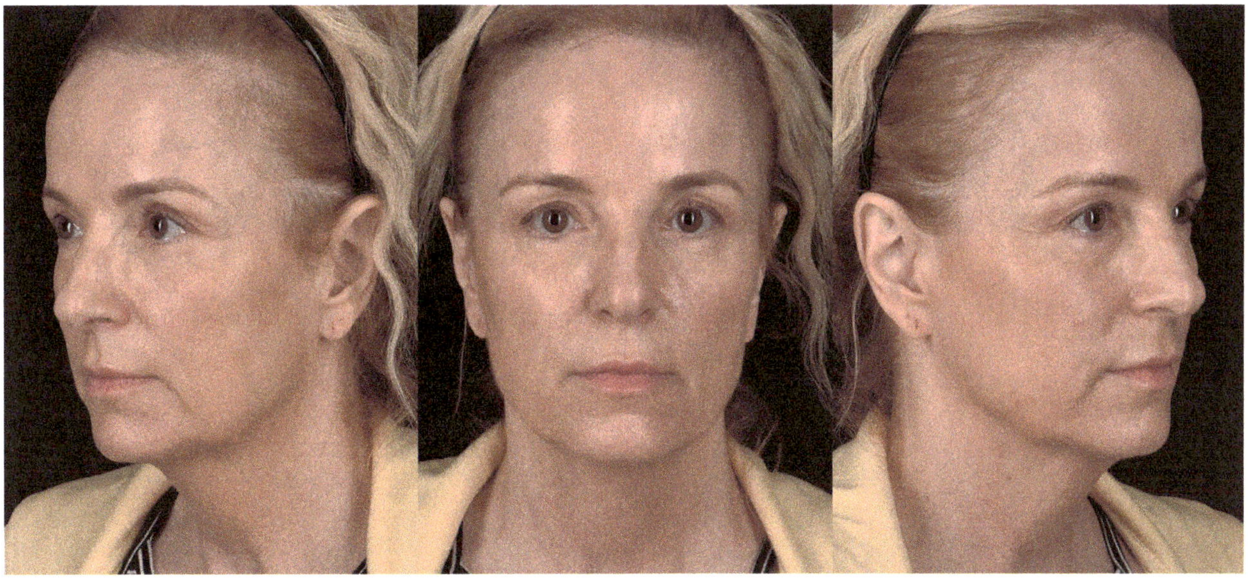

Fig. 10.1. This image shows the author's typical preoperative image poses. Other views and video footage are also frequently used for preoperative documentation as well.

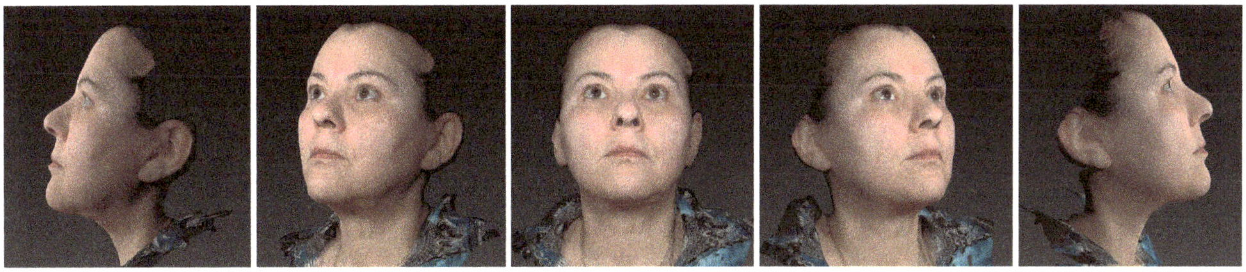

Fig. 10.2. This images shows 3D images from the Vectra photographic system.

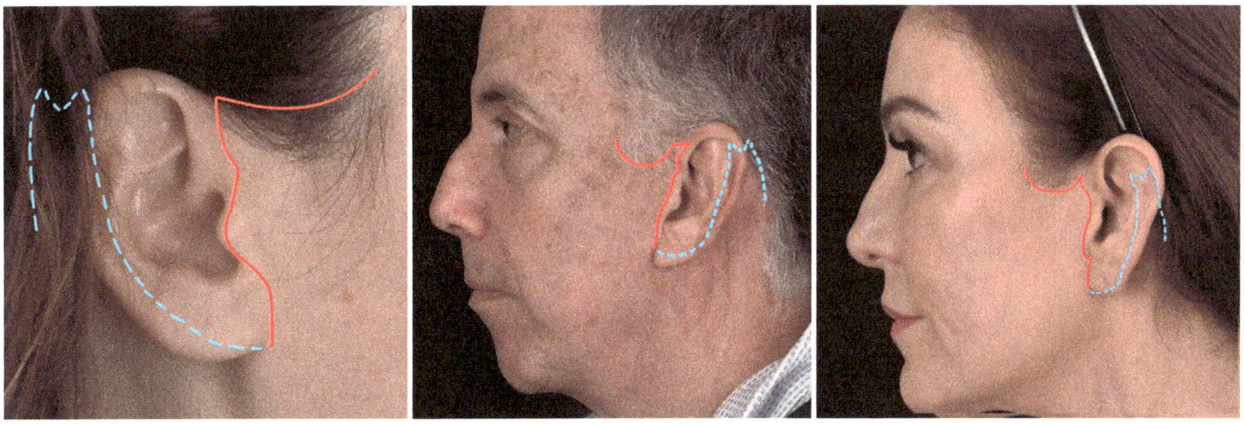

Fig. 10.3. The *left* image shows the author's preferred female facelift incisions, the *middle* image shows the author's preferred male facelift incisions, and the *right* image shows the author's alternate incisions used on some female patients.

is important to elicit as these procedures may make the skin flap and/or the deep plane dissection more challenging.

Patients on antiplatelet or blood-thinning medication, smokers unwilling to stop, and those with deteriorating health require special attention. These patients are at a high risk of nonoptimal postoperative outcomes and may be better managed conservatively.[6,7]

It is also imperative to categorize patients into those with realistic expectations and others who may require psychological assistance over surgical intervention. In psychologically appropriate patients, postoperative improvement in self-conscious sexual and bodily appearance is noted in validated quality-of-life surveys.

Preoperative Care and Anesthetic Considerations

Patients willing to stop smoking are advised to do so at least 2 months prior to the planned operation date. Those on medication or supplements that can alter coagulability are instructed to stop 2 weeks prior to rhytidectomy, if possible. These include vitamin E, fish oil, garlic, ginseng, aspirin, and nonsteroidal antiinflammatory medication.[5]

Prior to induction of anesthesia, patients are given intravenous antibiotics, dexamethasone, and tranexamic acid (TXA). In rarer instances, patients may be given oral sedative tablets to manage anxiety.

Anesthesia is managed through a combination of fentanyl and intravenous propofol, which is titrated to provide a consistent level of sedation. Patients who have no history of significant anxiety and have tolerated previous surgical or dental procedures are better candidates. The senior author prefers general anesthesia for his facelift patients as he finds it to be safer for control of the airway and for patient and surgeon comfort.

Infiltration prior to incision with lidocaine and epinephrine provides adequate local anesthesia, in addition to appropriate vasoconstriction. This combination provides a duration of 240 minutes. Although bupivacaine has a slower onset, the significant increase in duration of effect makes it an attractive option too. The success of these local anesthetics have made possible the option of rhytidectomy under local anesthesia, with comparable rates of postoperative complications.

Another consideration to note is the use of TXA. Its use within rhytidectomy is popular due to its antifibrinolytic properties by inhibiting conversion of plasminogen to plasmin. There are different applications reported, including intravenous administration, local infiltration, and TXA-soaked pledgets intraoperatively. The use of TXA corresponds with reduced surgical time and drier surgical dissection, significantly improved hemostasis and postoperative hematoma rates.

Surgical Technique

Planned Incisions

Tailoring surgical markings to an individual patient is important. The key principle is to camouflage incisions within the hairline, preauricular skin grooves, and natural creases. Although marking begins at the preauricular area, the incision follows a natural curve toward the tragus, lobule, and posteriorly into the hairline (Fig. 10.4).

Cutaneous marking for landmarks such as the angle of the mandible, potential course of the frontal branch of the facial nerve, and anterior border of the sternocleidomastoid muscle are made in certain cases, such as secondary surgery.

Although most females receive a posttragal incision, male patients often benefit from an incision anterior to the tragus to avoid transference of hair-bearing skin to undesirable locations. Patients with concerns surrounding hearing aid fit would also be good candidates for anterior tragal incisions. Similarly, there are slight alterations made if a patient has facial hair. Occasionally some midfacial skin can be removed without elevation or transformation of the hairline. In other instances, incisions can loop the area of hair and extend to the temporal scalp.

Particular attention is given to the lobule during marking. Following suspension sutures, the lobule will inevitably lie deep to the flap and require adequate skin excision for appropriate exposure. Slight, almost imperceptible, anterior rotation of the lobule aids with incision camouflage.

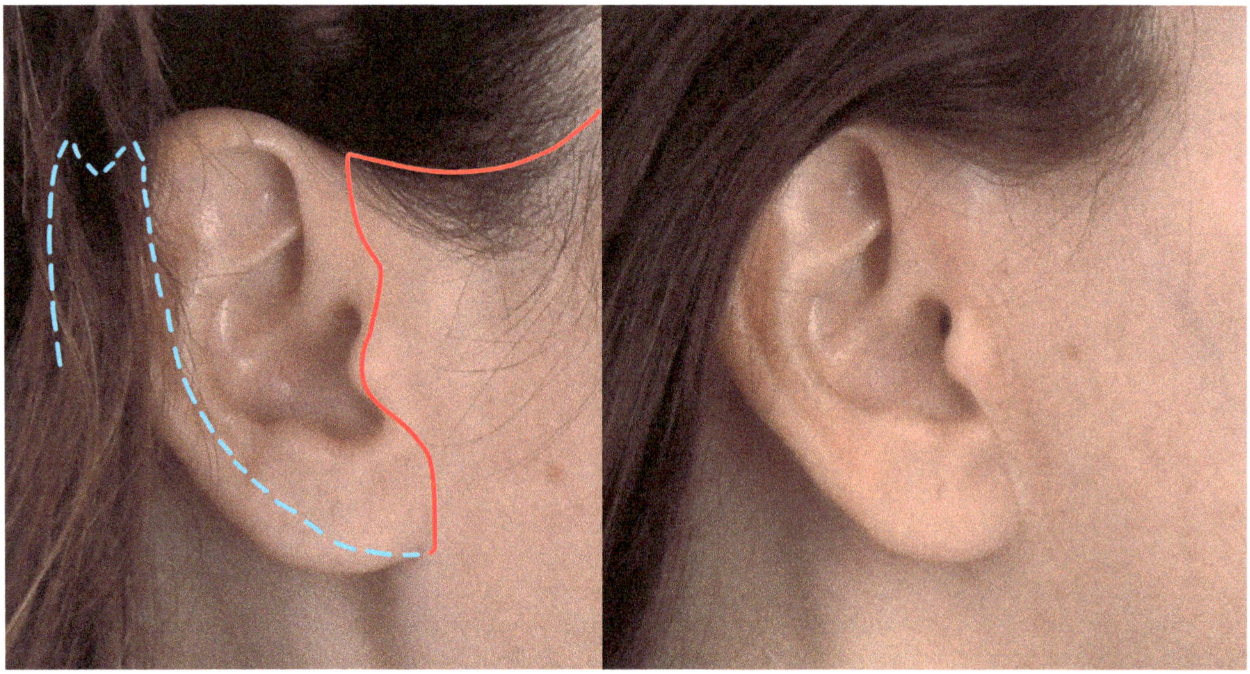

Fig. 10.4. The *left* image shows the patient surgical site before surgery, and the *right* image shows the healed scar with excellent aesthetics.

Procedure

Although there are numerous available techniques, including subcutaneous facelift, minimal access cranial suspension lift, SMAS-plication, lateral SMAS ectomy and subperiosteal facelift, this discussion will focus on the deep plane approach, which is the senior author's preferred approach.

Deep plane rhytidectomy was a modification first introduced over three decades ago by Hamra (Fig. 10.5).

The founding concept focused upon reversal of gravity-induced changes to deep soft tissues and resulted in dramatic improvements to an ageing face, while maintaining a natural appearance.

While initial subcutaneous dissection occurs, following several millimeters of exposure, the SMAS layer is incised. Although the plane of dissection remains sub-SMAS, there are particular landmarks in this layer used as reference points. These include the orbicularis oculi, zygomatic major muscle, and the zygomatic minor. Although the orbicularis oculi is not considered in conjunction with the flap, a section of soft tissue is incorporated for optimal results. The zygomatic major acts as a superior border indicator, and the zygomatic minor aids identification of the zygomatic-cutaneous ligament. As mentioned previously, it is necessary to release this ligament for adequate mobilization.

The facial flap, which involves skin, subcutaneous tissue, and fat pad, is then mobilized and positioned for optimal results. Closure is performed with nonabsorbable sutures to avoid unwanted skin reactions or scar inflammation.

The benefits of this approach include access to the facial ligaments and direct assessment of herniated fat pads. There is also reduced occurrence of perfusion-related complications due to improved retention of blood supply. Postoperatively patients notice results remain in situ longer than in techniques conducted above the deep plane. These potential benefits, coupled with operative experience, outweigh the increase in facial nerve damage.

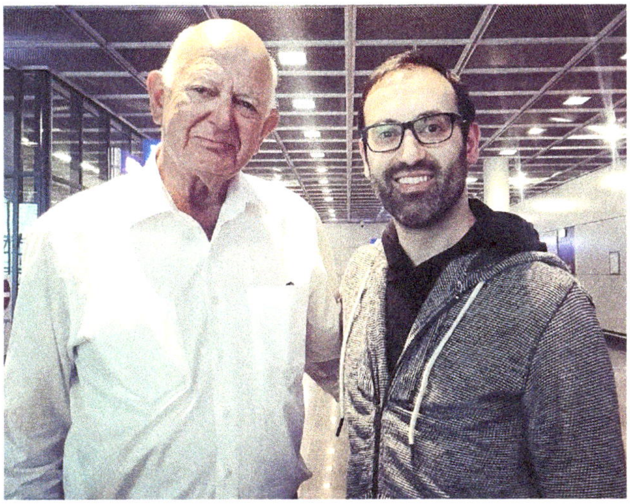

Fig. 10.5. Dr. Karimi (*right*) is shown with one of his mentors, Dr. Sam Hamara, who is considered by many as the father of deep plane facelift technique.

Complications

As with all surgical procedures, rhytidectomy has risks, with a figure of 4.5% typically reported. This figure is significantly increased in patients with high body mass index.

The most frequent complication is hematoma formation, with a range of 1%–15% reported. While drains are considered, there is a risk of introducing infection and displacement. Mild bleeding from the surgical site is not unusual in the initial postoperative period and responds well to pressure bandages. Small, nonexpanding hematomas can be treated with needle aspiration, antibiotic prophylaxis, and appropriate observation. Larger hematomas may necessitate reexploration and evacuation of blood.

Infection remains a risk in all surgical procedures, and post-rhytidectomy the common organism is *Staphylococcus aureus*.

Another stated injury involves sensory deficit and hypoesthesia in the distribution of the great auricular nerve. Seven percent of patients suffer with sensory changes; however, a majority resolve during the subsequent weeks and months.

Temporary or permanent facial nerve paresis or paralysis occurs in 0.5%–2.5% of patients. The most common branch is the marginal mandibular.

Skin flap necrosis secondary to vascular compromise can occur in 0.3%–3% of patients and requires prompt recognition and management. This can include warm compresses, massage, and topical nitroglycerine paste. Smoking and nicotine use increases the likelihood by approximately 12 times.

Despite optimal pre- and intraoperative procedures, undesirable scars can develop in patients. For hypertrophic scars, serial steroid injections may be necessary. Similarly, irregular contours and dimpling can occur; however, this typically self-resolves over the following months. In rare instances of persistent edema, local steroid injections can provide some level of benefit.

Finally, it is important to assess the patient systemically and address other complications including anesthetic risks, deep vein thrombosis, and pulmonary embolism.

Postoperative Care

Postoperative care is imperative for the success of rhytidectomy. The patient is monitored closely in the immediate aftermath of the operation and discharged to a caregiver when stable.

The patient is advised to have complete bed rest for the initial 24 hour period, except for walking to the bathroom, and to wear a circumferential compression dressing. They typically return 1 day postoperatively for removal of the compression dressing and any drains, and a slightly more comfortable compression strap is placed. This is worn for the first week continually and thereafter for a further week at night. Pain is managed with medications appropriately, and antibiotic coverage continues for 3–5 days. Postoperative patients are using less opioid analgesia in recent times, with the introduction of other pain controlling aids, such as cannabidiol oil and nonsteroid antiinflammatory medications. The senior author has his patients utilize cannabidiol oil (HealMD), Celebrex, and acetaminophen.

Patients should be advised that postoperative edema and tightness is common and usually reaches maximal point at 2 or 3 days, before slowly subsiding. During this recovery period, patients are advised to avoid bending over and to refrain from vigorous or strenuous movements.

With regards to diet, advice is given regarding a high-calorie, high-protein diet and plenty of fluids. This combination helps prevent nausea, in addition to promote ideal recovery.

Approximately 1 week postoperatively, sutures are removed, and thereafter adequate follow-up is planned to monitor surgical outcomes. Typically, at 2 weeks a patient can begin workouts at 50% exertion and may enjoy unrestricted exercise at 3 weeks.

Adjuvant Therapy

Although rhytidectomy continues to hold a prominent role in facial restoration, there are other adjuvant treatments utilized to improve postoperative outcomes. A multimodal approach is the gold standard with regards to management of the ageing face. These include the use of neurotoxins, facial fillers, polydioxanone threads, skeletal augmentation, skin resurfacing, and fat grafting.

The incorporation of fat grafting into rhytidectomy improves outcomes by a minimum of 6–12 months. The opportunity to address selective fat compartment volume restoration is appealing to any surgeon and has the ability to address soft tissue atrophy, while simultaneously minimizing patient recovery if each procedure was performed separately. Typically, this involves the malar and nasolabial locations (Fig. 10.6).

Laser resurfacing and skin tightening uses infrared light, which heats subdermal collagen and results in skin contraction. In isolation, it works well in a certain demographic of patients and in combination therapy provides an effective adjunct to rhytidectomy (Fig. 10.7). Chin implants can also increase the aesthetic benefit of rhytidectomy (Fig. 10.8).

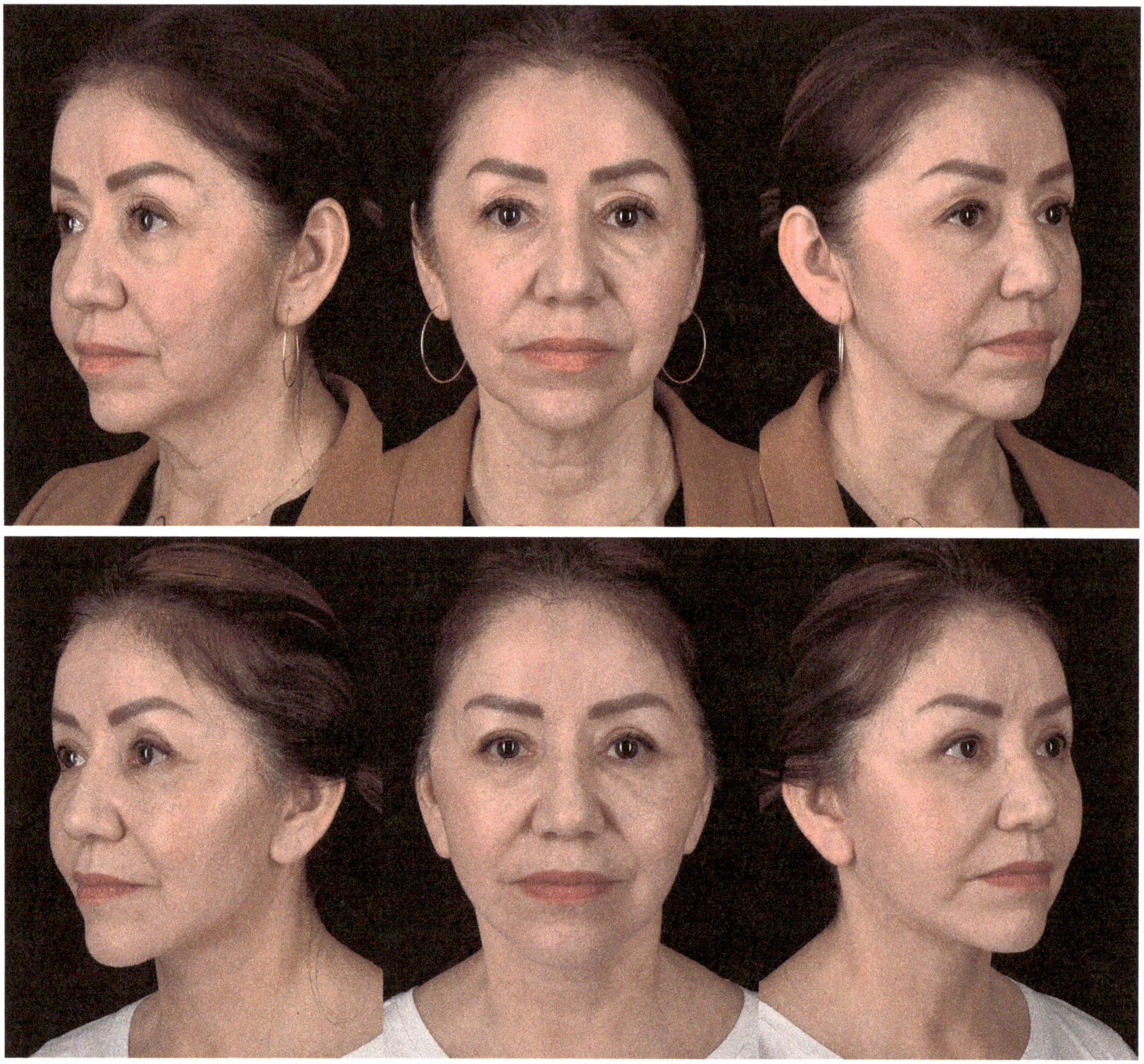

Fig. 10.6. The *top* images show the patient preoperatively, and the *lower* images show the patient after deep plane facelift with fat grafting.

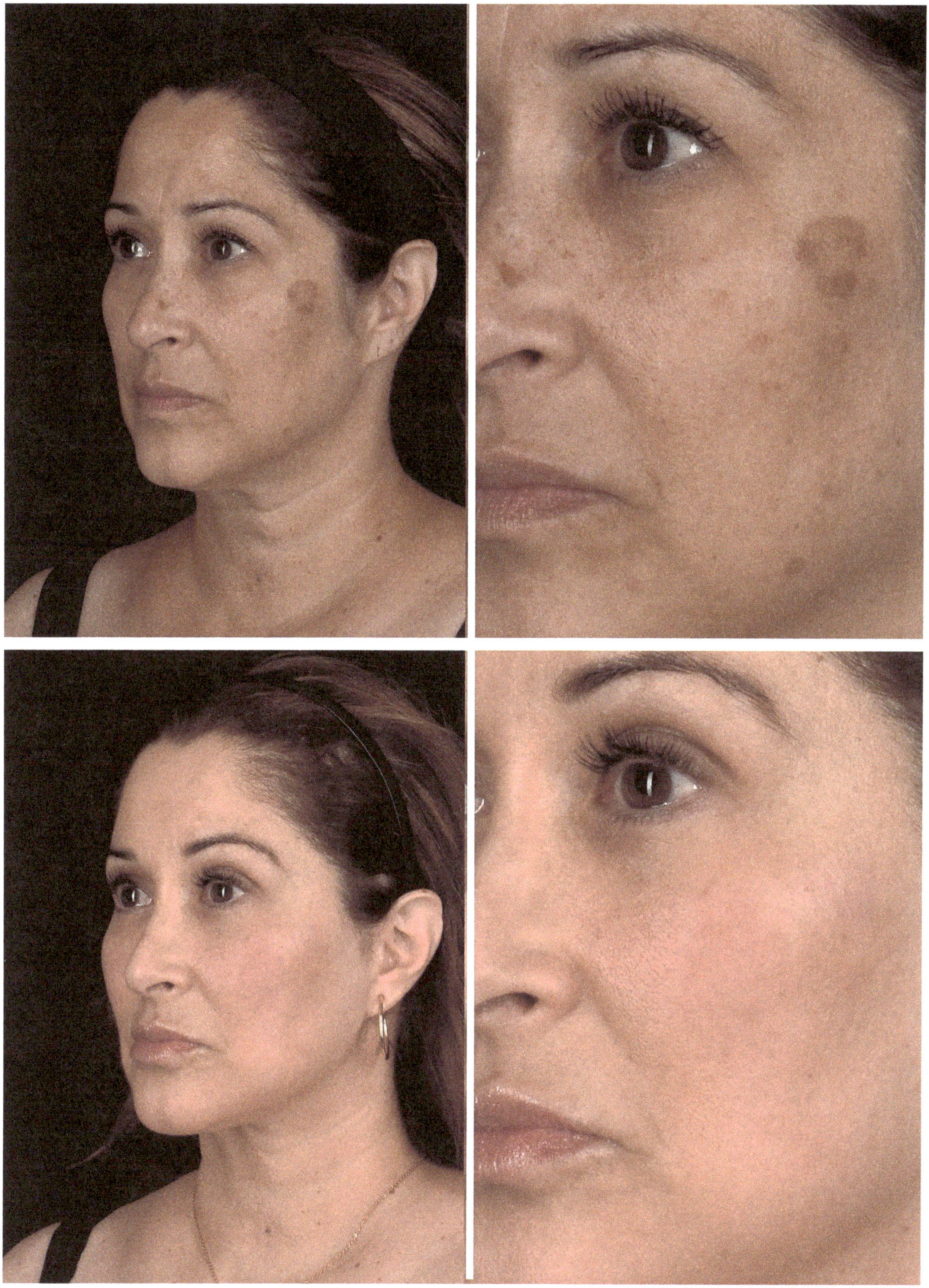

Fig. 10.7. The patient is shown before (*top*) and after (*bottom*) deep plane facelift with simultaneous laser skin resurfacing.

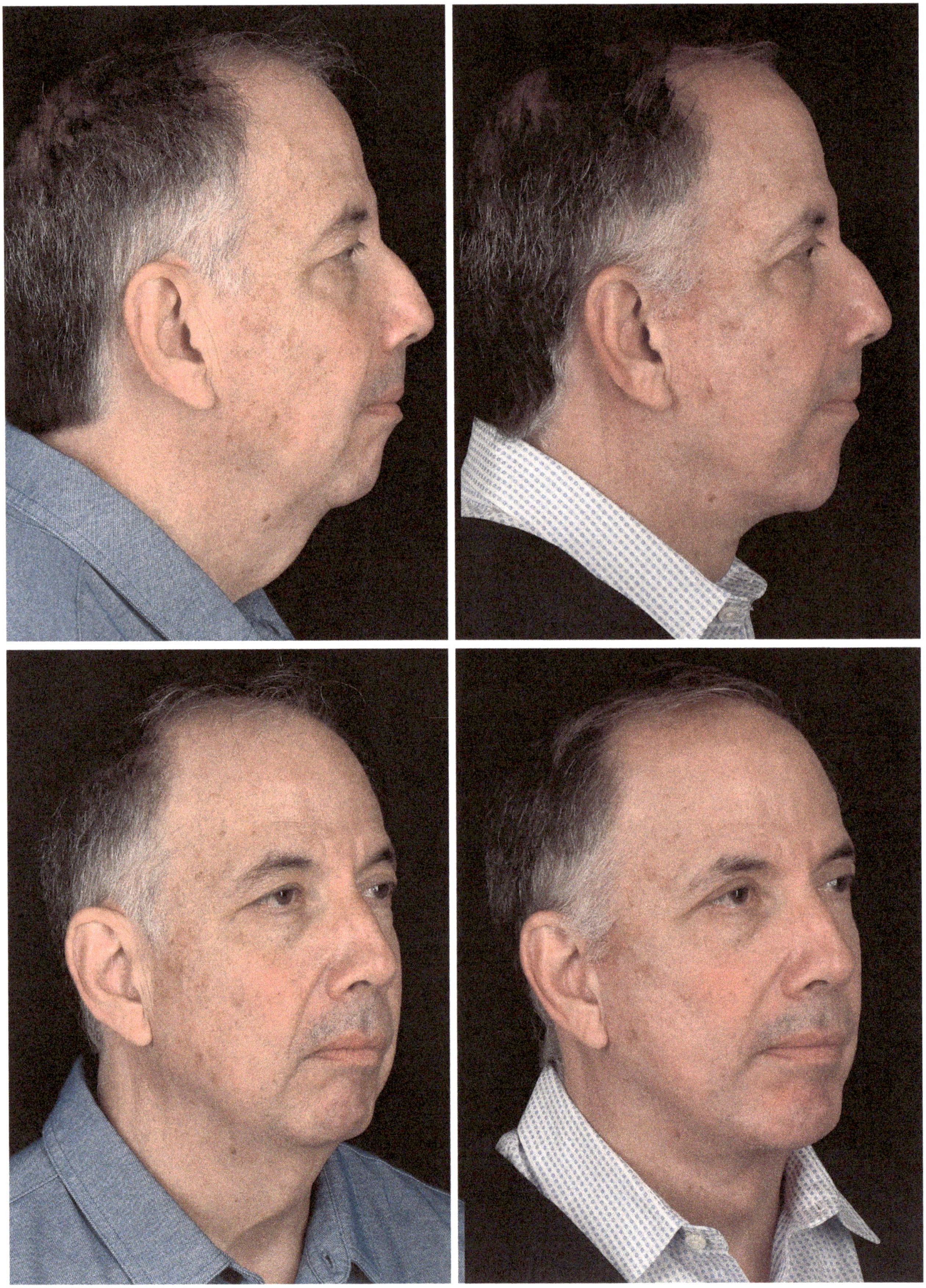

Fig. 10.8. This male patient is shown before (*top*) and after (*bottom*) deep plane facelift with simultaneous chin implant.

A facial plastic surgeon should utilize a combination of surgical treatment and relevant adjunct therapy. These treatments in isolation are effective, and if used appropriately, they augment and improve patient outcomes.

Summary

Although the notion of rhytidectomy has existed for over a century, it continues to evolve alongside surgeon knowledge, access, and treatment modalities. An effective outcome is based on both surgical skill in the operating room, in conjunction with appropriate and compassionate patient management. Although pitfalls still exist, there is no doubt about the safety of rhytidectomy in experienced hands.

References

1. Sykes JM, Riedler KL, Cotofana S, Palhazi P. Superficial and deep facial anatomy and its implications for rhytidectomy. *Facial Plast Surg Clin North Am.* 2020;28:243–251.
2. Surek CC, Moorefield A. Deep plane anatomy for the facelift surgeon: a comprehensive three-dimensional journey. *Facial Plast Surg Clin North Am.* 2022;30:205–214.
3. Perkins SW, Waters HH. The extended SMAS approach to neck rejuvenation. *Facial Plast Surg Clin North Am.* 2014;22:253–268.
4. Jacono AA, Talei B. Vertical neck lifting. *Facial Plast Surg Clin North Am.* 2014;22:285–316.
5. Rousso DE, Adams AS. Nuances in superficial musculoaponeurotic system rhytidectomy. *Facial Plast Surg Clin North Am.* 2020;28:285–301.
6. Waltzman JT, Zins JE, Couto RA. Face and neck lifting after weight loss. *Clin Plast Surg.* 2019;46:105–114.
7. Marcus BC. Rhytidectomy: current concepts, controversies and the state of the art. *Curr Opin Otolaryngol Head Neck Surg.* 2012;20:262–266.

Further Reading

Alexiades-Armenakas M. Laser skin tightening: non-surgical alternative to the face-lift. *J Drugs Dermatol.* 2006;5:295–296.

Beaty MM. A progressive approach to neck rejuvenation. *Facial Plast Surg Clin North Am.* 2014;22:177–190.

Carniol PJ, Ganc DT. Is there an ideal facelift procedure? *Curr Opin Otolaryngol Head Neck Surg.* 2007;15:244–252.

DeJoseph LM, Pou JD. Local anesthetic facelift. *Facial Plast Surg Clin North Am.* 2020;28:409–418.

Gerecci D, Floyd EM, Perkins SW. Incorporating midline platysmaplasty with lateral superficial muscular aponeurotic system facelifting. *Facial Plast Surg Clin North Am.* 2020;28:369–378.

Gupta V, Winocour J, Shi H, et al. Preoperative risk factors and complication rates in facelift: analysis of 11,300 patients. *Aesthet Surg J.* 2016;36:1–13.

Jacono AA, Alemi AS, Russell JL. A meta-analysis of complication rates among different SMAS facelift techniques. *Aesthet Surg J.* 2019;39:927–942.

Jacono AA, Rousso JJ. The modern minimally invasive face lift: has it replaced the traditional access approach? *Facial Plast Surg Clin North Am.* 2013;21:171–189.

Jacono AA. A novel volumizing extended deep-plane facelift: using composite flap shifts to volumize the midface and jawline. *Facial Plast Surg Clin North Am.* 2020;28:331–368.

Marcus BC. Rhytidectomy: current concepts, controversies and the state of the art. *Curr Opin Otolaryngol Head Neck Surg.* 2012;20:262–266.

Miller TR, Eisbach KJ. SMAS facelift techniques to minimize stigmata of surgery. *Facial Plast Surg Clin North Am.* 2005;13:421–431.

Mittelman H, Hershcovitch M. Management of the midface during rhytidectomy. *Facial Plast Surg Clin North Am.* 2015;23:195–200.

Molina-Burbano F, Smith JM, Ingargiola MJ, et al. Fat grafting to improve results of facelift: systematic review of safety and effectiveness of current treatment paradigms. *Aesthet Surg J.* 2021;41:1–12.

Moyer JS, Baker SR. Complications of rhytidectomy. *Facial Plast Surg Clin North Am.* 2005;13:469–478.

Niamtu J. Expanding hematoma in face-lift surgery: literature review, case presentations, and caveats. *Dermatol Surg.* 2005;31:1134–1144.

Quatela V, Montague A, Manning JP, Antunes M. Extended superficial musculoaponeurotic system flap rhytidectomy. *Facial Plast Surg Clin North Am.* 2020;28:303–310.

Rohrich RJ, Ghavami A, Constantine FC, et al. Lift-and-fill face lift: integrating the fat compartments. *Plast Reconstr Surg.* 2014;133:756e–767e.

Sarcu D, Adamson P. Psychology of the facelift patient. *Facial Plast Surg.* 2017;33:252–259.

Tiourin E, Barton N, Janis JE. Methods for minimizing bleeding in facelift surgery: an evidence-based review. *Plast Reconstr Surg Glob Open.* 2021;9:e3765.

Truswell WH 4th, Putman HC 3rd, Perkins SW, Johnson N. The superficial musculoaponeurotic system and other considerations in rejuvenation of the lower face and neck. *Facial Plast Surg Clin North Am.* 2018;26:135–161.

Zoumalan R, Rizk SS. Hematoma rates in drainless deep-plane face-lift surgery with and without the use of fibrin glue. *Arch Facial Plast Surg.* 2008;10:103–107.

CHAPTER 11

Minimally Invasive Management of the Neck Muscles and Cervicomental Angle Using a Percutaneous Suture Suspension System—MyEllevate

Gregory P. Mueller, Jonathan Cook, Jason N. Pozner, Barry DiBernardo

Chapter Outline

Introduction

Neck contours are determined as a result of multiple factors. Age, skin laxity, ethnicity, fat deposits, hyoid position, mandibular contour, submandibular gland prominence, and platysmal banding that all contribute to the appearance of the neck. Although the traditional surgical approach to facelifting can give an excellent degree of improvement for most patients, few are willing to have surgery when a minimally invasive approach might give results that are similar. Perceived risk, cost, and downtime are the major determining factors for many patients. The MyEllevate procedure was developed by Dr. Mueller after a decade of development, and he has refined the procedure so that he no longer opens the neck when performing facelifts and neck lifts.

Two variations of the procedure include the addition of thermal energy, such as radiofrequency, for further tissue tightening and minor periauricular skin resection in patients who have significant neck skin laxity. It can also be used as an alternative to traditional open neck maneuvers to address the underlying muscles and glands of the submental region in combination with facelifts and neck lifts. In many cases the procedure can be performed under local anesthesia. Steps in the procedure include marking, minimally invasive transection of the platysma muscle, followed by tumescent infusion. Liposuction is then performed if needed and undermining in the lower face and neck follows. Placement of a permanent suspension loop using a bidirectional threading rod whose tip is lighted to maintain a consistent depth is a key component of the procedure. Improvement in the cervicomental angle, definition of the submandibular shadow, correction of ptotic submandibular salivary glands, and improvement of mild to moderate skin laxity are the treatment goals.

The Theory and Background of MyEllevate

When I entered private practice, my patient population was focused on facial and neck contouring. I wanted to improve the patient experience, reduce visible incisions, and shorten the recovery period. Many of my patients were in their 30s and 40s, too young to need or qualify for the usual surgical approach. Many were men, whose potential for postoperative bleeding and hairline distortion as well as ingrown hairs in the submental incision steered me away from offering an open approach. There are many variables with open surgery, and the skin layer is destabilized with full detachment. This separation of the skin from the undersurface of the jawline can result in unpredictable healing and contour irregularities.

Initially I utilized a submental approach that I called the "trampoline" using a midline submental approach. Using a lighted fiber-optic retractor, I mobilized tissue down to the cervicomental angle. A 4-0 braided Ethibond suture was used to create an interlaced approximation of the medial platysma, in a manner similar to that of lacing up shoes. The crisscrossed suture matrix extended from the mentum back to the cervicomental angle. We evaluated the tensile strength of the retaining ligaments,[1] which withstood a 10 pound force prior to rupture. The Food and Drug Administration (FDA) requested these data compared with the tensile strength of the medial platysma borders when my self-funded company, Implicitcare, submitted a 510K application for the ICLED system in 2008, receiving FDA clearance in August 2009. This was the first and only patented light-guided technology for facial cosmetic procedures that utilizes the illuminated (fiber-optic lighted rod and suture) Suturod technology to accurately place a continuous suture in the subcutaneous space.

The trampoline procedure was hard to teach and did not produce consistent outcomes for all providers, so I began the search for a more effective approach. Some critiques were the inability of the anterior approach to address the cervicomental angle and ptotic submandibular salivary glands. In reviewing the literature, relevant articles included the experience of a surgeon who used transcutaneous braided Vicryl on a Keith needle to transect platysmal bands,[2] and Vince Giampapa and colleagues' work using an interlocking permanent suspension suture at the cervicomental angle anchored in the postauricular region.[3] Guerrerosantos[4] noted the use of a combination of purse-string suspension sutures with fat grafting for rejuvenation. Though my first percutaneous trampoline platysmaplasty was performed in October 2007, the platysma band division did not become a standard step in my procedural approach until 2012, when I learned that dividing the platysma bands at one level at the cervicomental angle followed by suture suspension that lifted and separated the edges was sufficient to help minimize the appearance of the bands.

In 2018, I began phasing out the trampoline platysmaplasty on my neck patients and adjusted the location of what I called the neck defining suture to enable it to become the workhorse addressing the comprehensive area of the jawline and neck region. This is what I eventually renamed the "MyEllevate" procedure. I learned from studying oVio360™ dynamic images how I could adjust the location and tension of the system to improve outcomes. This modified and simplistic MyEllevate procedure involved identification of the medial platysmal bands while the patient was in the upright position preoperatively. Local anesthesia with epinephrine was administered anterior and posterior to the isolated bands before transcutaneous application of the braided Ethibond suture that is attached to the 9 inch fiber-optic Suturod for muscle transection. Tumescent anesthesia was infused, and 20 minutes was allowed to pass prior to liposuction and undermining. The ICLED light-guided suture delivery system was then used to pass the suture for suspension through nine access ports. The suture was anchored in the postauricular mastoid region using the dense dermal-retaining ligaments prior to tying with the patient's head in an elevated position.

One concern at this point was that about 50% of the bands recurred at 1 month, probably from muscle fibers reconnecting. On one patient I used a cervical collar to keep the neck elevated and muscle ends distracted. This approach seemed to work well with only a 5% recurrence rate. When revising recurrent platysmal bands, I found that once the bands are cut, you must resuspend the neck or recurrent platysmal bands will appear shortly afterward. Cadaver studies have revealed that the suture suspension lifts and separates the freshly cut platysma borders helping to prevent reconnection. A limitation of the procedure is that lateral platysmal bands are unable to be addressed. I did transect lateral bands in about five patients but don't do it anymore. Large vessels could be damaged, and subsequent ptosis of the submandibular salivary glands could be a consequence.

Addressing submandibular salivary glands can be a challenge. Few surgeons address ptosis of the glands, even with open techniques. The Giampapa suture did help to elevate ptotic glands. The glands do need to be soft and mobile, not large and stiff, to be corrected with the MyEllevate method.

One of the big improvements that I made recently was the position of the #1 and #9 suture ports. This used to be located centrally at the cervicomental angle. I moved it anteriorly to the midpoint between the chin and the cervicomental angle. This results in flattening of the submandibular area between the chin and the cervicomental angle. The location of this midline crossing should always be placed midway or more anterior. Placing the suture strands at the cervicomental angle frequently results in a skin fold as vertical neck skin gets recruited upward. There is also a lack of support just under the chin if the suture is not placed in a more anterior position.

Patient Assessment and Evaluation: Who Is a Good Candidate?

A comprehensive medical history is required to determine if a patient is suitable for any cosmetic procedure. Any anatomic alteration of the neck due to trauma, previous surgery, or history of malignancy should be considered. The presence of any congenital or autoimmune conditions, especially those that involve the skin, should be taken into account so that risk assessment of surgery or alternatives can be completed. The history should include a log of prior complications, poor wound healing, excessive scarring, smoking, or a history of recreational or problem drug use.

Understanding the exact nature of patient expectations should always be a priority. Percutaneous suture suspension is most effective for younger patients who present with good skin quality and minimal excess skin. It is an excellent option when patients also have identifiable platysma bands and desire a short recovery time. Because it does not target facial laxity, it is not a substitute for a facelift. The aesthetic improvement created by this procedure is observed as increased definition along the mandibular angle and the upper half of the neck, with less lifting seen in the lower half of the neck. Although some patients may notice mild improvement in the jowls, patients bothered by jowling should be directed to more traditional facelifting techniques.

Markings

While sitting upright in the preoperative area, patients are asked to flex the platysma muscle by actively engaging the lower lip depressors and showing the lower teeth. In most patients, one or two dynamic anterior platysma bands are identified and marked. Puncture sites are marked in the midline and then 2 cm lateral to each band at the level of the desired cervicomental angle. These punctures represent the level of the platysma band division and the sites of insertion of the rod and attached suture (Fig. 11.1).

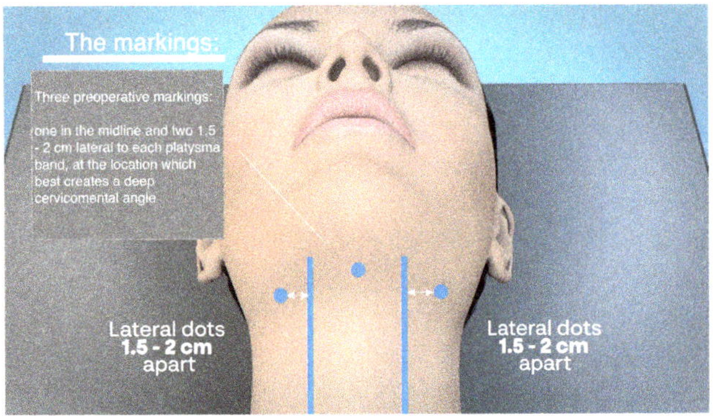

Fig. 11.1. Preoperative markings. Three access sites are marked for platysma band division and insertion of the rod and attached suture.

Anesthesia

Local anesthesia is injected superficial and deep to the platysma bands (9 mL of 1% lidocaine and epinephrine [1:100,000], 1 mL sodium bicarbonate). Access to the anterior platysma border is achieved by pinching the skin and underlying muscle band during active contraction of the muscle and distracting it away from deeper structures. Care is taken to only inject 2–3 mL of the local anesthetic into the underlying muscle band and subcutaneous space to prevent distortion of anatomy. Additional access sites for the injection of tumescent fluid, tunneling, and liposuction in the submentum, as well as the right and left earlobe junctions, receive 1 mL of local anesthetic each. Lastly, approximately 4–5 mL of local anesthetic is injected over the mastoid fascia bilaterally.

Following division of the platysmal bands, the entire neck region is infiltrated with 250–500 cc of tumescent solution (1 L normal saline with 50 mL of 1% lidocaine and 1 mL of 1:1000 epinephrine). This is best accomplished using a spatulated cannula. Larger volumes of tumescent solution may be used in patients undergoing simultaneous liposuction or subcutaneous energy-based tightening. After allowing adequate time for maximal epinephrine effect, and after performing any liposuction or tightening adjuncts, the suspension suture is placed.

Undermining

Beginning during infiltration and continuing during liposuction (when performed), the skin of the neck is extensively tunneled with a spatulated canula. This is essential to facilitate passage of the surgical suture, to create space for the passage of energy devices (when used as adjuncts for skin tightening), and to facilitate redraping of the skin following the procedure. High-volume tumescent infiltration coupled with extensive tunneling ensure that the permanent suture material will be safely and accurately placed directly on the surface of the underlying muscle. It also ensures that skin dimpling will be prevented, and inadvertent intradermal placement of the suture material will be avoided.

Description of Procedure

Division of Platysma Bands

Using the 2 mm puncture device, access sites are established at the previously marked locations, medial and 2 cm lateral to the identified platysma bands. The included clearing tool is used to bluntly dissect deep and through the platysma bands. The rod and attached suture are introduced through the midline puncture, passed through the edge of the platysma band, and then reversed in direction back through the subcutaneous space, advancing along the anterior surface of the muscle. This maneuver enables the suture to surround the platysma band. The suture material itself is then used in the same manner as a Gigli saw, moving back and forth to cut the platysma band (Fig. 11.2).

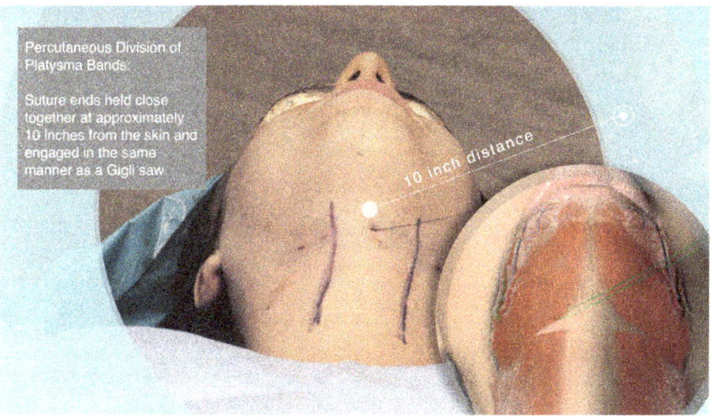

Fig. 11.2. Percutaneous division of platysma bands.

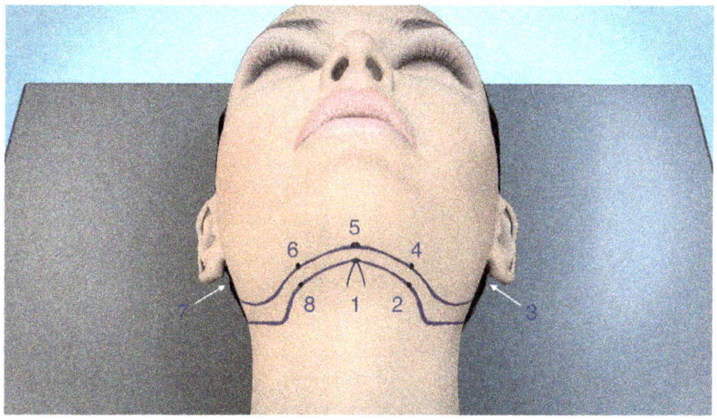

Fig. 11.3. Eight puncture sites are required for insertion of percutaneous suture suspension. The numbers correspond with the course of the suture suspension loop.

Placement of the Suspension Suture

A template is utilized to identify the positions of the remaining access sites for placement of the suture rod. As mentioned previously, after dividing the platysmal bands, we infiltrate the neck with tumescent local anesthesia.

Using the 2 mm puncture device, a total of eight access sites are created for the light-guided Suturod (Fig. 11.3). One access site is located behind each the ear, overlying the mastoid fascia located just posterior to the superior border of the soft earlobe/cartilaginous ear junction; these permit access to the mas toid-cutaneous and platysma-auricular ligaments, which serve as anchor sites for the suture suspension. The remaining six sites are located just underneath the mandible and midway between the chin and the cervicomental angle and serve as pivot points for continuous passage of the suture. A dermal clearing tool is inserted at each access site to release dermal attachments. This clearing helps prevent inadvertent intradermal placement of the suture material that would result in suture extrusion. The light handle is then attached to the Suturod to provide transillumination to guide the surgeon regarding depth and direction of travel of the illuminated rod and suture.

The light guide is inserted through the posterior midline puncture until a dull yellow spot is observed in the subcutaneous layer, confirming the correct depth of travel (Fig. 11.4). As the rod is passed underneath the skin, the surgeon observes the light; if it suddenly changes to dull red, this indicates that the rod has passed deep to a segment of the platysma muscle. While passing the Suturod through each access puncture, care is taken to not fully remove the rod from the subcutaneous space, ensuring that the continuous suture is delivered at the correct depth, which is directly on the underlying muscle.

Once the suture reaches the postauricular access point, the Suturod is rotated 45 to 90 degrees to engage the mastoid-cutaneous and platysma-auricular ligaments that serve as superolateral anchor points. The remaining holes are then used to advance the suture back to the midline, to exit through the anterior midline puncture site, anterior to the puncture where it was first inserted. The suspension suture is secured by tying the suture ends together in the usual fashion (Fig. 11.5). The knot is pushed deep into the subcutaneous space using the

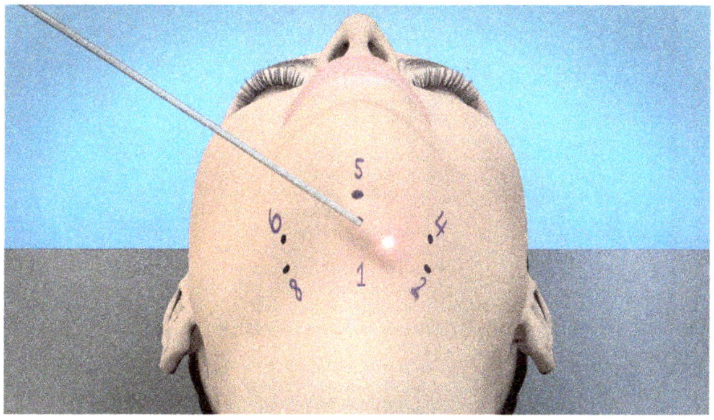

Fig. 11.4. Light guide insertion through the midline puncture. A bright yellow light indicates correct placement of the rod in the subcutaneous layer.

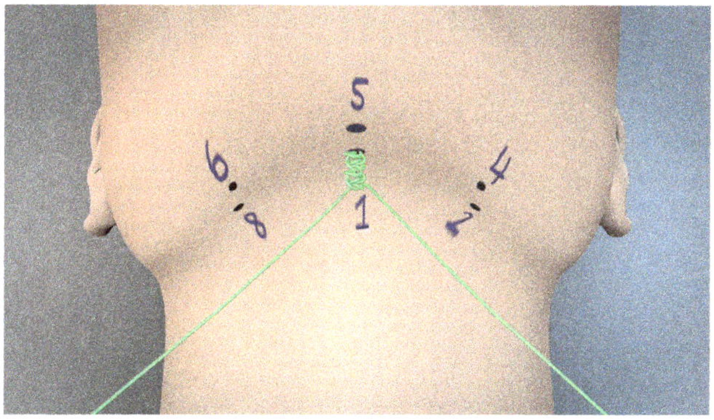

Fig. 11.5. Securement of suture suspension at the cervicomental angle. The knot is subsequently retracted into the subcutaneous space.

Suturod. A chin strap and a soft cervical collar are applied to the patient.

Concomitant Procedures

We routinely employ liposuction and adjunctive procedures for skin tightening, where indicated. We find that most patients benefit from some degree of liposuction to define the jawline and evacuate excess preplatysmal fat. In cases where there is no fat needing removal, extensive tunneling/undermining is still required to elevate the skin and to create the space to construct the

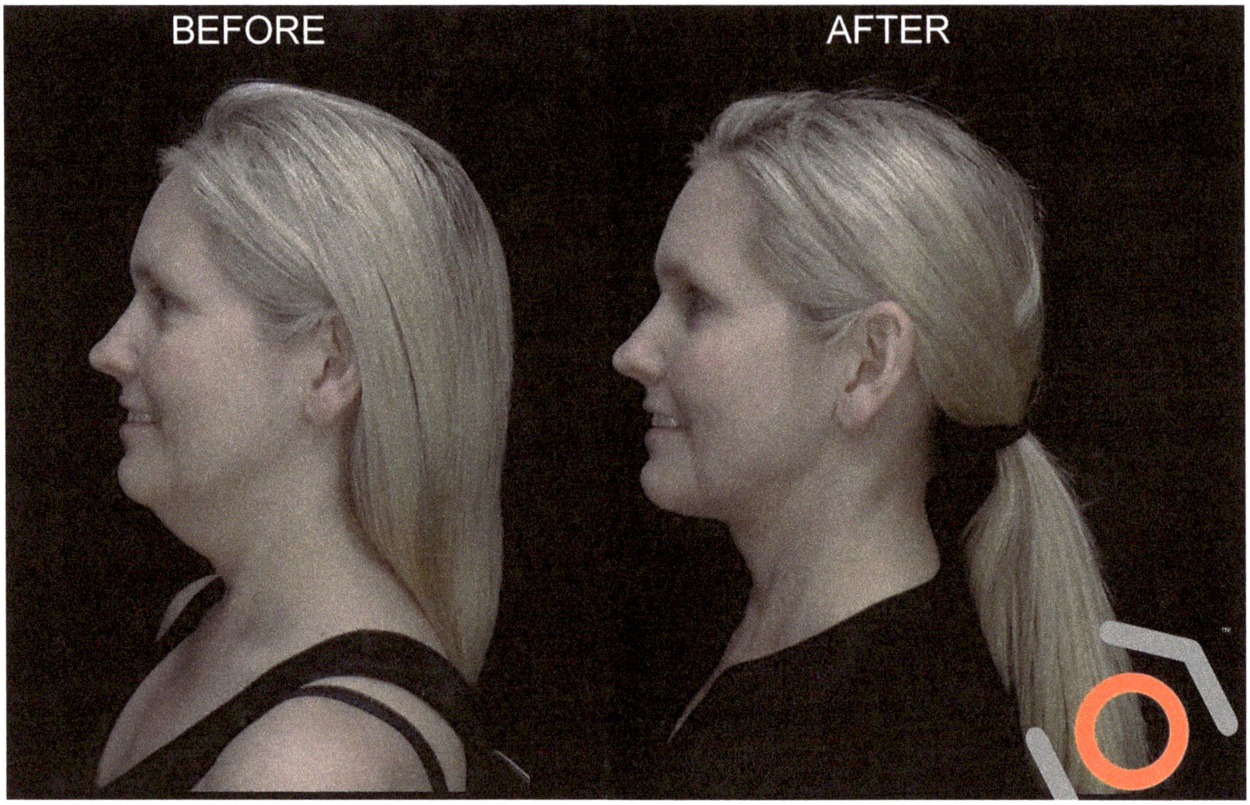

Fig. 11.6. This 52-year-old female presented with an obtuse cervicomental angle and ptotic submandibular glands. She underwent light-guided percutaneous neck suspension with liposuction and PrecisionTx laser. Preoperative (*left*) vs. 5 years and 9 months postoperative (*right*).

MyEllevate suture suspension. The tumescent fluid combined with tunneling also facilitate the use of energy-based skin tightening technologies. Accurate and precise delivery of the suture material onto the muscle also relies on voluminous tumescent fluid and comprehensive tunneling. Smooth redraping of the skin is also ensured with this approach.

In our large study,[5] in conjunction with the light-guided percutaneous neck rejuvenation (Fig. 11.6), 97% of patients elected to undergo concurrent neck therapy, which primarily consisted of energy-based subcutaneous tissue tightening with or without submental liposuction (Figs. 11.7 and 11.8).

Postoperative Care

Patients are placed into a soft cervical collar, which is left in place for 10 days. This is removed only for showering to reduce the risk of recurrent platysmal banding and also to reduce swelling. As part of the postoperative protocol, patients are instructed to avoid vigorous activity and to sleep with their head elevated for several days to further reduce swelling. They are also directed to massage any lumps and bumps that may appear and are reassured that these will go away on their own. We recommend minimal activity for at least 10 days after surgery.

Complications and Prevention

In our study reviewing 391 patients,[5] we found that the most common adverse event was recurrent platysma banding (4.6%) followed by residual skin laxity (1.8%). Additional, rarer complications were short-lived transient marginal mandibular neuropraxia (1%) and infection (1%). There were two small seromas in patients who also received AccuTite radiofrequency treatment. Both were successfully aspirated in the office. No postoperative hematomas or bleeding complications were noted.

One complication that could occur is rippling of the skin, which may result from either overresection of preplatysmal fat during liposuction or selecting a patient with excessive skin laxity who would be better served with a traditional excision procedure.

Pearls and Pitfalls

The most important pearl has already been discussed but deserves repeating: patient selection is essential. Patients without excess skin laxity or excess jowling will do best, as these problems are incompletely corrected by this procedure. It is an important point to recognize that percutaneous suture suspension can add further definition to the jawline in patients who are otherwise good candidates for submental liposuction alone. We find this to be especially true in younger patients, whose skin will contract well with or without the use of energy, and who are looking to achieve a chiseled or sculpted jawline.

It is important to tighten the suture enough at the end of the procedure. There is a tendency to hesitate when tying the suture which results in dimpling and wrinkling of the skin; however, this is exactly the end point that should be reached. The rippling invariably settles out when the distended submental tissue has absorbed the tumescent fluid and the postoperative edema subsides. One

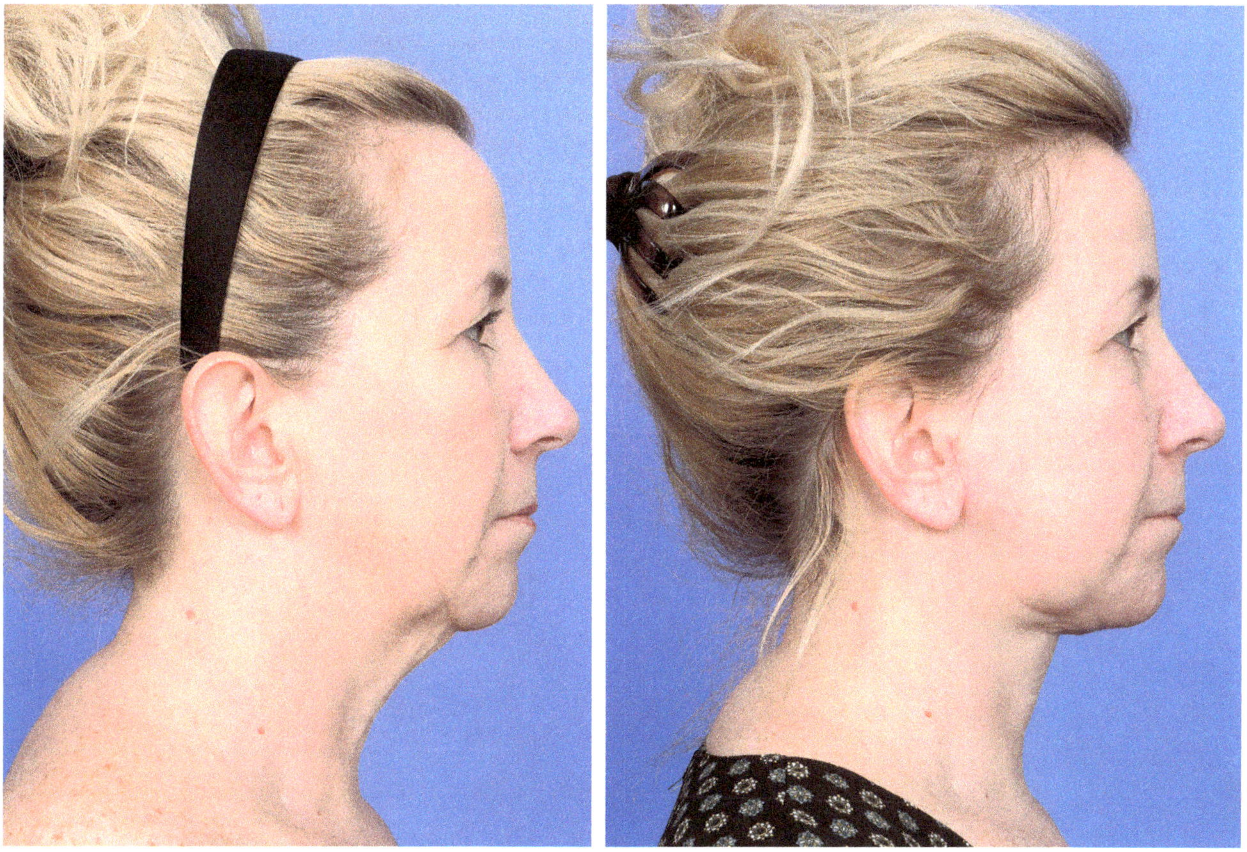

Fig. 11.7. This 56-year-old female sought a more defined jawline and skin tightening. She underwent a MyEllevate Plus procedure (minor skin excision with preauricular incision). *Right* photo taken at 2 months postoperatively.

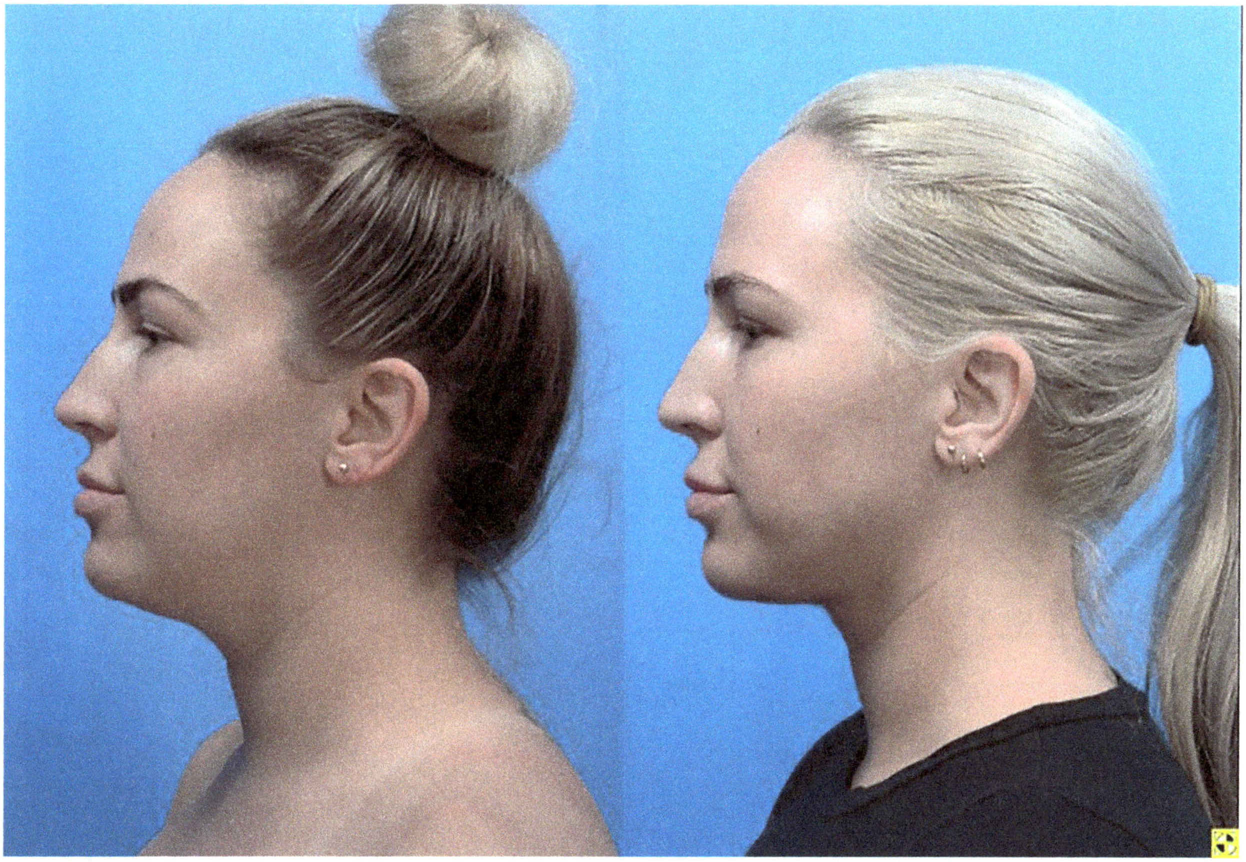

Fig. 11.8. This 43-year-old female seeking an improved jawline appearance received the MyEllevate procedure. Photos before vs. 1 month after MyEllevate.

final pearl is to avoid skeletonizing the neck through overresection of fat during liposuction. A small amount of subcutaneous fat in the submental area is important to camouflage the deep structures of the neck and to prevent postoperative skin rippling.

Conclusion

In the appropriately selected and counseled patient, MyEllevate is a safe and viable option for improving neck contours. The division of platysmal bands through a minimally invasive technique is a major advance in the treatment of these patients. In our experience, the technique works best in younger patients and when combined with energy-based skin tightening and liposuction. Importantly, this technique does not address excessive skin laxity, and as such, it is not a substitute for skin excision. However, in the appropriate patient, results are very good with a low risk of complications.

References

1. Mueller GP, Leaf N, Aston SJ, Stone CW. The percutaneous trampoline platysmaplasty: technique and experience with 105 consecutive patients. *Aesthet Surg J*. 2012;32:11–24.
2. Shiffman M, Mirrafati S. Scarless platysmaplasty for platysmal bands. *Indian J Plastic Surg*. 2004;37:60–63.
3. Giampapa V, Bitzos I, Ramirez O, Granick M. Suture suspension platysmaplasty for neck rejuvenation revisited: technical fine points for improving outcomes. *Aesthetic Plast Surg*. 2005;29:341–350; discussion 351–352.
4. Guerrerosantos J. Evolution of technique: face and neck lifting and fat injections. *Clin Plast Surg*. 2008;35:663–676, viii.
5. Gomez DA, James IB, Turer DM, et al. Light-guided percutaneous neck rejuvenation with division of platysma bands and suture suspension: a multicenter retrospective study. *Aesthet Surg J*. 2023;43:393–404.

CHAPTER 12

Facelift Complications: Recognition, Treatment, and Prevention

Joe Niamtu, III

Chapter Outline

"I remember all of my complications but forget most of my successes." Someone once said that "we learn more from our failures than we do from our successes" and nowhere is this truer than in surgery. In this chapter I have attempted to chronicle some of the most common and some of the most uncommon complications seen in a busy facelift practice. Although many of the complications shown in this chapter are mine, many of them are from patients that I have seen that were operated on elsewhere by other surgeons. This chapter represents over two decades of personal facelift experience and over 1600 facelift and neck lift cases. If you have followed my writings, you are aware that I never use old material for new editions of a textbook. This particular chapter has less updating due to the fact that complications do not change that much and the cases I present are classics for complications and treatments. Regardless, I have updated much in this chapter. As I went through each picture, I searched my collection to see if I had a new or better picture for specific complications. In 75% of the cases, I did not have more recent pictures. As I finished the revision of this chapter, it occurred to me that the majority of my complications were during the earlier part of my career. This would be expected in a surgeon's learning curve, but I am also a consummate photojournalist. By this, I mean that from day one, I took pictures of just about every procedure I performed. For this reason, I had more pictures than the average surgeon. In any event, it is personally a good feeling to see that many of these complications were rare.

Anyone who operates will have complications, and they can be minor or as severe as death. I've always been honest about my complications as they are a very important teaching tool. Surgeons that deny having complications either are not telling the truth or do not have busy practices. The number of complications that a surgeon experiences is also related to the volume of surgery they perform. A surgeon that does 10 facelifts per year will statistically see fewer complications or sequela than a surgeon who performs 100 facelifts a year. If you are busy and practice long enough, you will sooner or later see it all!

Most of these complications boiled down to statistic intervals and are predictable. In other words, if a practitioner does 100 facelifts, they may have a 1% hematoma rate, for example. For most surgeons, their victories greatly outweigh their defeats but nonetheless, there is a lot to be learned from our defeats. Anyone reading this book can see I have meticulously documented all of my cosmetic surgery experiences with high-grade, high-quality pictures. These pictures have proven invaluable for teaching, learning, and publishing, and I would implore all surgeons to continually keep their camera at their side and photograph the good, the bad, and the ugly, as it will be useful in your career and the careers of others.

No surgeon wants to experience complications; facelift complications carry the added burden of being visible. Some complications that involve breast surgery, abdominoplasty, and so on could be severe but are hidden during their resolution. There is no hiding most cosmetic facial complications. Cosmetic facial surgery complications therefore have a larger physical and emotional impact on the patient, the surgeon, and the staff.

This chapter will review common facelift complications but by no means covers every single potential problem. Facelift complications can be broken down into three main phases: preoperative, intraoperative, and postoperative. Complications can be a result of the surgeons' technique, the staff's instructions or lack thereof, and the patient's compliance or lack thereof. Understanding all of this, one can be a highly qualified surgeon and have a tremendously compliant patient, but the force known as Mother Nature can intervene and cripple the process. Finally, there can be "preoperative complications," which in reality are caused at or after surgery, due to a lack of proper preoperative attention to the patient's medical status and related factors.

As this chapter describes a plethora of complications, they are the downside of cosmetic surgery for both the surgeon and patient. They can lead to unhappy patients, damaged reputations, and lawsuits. Many questions arise when complications are incurred. One of the most common is "Who will pay to fix the complication?" This is an uncomfortable question as it may not be the fault of the surgeon or the patient. Surgeons have to weigh the pros and cons of doing free revision surgery versus the patient going to a competitor or, worse, an attorney. The informed consent must cover such matters, and as uncomfortable as it may be, they should also be verbally discussed before surgery.

Preoperative Complications

The phrase "preoperative complication" does not register correctly with most people because how can you have a complication when you haven't operated on the patient yet? The answer to that is that you may have chosen the wrong surgical candidate, and problems with this case are going to manifest after surgery. Astute and experienced surgeons may have seen red flags preoperatively that would portend problems with this patient after a surgical procedure. Obviously, no surgeon can predict physical or healing problems; however, they certainly may be able to predict patients that are not suitable for surgery for many various reasons and a perfectly executed surgery with perfect healing can be a nightmare on the wrong patient. Specifics on red flags and patient selection are discussed in Chapter 4 of this text.

Failing to recognize preoperative blood pressure or other vital signs can also lead to intra- and postoperative problems.

Intraoperative Surgical Complications

As the name implies, these are problems that occur during the surgical procedure. They may or may not be an actual "complication" but needless to say, they can "complicate" surgery.

Anesthesia

Regardless of the type of anesthesia used for surgery, the patient needs to be safe, comfortable, and homeostatic. A hypertensive patient can bleed. A stimulated patient who feels pain can move, have elevated blood pressure, or even remember the surgery. A patient with unstable vital signs can die. Anesthesia is a critical part of the surgical experience, and it is up to each surgeon to ensure that providers use safe and effective techniques. Anesthesia considerations are also very relevant in the postoperative period, especially if the patient has nausea and vomiting and is retching. Not only is this a terrible experience, but it elevates blood pressure, which can lead to hematoma.

Bleeding

Hemostasis is a prime consideration of any surgery including facelift surgery, and careful attention to bleeding must be observed throughout the entire procedure (Figs. 12.1 and 12.2). Although rare, extreme interoperative bleeding could lead to hypovolemia, hospital admission, and death.

Control of bleeding must begin in the preoperative history and physical discovery phase. It is important to rule out any bleeding or coagulation disorders as well as hypertension. Patients that are motivated to have cosmetic surgery will frequently downplay their medical problems for fear of having the facelift canceled, so it is imperative that the surgeon and staff press on for details that may lead to bleeding problems.

Intraoperative bleeding can vary from being a minor nuisance to a major problem period, as stated so many times in this book; any surgeon attempting facelift or eyelid surgery must have some type of cautery system available. Some patients inherently bleed more than others without the presence of any discernible pathology. Although most anatomy is predictable, some patients exhibit larger or more concentrated vasculature (Figs. 12.1 and 12.2).

Controlling intraoperative bleeding can slow a typical facelift down and add an hour to a case. As stated, the preoperative control of bleeding is also very important. Patients that have a tendency for hypertension are given 0.1–0.2 mg of clonidine before the case and occasionally after the case. Controlling hypertension is probably the single most important means of controlling bleeding. This includes the preoperative intraoperative and recovery and

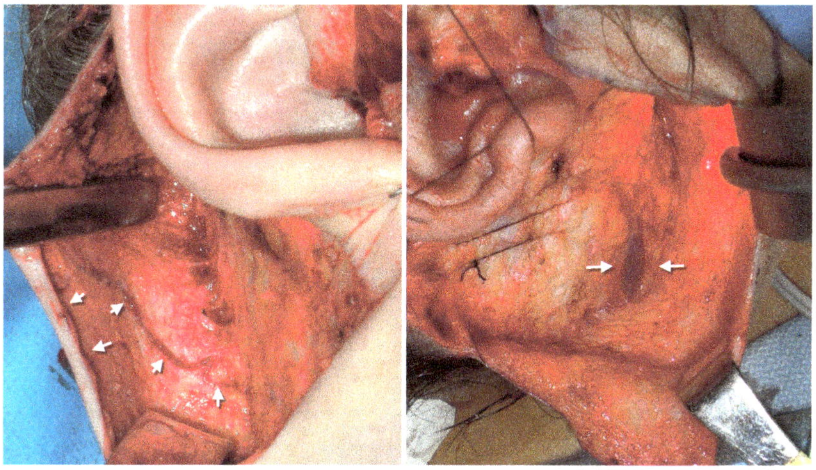

Fig. 12.1. Bleeding is encountered in any surgery but the vascularity of the head and neck is significant and surgeons should always be anticipating, avoiding, and treating small (*arrows*, *left* image) or larger blood vessels such as the external jugular vein (*arrows*, *right* image).

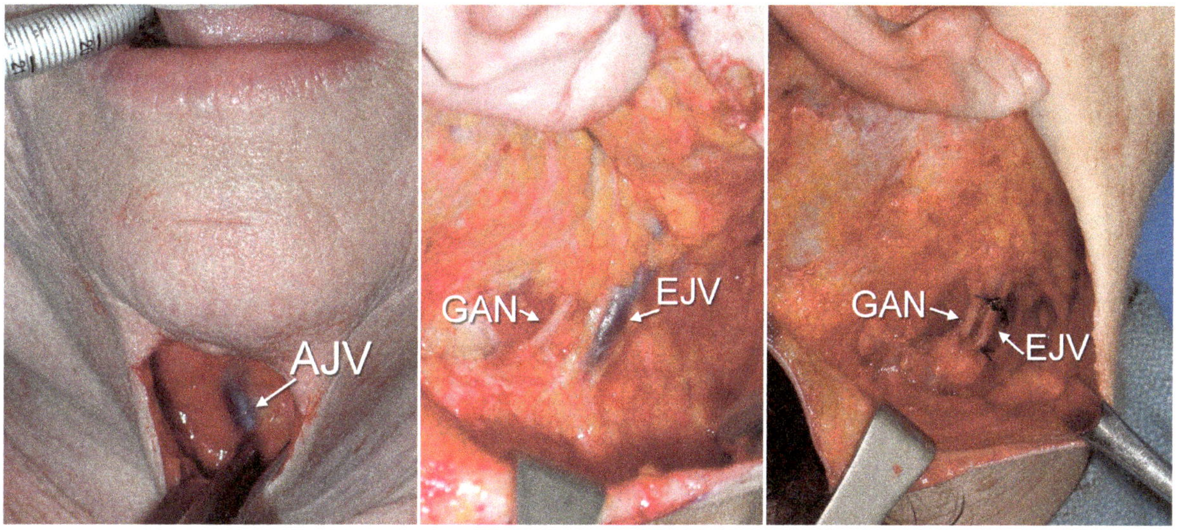

Fig. 12.2. The *left* image shows one of the paired anterior jugular veins (*AJV*). The middle image shows the greater auricular nerve (*GAN*) in close approximation to the external jugular vein (*EJV*). The right image shows the GAN in close approximation to the surgically ligated EJV, which was inadvertently lacerated during surgery. Note that the GAN and EJV are generally in close proximity to each other at Erb's point.

postoperative phase of the procedure. Bleeding must be controlled from the onset of the first incision as "catching up" can be hard to do as more tissue is disrupted.

The biggest game changer in my career has been the incorporation of tranexamic acid (TXA) in facelift procedures. This can be given 1 g IV at the beginning of the case; it can be mixed with the tumescent anesthesia and is also can be used for topical hemostasis throughout the case. You are reading the fifth chapter I have written on facelift complications, and this is the first text where I do not have a recent postoperative hematoma to show. I attribute this largely to the use of TXA. I have not had a "return to the operating room" hematoma over the 4 years I have been using TXA.

TXA is an antifibrinolytic agent and prevents the breakdown of blood clots. TXA is a synthetic analogue of lysine and inhibits fibrinolysis by competing with fibrin for the lysine binding sites in plasminogen. TXA inhibits the capacity of plasminogen and plasmin to bind to fibrin, hence preserving blood clots from plasmin-mediated lysis.

Few cosmetic surgical experiences are more stressful than dealing with a postoperative expanding hematoma in the middle of the night. This is something that must be planned for in advance and anticipated for each case. Most novice surgeons have found themselves in the precarious position of having to take a patient back to the office surgery center after hours and the stress of not being to reach their staff, the surgical instruments are still dirty in the sink, the anesthetic medications are locked up, and the surgeon is alone with an anxious patient and family. An ounce of prevention is definitely worth many pounds of cure in this situation. The key is to anticipate the complication. This involves having staff on call to respond, having sterile instruments available, and having access to anesthetic and medications and personnel. Having a proactive plan for dealing with hematoma or other emergent complications is a significant necessity.

Expanding Hematoma

An expanding hematoma is a collection of blood under the flap and considered a facelift emergency. Because the bleeding is continuous and the flap is sutured, the system becomes pressurized, which can occlude the delicate vessels of the dermal plexus and lead to skin necrosis and in severe cases airway compromise, which could result in death. Search of the facelift literature will show a hematoma rate from 0% to 15%. I personally believe that if a surgeon performs facelift surgeries, he or she will eventually experience postoperative hematoma. Expanding hematomas can occur intraoperatively or on the table during anesthesia emergence and in the postanesthesia care unit or at home after the patient is discharged (Fig. 12.3).

Hematomas can be further classified into minor and major. A minor hematoma is nonexpanding and represents a collection of blood that is stable. As explained earlier, an expanding hematoma is dynamic and continues to bleed and puts pressure under the flap. Hematomas are more common in male patients and usually occur within the first 12 hours after surgery. Although I have treated hematomas that occurred in the early hours after facelift surgery, the vast majority occur late at night and require an urgent return to the office. In some cases, the hematoma would have been recognizable earlier; however, the patient or the caregiver did not recognize the signs or symptoms. For this reason, it is very important to instruct the patient and caregiver about signs and symptoms of hematoma formation as well as things to avoid to prevent hematomas. It is also important for the surgeon or staff to check in with the patient in the evening of surgery to make sure there is no unusual swelling, pain, or bleeding (Fig. 12.3). Videoconferencing applications and smartphone cameras have made this much easier.

As stated earlier, most hematomas are usually in some way related to hypertension. They can also be related to extrinsic activity that causes the blood pressure to spike or Valsalva pressure increases to the head and neck. This would include coughing, clearing the throat, retching, vomiting, bending, straining with a bowel movement, and excessive talking or chewing. Postoperative patients often take narcotic pain medications that can cause severe constipation. Straining to evacuate the bowels can elevate blood pressure enough to produce significant bleeding. All patients that are given narcotics should be given written

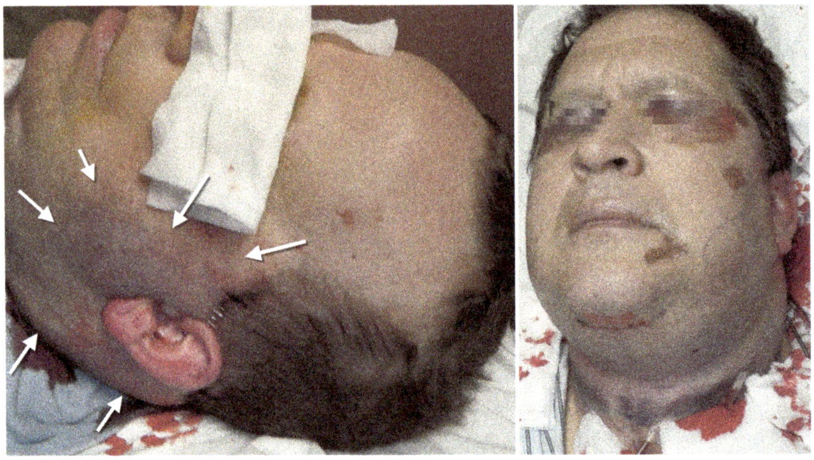

Fig. 12.3. The *left* image shows an intraoperative hematoma where the first side bled while the second side was being operated on. Another patient, shown on the *right*, developed postoperative hypertension and a left-sided hematoma in the postanesthesia care unit. He returned to the operating room for evacuation and hemostasis. The full neck and loss of mandibular border are common signs of hematoma.

information about simultaneously taking a stool softener and over-the-counter laxative such as MiraLAX. Adding a fiber source such as Metamucil rounds off this triad of over-the-counter medications to prevent constipation.

Hematomas can also occur from intrinsic factors such as coagulopathy or taking medications that affect the coagulation cascade. The major signs and symptoms of expanding hematoma formation include a rapid onset expansion on one side of the facelift associated with pain and bleeding from the incision sites. Expanding hematoma can grossly distort the face and a common finding is loss of the definition of the inferior border of the mandible (Figs. 12.3–12.6). I explain to patients that an expanding hematoma looks like a water balloon on the side of their face. The patient usually knows something is awry and often has a feeling of uneasiness or doom. The patient also may have difficulty closing their mouth due to the fact that the pressurized clot expands into the buccal space pushing the oral mucosa between the upper and lower teeth. Although many hematomas are unilateral, they can cross the midline and become bilateral. These situations have been known to cause fatal airway obstruction.

This is an extremely stressful experience for patient, caregiver, and family. When the patient arrives at the office, they

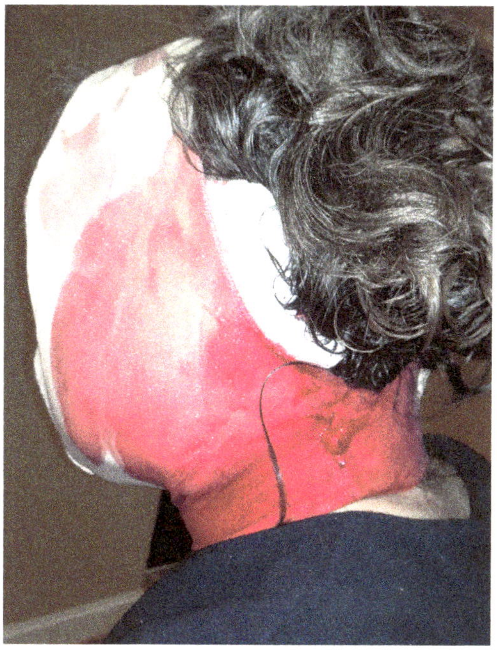

Fig. 12.4. This patient is shown approximately 12 hours after her comprehensive facelift and neck lift. Her caregiver called complaining of bleeding, which turned out to be an expanding hematoma. Most hematomas will bleed through bandages, but not always.

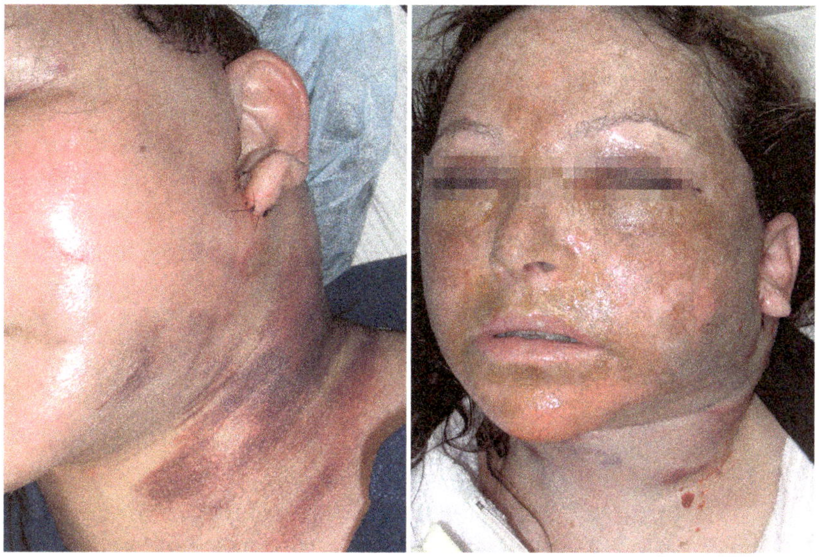

Fig. 12.5. Two patients are shown with postoperative expanding hematomas. The patient shown on the *left* has a smaller collection of blood than the patient on the *right*. Expansive distortion of the face and neck with the loss of mandibular border definition are common signs.

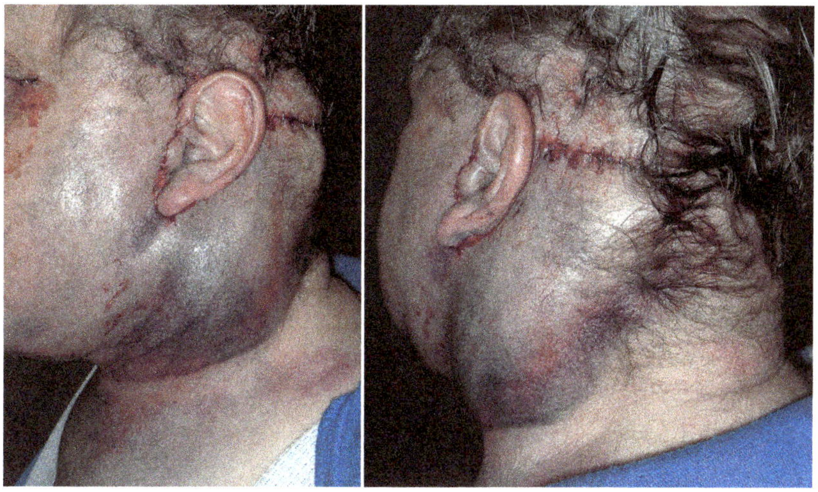

Fig. 12.6. This patient is shown the night of surgery and presented with an extremely large pre- and postauricular expanding hematoma.

and their caregivers or family must be reassured that as bad as this situation appears clinically, it will be rapidly treated, and the patient will recover without consequence to the final result. This is also an extremely stressful situation for the surgeon and the staff. Since most hematomas occur within the first 12 hours, this usually happens late at night after the office is closed, and it is sometimes difficult, if not impossible, to rally your staff and anesthesia provider. This is a problem for surgeons with office surgery centers. In the event the surgeon does not have the correct staff in anesthesia, the other option is transfer to the hospital for emergency decompression of the hematoma. Although this is an option, it will incur hospital fees that will probably not be covered by insurance as well as put your complication in a public venue.

Very small and inactive hematomas may respond to evacuation and pressure (Fig. 12.7). It is tempting to try this instead of reopening the surgical sites and exploring the face, but frequently it will just delay the inevitable. If aspiration and pressure is attempted, it is important to keep the patient in the office for at least an hour to verify hemostasis. The last thing you want to happen is to return to the operating room twice in one night!

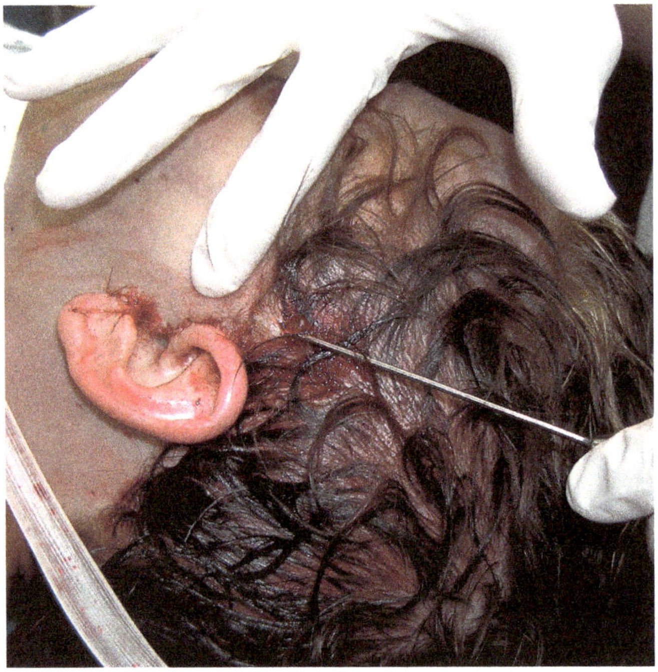

Fig. 12.7. A small, inactive hematoma may respond to aspiration with a blunt liposuction cannula and compression. If there is any doubt about active bleeding, then the incisions need to be opened and the surgical sites explored.

If a patient has a significant hematoma, it should be considered an emergency. In the rare case that the patient is undergoing respiratory distress, all staples and sutures should be immediately removed and the clots evacuated to relieve the pressure. In the 12–15 hematomas that I have treated out of 1600 lifts, only one of these patients experienced the feeling of difficulty breathing but his vital signs were never compromised. Death has been reported from respiratory failure due to bilateral hematoma, so it is a situation never to be taken lightly.

Treatment of a major expanding hematoma requires removing the sutures or staples and opening the flaps to explore and control bleeder(s). Generally, these patients are scared, agitated, and uncomfortable, and treatment is difficult without IV sedation or general anesthesia, as further manipulation and discomfort worsens the experience and increases blood pressure. In addition the rare but possible situation of airway compromise may require advanced airway techniques. Although any bleeding vessel or tissue can lead to a hematoma, it is rare (in my experience) to find a single, isolated bleeder during exploration (Fig. 12.8). Almost always, the surgeon will find several major bleeding points and scores of minor bleeding points when the flaps are opened and inspected. It is a demanding task and every surgeon is reluctant to remove the artistic suture closure that they performed earlier that day, but it is imperative to have access to control the bleeders. If there is any doubt that the bleeding maybe bilateral, then all lesions must be opened, and all surgical sites must be examined for bleeding. As stated earlier, going to the office in the middle of the night to treat a hematoma is stressful enough—having to return several hours later and repeat the process would be intolerable.

After the sutures or staples are removed, the surgeon most commonly encounters a currant jelly blood clot throughout the entire surgical site (Fig. 12.9). Most hematomas I have treated have been unilateral.

As the clots are removed, the surgeon is usually confronted with multiple bleeding points. Confined bleeding as seen in expanding hematoma is an irritant to the underlying tissue and encourages global bleeding and oozing of the entire raw surfaces. In some cases, the surgeon may see bleeding in an area that bled during the

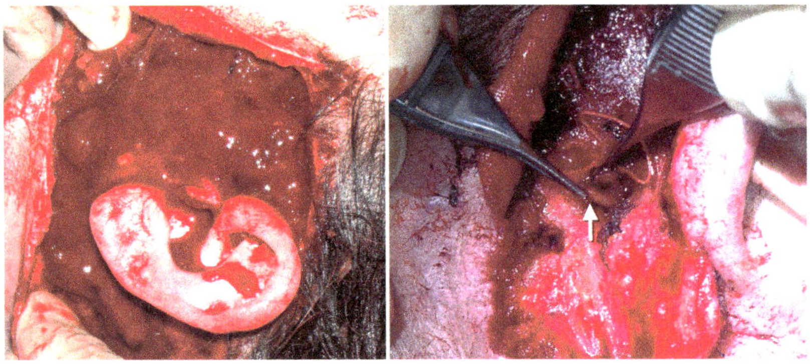

Fig. 12.8. The *left* image shows bright red blood and active bleeding from an expanding hematoma. The source of the bleeding was identified as the superficial temporal vein shown by the *arrow* in the *right* image. The vein was cauterized, and bleeding was controlled.

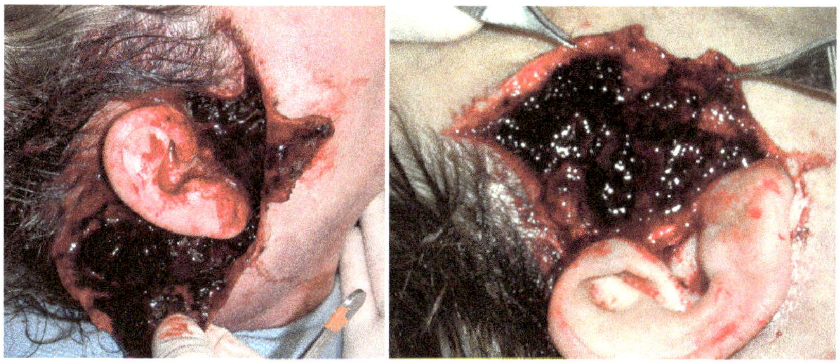

Fig. 12.9. Two different patients are shown with "currant jelly" blood clots after reopening the surgical sites.

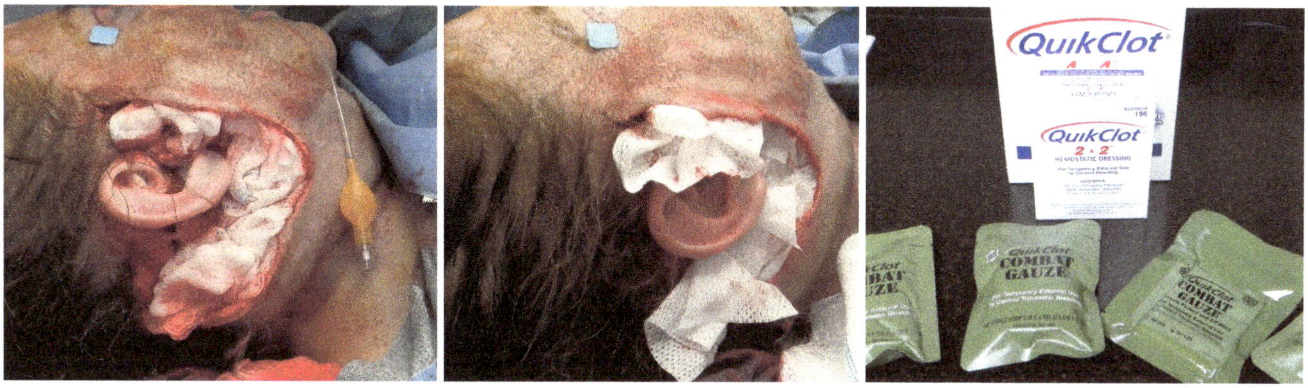

Fig. 12.10. The author treats hematomas by repeated packing with chilled saline gauze, hydrogen peroxide–soaked gauze, and hemostatic gauze. The *left* image shows the chilled saline gauze in place, and the *middle* image shows the hemostatic gauze packing. The *right* image shows the combat gauze product. Exploration and hemostasis are performed between packings until the bleeding is controlled.

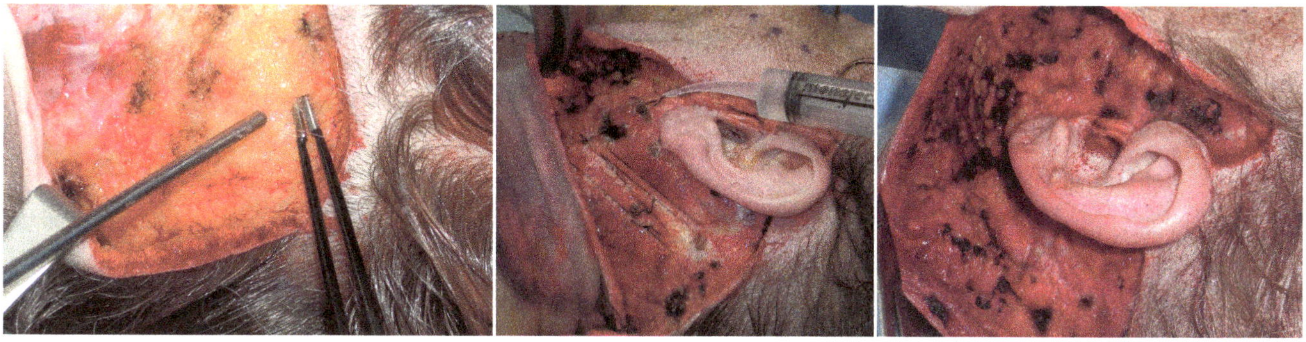

Fig. 12.11. The *left* image shows bipolar forceps that are used for hemostasis. The *middle* image shows hydrogen peroxide irrigation to identify and control small bleeding points. The *right* image shows the many bleeding points that were cauterized to stop the bleeding and control the hematoma.

initial surgery and was aggressively treated. More often, the bleeding occurs at sites that did not present any significant hemorrhage during the initial procedure. When the flaps are opened, the clots removed, and the tissues inspected, the common surgeon's response is "everything is bleeding," and it usually is.

Critical blood loss is usually not a problem with postfacelift hematoma but could be a possibility and must be monitored. The treatment to this point can be very intimidating if not frightening to the novice surgeon facing their first hematoma. Initially it may seem that the bleeding will never stop, and the surgeon can feel doomed. This is when the "inner surgeon" must kick in and manage the situation in a controlled manner with a cool head and manage the staff similarly. Anesthesia must control blood pressure as the first item of action. The first step after opening the incision is to remove the clotted blood with fingers and suction. This may aggravate bleeding. After the clots are removed, all flaps are packed with chilled saline (Fig. 12.10, *left*). This is kept on hand in the medical refrigerator for such purposes. One gram of TXA is given IV and another gram is mixed with 250 mL of saline to use with gauze packing and irrigation. This could also be mixed with the chilled saline solution. After 5–10 minutes, the gauze is replaced, and visible bleeding points are cauterized with bipolar forceps. I then repack the surgical sites with hydrogen peroxide–soaked gauze for further hemostasis. This gauze is left in place under compression for another 5–10 minutes. After removing, exploration and cauterization is continued, and I perform a third packing with hemostatic gauze (quickclot.com) (Fig. 12.10, *middle* and *right*). This is also known as "combat gauze" and is used by all five branches of the military for battlefield hemostasis.

The repetition of packing, exploring, and cauterization is repeated until all the bleeding is controlled (Fig. 12.11).

- Educate staff, patients, and caregiver to recognize postoperative expanding hematoma.
- Be prepared with instruments, medications, anesthesia, staff, and emergency airway for possible return to operating room.
- If present, treat immediately; it is an emergency.
- Be prepared; anesthesia or pain control will be required.
- Aspiration and compression for smaller hematomas can be attempted.
- Control blood pressure intra- and postoperatively.
- Use tranexamic acid intravenously and topically.
- Open incisions on affected side and manually evacuate clots.
- Pack in succession with chilled saline, peroxide, and/or tranexamic acid-soaked gauze and hemostatic gauze.
- Cauterize any bleeding areas between packings.
- After hemostasis, irrigate with H_2O_2 and reclose incisions with drain insertion.
- Apply pressure dressing.
- If unable to control bleeding, draw labs, pack with hemostatic gauze, place temporary staples.
- Transport to hospital.

Table 12.1. Postoperative expanding hematoma.

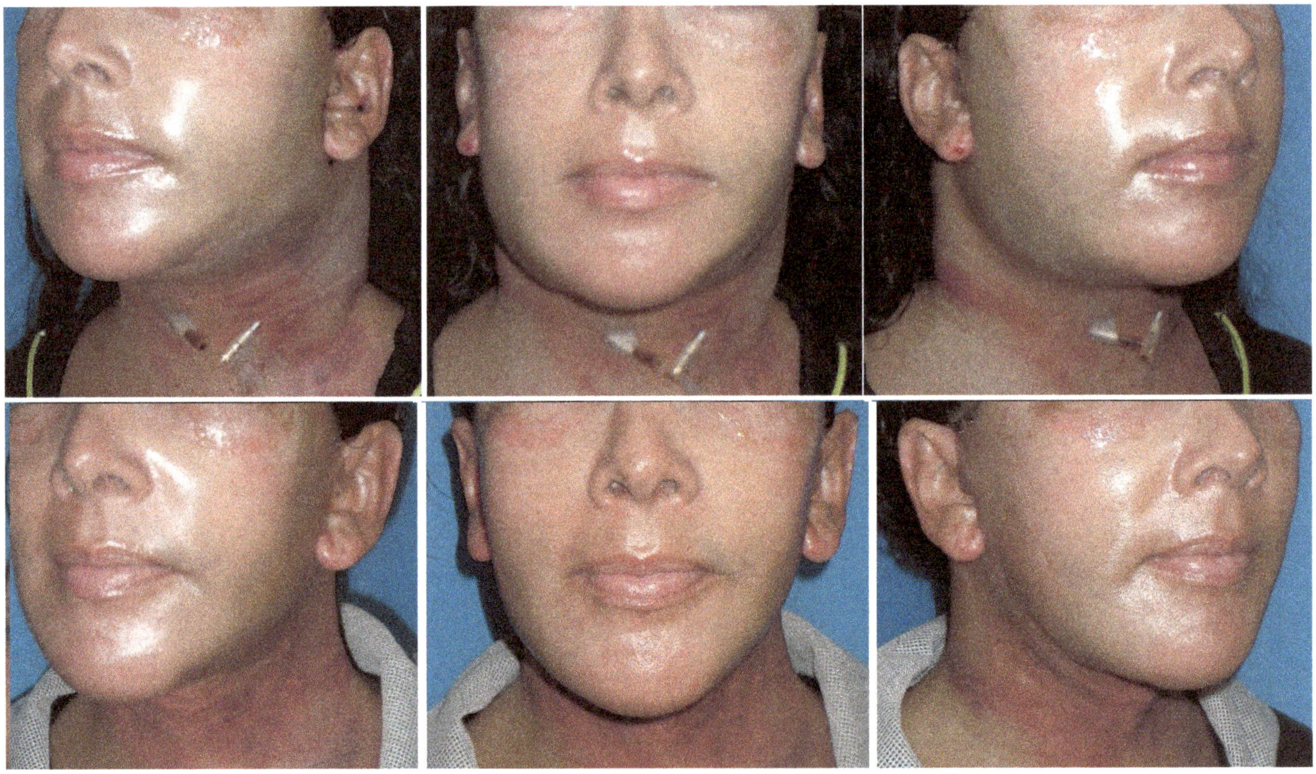

Fig. 12.12. The *top* images show a patient with a bilateral expanding hematoma the evening of her facelift surgery. The *bottom* images show the same patient then next morning.

In an optimal situation anesthesia support is available and the blood pressure is lowered during the hematoma treatment. If this is the case, it is important to return the patient to a normotensive state before reclosing the incisions, to verify that the increased blood pressure does not aggravate cauterized areas or produce new bleeding points. Topical thrombin is also used by some surgeons to control bleeding. If the aforementioned steps do not produce hemostasis, then the surgeon must consider external factors such as a bleeding diathesis. Appropriate labs should be drawn, and the patient should be transferred to a facility suitable for the diagnosis of bleeding disorders and the administration of blood factors. In my experience, this is exceedingly rare as significant hemorrhage would have occurred during the initial procedure. This entire scenario enforces the point that no surgeon should undertake surgical procedures when they cannot manage the complications. Table 12.1 shows some suggested steps in the emergent treatment of expanding hematoma.

As bad as most hematomas appear after the skin closure is removed and the hematoma treated, I am always amazed by how well the resutured incisions heal (Figs. 12.12 and 12.13). No patient I have treated for hematoma by reopening and reclosing the incisions has ever had significant postoperative scarring.

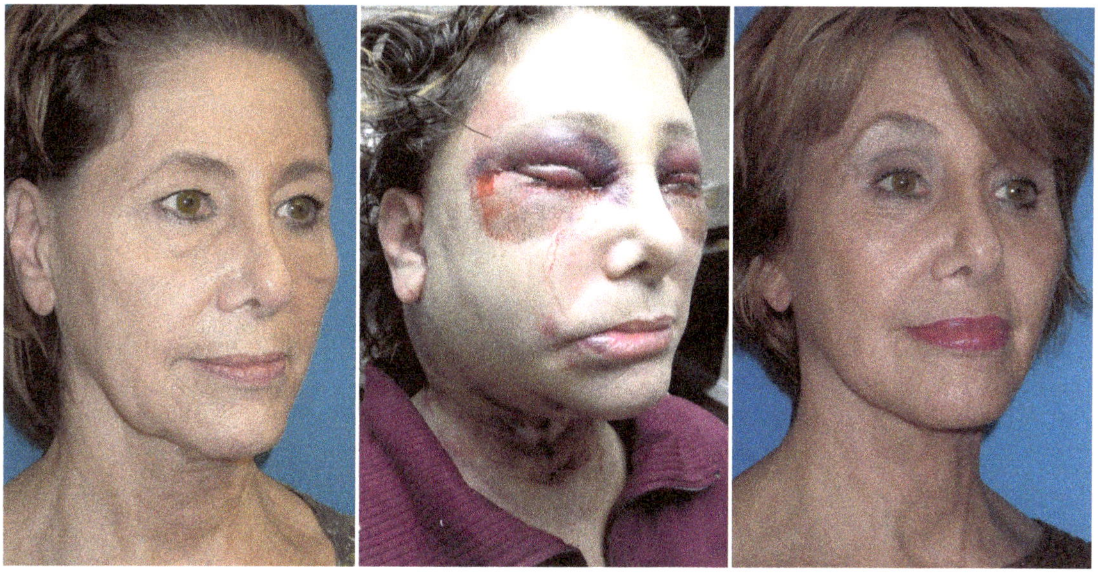

Fig. 12.13. This patient is shown before surgery (*left* image), the night of surgery with right expanding hematoma (*middle image*), and 6 weeks after surgery with normal healing and good aesthetic result (*right* image). Significant or permanent damage to the flaps is unusual.

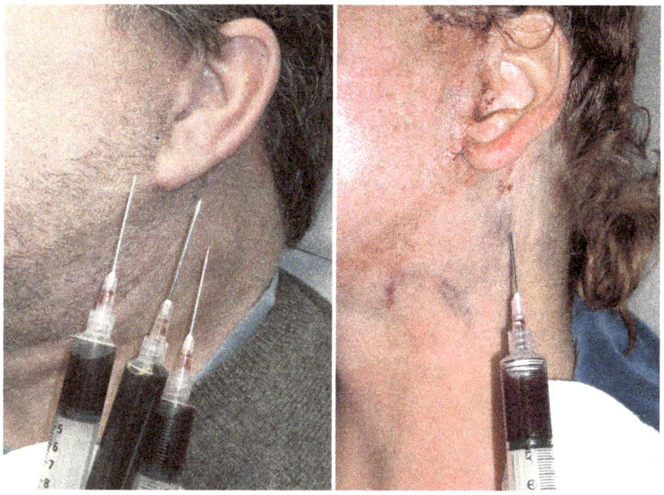

Fig. 12.14. These images show two different patients that required seroma aspiration after treatment of expanding hematoma. There will always be some remnant clot with breakdown when treating a hematoma, so the surgeon and the patient should understand that there will most likely be seromas to drain.

After the bleeding is controlled, the wound is closed in the same manner it was originally. A light compression dressing is placed on the patient and they are discharged and seen the following day. Drain placement is up to the surgeon and may be useful as posthematoma seroma formation is very common. Even though all the clotted blood was removed, some will remain, and this plus the trauma of two surgeries in a single day will contribute to seroma formation as the clots are metabolized. This requires needle aspiration. Some seromas will resolve after a single aspiration and some may require aspiration daily or every other day for several weeks (Fig. 12.14).

I believe regardless of hematoma, some patients form much more fluid than others during healing. Regardless of the cause, a seroma will delay healing and can serve as a culture medium for infection or it can organize into scar tissue that can leave irregularities that are difficult to resolve. All fluid collections present after facelift surgery should be aspirated.

Proponents of postoperative drains claim to experience less seroma formation. To be clear, the presence of a drain and or a tight pressure dressing will not prevent hematomas.

Significant ecchymosis is also common after hematoma.

Although most critical hematomas occur early in the postoperative experience, in rare instances they can spontaneously occur at a later date. I have seen several patients with normal postfacelift healing develop spontaneous minor hematoma several weeks after surgery. Possible causes include overexertion, a cauterized vessel that becomes disrupted, or a suture that erodes into a vessel.

Seromas are not true active bleeding or clotted blood but rather serum from the healing process and blood breakdown products. They are initially dark, then change to a serosanguinous color, and finally change to a more amber color, and they usually do not pose a threat other than delayed healing. The newer technology of portable or hand held ultrasounds has allowed surgeons to quantify the presence of seroma or hematoma (Fig. 12.15). Seroms fluid can be extremely irritating to the overlying tissues and can set off a fibrotic inflammatory process that causes induration and "washboard" corrugations of the surrounding skin. This is something that is extremely bothersome to the patient and can take months to resolve. This will be covered in depth later in this chapter. The take-home point here is that seromas can be bad and lead to prolonged healing problems, so the doctor and staff must be on alert for retained fluid in the face or neck and evacuate it immediately. Unrecognized seromas can organize and cause a permanent fibrosis, lumps, bumps, or ridges. Seromas do not necessarily only happen after hematoma.

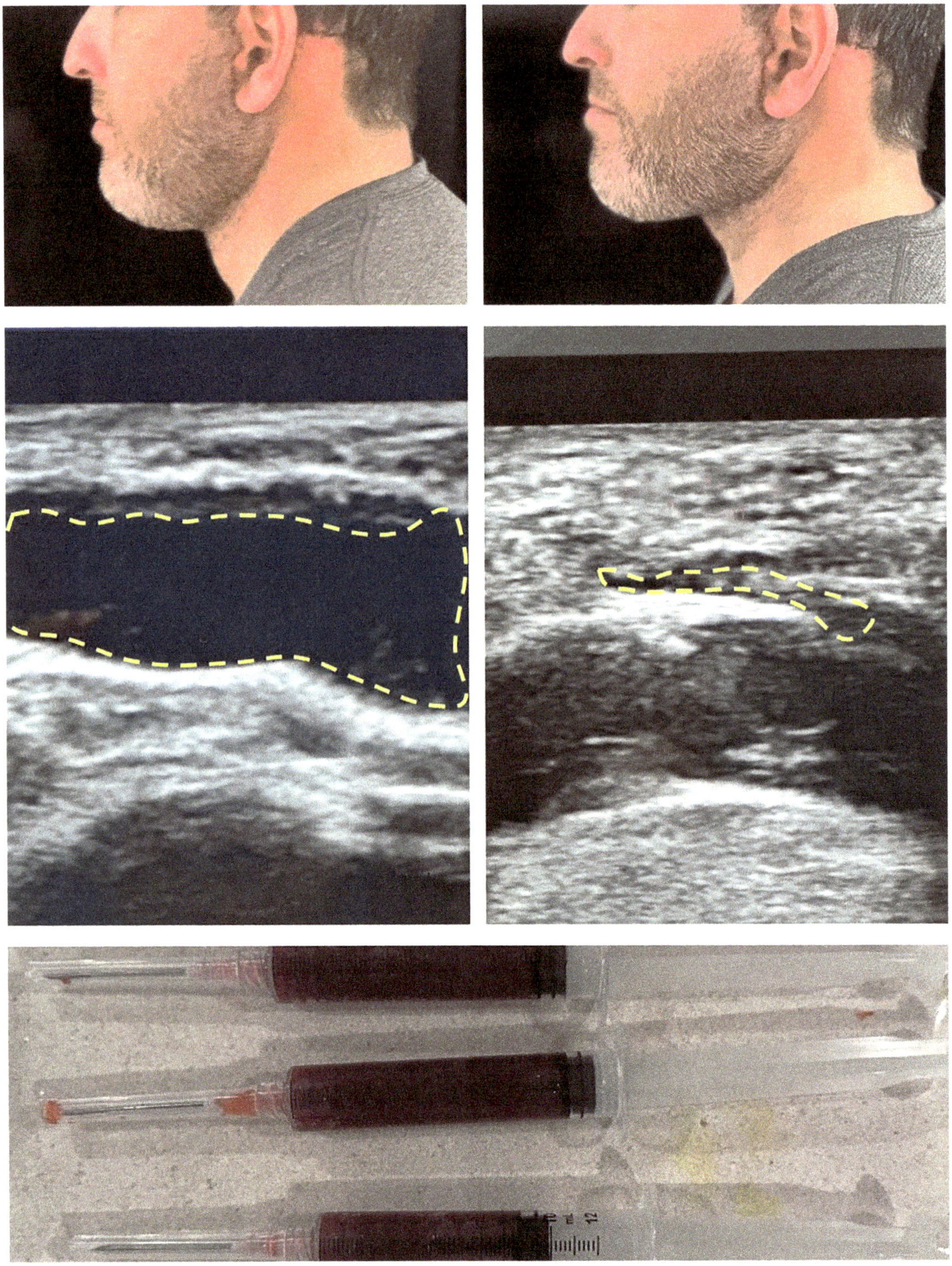

Fig. 12.15. The *upper left* image shows a patient 5 days after deep plane face and neck lift with submental fulness from a suspected seroma. The *top* picture in the *center* image shows an ultrasound image confirming a large seroma in the submental and later cervical regions (*large dotted yellow line* identifies the seroma space before aspiration). The *upper right* image show the patient immediately after aspiration of a 30 mL. In the *center* picture, the *dashed yellow line* shows the seroma after aspiration and the *bottom* images show the aspirate. (Photos and ultrasound treatment by Marcie L. Rabin, MD.)

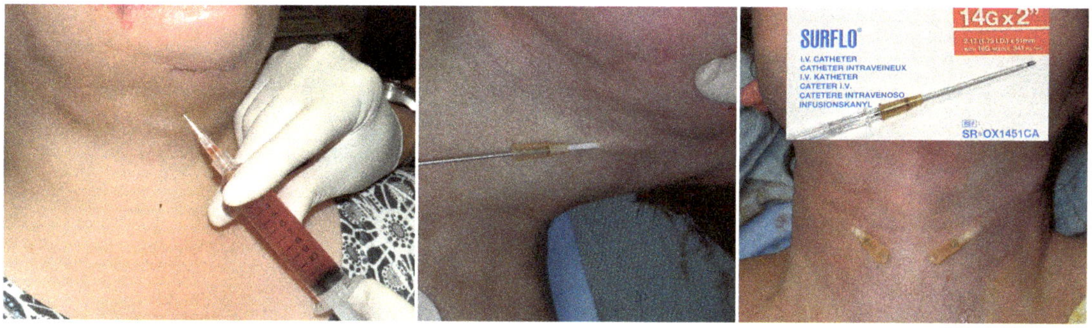

Fig. 12.16. Not all seromas are related to hematomas, and they can commonly occur after facelift surgery. They must be drained and can be cannulated with a 14 gauge angiocatheter, which is taped in place for several days until drainage stops. For much of my career I routinely placed two angiocatheters at the end of the facelift procedure and removed them several days later. I still do this on occasion. This "poor man's drain" is not under suction but still can drain impressive fluid from passive dependence.

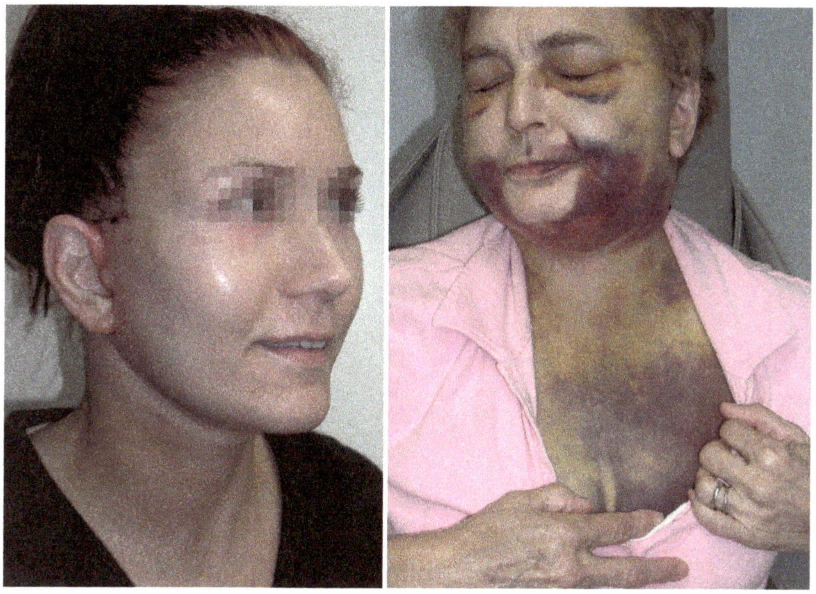

Fig. 12.17. In the *left* image shows a patient in her 40s 24 hours after comprehensive facelift and neck lift, and the *right* image shows a patient in her 70s at 24 hours after the same procedure.

Almost all hematomas will lead to seroma formation in the healing phase, but other patients will simply develop spontaneous seromas without having a hematoma (Fig. 12.16).

Postoperative Edema and Ecchymosis

Swelling and bruising are common with all facial procedures due to the increased vascularity in the region. I explain to patients that although I can speak with extreme accuracy about anatomy, anesthesia medications, incisions, and so on, the biggest unpredictability in facelift recovery is swelling and bruising. The variability is impressive as some patients recover with virtually no edema or ecchymosis, but other patients have significant swelling and bruising (Figs. 12.17 and 12.18). Again, these can be from extrinsic or intrinsic factors. Undiagnosed Von Willebrand disease is an example. Other patients were not compliant in stopping aspirin, fish, or krill oil or other medications or supplements that can affect clotting. A large component of swelling and bruising is also procedure dependent. A patient that has a facelift only will usually have less swelling and bruising than a patient that has a facelift with simultaneous brow lift, four-quadrant blepharoplasty, cheek implants, chin implant, and laser.

Swelling and bruising do not inherently cause problems other than they frequently make the patient feel that something is wrong or that something was done improperly by

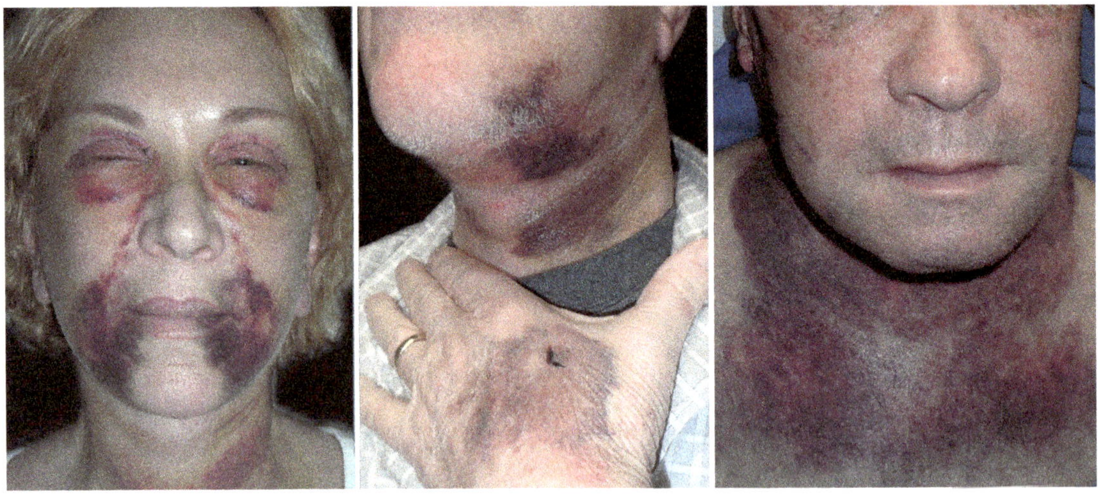

Fig. 12.18. Three patients are shown with various degrees of swelling and ecchymosis. All three of these cases are atypical but possible, and all three of these patients probably have some borderline coagulopathy. The patient on the *left* has dependent ecchymosis as the central face was not included in her operation. The patient in the *middle* picture had unusual bruising, but his IV site was also extremely bruised, indicating that the patient has a higher proclivity toward ecchymosis. The patient on the *right* had extreme and unusual bruising after facelift and neck lift and treatment of a postoperative hematoma.

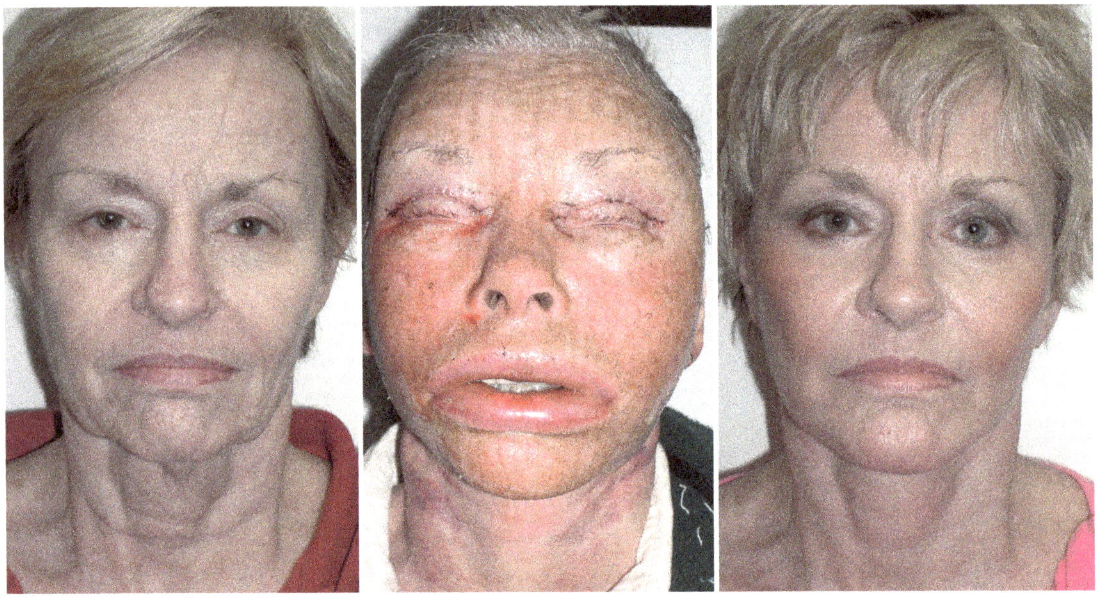

Fig. 12.19. This patient is shown before surgery (*left* image), the second postoperative day after multiple cosmetic facial procedures including facelift, browlift, blepharoplasty, facial implants, and simultaneous laser skin resurfacing (*center* image). The *right* image shown 8 weeks later with a normal result.

the surgeon. On the other hand, they also can tax the reputation of a surgeon when friends of the patient see severe swelling and bruising. The bottom line is it is not a good situation for anyone, and any steps that can be taken to mitigate swelling and bruising are important in the recovery process. Some surgeons recommend Arnica Montana preparations and other topical treatments. I have never seen a significant difference in swelling or bruising when I tried these preparations, although some doctors and patients swear by them. Gentle handling of the tissues and making sure the patient is not taking anything that affects their coagulation is time well spent. Preoperative screening for any type of disease entity that would worsen their swelling and bruising is also standard of care. A recent personal informal survey of 15 respected multispecialty facelift surgeons confirmed that none of them perform routine preoperative coagulation studies (prothrombin time/partial thromboplastin time), but all of them have their patients refrain from aspirin, vitamin E, and fish and krill oil.

Bruising generally is not in itself problematic, but significant edema can put pressure under the flaps and lead to tissue necrosis or scar problems from the sutures being under tension.

Postoperative edema can also be impressive in some patients and extremely disfiguring; it is important to let patients know that this will not affect their outcome (Fig. 12.19). I place all of my surgery patients on a nontapering regimen of prednisone. Preoperatively, all patients receive a prescription for 15 tablets of

20 mg prednisone. They are instructed to take three tablets (60 mg) as a single dose, beginning the first postoperative day and continuing until finished. I have found this regimen much more effective and dramatic than common tapering dose packs.

Extended swelling can be very problematic for patients who are trying to get back to work or to play. One of the biggest causes of patient anxiety and dissatisfaction is when they have a problem and they are not offered any options for treatment. If a patient complains of a significant problem, the surgeon must suggest some form of treatment, otherwise the patient may lose confidence and possibly seek treatment elsewhere. Sometimes reassurance is all that is necessary. Preoperatively I tell my patients that healing can take a full year to be complete. Knowing this preoperatively helps set the stage for postoperative problems.

Everyone reading this text understands the fact that in some cases there really is *nothing* to be done that would make a huge difference other than the passage of time. Having said this, the ability to offer the patient some type of treatment will go a long way in relaxing them and maintaining their confidence in your care. Reassuring the patient that you realize their problem and have seen it before and will provide the necessary treatment can assist in relaxing the patient. It may also involve recommending light cardio exercise, prescription of steroids, or lymphatic massage. The goal is to do something! Doing nothing merely exacerbates the patient's anxiety and dissatisfaction. Sometimes treatments can even be placebo oriented but still make the patient feel that their concerns are being addressed. All of this patient anxiety has become much worse since the introduction of the Internet. It is so common for patients to have some minor situation and go online only to see misinformation or unrelated information that further fuels their anxiety.

One of the best investments I have made is a $2500 ultrasound machine (Fig. 12.20). We use this frequently on many types of swelling or inflammation. Many facial surgery patients will experience normal swelling but an abnormal psychological response to it. They can become very impatient and even more impatient if they feel that nothing is being done to improve their condition. In rare cases, a lack of action may prompt patients to seek a second opinion. Any patient that has swelling, whether usual or not, will benefit from in office ultrasound treatments. Ultrasound treatment generates deep heat, is totally noninvasive, can be performed by staff, feels good, and can reduce edema. Whether the patient actually experiences any significant improvement from the treatment is secondary as they feel treated and this helps endure the passage of time for further healing. What is most important is that the patient feels that something is being done to improve their situation. Sometimes it is the ultrasound that reduces the swelling, and sometimes it is the psychological or placebo effect that makes them feel better. We do not charge for these treatments and they only take about 10 minutes and are performed by staff. We especially use this treatment for postfacelift patients that are 2–4 weeks out of their procedure but still manifest isolated submental or neck swelling. This device is also extremely useful for patients that develop fibrosis or banding in the submental in cervical regions, which will be discussed later in this chapter. Obviously, all of these problems should be discussed in the verbal and written informed consent. It is important to not only discuss the fact that swelling and bruising can occur, but it may be extended for weeks or months in some patients.

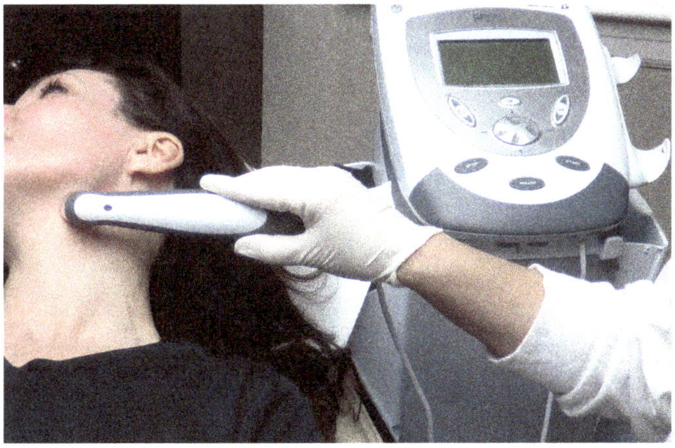

Fig. 12.20. A portable professional ultrasound machine is a useful addition to any cosmetic surgery practice and is useful in treating inflammation, swelling, and fibrosis.

Neurologic Complications

Motor Nerve Injury

Motor nerve damage is one of the most feared complications associated with facelift and neck lift as well as other cosmetic facial surgical procedures. Unlike many of the complications discussed previously, permanent nerve damage can be disabling for the patient and has far-reaching effects on the surgeon as well, sometimes leading to damage of reputation and litigation. All facial nerve branches (temporal, zygomatic, buccal, marginal mandibular, and cervical) can be temporarily or permanently affected by facelift surgery.

Nerve injury can result from a variety of things, including direct injury (clamps, needles, scalpels, and scissors), neuropraxia (stretching from overaggressive retraction), thermal injury from cautery, or compression injury from sutures, edema, hematoma, and other causes. This is very disconcerting for the patient and surgeon in the early postoperative period. It is a bad feeling to have an awesome facelift result with a partially paralyzed face. Even though most of these will spontaneously resolve within weeks or months, the interim is very stressful for all parties involved. I think surgeons lose a few days off of their life span for each major complication they incur! The gradual return of function to the affected area is seen and greeted with relief. Patients should be reassured that the nerve weakness is likely temporary but advised (hopefully preoperatively) that return of full function cannot be guaranteed. In the 1600 facelifts I have performed over the past 20 years, I have experienced two permanent motor nerve injuries. When I began doing deep plane facelifts and neck lifts, I began seeing more lower lip weakness, which is explainable due to the proximity of the dissection to the nerves. Although I see more nerve paresis with deep plane techniques, they have all healed over several weeks or months (Figs. 12.21–12.25).

The marginal mandibular nerve is the most commonly injured motor nerve in facelift surgery. Motor nerve injuries that do not seem to improve at all or those that are severe and include multiple nerve branches should be evaluated after 90 days by a surgeon experienced in microneurosurgery. I have seen sensory or motor nerve injuries that took a year to improve. The buccal and zygomatic branches have numerous anastomoses, and for this reason, a permanent injury from a distal injury is rare, but this also makes it difficult to characterize the exact nerve injury.

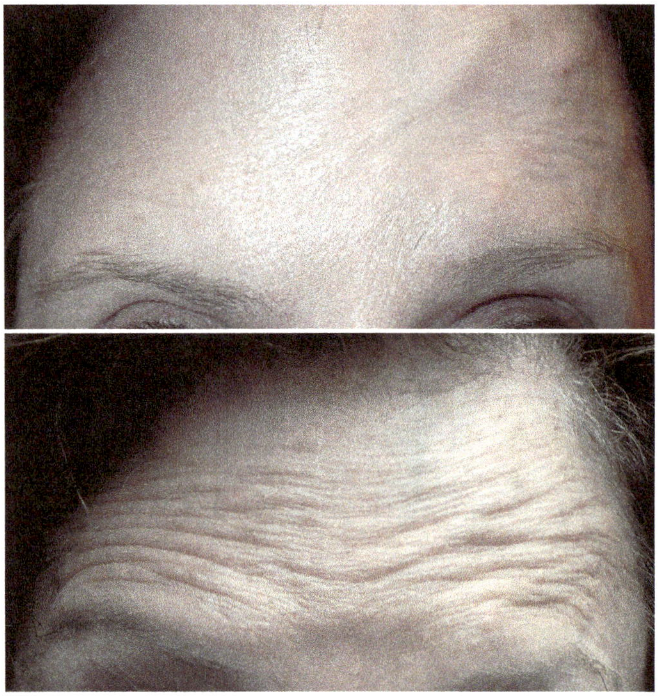

Fig. 12.21. This patient exhibits a right frontal branch injury after surgery (*top* image) and return to normal 4 months postop (*bottom* image).

Rami of the zygomatic branch of the facial nerve innervate the lower portion of the orbicularis oculi and if injured can affect lid closure. This is an unusual injury and is shown in Fig. 12.25 (*upper right* image).

As stated, the marginal mandibular branch is a commonly affected motor nerve in facelift surgery and can be damaged during dissection, submental liposuction, and chin implant surgery. When a patient with damage to this nerve smiles or rolls their lower lip down, the affected side does not depress, owing to the loss of innervation of the depressor anguli oris and/or the depressor labii (Figs. 12.23–12.25). Sometimes this can also be related to a cervical nerve injury in that the platysma also depresses the lip or corner of the mouth in many patients. In these patients, the motor function of the platysma would likely be involved. When the lip is affected from a marginal mandibular nerve injury, the normal side can be treated with a small amount of neurotoxin to even out the asymmetry.

Most patients are content to wait for the nerve function to improve. Showing them progress pictures over several months can confirm their improvement and relax nervous patients. Also, showing them pictures of other patients with similar injury (or from this text) and resolution reinforces their patience to "wait it out."

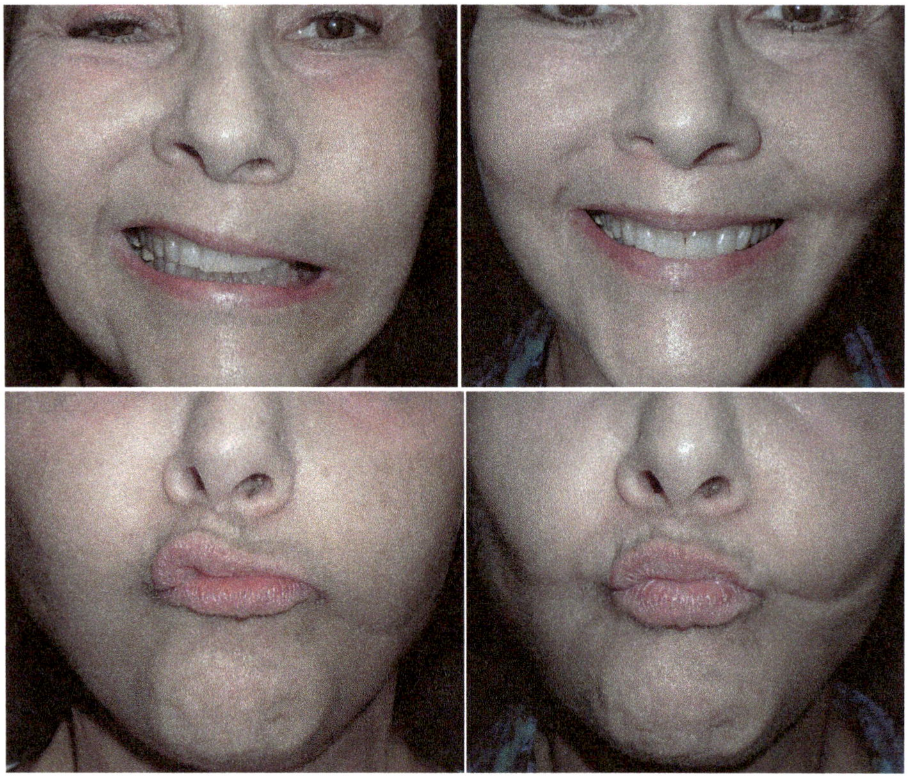

Fig. 12.22. This patient exhibits a left zygomatic and buccal branch injury after facelift surgery. The *upper right* image shows the inability to close the left eye or elevate the cheek, lip, or nostril on the left side. The *upper right* image show return to normal nerve function 90 days later. The lower left image shows the patient trying to pucker postinjury and normal animation at 90 days.

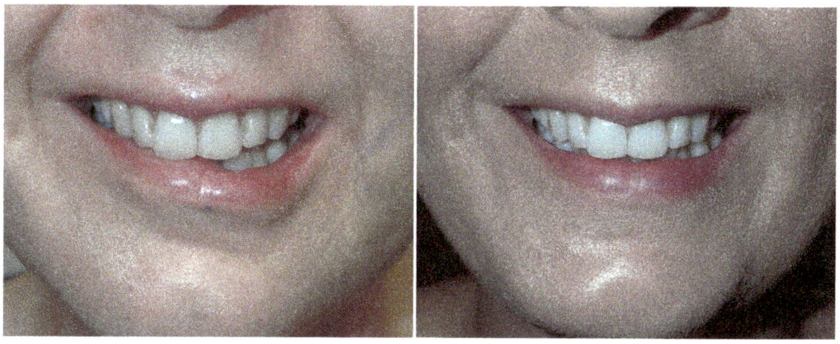

Fig. 12.23. This patient is shown with a lower left marginal mandibular nerve injury after facelift surgery and normal animation 4 months later.

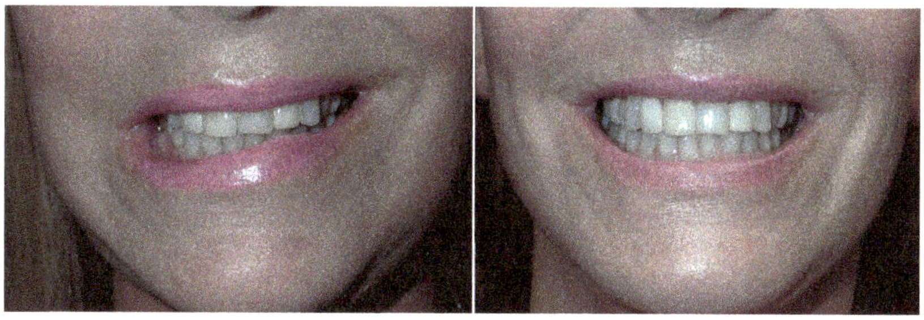

Fig. 12.24. This patient is shown with an upper right buccal branch injury and a lower left marginal mandibular branch injury. She is shown 3–4 months after surgery with total return of both deficits.

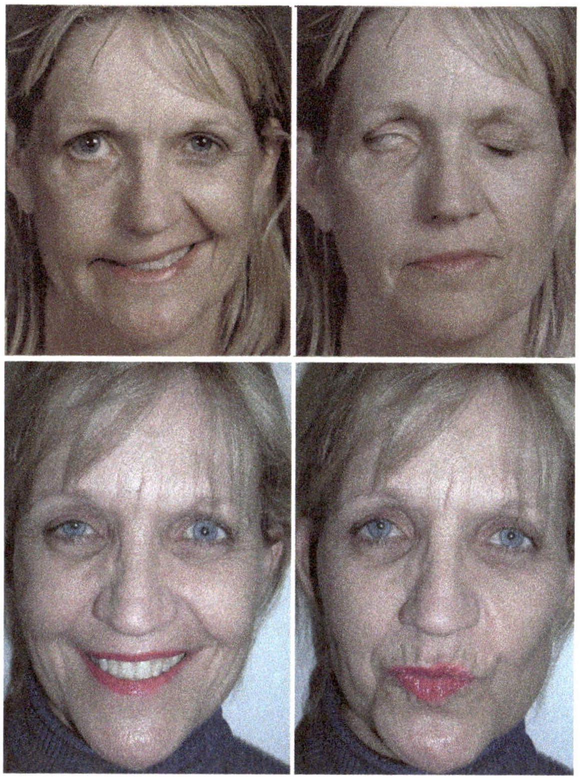

Fig. 12.25. This patient underwent facelift surgery by a plastic surgeon from another office and sustained a total facial nerve injury, which is unusual in facelift surgery. She underwent nerve repair by a nerve specialist and regained most of her function.

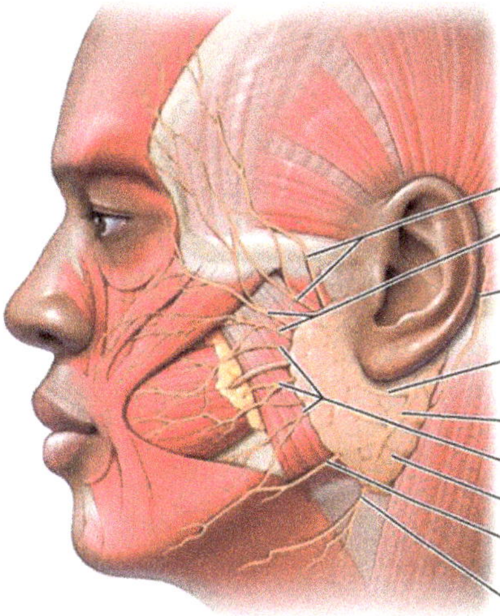

Fig. 12.26. This diagram shows the common location of the facial nerve branches.

The facial nerve branches are rarely in jeopardy until exiting the parotid gland and crossing the masseter. Novice surgeons should stay over the gland in the safe zone (Fig. 12.26).

Total main facial nerve trunk injury is rare in facelift surgery as it is protected by the parotid gland but has been documented. Injury to the frontal branch is less frequent. I have seen temporary forehead paresis from cauterizing a bleeder in the temple.

An even rarer motor nerve injury that has been documented with facelift surgery is damage to the cranial nerve eleven, the spinal accessory nerve. This nerve innervates the sternocleidomastoid and trapezius muscles, which assist in turning the head and shrugging the shoulders. The spinal accessory nerve exits on the posterior border of the sternocleidomastoid muscle at Erb's point (the same level of the greater auricular nerve [GAN]) and enters the posterior triangle (Figs. 12.27 and 12.28).

Technically, Erb's point was classically described as a point where the cervical plexus exits from behind the posterior border of the sternocleidomastoid muscle. The four cutaneous nerves of the cervical plexus are the lesser occipital nerve, great auricular nerve, transverse cervical nerve, and supraclavicular nerve. The scientific literature has many different descriptions of Erb's point, and many articles describe the spinal accessory and GAN emerging from Erb's point, and this description will be used in this text.

At the point where the posterior platysma terminates, and the nerve is only protected by skin and variable amounts of subcutaneous fat and fascia and is vulnerable. Although injury is rare, all surgeons should keep in mind that an errant liposuction cannula or tumescent needle, aggressive retraction, or lateral thermal damage from cauterization could injure this nerve. Fig. 12.27 shows a patient with a spinal accessory nerve injury. The patient healed uneventfully from her facelift, and at her 3-month visit was happy with her result. On her way out of the office in the hallway, she was asked if she had any other problems. She thought for a moment and mentioned in passing that she was experiencing shoulder pain. Examination showed decreased range of motion and inability to abduct the affected side and confirmed by electromyography (EMG). Although the deficit and pain were slowly improving, a microneurosurgeon advised exploration and repair. Although waiting for increased function was an option, postponing the surgery could have closed the window of time for optimal treatment and nerve recovery; therefore, the decision was made to explore and repair. Exploration showed a neuroma, which was removed (Fig. 12.28), and primary nerve repair was performed, and the patient regained normal function (Fig. 12.27, *lower* image). Fig. 12.28 (*left*) shows an outline of the incision used to treat the neuroma at the level of the injury. This location should be committed to memory as this is an approximation where the nerve is in jeopardy. Anytime dissection of manipulation is extended into the posterolateral neck, the surgeon must remain vigilant (Fig. 12.29). When I perform my preoperative evaluation on patients, I test their entire facial nerve function by having them raise their eyebrows, close their eyes, smile, pucker, flex their platysma, and also raise their shoulders to evaluate the spinal accessory nerve. Patients can have damage to this nerve and not even realize it until pain becomes an underlying problem. This pain can be manifested as shoulder pain from using accessory muscles to try to compensate for the denervated musculature. As stated, most facial nerve motor injuries heal spontaneously. Some physical therapists perform electrical nerve stimulation for facial motor nerve injuries, and this can accelerate return of function in some cases. It is a simple procedure, but not all physical therapists perform it. I am lucky to have a local physical therapist who performs electrical nerve stimulation. It is covered by insurance in my experience and provides the patient with the understanding that "something is being done" to improve their situation.

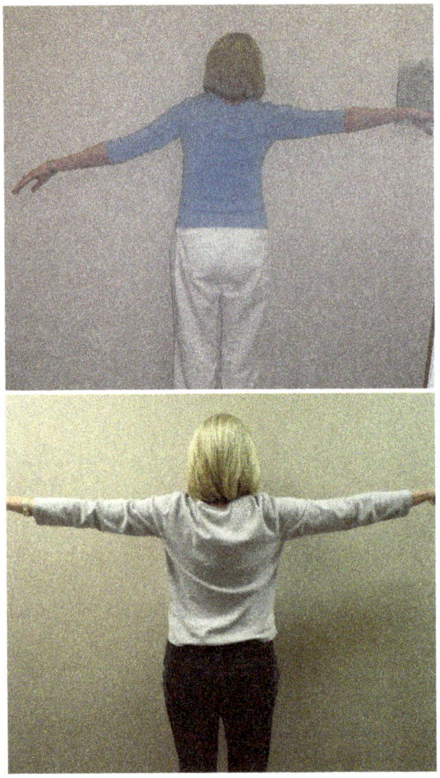

Fig. 12.27. This patient is shown 90 days after surgery with a spinal accessory nerve injury (*top* image) and full function a year later after removal of a neuroma and microneurosurgical repair (*lower* image).

Sensory Nerve Injury

Although no level of nerve injury is intended, or acceptable, sensory nerve injury generally carries less severity than their motor nerve counterparts. With motor nerve injury there is functional disability, which is very visible and can affect everyday tasks such as eating, animation, and corneal hydration. Sensory nerve injury, although unpleasant for the patient, is not generally visible to others. Having said that, a patient trying to drink coffee or eat with a lip paresthesia will frequently drool, drop food, or unknowingly have residual food on their lip.

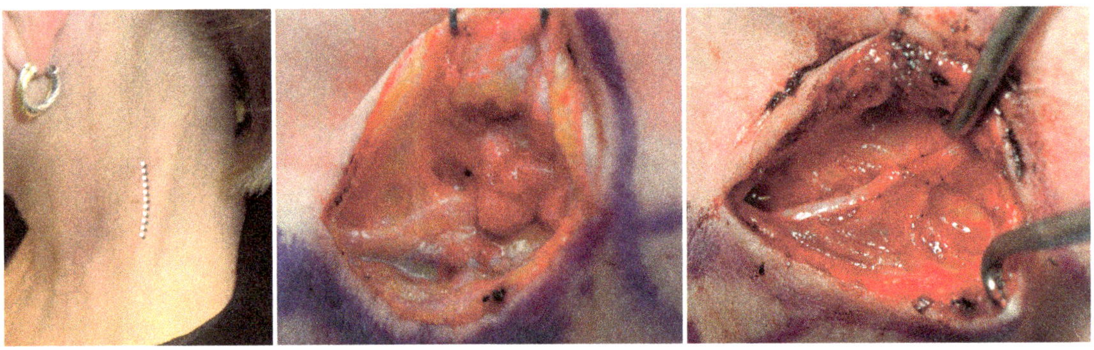

Fig. 12.28. The *left* image shows the patient's neck and incision line that was made to explore the nerve injury. The *middle* image shows a large neuroma that had formed, and the *right* image shows the nerve after neuroma removal and microsurgical repair.

The mere act of undermining the dermis from the deeper tissues will denervate the superficial sensory nerves, so all postoperative facelift patients will have a component of temporary paresthesia. The superficial sensory nerves regenerate, and feeling usually returns to normal over several weeks or months. It is not uncommon for some areas of the face to remain numb up to a year. Without a significant main trunk nerve injury (infraorbital, mental, GANs), the loss of feeling almost always returns. It is really important to underline this in your written and oral informed consent. If a patient understands they may be numb for a year and their feeling returns in 3 months, you are a hero. If you tell them the feeling will return in 3 months and it takes a year, you are a zero! If there is one thing that I have learned over the years, it is to always overestimate anticipated recovery with patients. Some surgeons sugarcoat recovery in an effort to promote a case. Patients feel very betrayed if their recovery is underestimated.

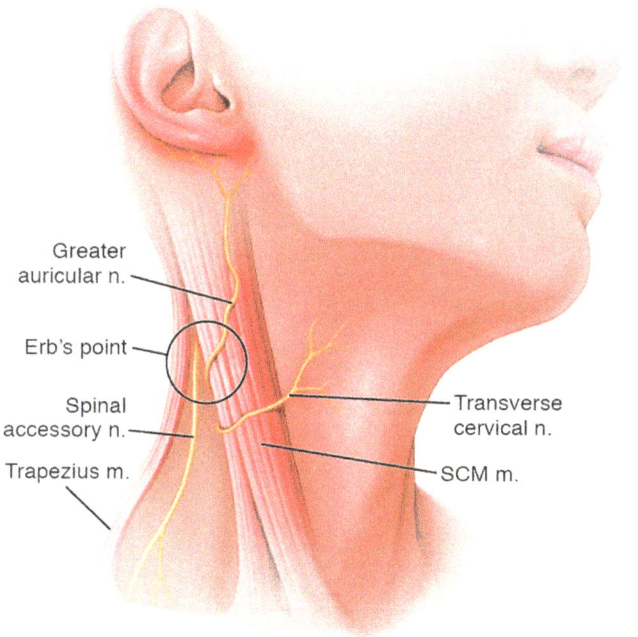

Fig. 12.29. The spinal accessory nerve (motor nerve) traverses the posterior border of the sternocleidomastoid muscle in relatively close proximity to the greater auricular nerve (sensory nerve). The *blue circle* illustrates this danger zone, which should be imprinted in every surgeons' mind. *n.*, Nerve; *m.*, muscle; *SCM*, sternocleidomastoid muscle.

The GAN is the most commonly injured sensory nerve in facelift and neck lift surgery. As shown in the earlier part of this chapter, this nerve can be extremely superficial and is subject to injury (Fig. 12.29). For this reason, all dissection below the inferior board of the mandible should always be performed with direct vision to prevent injury. The nerve is especially vulnerable at the described 6.5 cm inferior to the external auditory canal and when the nerve crosses the belly of the sternocleidomastoid muscle. If the nerve is inadvertently transected, it is repaired with 7-0 Prolene suture (Fig. 12.30). If for any reason it cannot be repaired, the stumps should be tagged with a permanent suture for later identification for secondary repair. The GAN has an anterior and posterior branch. Damage to this nerve can produce paresthesia or anesthesia in dermatome, which includes the skin over the mastoid, posterior and anterior ear, external acoustic meatus, and parotid gland (Fig. 12.31). Anatomically in facelift surgery the GAN and external jugular vein (EJV) are both vulnerable in close proximation (Fig. 12.32).

A damaged or repaired GAN can also develop a neuroma, which manifests as an induration palpable through the skin over the area of the nerve. A GAN neuroma can be painful and when compressed by the examiner can radiate pain into the associated dermatome. MRI scan and nerve conduction studies are useful for diagnosis.

The transverse cervical nerve horizontally crosses the sternocleidomastoid muscle inferior to the GAN and provides sensory innervation to the skin over the anterior triangle of the neck (Fig. 12.19). This nerve can also be damaged in a low inferior cervical dissection.

External Jugular Vein

Although the EJV is a large vessel present on both sides of every facelift, it is only occasionally encountered during dissection. Some patients have large, distended, and superficial EJVs, which

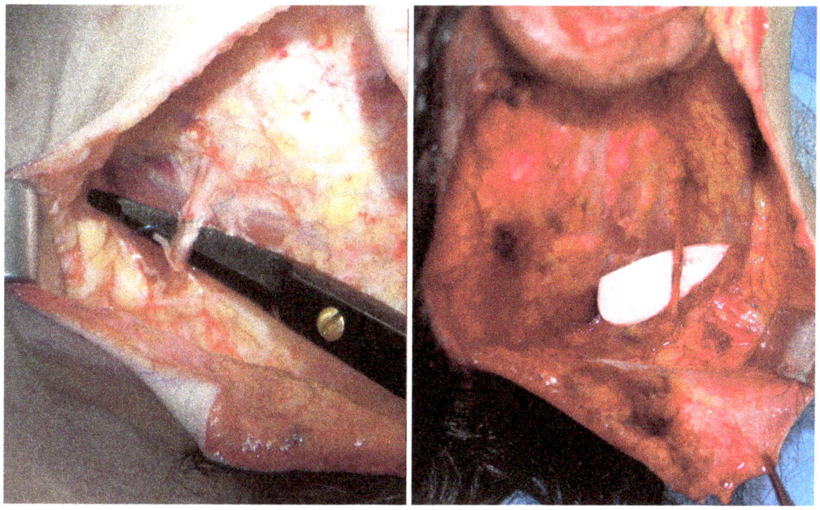

Fig. 12.30. Two cases of inadvertent transection of the greater auricular nerve and repair are shown in the *left* and *right* images. The repair is made with loupes and 7-0 Prolene suture. The suture ends are left long to identify the repair location in the rare instance that future surgery is required.

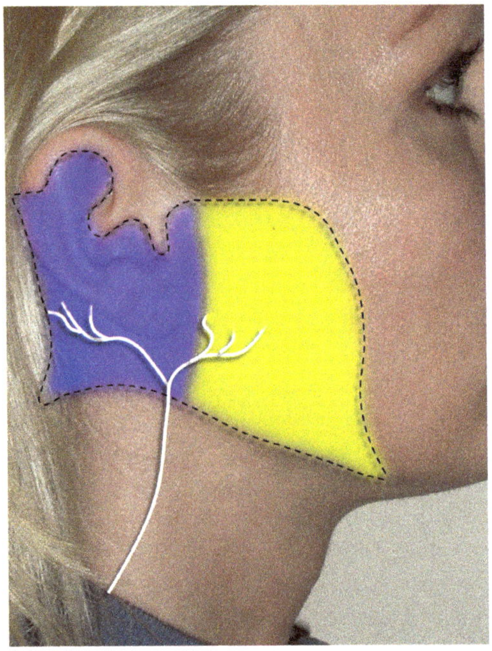

Fig. 12.31. This image illustrates the approximate dermatome of the greater auricular nerve.

can be encountered in normal dissection or from novice surgeons entering too deep of a plane. Generally, the EJV crosses the sternocleidomastoid muscle at a similar level as the GAN and then runs parallel to the GAN.

The vessel can be damaged with blunt liposuction cannulas or punctured or transected with scissors, sharp tumescent anesthesia needles, instruments, or suture needles. When suturing the posterior platysma border to the mastoid fascia, the surgeon should be vigilant to avoid puncturing the EJV. The suture needle must be placed either medial or lateral to the vessel. In the case of bleeding while suturing in or around this area, the stitch should be removed, and the area should be inspected for possible EJV perforation. In the case of nick, puncture, or transection, brisk bleeding can occur from the EJV. A high-volume suction (tonsil suction) is used to clear the area while the assistant exerts pressure on the neck skin to compress the bleeding vessel. Confirmed bleeding necessitates EJV ligation with permanent suture, and the surgeon must be sure that the bleeding is controlled before wound closure (Figs. 12.33 and 12.34). This is another situation that can be very traumatic for the beginning facelift surgeon, but if the surgeon keeps calm and collected and has

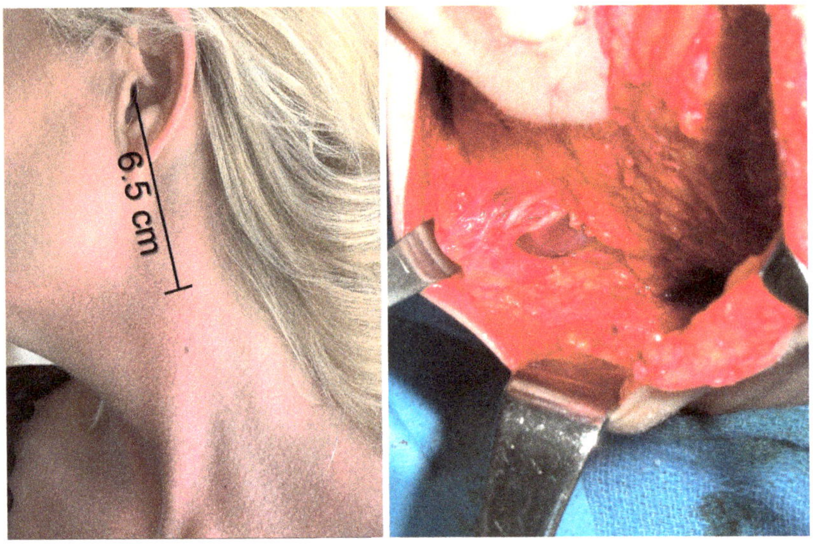

Fig. 12.32. The *left* image shows the approximate measurement of the greater auricular nerve and external jugular vein crossing the lower sternocleidomastoid muscle. The *right* image shows an intraoperative picture of both structures, which are vulnerable in facelift surgery.

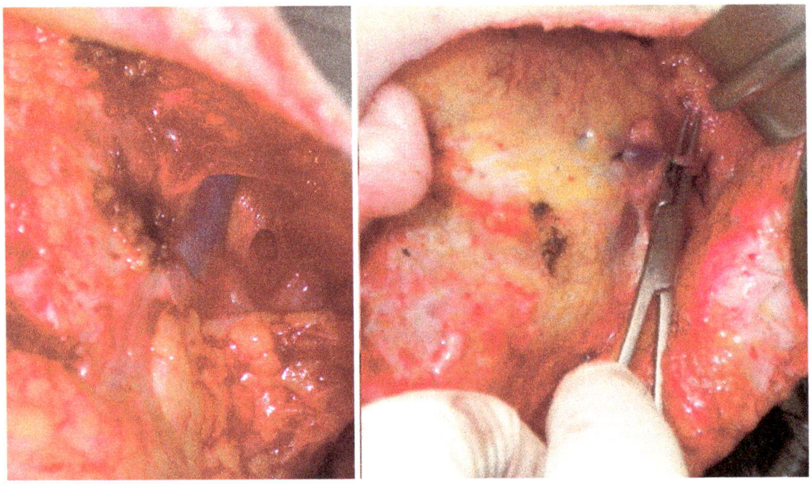

Fig. 12.33. The external jugular vein can be encountered during facelift dissection. The external jugular vein can be the size of an index finger (*left* image) but when ligated will become much smaller (*right* image).

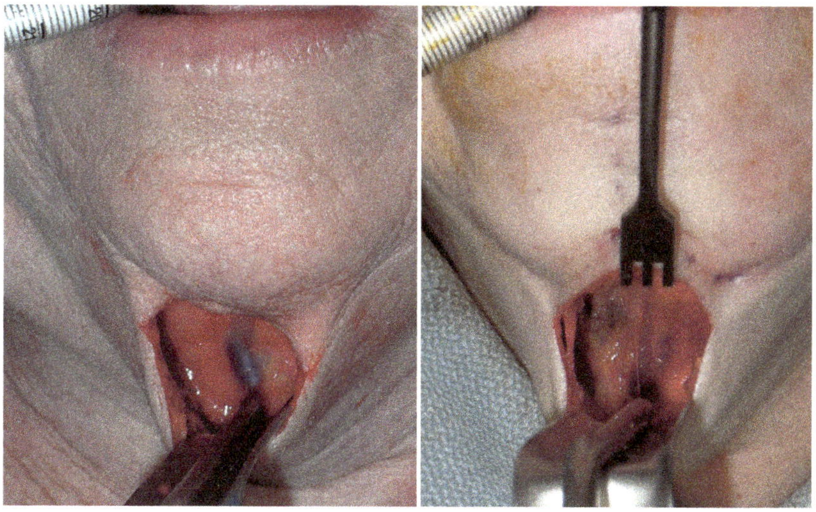

Fig. 12.34. The anterior jugular veins branch from the external jugular vein to the submental midline and can cause brisk bleeding if inadvertently lacerated. Hemorrhage is controlled with ligatures or bipolar cautery, depending on the caliber of the vein.

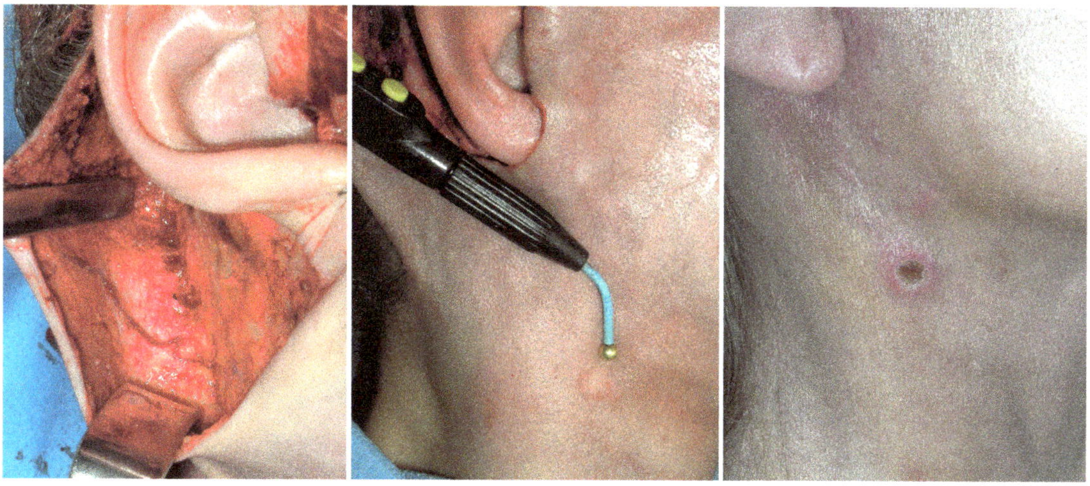

Fig. 12.35. A small area of flap necrosis is seen after cauterizing the flap with a ball electrode to control a bleeder. The *left* image shows a typical flap vessel, the *middle* image shows what the device would look like under the flap, and the *right* image shows the damaged area at 7 days. Most small vessels like the one shown do not need cauterized unless they exhibit arterial pumping. The lower energy settings should be used when cauterizing the underside of a flap with Bovie or bipolar forceps.

access to adequate suction, the bleeding is easily controlled by ligation sutures. If the vein cannot be significantly accessed through the flap, an incision through the neck flap would be in order, but this would be an uncommon situation. This is another example of the fact that no surgeon should undertake an operation where they cannot manage the common complications.

Flap Viability Complications

Successful facelift surgery is contingent upon survival of the vascularized lipocutaneous flaps. Tragic outcomes can occur if the blood supply is compromised. Although small areas of necrosis may heal without scarring, large areas of flap necrosis and tissue loss can lead to massive scarring requiring skin grafts and disfigurement and can seriously affect the quality of life of the patient. Compromise of flap vascularity can result from a number of causes, including but not limited to rough handling of the flap during surgery, excessive retraction, making the flap too thin, burning the flap with lateral heat damage from cauterization (Fig. 12.35), tight bandages, patient applications of heat or cold, and sometimes from no apparent cause at all.

Smokers may have a higher incidence of flap viability problems. In other cosmetic surgeries such as breast surgery or abdominoplasty where flap necrosis is much more common, the outcome may have less impact because it can be hidden by clothing. There are many more emotional implications when this occurs on the face as it cannot be hidden and is visible during the entire healing and any scarring would be visible as well. When patients come to a cosmetic surgeon for rejuvenation and they end up with permanent scarring, the outcome is not good for either party.

Decrease in flap perfusion can sometimes be seen within 24 hours of surgery or may not manifest until 10–12 days postoperatively. Although dusky flap skin color can be an ominous sign portending necrosis, sometimes the dusky color is only a result of bruising (Figs. 12.36 and 12.37).

When pressing a finger on a dusky flap, capillary refill (momentary blanching and return to normal color) is a positive

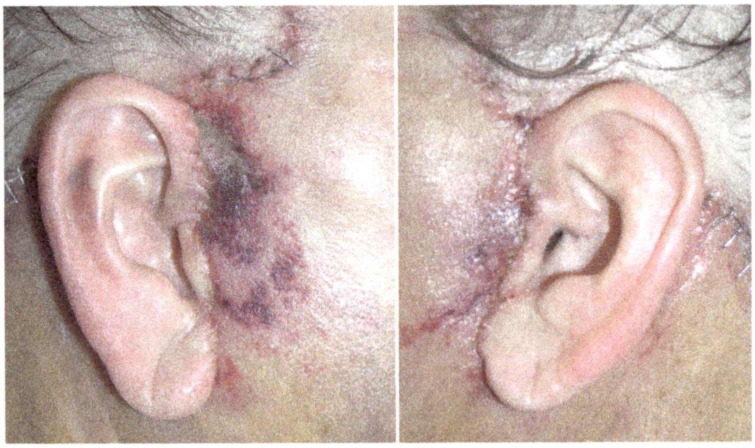

Fig. 12.36. This image shows another patient who presented 5 days after surgery with dusky areas on the preauricular flaps with very minor breakdown as shown in the left preauricular region. This case did not progress, and the patient had no significant breakdown and no scarring.

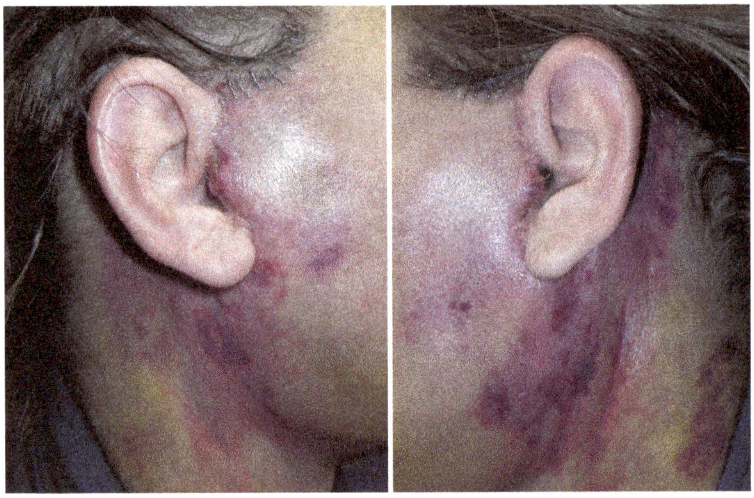

Fig. 12.37. These images show a "dusky" region on all the flaps that resembled early flap vascular compromise but represented only ecchymosis, and the patient healed uneventfully.

sign of blood flow (based on refill time in seconds) but is not a guarantee that the flap will not become compromised.

Many surgeons advocate topical nitroglycerin treatment for impending vascular compromise. Although I have never seen any scientific evidence that it is effective, I do have patients apply a small amount of nitroglycerin over the dusky areas every 8 hours. A small amount will go a long way in the patients instructed that if they develop headache, they are using excessive amounts and need to reduce the amount. It is important to follow patients with suspected vascular compromise very closely, and these patients need to be seen several times a week to assess the risk or progression of skin necrosis.

Hyperbaric oxygen treatment (HBO) is an appropriate therapy if the surgeon is highly suspicious of significant impending flap necrosis. This can be a scary proposition for the patient who at the point of the conversation does not realize how much damage can ensue from major flap loss. The patient can be scared, confused, and worried about the cost and necessity of the suggested HBO treatment. HBO treatment can be very expensive, but in the cases I have experienced, it was covered by insurance with the diagnosis of "failed flap." The cases that I referred to the local wound care center were told that they would require 30 days of treatment, but every case improved within 10–12 days of HBO treatment. In over 1600 facelifts I have only ever referred four patients for HBO therapy for flap necrosis and one case was diagnosed with pyoderma gangrenosum. One patient decided not to have the treatment because they would have to quit smoking. Some cities have numerous HBO treatment centers in hospitals or are privately owned in the community and getting a patient in treatment is expedient and affordable. Unfortunately, many cities (including Richmond, Virginia) have very few centers that get very booked up, and getting a patient immediate treatment can be impossible. Not all instances of assumed duskiness will portend absolute of necrosis. I have seen several patients where minor hypoperfusion only resulted in some superficial epidermal sloughing and other cases where I assumed the blood supply to the flap was compromised and it only turned out to be bruising and the patient healed totally normally (Figs. 12.36 and 12.37). Generally, the compromised tissue begins to take on a dusky or violaceous color in the first few days postoperatively. The decrease in blood supply and resultant duskiness can be seen as early as 24 hours or as late as 1 week. In most cases, significant breakdown will manifest signs within the first 10 days and usually earlier. Figs. 12.38 and 12.39 show cases of mild skin necrosis that did not progress beyond the pictured state.

In rare cases, massive tissue loss can occur causing wounds that take months to heal. Figs. 12.40 and 12.41 show cases of significant necrosis from loss of blood supply to the skin and resultant healing.

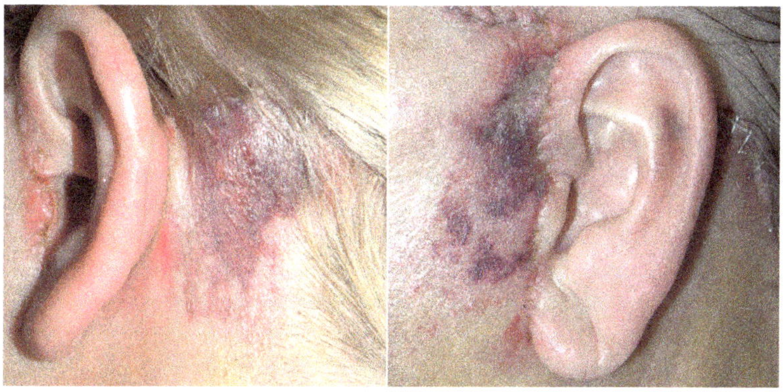

Fig. 12.38. This image shows early flap breakdown. Decreased blood supply of this nature may experience mild necrosis and heal uneventfully.

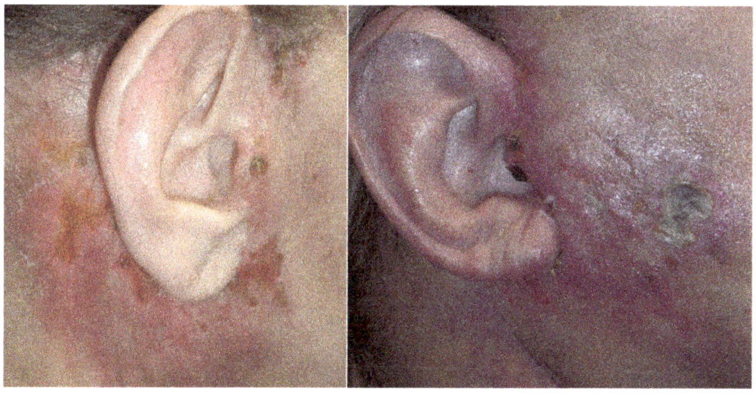

Fig. 12.39. These two different patients show early moderate necrosis. At this stage, the tissue destruction may be limited or progress to involve large portions of the flaps. By this stage (if not earlier), arrangements for expert wound care and hyperbaric oxygen treatment should be in play.

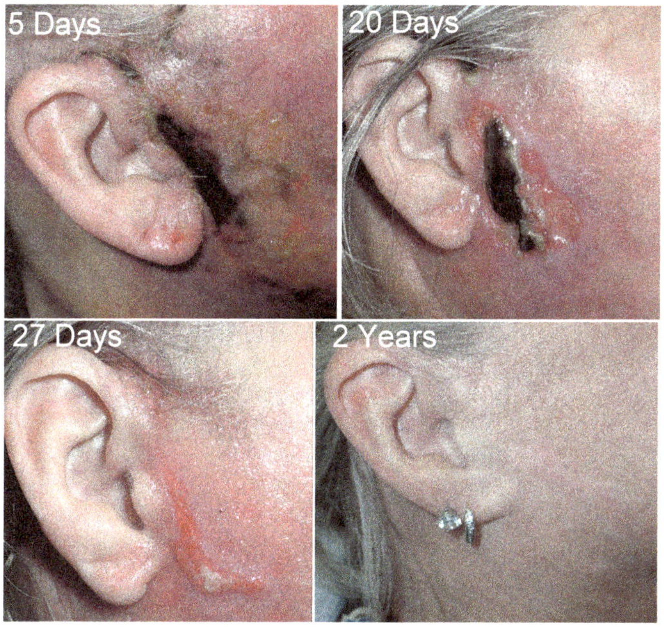

Fig. 12.40. This image shows flap breakdown that requires intense wound care and hyperbaric oxygen treatment and intensive wound care.

Fortunately, most flap necrosis occurs on the superior portion of the posterior flap. Although no level of skin necrosis is desirable, it is much better to have this happen in the posterior region as it is much easier to camouflage during the healing phase for females with long hair (Figs. 12.42 and 12.43). As bad as skin necrosis can appear, it generally heals well in the posterior region. Patients are extremely anxious about skin necrosis, and I think it helps them considerably to see pictures showing similar cases of skin necrosis with acceptable healing. Some breakdown will heal with little sign of scarring, but other breakdown can heal with hypertrophic scarring, hair loss, and hyperpigmentation.

Wound Care for Necrotic Skin

Small areas (the size of a dime to a quarter) will generally scab over and granulate from the base and do not require intensive wound care other than keeping the site clean and the scab moist. This can be done simply by soaking with hydrogen peroxide (H_2O_2) and hypochlorous acid until it resolves (note: some wound care specialists do not recommend hydrogen peroxide, but I use it routinely). Larger areas of skin slough and necrosis require treatment with antibiotics and more intensive wound care. I personally prefer BID wound care consisting of irrigation with hypochlorous acid, which is a pH balanced wound care agent with powerful antimicrobial, antibiofilm, and wound healing potency and antiseptic solution such as Vashe (urgomedical.us) or Phase One (phaseonehealth.com) (Fig. 12.44). The availability of these hypochlorous acid preparations have been welcomed in wound care and infections.

Wounds can also be treated with saline soaks and hydrogen peroxide. After this "wet" wound care, continual application of some type of wound treatment is performed. Numerous topical applications are available, and I have used (or seen the following used) Silvadene, Biafine, MediHoney, DermaWound, Stratamed, Altrazeal, Santyl, Neosporin, Curad Oil Emulsion Dressing, which have been effective in my experience (Fig. 12.45). Stratamed (stratamed.com) is a newer silicone gel wound dressing that has been approved by the Food and Drug Administration to place

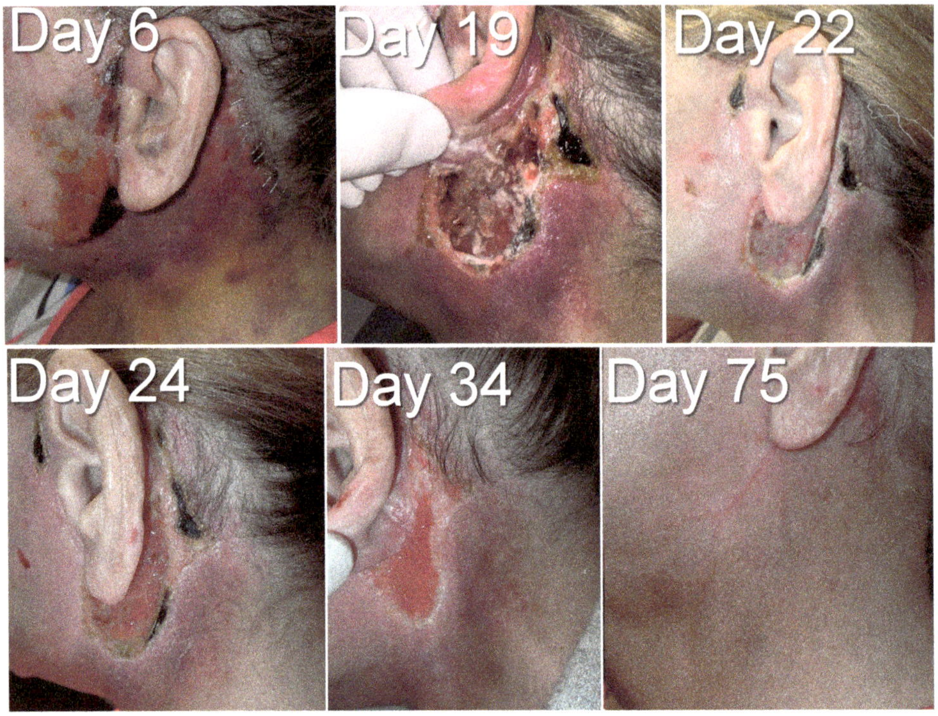

Fig. 12.41. This patient is shown during her flap breakdown and healing over 10 weeks with intensive wound care and hyperbaric oxygen treatment therapy. This patient was a smoker and had severe flap breakdown with abdominoplasty surgery and knee replacements. Unfortunately, she did not inform us of her previous wound breakdown experiences.

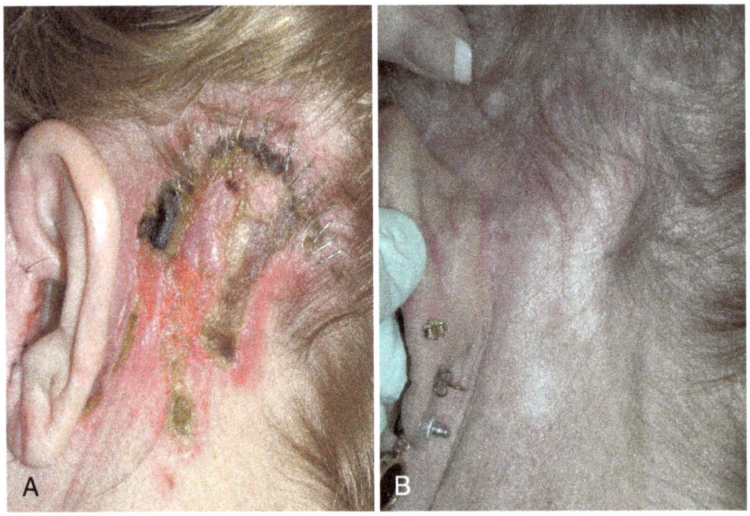

Fig. 12.42. This image shows significant posterior auricular flap breakdown with full healing at 12 weeks. Fortunately, most of these cases heal with acceptable scars although hypopigmentation can be problematic.

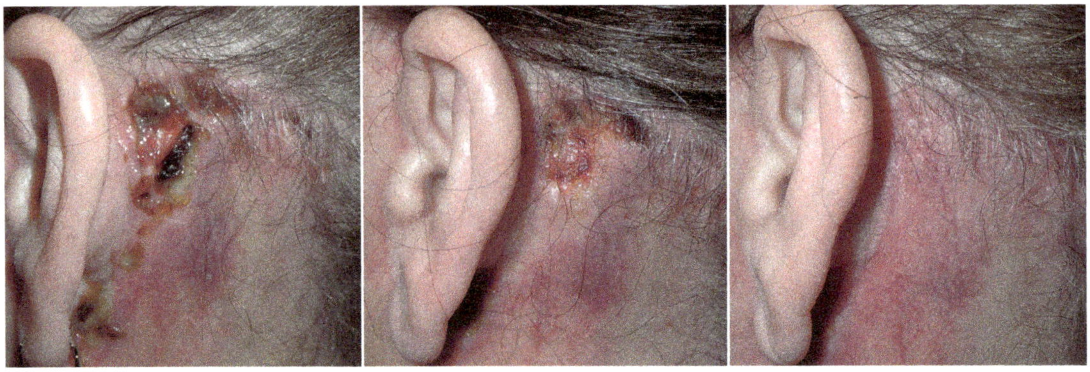

Fig. 12.43. This patient with post facelift wound breakdown is shown at 2 weeks, 6 weeks, and 8 weeks.

directly on raw wounds. I have had impressive results using this on wounds that heal with improved scarring Fig. 12.46.

Any other burn or wound preparation that is suitable for raw skin is also appropriate, and many different brands exist and are surgeon preference. It is important to point out that professional opinions differ on how to treat full-thickness wounds. As I prefer to leave the eschar in place, but other surgeons may denude a scabbed surface. I do debride the eschar when the edges begin to evert. I generally treat the tissue loss with open treatment, but others may choose to occlude the region. Although I have never had personal experience with them, portable wound vacuum systems can be used on facial skin necrosis (Fig. 12.47). I have only treated flap breakdown with open techniques but find various wound meshes, Mepilex, SecondSkin, MediHoney, or Telfa useful to protect the wound.

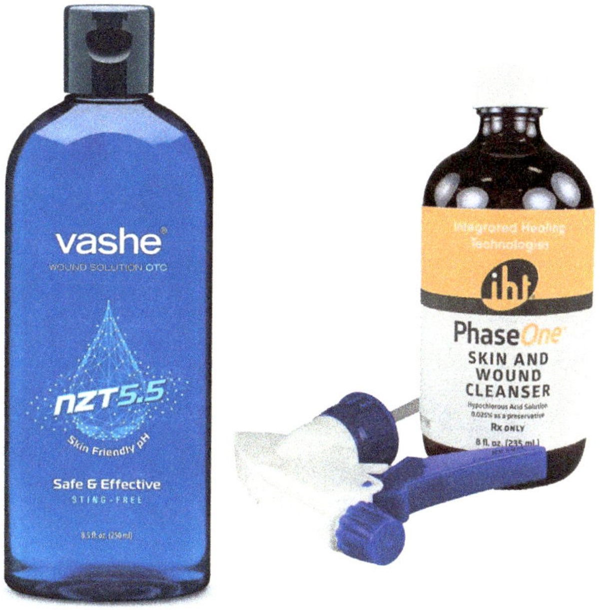

Fig. 12.44. This image shows two popular brands of hypochlorous acid would care products.

If patients have a competent caregiver that can manage the granulating wound, then home treatment is an option with regular office visits. If the patient does not have competent support, then the patient should return to the surgeon's office for daily wound care. Some localities have dedicated wound care centers that offer not only HBO, but professional wound care managed by a physician and nursing staff. These services may be covered by the patient's insurance if coverage includes the "failed flap" diagnosis as previously discussed. As the wound matures, the healing proceeds from all surfaces but basically the wound contraction occurs from the periphery and the edges heal toward the center. The central necrotic area gradually becomes smaller until the entire surface is reepithelialized and the eschar shrinks and the scab edges evert.

As the eschar shrinks, I trim the edges but do not disrupt the main attached eschar (Fig. 12.48). It is important to understand that this eschar (in my opinion), albeit it unsightly, is "nature's Band-Aid" and the wound will heal best with this "scab" intact. This is especially important for patients that pick at their wounds. Each week, the eschar will evert on the edges, and this lifted portion of dead tissue can be trimmed away. This exposes peripheral areas of granulation tissue that epithelialize, and the eschar again everts at its edge. This continual process of cleaning, dressing, and debriding is continued until the epithelial coverage is complete. The patient is kept on antibiotics for the first several weeks, but they are not continued for an extended time unless infection is a contributing factor. The wound should be irrigated with a hypochlorous solution several times a day, and home care spray kits are available for patients. If the wound becomes malodorous or exudate increases, cultures should be taken and antibiotics appropriately prescribed. Maturation and healing of a larger area of necrosis may take weeks to months to granulate and reepithelialize. This treatment will usually produce an acceptable scar that may need no further treatment. Residual scars can be improved with CO_2 laser resurfacing in some cases. It is important to remember that the wounds heal from the base up, and

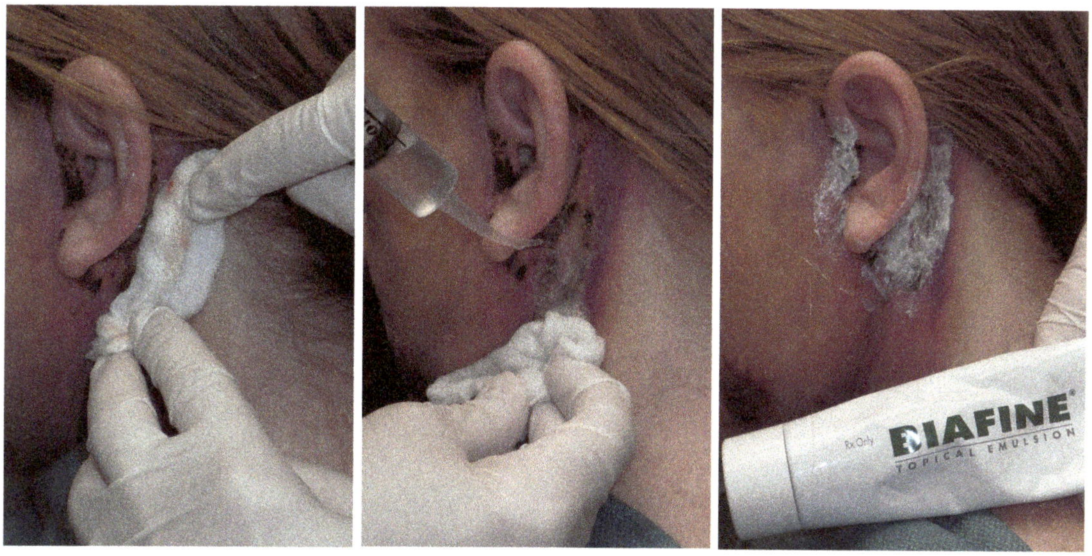

Fig. 12.45. The *left* image shows saline soak, the *middle* image shows hypochlorous acid lavage, and the *right* image shows a topical wound cream on the areas of breakdown. This treatment is usually performed once a day.

in my opinion, leaving the eschar intact is preferable to removing it. In severe cases, epithelialization may not proceed, and the defect is taken over with fibroblasts instead of epithelium. In these unusual cases, skin grafts may be necessary.

HBO can make a significant difference in the healing time and result, and I have used it on several occasions (Fig. 12.49). The accelerative effects of HBO can be phenomenal.

Loss of flap vitality can occur from increased pressure and excessive tension while retracting the flap during the placement of key sutures (Figs. 12.49 and 12.50).

Finding an HBO facility is usually not difficult as most major hospitals have wound care centers. Getting it covered by insurance may be trickier. In the past I have had three patients that were qualified for insurance as a "failed" flap but one that insurance refused. The other big problem is that it may take several weeks for insurance verification to go through, which interrupts valuable treatment time. Some cities have true medical grade HBO facilities that are stand-alone facilities and charge about $100 per treatment. As long as they are getting actual medical grade HBO, this can be a distinct advantage from going to a hospital environment. One caveat is that some spas and so on advertise HBO therapy but have inexpensive, nonmedical grade chambers.

Necrosis can also be caused by factors other than flap blood supply. If necrotic, nonhealing wound breakdown occurs after surgery, rare healing problems such as pyoderma gangrenosum should be ruled out.

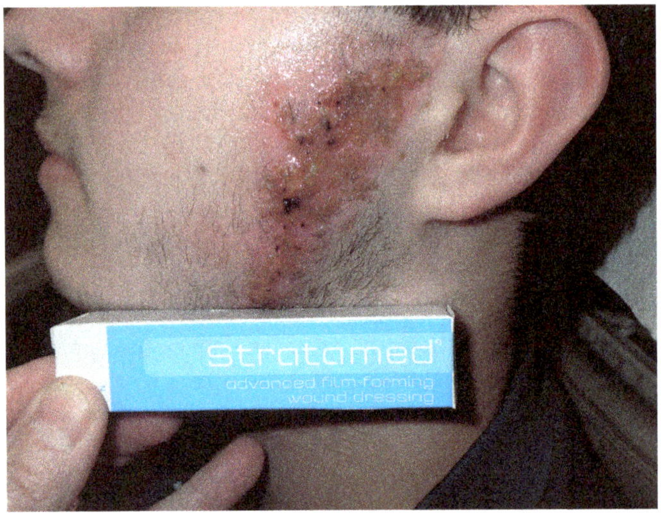

Fig. 12.46. Stratamed clear silicone gel that can be applied to raw wounds is approved by the Food and Drug Administration.

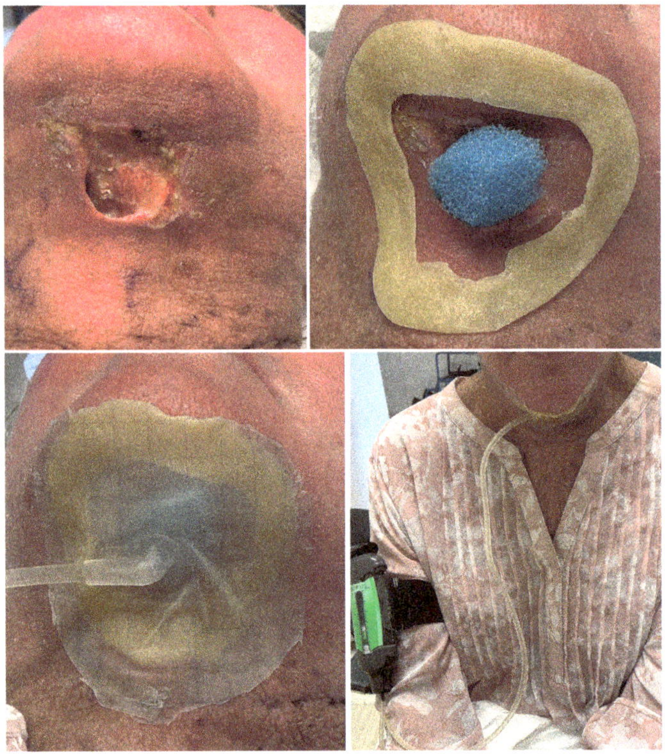

Fig. 12.47. This is not one of my cases but loaned from a colleague. The *top left* image shows submental wound breakdown from another surgeon. The *upper right* image shows seal portion of the drain, and the *lower left* image shows the drain in place. The patient is shown with the portable unit secured with an arm band in the *lower right* image.

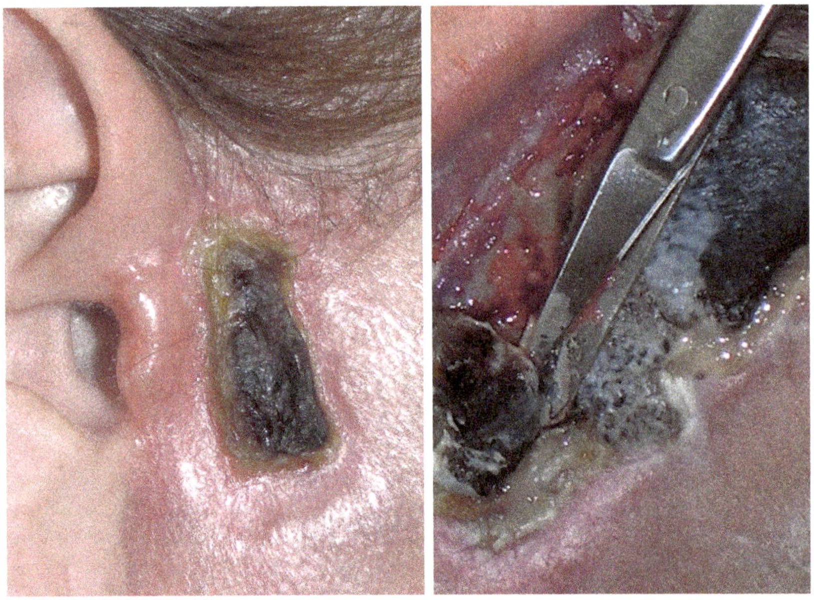

Fig. 12.48. The *left* image shows a postauricular eschar from skin necrosis, and the *right* images show the everted edges of the eschar being trimmed.

When the flaps are placed under the required tension, the surgeon should look for blanching, which could indicate vascular compromise. Although experienced surgeons may suspend flaps with minor blanching, this should be a warning sign for novice surgeons. In smokers or patients with other possible vascular compromise, tension should be adjusted to prevent flap blanching (Fig. 12.51).

Compression from overly aggressive skin pull, overly tight bandages, or even the patient's head position following surgery can impede flap vascularity (Fig. 12.52).

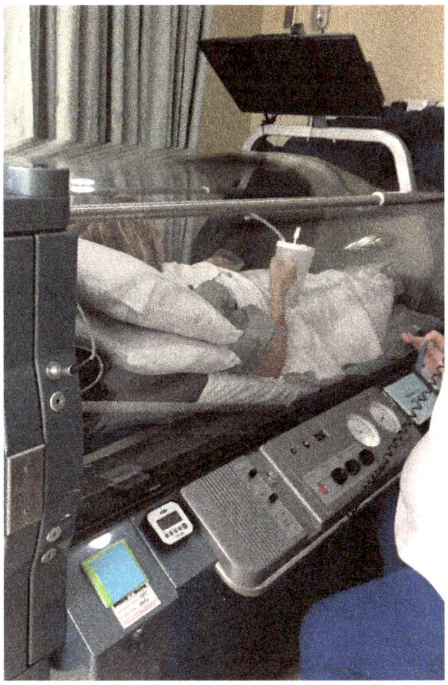

Fig. 12.49. Modern hyperbaric chambers are comfortable and less claustrophobic. Patients can watch movies and drink beverages.

Head position in the early postoperative period is controversial. Most surgeons ask their patients to sleep in an elevated position. Recent thinking has many surgeons recommending their patients *not to* sleep elevated as it can decrease drainage to the unoperated lymphatics, as well as all the neck to flex, which can cause dependent swelling and or neck ringlets between the skin folds. Many patients have difficulty sleeping in an elevated position and become sleep deprived. I tell my patients to sleep in whatever position is most comfortable for them so they can actually sleep. Some surgeons recommend the horseshoe-type airline pillow for the first week or two after facelift surgery. I have had positive experiences with these in some patients but did see one patient that experienced abrasions from the wings rubbing against the cheeks.

Any situation that places pressure on a healing flap may cause wound breakdown. Eyeglasses can be problematic for some patients after facelift surgery as the earpieces may lie over incisions (Fig. 12.53). I discuss this with patients preoperatively and recommend that they use an old pair of glasses that they can bend the temple and earpieces to lie passively and not compress suture lines.

Neck and Submental Irregularities

Contour irregularities of the neck can occur in healing facelift patients, frequently in the form of edematous, fibrotic indurated skin rolls in the neck that can develop early in the healing process. This accordion skin redundancy is also referred to as "washboard" neck or "scrotal" neck. Some patients have preexisting deep horizontal neck rhytids (neck rings) and are predisposed to developing rolls and induration during healing (Fig. 12.54). Indurated rolls and banding can develop from

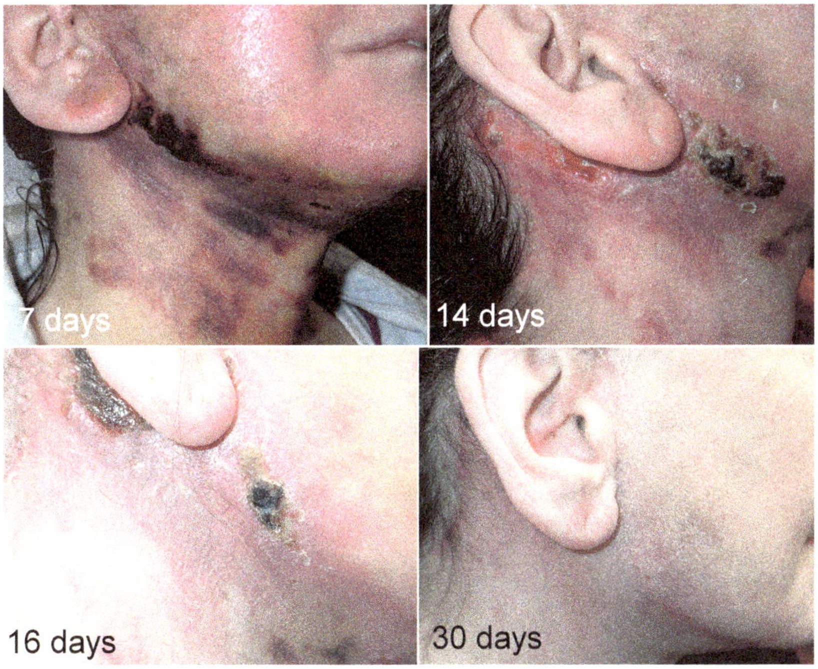

Fig. 12.50. This patient underwent hyperbaric oxygen treatment therapy, which accelerated healing.

inflammation to the area from healing problems, hematoma, seroma, or by trapping clotted blood within the skin rolls, especially in patients that rest or sleep with their necks flexed. In addition these ringlets being etched into the dermis will not resolve with facelift and neck lift. It is important to explain this preoperatively with patients that have these ringlets. Fibrotic folds can also form when the skin protrudes through layers of a postoperative dressing (Fig. 12.55).

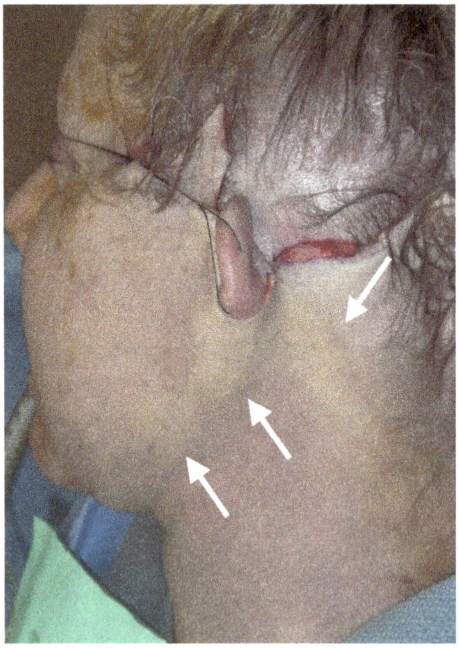

Fig. 12.51. This image shows blanching from flap traction during key suture placement. This may be a sign of excessive pressure placed on the tissue and therefore the suture tension is adjusted to reduce blanching. The *arrows* point to the blanched areas.

In the postoperative period, many patients have nothing else to do besides look at their tablet, phone, or computer. They may look in the downward position for extended periods of time. This can create "rolls" of skin and edema or blood can settle in these rolls causing fibrous banding. I refer to this as "tech neck" (Fig. 12.56). It is important to stress this in the postoperative instructions, and some patients may need to wear a rolled-up towel (or loose-fitting airline pillow) around their neck as a reminder and "brace" to discourage flexion. Obviously, any support must not be tight or impede blood supply. Although these irregularities will usually resolve with time, patients can become very disconcerted with their appearance, and their circle of friends see a result that can affect one's reputation and brand.

Banding can result in several large, thick bands or numerous thin bands (Figs. 12.57–12.59). Proponents of postsurgical drains feel that banding is reduced or eliminated with drainage. Wearing a compressive head and neck wrap for the first week may also assist in keeping the area flat. In my personal experience most banding is caused from inflammatory changes after seroma formation. For this reason, all seromas must be drained as soon as possible and as often as necessary.

Massage and ultrasound treatment are very helpful (Fig. 12.60). I have earlier referenced my in-office ultrasound device, which is very useful for this type of situation. Patients can also be referred to physical therapists that perform ultrasound

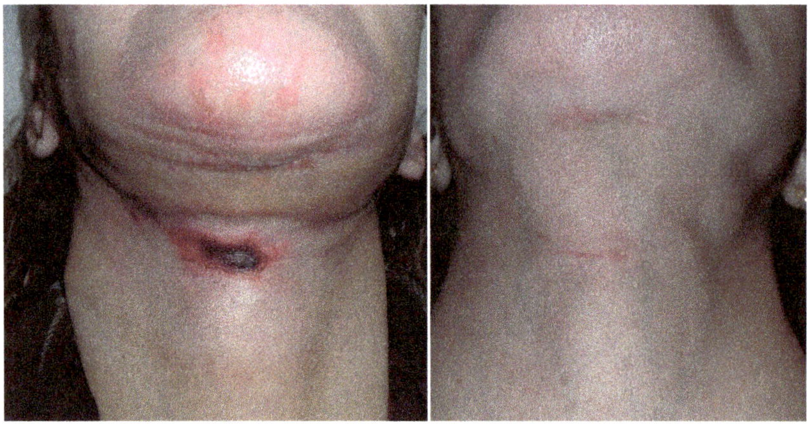

Fig. 12.52. This patient is shown 5 days after facelift with skin breakdown from an overly constrictive elastic facelift dressing (*left* image). It is imperative to make sure that any bandage or dressing are not overly tight. The *right* image show healing at 6 weeks after surgery and wound care.

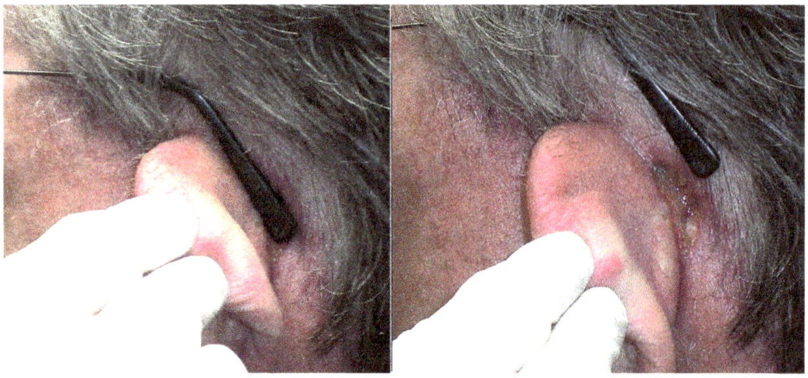

Fig. 12.53. This patient developed pressure necrosis from eyeglass compression over the incision.

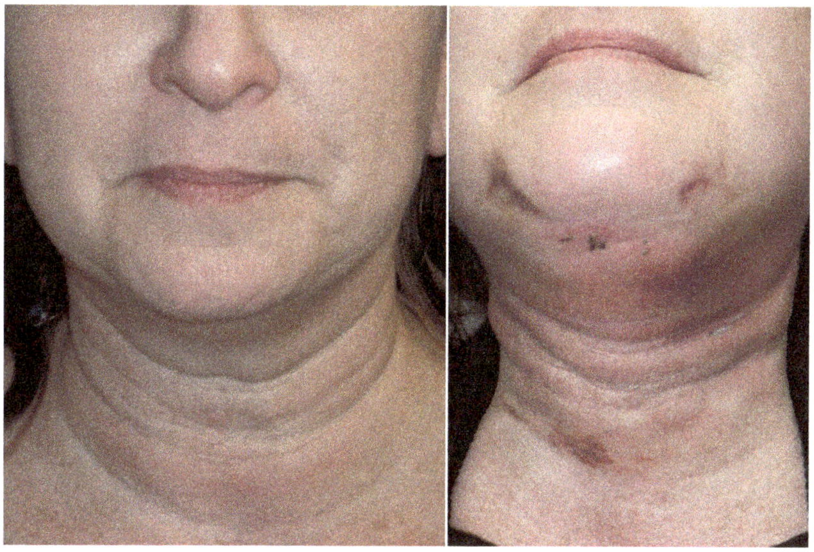

Fig. 12.54. Some patients have well-delineated, deep dermal ringlets on their neck, and these can entrap blood and serum when the patient maintains a flexed posture, thereby creating fibrous bands.

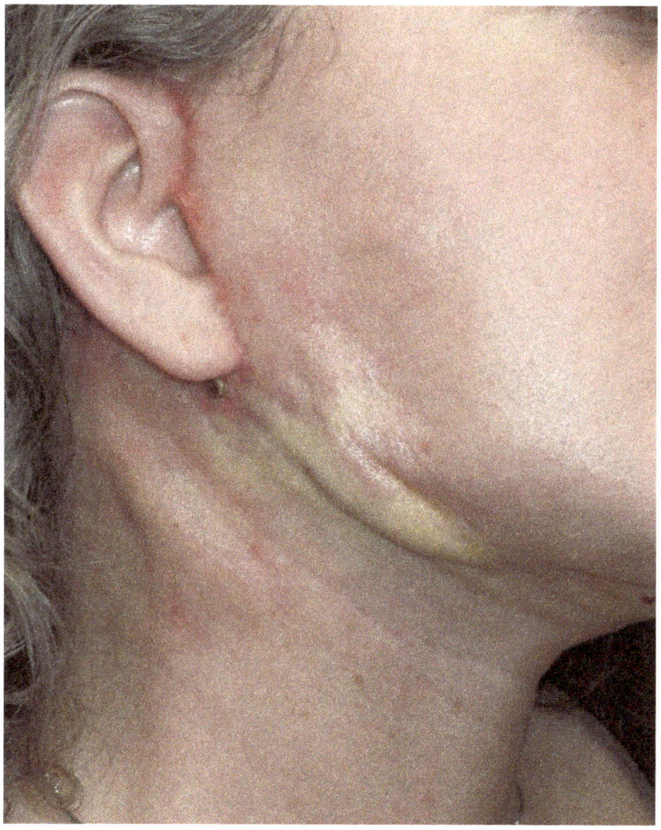

Fig. 12.55. This patient has a gauze wrap as a postfacelift dressing and a portion of the skin protruded out between layers of the bandage. This caused inflammation and folds.

therapy. Massage or lymphatic massage is also helpful. The patient needs to perform massage numerous times throughout the day. This can be finger massage with a moisturizer lubricant. The massage should be a form of stretching to distract the irregularities and also in a circular or kneading motion. Using the nonbristle end of an ultrasonic toothbrush is a "poor man's ultrasound" but in my opinion can be effective (Fig. 12.61).

In stubborn cases I use prednisone (60 mg per day for 5–7 days) and many surgeons use Singulair (montelukast) 10 mg orally once daily for antiinflammatory effects.

Monthly intralesional injections of triamcinolone 10 mg/mL or 5-flurouracil are also useful adjuncts to soften bands by reducing inflammation (Fig. 12.60, *left*). If severe, I may inject every 3 weeks for several sessions. These medications may be mixed together (0.5 cc of each) and injected, or the surgeon can alternate using one medication 1 month and the other medication the next month. 5-Flurouracil is more painful on injection, so mixing them together is an effective strategy. When using any injectable steroid, it is important to keep the medication intralesionally as it can produce divots from subcutaneous fat necrosis. Oral steroids may also be helpful to reduce inflammation. The neck is generally still numb in the early phases of recovery, and these bands can be injected painlessly with a dilute steroid injection (Kenalog 10 mg/mL) with a 32 gauge needle.

Submental and cervical neck banding can also occur from multiple situations or sometimes appear and disappear as part of normal recovery. One cause is overly aggressive liposuction where dermis heals to the platysma muscle without the cushioning interface of fat. "Bowstringing" is another phenomenon that can produce longitudinal fibrous bands in the healing neck. This is discussed in Chapter 6 in the platysmaplasty section. When performing a platysma plication from the mandible to the cricothyroid region, a long suture line is created. When the patient is supine on the operating table, this may lie passively in place. When the patient assumes the upright position and animation or neck extension, the suture line can be put under tension and protrude as visible banding through the skin (Fig. 12.62). Placing cutbacks or releasing incisions at the level of the hyoid or cervicomental junction helps break up the long suture line and allows this area to settle posteriorly, therefore having a superior and inferior part of the platysma plication that will not result in a single longitudinal band because the center is relaxed. As illustrated in Chapter 6, extending the

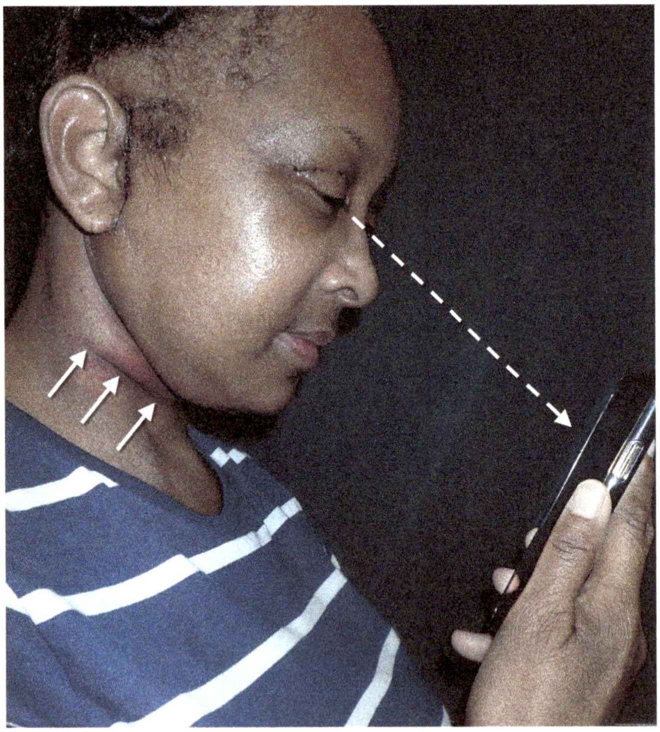

Fig. 12.56. "Tech neck" is a term for inflammatory, fibrotic neck rolls that can develop from flexion postures that encourage a stasis of blood, serum, or lymph fluid that can become organized into banding. The *solid arrows* point to the inflamed neck banding and the *dashed arrow* shows the flexion posture while looking down at a smartphone. Brief and intermittent flexion is acceptable, but sustained neck flexion can encourage fluid stasis and contribute to fibrous bands.

patient's neck intraoperatively when the platysmaplasty is completed can show a bowstring, which can be dealt with immediately by making cutbacks. Longitudinal neck bands can also be caused by untreated platysma bands, in which case may require further surgery to correct. Longitudinal neck banding, especially when visible during neck extension, may simply occur from swelling and inflammation and will improve with healing.

If this banding is platysma muscle, neurotoxin injections may improve the band and allay patient worry (Fig. 12.63).

Although heat may be helpful, I never recommend heat for postfacelift patients for the first several weeks due to the injury potential as will be explained in this chapter. Minimally invasive therapy and recovery time will usually resolve such banding, although in some cases it can be permanent and require a surgical revision.

Although it may be tempting for the surgeon to consider surgical intervention in the early stages of banding, this is generally a poor idea as it can accentuate the inflammatory process and cause further fibrosis. I would suggest exhausting all conservative therapies over 3 to 5 months before considering a surgical revision. In selected cases I have been successful with minimally invasive transection of the longitudinal bands under local anesthesia. Initially I inserted an eleven blade subcutaneously to transect the bands but have switched to an 18-guage NoKor needle, which is much smaller and leaves a puncture wound instead of an incision scar (Fig. 12.64, 12.65). I have treated several patients in this manner, and it required two to three appointments to totally correct

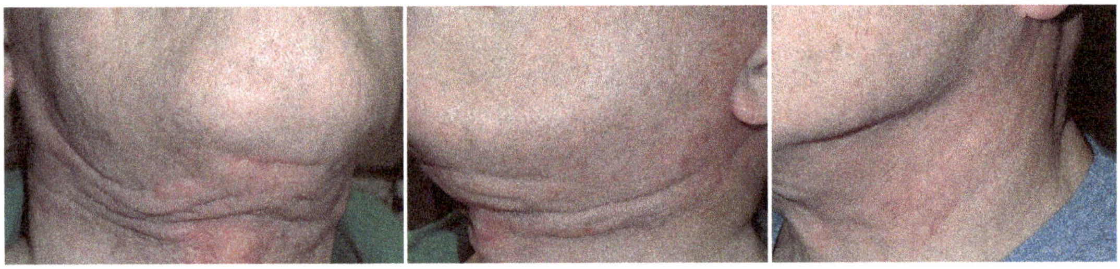

Fig. 12.57. The *left* and *middle* images show an example of "washboard neck," and the *right* picture shows the patient 5 months later after ultrasound, massage, triamcinolone, and 5-flurouracil injections. These contour defects can be very resistant to treatment and last for months but in my experience always resolve.

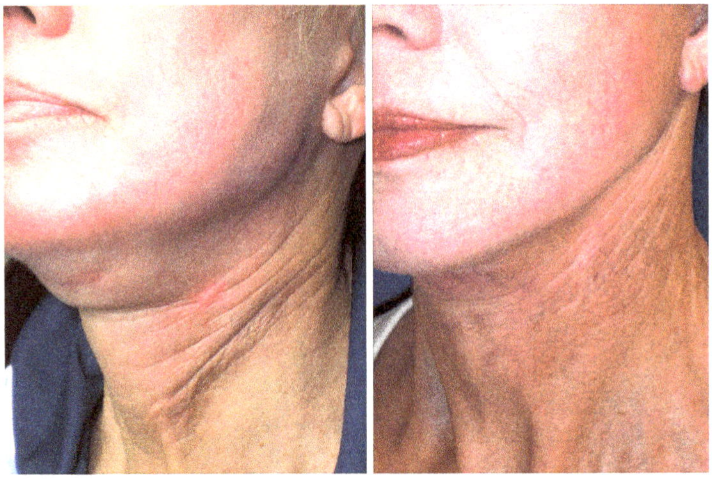

Fig. 12.58. An additional case of washboard, or scrotal, neck is shown on the *left* image. The *right* image shows the patient after 8 weeks of conservative treatment. Notice the patient's existing horizontal neck rhytids contribute to banding by trapping fluid, due in part to the natural separation between bands.

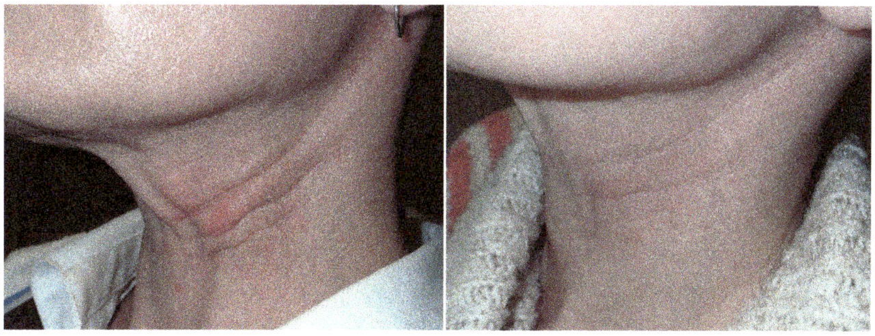

Fig. 12.59. This patient is shown 6 weeks after facelift and neck lift with fibrotic horizontal bands after a seroma (*left*). She is shown 90 days later (*right*) after steroid and 5-fluorouracil injections and ultrasound treatments from her physical therapist.

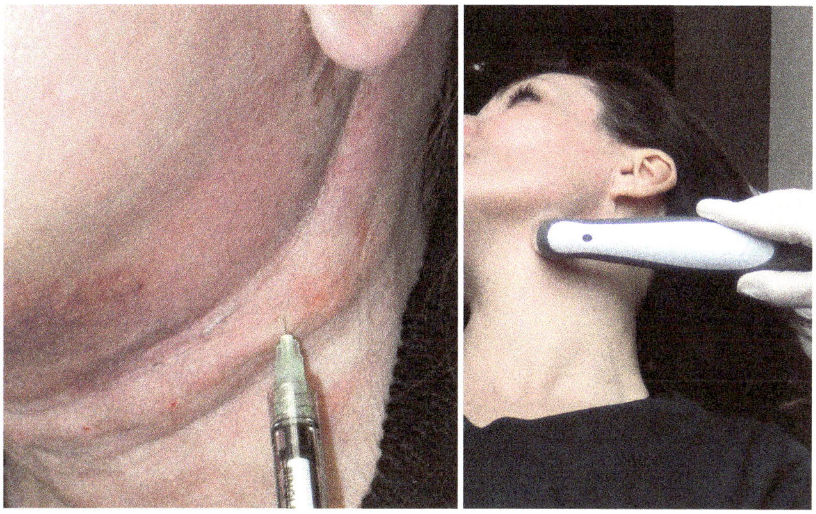

Fig. 12.60. The *left* image shows steroid injection to fibrous bands, and the *right* image show an in-office ultrasound treatment.

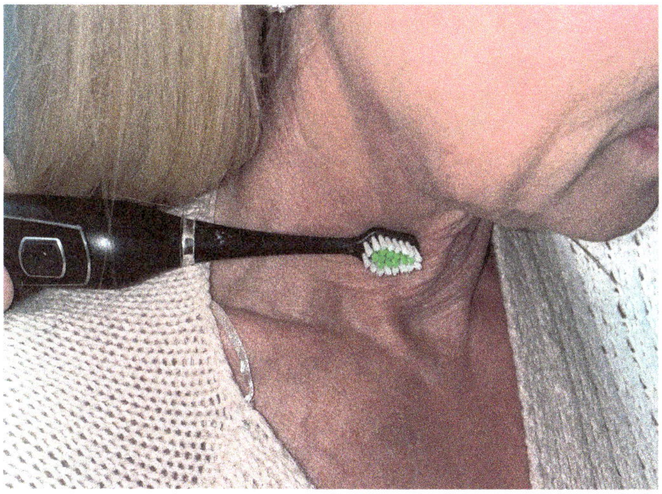

Fig. 12.61. The back side of an ultrasonic toothbrush can be effective in massaging fibrotic bands.

the banding. The recovery is minimal, and this has proven to be an effective treatment in the handful of cases I have treated. Once again, it is a mistake to attempt to reopen the neck in the early stages of banding or fibrosis. The temptation to fix the problem exists but can worsen the situation. With any unanticipated post-surgical problem, reassuring the patient is paramount, otherwise they may seek another surgeon.

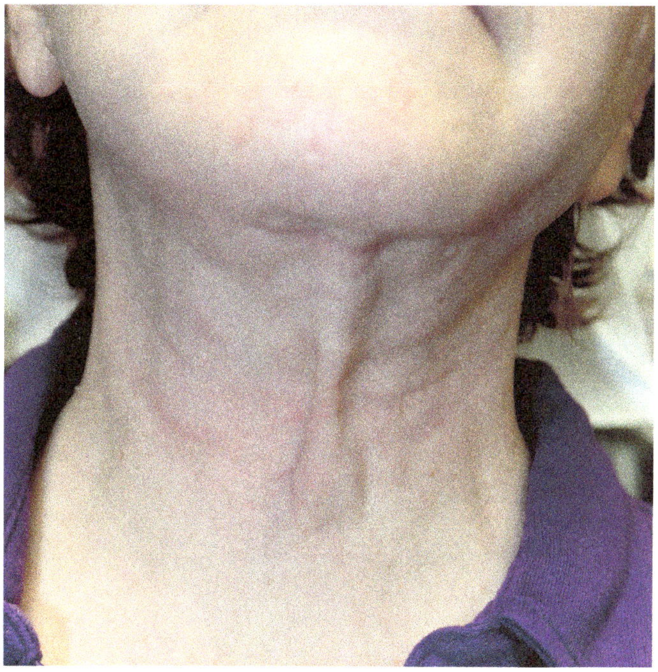

Fig. 12.62. This patient shows postoperative longitudinal neck bands that can result from inflammatory fibrosis or from bowstringing where the platysma plication sutures are not released with cutbacks. Although it may heal spontaneously, severe cases may require surgical revision.

In the continuation of discussion of submental problems, excessive submental fat removal was referenced earlier in this chapter and judicious liposuction is important, as overresection of fat is an extremely noticeable deformity that is difficult to correct (Fig. 12.66).

Other neck and submental irregularities after facelift surgery include protrusive digastric muscles and submandibular glands (Figs. 12.67–12.69). These regions may not be apparent preoperatively as they are covered with fat or loose tissue but may be apparent on thin patients or those with hypertrophic glands or muscle. Many patients realize this is normal tissue and are not bothered by these bulges, but other patients become quite concerned. This condition should be discussed preoperatively especially with patients that have obvious submandibular gland protrusion. In terms of treatment the superior lobe of the gland can be reduced during surgery, but this is not a procedure for the novice surgeon as critical nerves and large-gauge vessels are associated with the submandibular gland and is discussed in the deep neck lift and submentoplasty sections of this book. Intraoperative submandibular gland reduction has become a popular procedure with deep plane neck lifts. Suture suspension of ptotic glands is also a procedure favored by some surgeons and is described in the facelift literature.

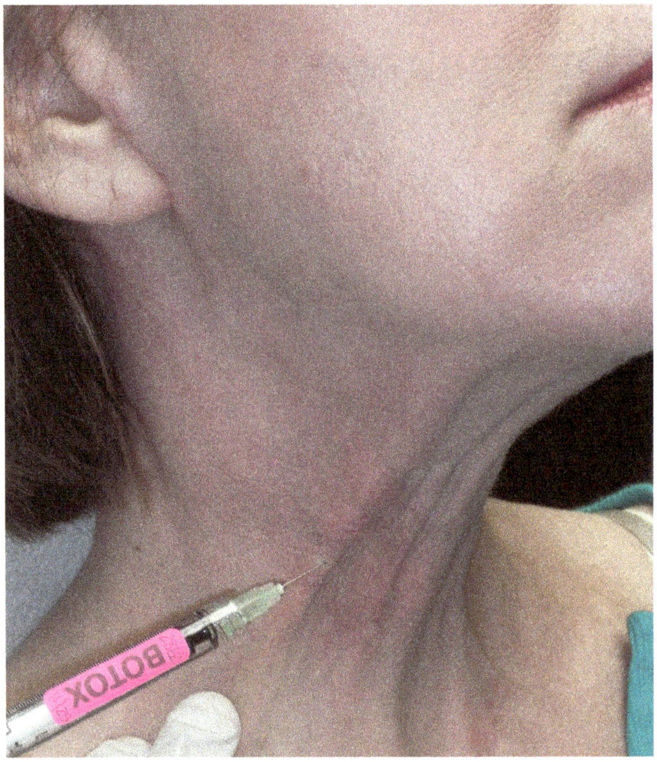

Fig. 12.63. Longitudinal neck bands may be improved with neurotoxin injection if there is truly a muscular component to the banding. This can be a useful adjunct in the early treatment of the bands where 10–20 units of onabotulinum toxin A is injected in the muscle along the band.

Some surgeons address the gland in a secondary procedure, and botulinum toxin injections have been reported as effective in reducing the size (Fig. 12.70). Small amounts of botulinum toxin A can also be used to reduce the digastric muscle size.

Salivary Gland Fistula

Surgical manipulation at or about the regions of the submandibular and parotid gland can result in fistulas or sialocele (Fig. 12.71). Parotid gland fistula is a well described but uncommon complication of facelift surgery. This can occur from inadvertent laceration of the gland or placing a suture too deep and disrupting the glandular tissue. I have not experienced a significant case of this, but have a colleague who had a case of devastating tissue loss from a major parotid fistula that compromised the flap in the same manner as a hematoma does.

Generally, a parotid or submandibular gland fistula is self-limiting and can resolve spontaneously. If a collection of saliva is suspected, needle aspiration of saliva is performed, and pressure is applied over the affected region. In minor cases, the fistula will only be apparent at mealtime from increased salivation and will wane after eating. I have only had a single parotid fistula in over 1600 facelifts and it was minor. The patient developed swelling within the first 10 days of facelift. Aspiration showed a clear fluid with the appearance of saliva.

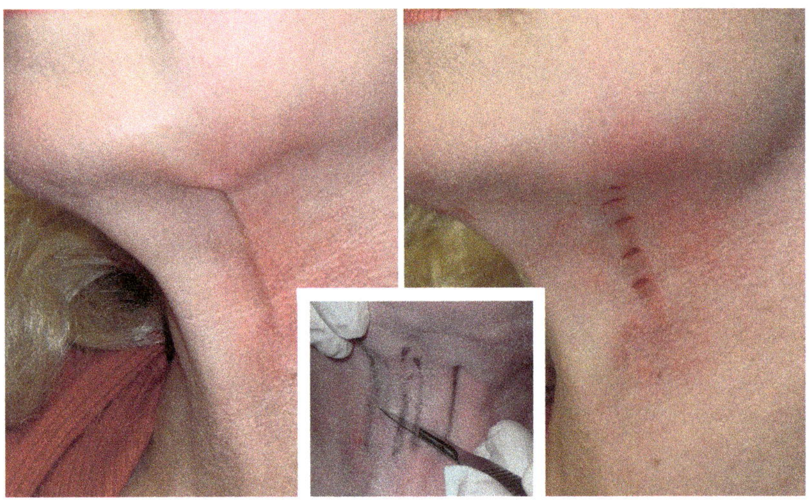
Fig. 12.64. These images show the author's original band transection technique with an eleven blade. Obviously, the blade would be placed subcutaneously and is only shown outside the skin for purposes of illustration (*inset*).

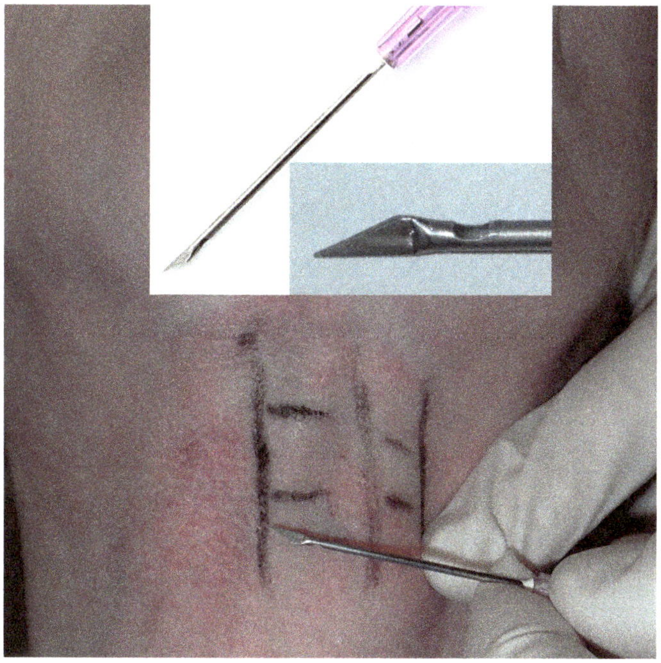

Fig. 12.65. A less invasive means of transecting bands is to use a Becton Dickinson 18-gauge Nokor needle has a mini "scalpel" on the tip (*inset*). This works well for transection or subcision with minimal or no scarring.

The patient was placed on scopolamine patches for the vagolytic antisialagogue effect, botulinum toxin A was injected in the area of the swelling to decrease salivation via acetylcholine inhibition, and a pressure dressing was utilized. The patient was also placed on a bland diet to avoid foods that would stimulate salivation such as citrus or sour item. This combined therapy halted the fistula in a matter of several days. Laboratory testing for the presence of salivary amylase is an option if the surgeon is unsure if the fluid collection represents saliva. In severe cases that do not respond to conservative treatment, surgical intervention may be necessary to drain the fistula and remove offending sutures.

Well-known London facial plastic surgeon Dominic Bray, MD, uses a silastic bolster, which is simple technique for the surgeon and well tolerated by the patient. This technique is used along with aforementioned conservative treatments. A rolled gauze or cotton roll is affixed over the area of drainage using 4-0 silk suture. A Tegaderm (www.3M.com) transparent film dressing places pressure over the fistula and allows monitoring of the underlying skin either in person or with virtual consultation (Fig. 12.72). The bolster and dressing are painless and well tolerated. The bolster is removed 5 days after complete resolution of swelling.

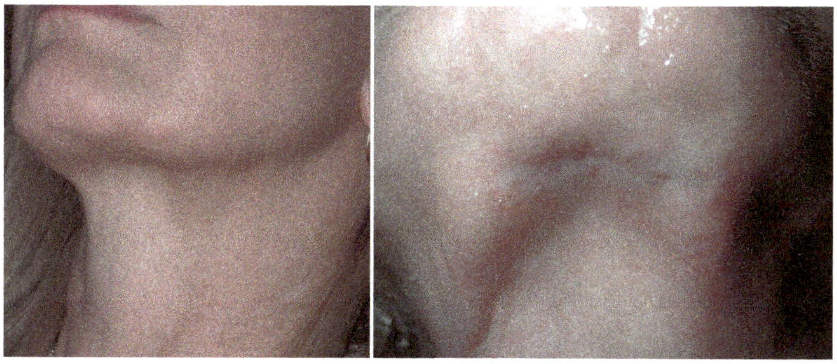

Fig. 12.66. These patients were treated by other surgeons and presented with a "cobra deformity" of the submental region from excessive liposuction and deep fat removal. Several sessions of fat transfer were required to improve this defect.

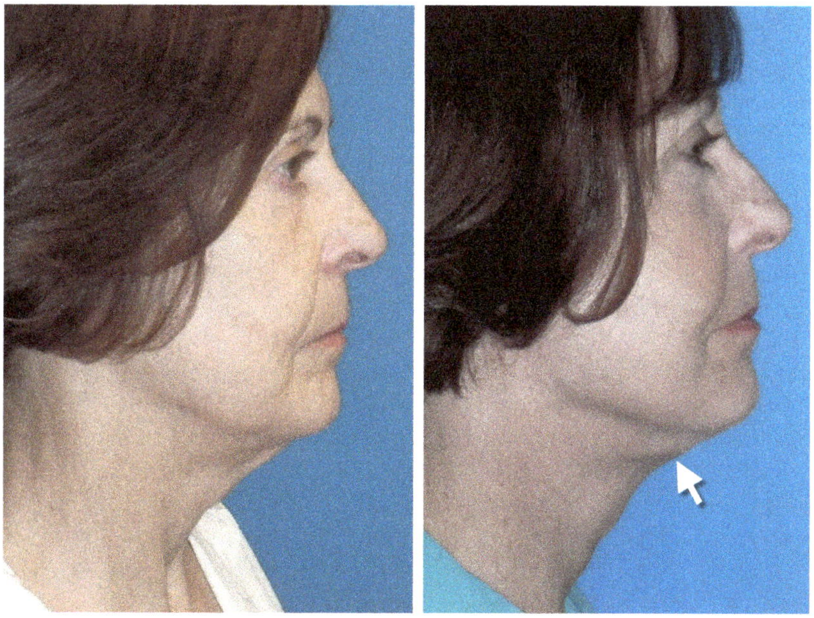

Fig. 12.67. This patient is shown before surgery in the *left* image and after surgery in the *right* image. Her digastric muscle hypertrophy is noticeable in the postoperative (*right*) picture. Patients may not notice muscle or gland hypertrophy preoperatively because it is hidden by sagging skin or fat and does not become noticeable until the postoperative period.

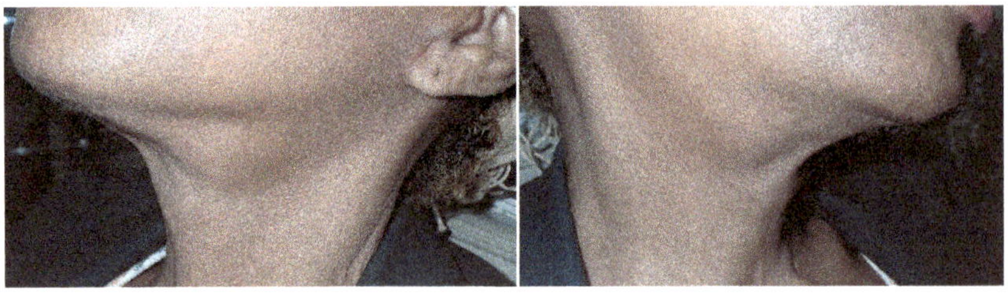

Fig. 12.68. This patient is shown after surgery. The round bulges under the inferior border of the mandible represent ptotic submandibular glands.

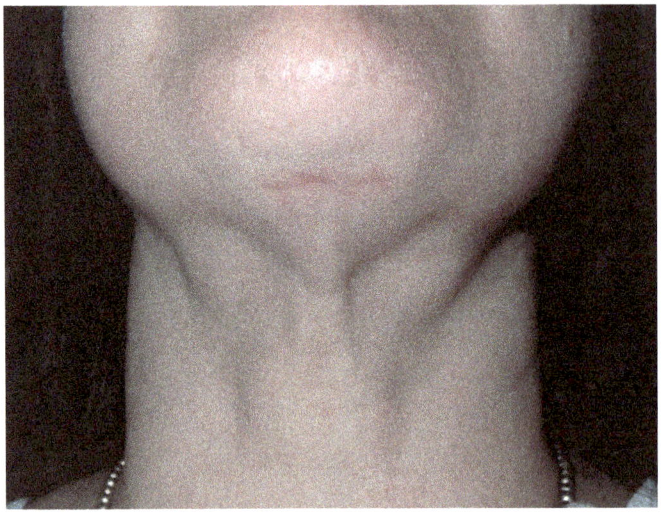

Fig. 12.69. This image shows a case of postoperatively visible submandibular glands. This patient also has a component of fibrotic swelling in the submental region.

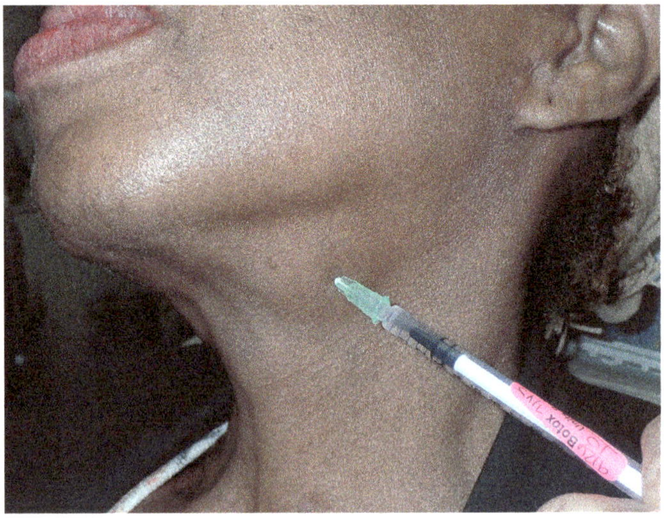

Fig. 12.70. This image show a dose of 20 units of Botox injected into a hypertrophic left submandibular gland, which was prominent after facelift surgery.

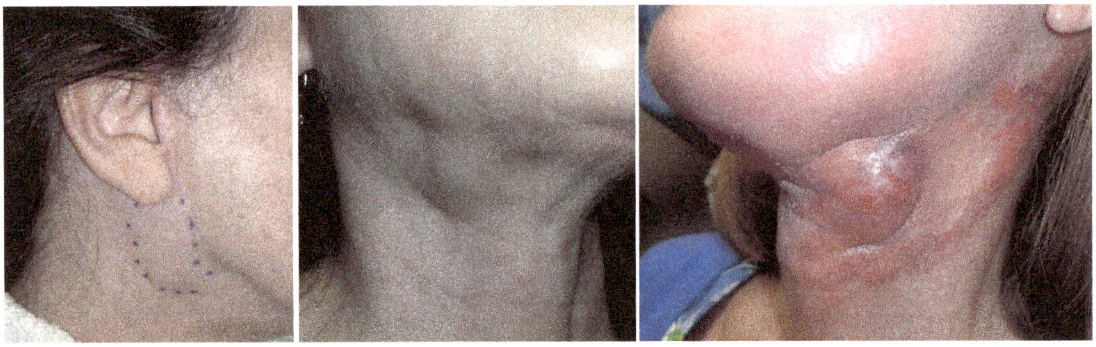

Fig. 12.71. The *left* and *center* images show minor submandibular gland sialoceles. The *right* image shows a major sialocele with skin changes that required immediate and aggressive drainage and treatment. All of these cases occurred after submandibular gland reduction in conjunction with deep plane neck lifts.

Suture Complications

The use of sutures is obviously an important part of facelift and neck lift surgery. There is always some controversy between using permanent versus resorbable sutures and, in the interest of efficiency, sutures that tie well and stay tied are a distinct advantage. In my several decades' experience with facelift and neck lift surgery I used silk or braided nylon sutures and saw a fair amount of suture extrusion or localized suture infection (Fig. 12.73). For the last 15 years I have used only 2-0 Vicryl sutures for deep suturing of the platysma and superficial musculoaponeurotic system (SMAS) and have never had a problem with this material.

Some surgeons only advocate permanent sutures with facelifts, stating their result will be permanent. It is important to understand that platysma and SMAS and platysma sutures are very important in the initial healing phase as they keep suspended tissues in place. After healing begins and progresses, all of the dissected surfaces will "scar down" and form an adherent interface between the tissue layers. This process occurs and is probably established by 6 weeks and complete by 90 days. When the healing process is completed and organized, the tissues are stable and there is no benefit of sutures. This can be verified by the fact that reentry into a facelift will oftentimes show loose sutures from previous procedures (Fig. 12.74).

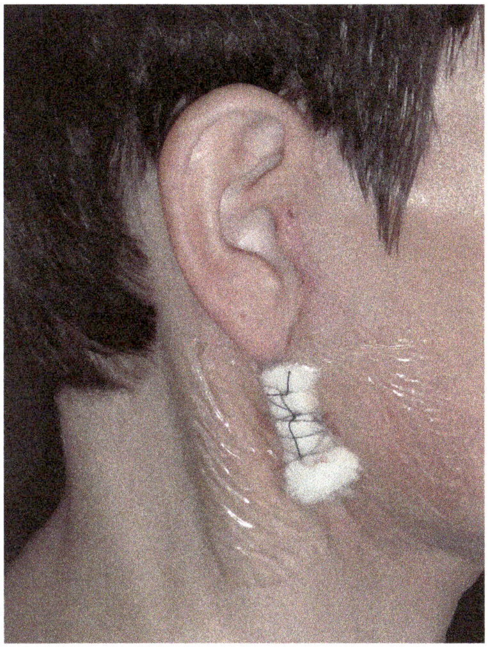

Fig. 12.72. This images show a silastic bolster placed over the salivary fistula and compressed with a transparent film dressing. (Courtesy Domenic Bray, MD.)

Between scarification, suture stretching, and continued tissue aging, it is doubtful that any permanent sutures are really permanent.

Complications of the Hair and Hairline

Working with the hair and hairline is an integral part of facelift surgery and must be managed correctly for natural outcomes. Even small changes in the patient's natural hairline can be problematic.

As stated often throughout this chapter, the hair follicles must be managed with care as they are easily damaged. Hair loss can occur from poor incision design, excessively superficial dissection under hair-bearing skin, suture tension, flap devitalization, and direct follicular damage from cautery and other insults. Finally, the administration of general anesthesia and surgical procedures in general have been implicated in transient hair loss from its stress on the body. Telogen effluvium, which is sometimes referred to as "hair shock," is a condition in which generalized hair loss occurs over the scalp after things that trigger the body's stress response; causes can include acute illness,

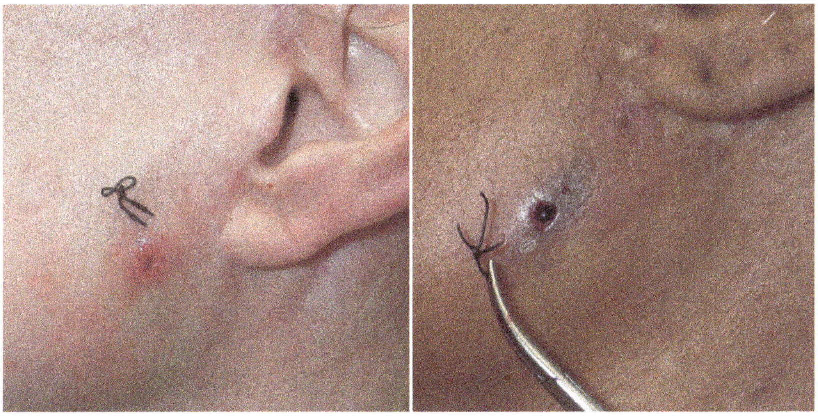

Fig. 12.73. The *left* image shows a suture infection and extrusion with silk suture and the image on the *right* shows the same situation with a braided nylon suture.

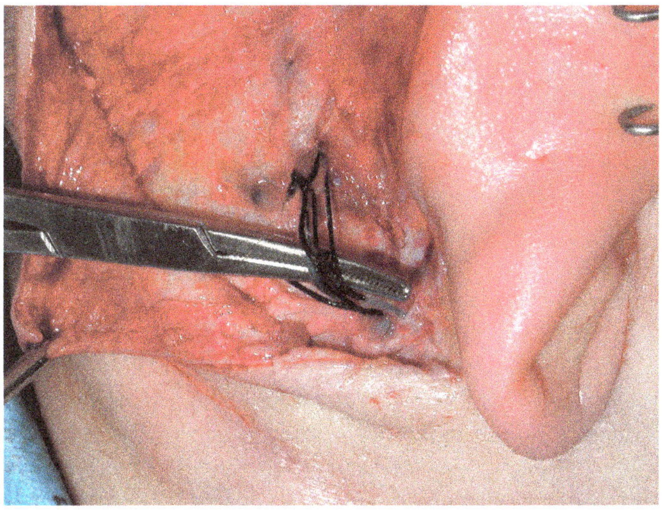

Fig. 12.74. This image shows a revision facelift with loose sutures that were placed a decade earlier. This is a situation I have witnessed many times. To think that a suture that is placed taut will remain that way with aging and further ptosis is unrealistic.

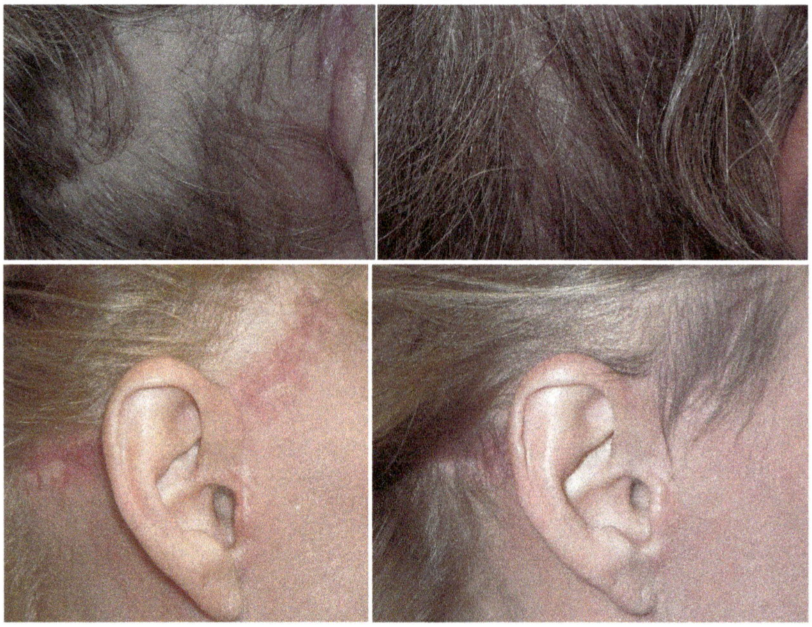

Fig. 12.75. The *top* images show an area of hair loss at the posterior incision and the same patient 4 months after surgery. The *bottom* images show a patient 6 weeks after facelift surgery with a methicillin-resistant *Staphylococcus aureus* infection and resultant hair loss. She is shown 6 months later with regrowth.

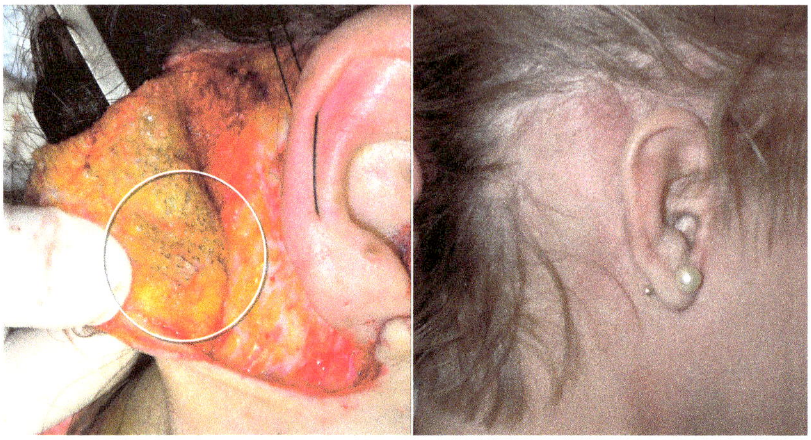

Fig. 12.76. Hair follicles can be seen on the posterior auricular flap (*circle*, *left* image). Excessively thin flap dissection or excessive heat from cautery may damage the follicles. The *right* image shows a patient with hair loss after facelift.

major surgery, severe trauma, chronic illness, changes in diet, and a variety of medications (Fig. 12.75). Since general anesthesia and surgery are usually concomitant, I do not believe there is any proof that the anesthesia in and of itself can cause hair loss. Generally, this condition is transient and will improve over several months, although it could be permanent depending on the extent of follicular damage.

Thermal damage to hair follicles from cauterization can also contribute to temporary or permanent alopecia (Fig. 12.76).

Pressure alopecia is another problem that can be experienced with facelift and neck lift surgery. Anytime the head is in a position where localized pressure occurs over several hours, hair loss is possible (Fig 12.77).

This can be a transient experience and self-corrects over time. Although quite rare, cases of permanent hair loss can occur from facelift surgery, and follicular grafts may be necessary to correct the isolated areas of alopecia (Fig. 12.78). Experienced hair transplant surgeons are well versed with postfacelift hair replacement as it is a common problem.

Postfacelift Infections

Due to the rich vascularity of the head and neck region, postfacelift infections are unusual. In over 1600 facelift surgeries I have never experienced a severe infection that required hospitalization or progressed to a life-threatening situation. Although full-blown purulent abscess formation after cosmetic facial surgery and facelift is rare, minor infections can be seen. I have seen several staphylococcus or MRSA (methicillin-resistant *Staphylococcus aureus*) infections that colonized over undermined flaps. These present as white papular lesions over violaceous-colored skin (Fig. 12.79). The violet skin color seems to be a common denominator of these Staph infections. Although they look quite ominous, they generally respond

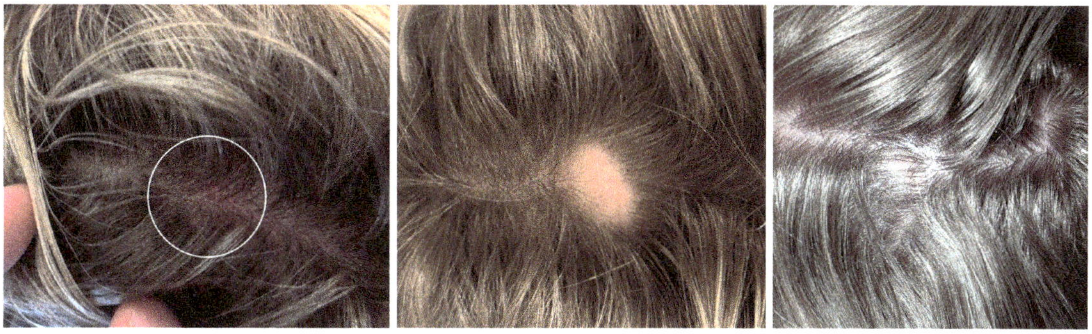

Fig. 12.77. This patient reported pain on her scalp the day after facelift surgery. The area looked normal except for some pinkness (*circle*, *left* image). The patient presented 6 weeks later with a 2 × 2 cm bald spot (*middle* image). The *right* image shows improving hair regrowth at 4 months.

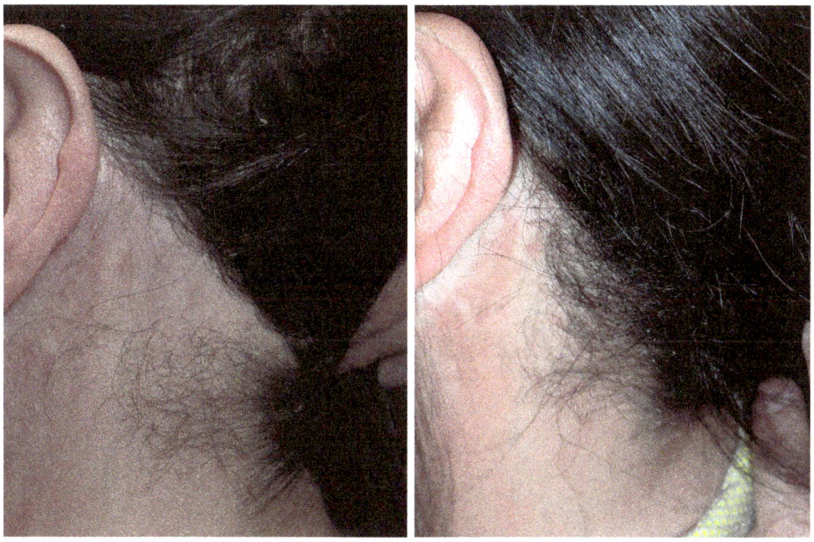

Fig. 12.78. Out of over 1600 facelifts performed, I have seen several patients with substantial hair loss from routine surgery. The *left* image shows the hair loss on the posterior flap presumably from the trauma of raising the flap. The *right* image shows the patient after follicular grafting to the area.

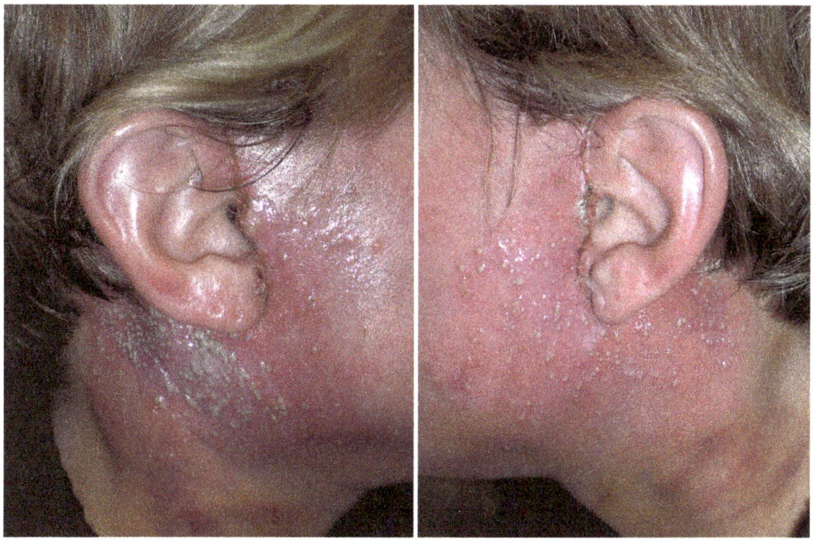

Fig. 12.79. This patient presented with a culture-proven methicillin-resistant *Staphylococcus aureus* infection. The lesions were drained by puncture with an 18 gauge needle. The patient responded to trimethoprim and sulfamethoxazole (Bactrim DS) and topical mupirocin (Bactroban).

well and quickly to topical and oral antibiotics. Most MRSA infections I have encountered have been sensitive to clindamycin, levofloxacin, ciprofloxacin, trimethoprim/sulfa, and vancomycin. Another common denominator with these infections is that they may cause postinflammatory hyperpigmentation after healing.

Staphylococcus infections are the most common type of infection after surgery given in part to the fact that *S. aureus* is part of normal skin flora. I have also encountered less common infections such as Corynebacterium, Pseudomonas, and Mycobacterium (Figs. 12.80) as well as clinical conditions thought to be infection that proved to be otherwise.

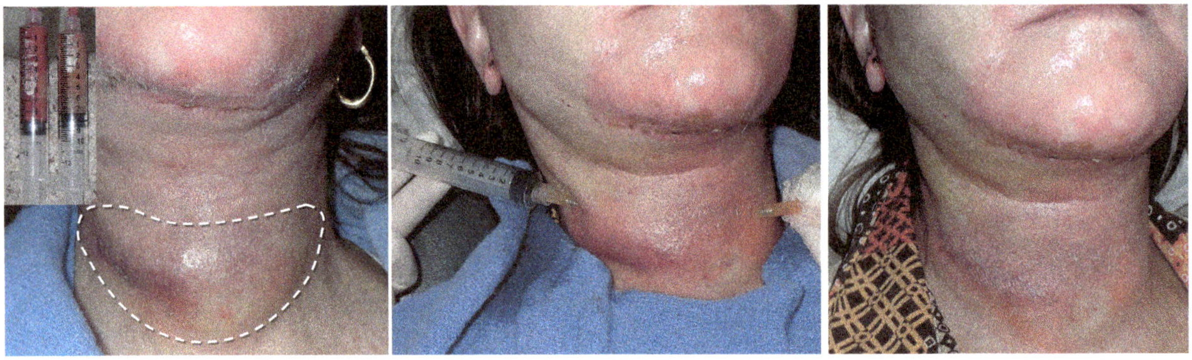

Fig. 12.80. This patient presented with a neck abscess 6 days after deep plane face and necklift (*left* image). 16 ml of mucopurulent puss was aspirated (*inset left* image). The abscess was then irrigated by placing a 14 gauge angiocath as an exit port and flushing the pocket with clindamycin solution followed by several flushes with hypochlorous acid solution (Phase One) (*center* image). The *left* image shows the patient 5 days later after two flushing sessions. Culture results showed *Corynebacterium*.

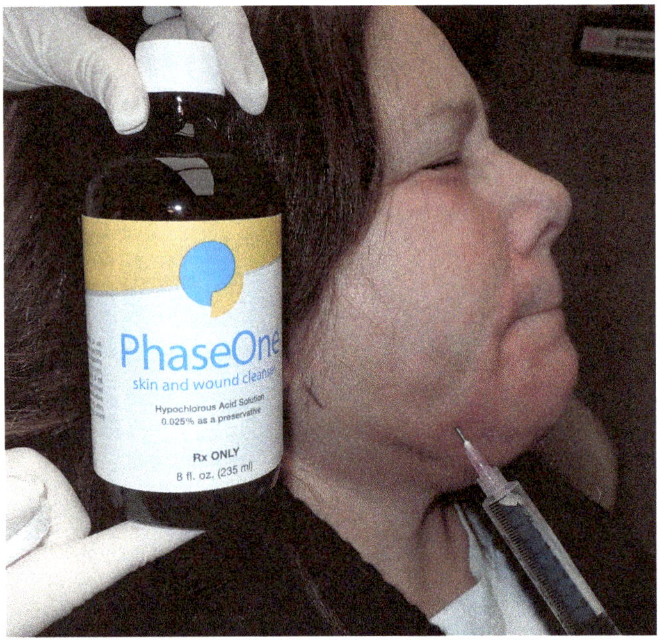

Fig. 12.81. This image shows hypochlorous acid irrigation after incision and drainage of postfacelift abscess.

I recently saw a postfacelift patient with a purulent abscess, which was drained and cultured. At the time of drainage (but after culture), the wound was irrigated with hypochlorous acid (Fig. 12.81). Interestingly, the cultures never identified an organism. The patient had been placed on oral antibiotics several days before drainage, which may account for the culture result.

In my 20-plus-year facelift experience I have also seen minor localized infections.

Sleeping with pets is problematic as they can be vectors of numerous microbes and diseases, especially MRSA. Patients with any open wounds should not have close contact with their pets until healed, especially sharing a bed. Mycobacterium infections or other infections can also occur from contamination from the patient's home such as contaminated shower heads. Patients with hearing aids should routinely cleanse their device and ear canal as Pseudomonas is a common inhabitant of the ear canal (Figs. 12.82–12.84).

Wound Dehiscence

Any sutured wound has the ability to dehisce and spread apart. This is more common in eyelid surgery, and actually in my

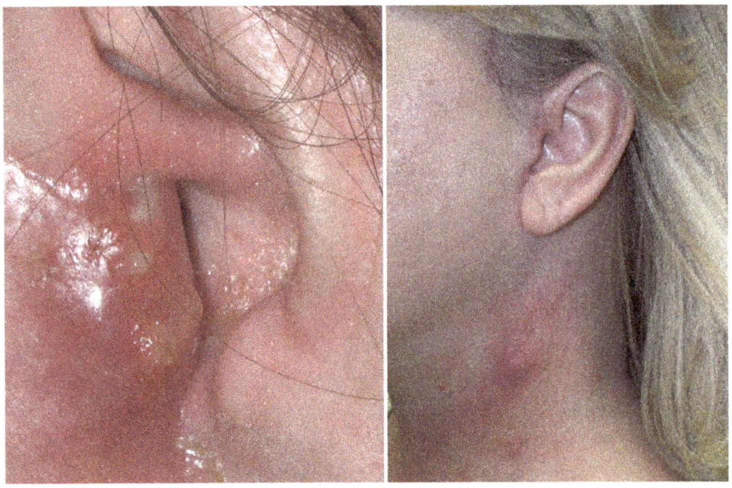

Fig. 12.82. The *left* image shows a pseudomonas infection. This bacterium is a common inhabitant of the ear canal and can manifest on the face. The *right* image shows a mycobacterium infection that was treated successfully with antibiotic therapy.

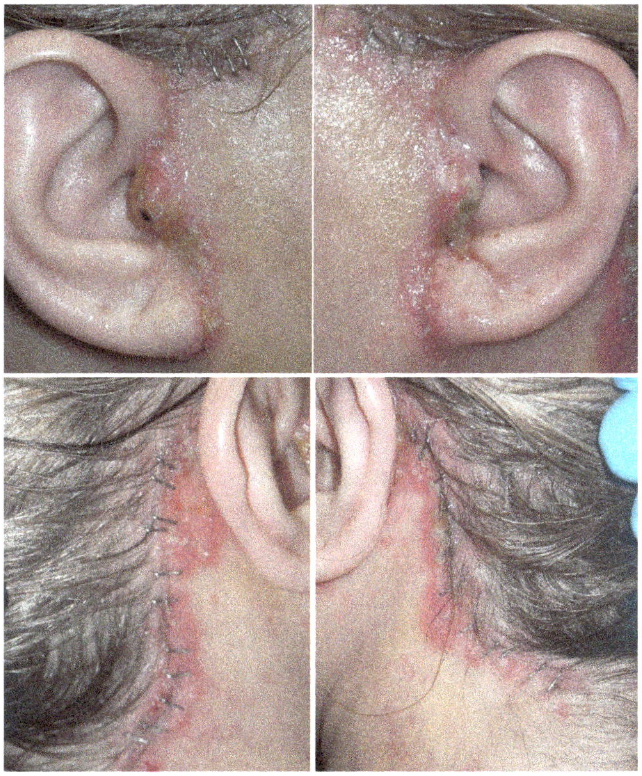

Fig. 12.83. This patient developed inflammatory reactions on her suture lines, which early on were thought to be skin infection but later turned out to be allergy to triple antibiotic ointment.

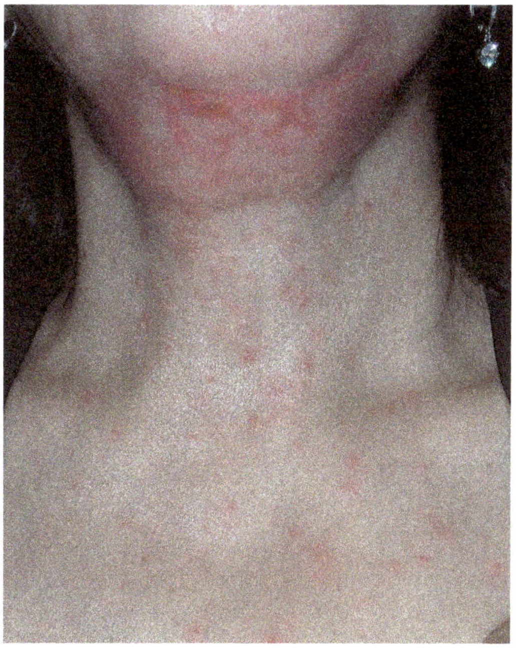

Fig. 12.84. This patient presented approximately 1 week after facelift and neck lift surgery with a diffuse rash of the neck and upper chest resembling with a skin infection. Cultures did not show any causative agent. The rash mysteriously improved over several days, and it was discovered that the patient had some type of reaction from a wool scarf that she was wearing during her recovery.

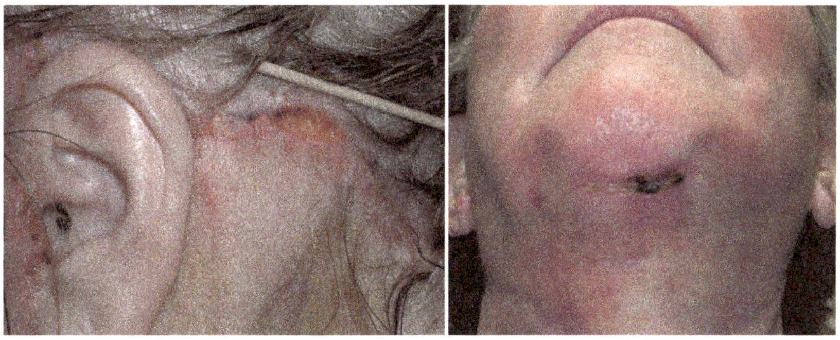

Fig. 12.85. Wound dehiscence can occur at any suture site. Small areas will granulate, and larger areas can be treated in the early stages with surgical prep and resutured (if not under excessive tension). This patient on the *left* is shown 2 weeks after surgery, and the patient on the *right* is shown at 3 weeks after and did not report the complication earlier.

experience is less frequent with facelift surgery (Fig. 12.85). Wound dehiscence could be an indication that the skin was closed under excessive tension or merely suture failure. If the wound was not closed under excessive tension, it can be disinfected and reclosed in the early phases of healing period; otherwise, it would require healing by secondary intention.

Accidental Burns

Although some surgeons recommend ice or heat at some time in the early postoperative period, I do not. The skin is numb and applying heat or ice without the patient's ability to feel the area can cause burns, and I have seen this many times. People disobey postoperative instructions and I have seen five or six patients cause significant self-inflicted burns from heating pads, hot water bottles, microwave heating devices, excessively hot tap water, curling irons, and hair driers (Figs. 12.86–12.91). Although some surgeons recommend ice applications, I feel this can limit blood flow to the fragile flap and do not recommend it.

Regardless of how many times patients are warned about using heat or ice over undermined facelift flaps, they seem to find a way to burn themselves! I actually had a patient who had a new hot water tank installed in her home and blistered her facelift from excessively hot tap water. Due to the fact that the undermined flaps are numb for several weeks or longer, the patient cannot judge the intensity of the heat or cold source. Although ice can discourage swelling and controlled heat can lessen swelling, I don't suggest the use of either because of the potential for burns that can lead to permanent scarring. Hair dryers should be used on low or cool settings, and heating pads

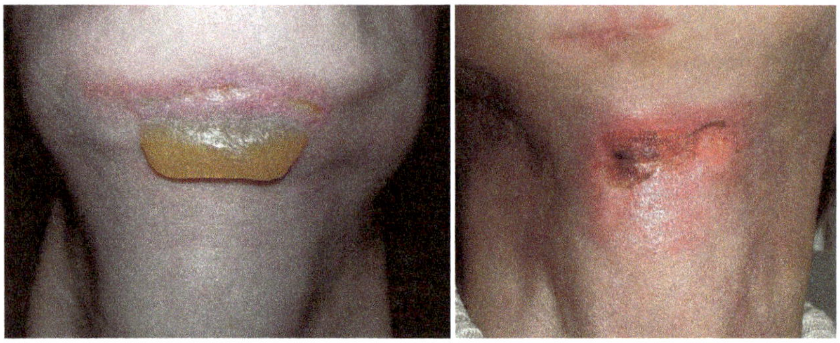

Fig. 12.86. These images show two different patients who burnt themselves with microwave heating devices in the early postoperative stages. Although these generally heal well, they can cause significant setback and sometimes permanent scarring. It is imperative that your patients understand what not to do.

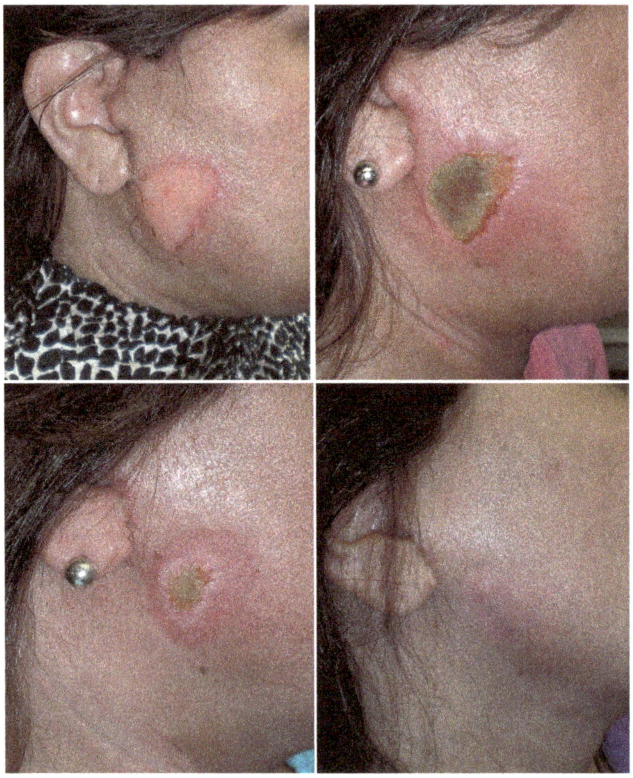

Fig. 12.87. This patient sustained a full-thickness burn from a heating pad and is shown in the *upper left* image at 8 days after surgery (24 hours after the injury). The *upper right* image shows the patient at 23 days after her burn. The *bottom left* image shows the patient approximately 60 days after her injury, and the *bottom right* patient shows the patient 6 months later after multiple sessions of CO_2 laser resurfacing to improve the scar.

should be tested on normal skin and not worn excessively. I feel better if patients do not use ice or heat.

Flap injuries that resemble burns can also be the result of patient behavior in the postoperative period (Fig. 12.92).

Complications Involving the Ear and Earlobe

As discussed, many times in this text the aesthetics of the earlobes after facelift surgery are a prime concern and are subject to a number of intra- and postoperative problems. The postfacelift earlobe is vulnerable, and a relatively common problem that occurs usually in the first week of recovery is detachment of the sutured earlobe from the cheek skin. Earlobe detachment is multifactorial and can occur from careless use of dressings, injury while cleaning the region, rolling over in bed, and more commonly tearing the earlobe while taking pullover clothing on and off (Fig. 12.93). It is important to inform the patient and the caregiver in the consent process but also postoperatively not to use shirts, blouses, and other articles of clothing that require pulling over their head. It is very common to detach one or both lobes doing this (especially during removal), and button-up clothing should be used in the first several weeks after surgery. Minor detachment of several millimeter will reattach by keeping the area clean and usually will require no further treatment.

Larger tears can be cleaned, prepped, and reclosed in the first 4–6 days after the facelift surgery if the surfaces have not granulated. If the surfaces are minimally granulated, they can be surgically freshened and reattached. If the wound is granulating and contracting, it should be allowed to fully heal and revised at a later date (Fig. 12.93, *right*, and 12.94). When repairing an unattached lobe, it may be advisable to apply several Steri-Strips from the lobe to the cheek for further reinforcement during healing.

Small irregularities after facelift surgery can detract attention from an otherwise satisfactory case. One of the small things that bothers patients are contour irregularities at the posterior auricular sulcus suture line (Fig. 12.95). This can occur from inattention to wound closure when suturing. In addition the posterior auricular region lies over the mastoid area, which does not have abundant subdermal tissue, and wound contraction can occur. Finally, the sulcus is concave, and incisions are more prone to healing issues when closed over concavities. Irregular or hypertrophic tissue can easily be recontoured with simple excision or laser or radio wave tissue ablation (Fig. 12.96). Using a subcuticular running horizontal suture provides wound eversion and, in my experience, a more aesthetic closure (Fig. 12.97). As stated earlier, some surgeons prefer placing the postauricular incision several millimeters superior to the sulcus. I have not found this to be a solution for postsurgical irregularities and feel that careful closure will reduce this problem in most patients.

Earlobe malposition is very problematic for the patient and surgeon, as alluded to many times in this chapter. The "pixie" or

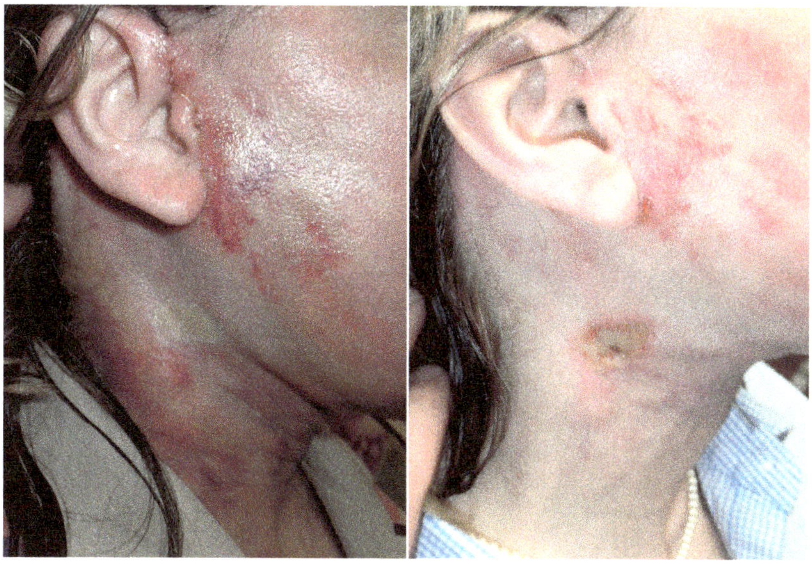

Fig. 12.88. This patient burned her numb skin with a curling iron and is shown 24 hours after injury (*left*) and 1 week later (*right*).

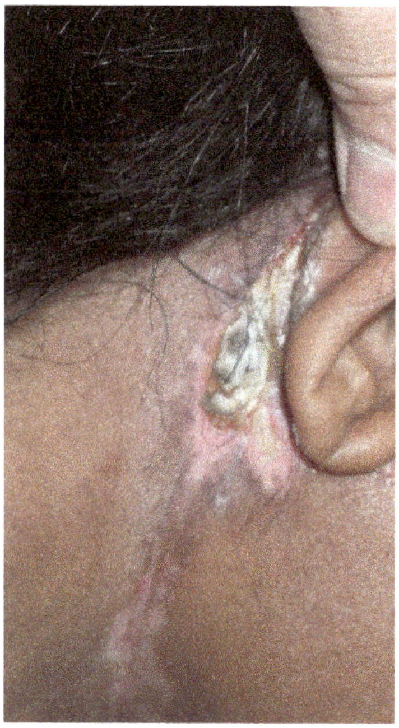

Fig. 12.89. This patient had been putting warm compresses on her skin. She recently purchased a new water heater that produced higher temperatures than the previous one and brunt herself.

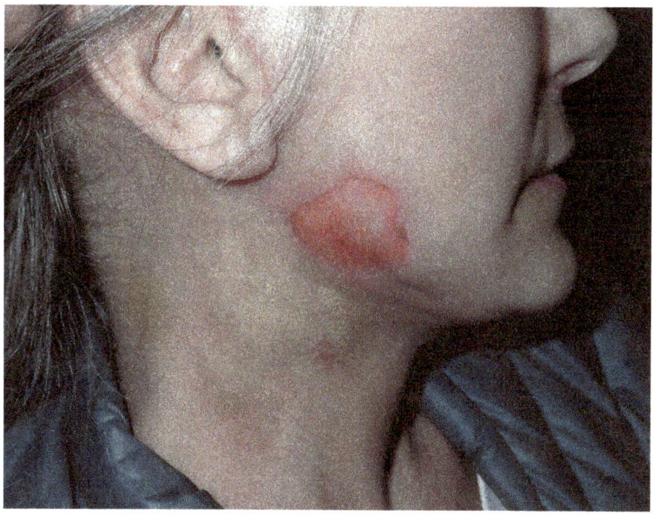

Fig. 12.90. This patient is shown 5 days after a thermal burn from an electric heating pad.

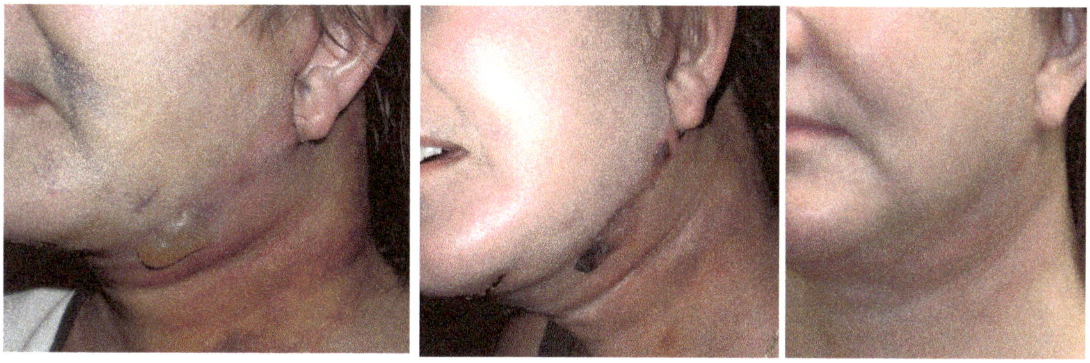

Fig. 12.91. These images show a burn from an electric heating pad (24 hours, *left*), 1 week (*center*), and 90 days later (*right*).

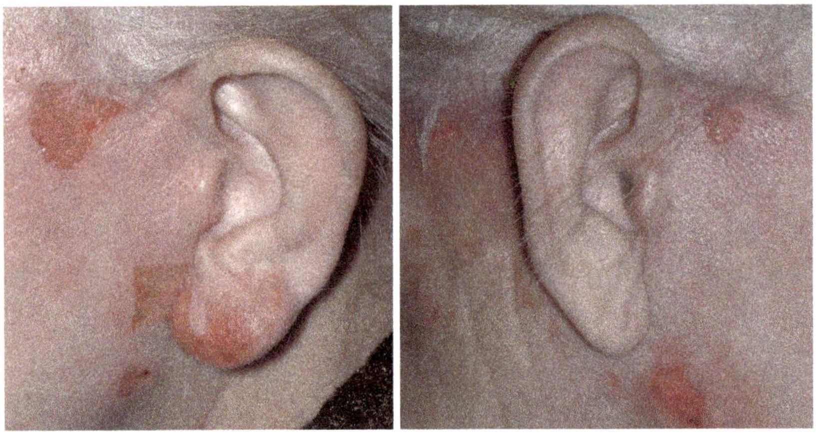

Fig. 12.92. This patient presented with burnlike lesions bilaterally approximately 5 weeks after facelift surgery. The patient admitted to scratching and picking at her skin because it was itching in response to "things crawling beneath her skin."

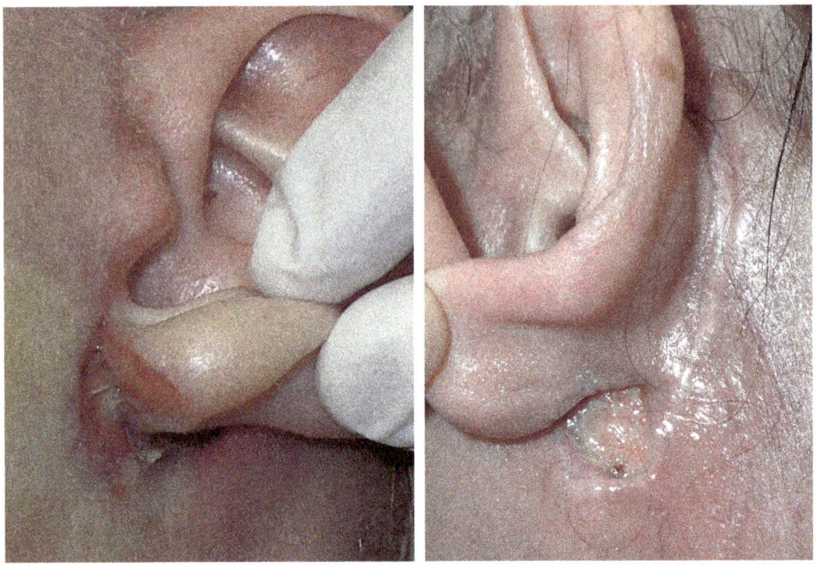

Fig. 12.93. The *left* image shows a detached lobe at 8 days, and the *right* image shows a granulating detachment in another patient at 3 weeks.

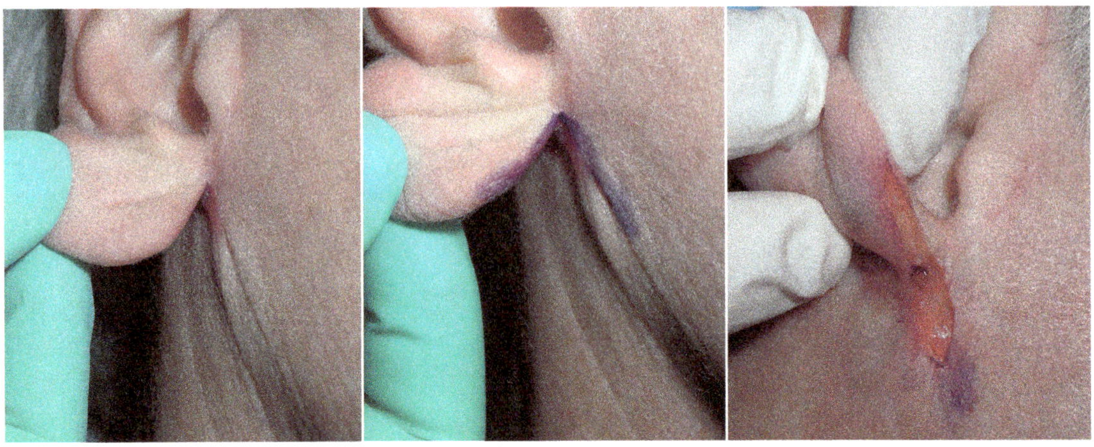

Fig. 12.94. This patient sustained a large detachment of the entire earlobe, which was allowed to heal and surgically repaired at a later date. The *left* image shows the healed detachment, the *center* image shows the proposed skin excision for repair, and the *right* image shows the excised scar just before resuturing and reattachment.

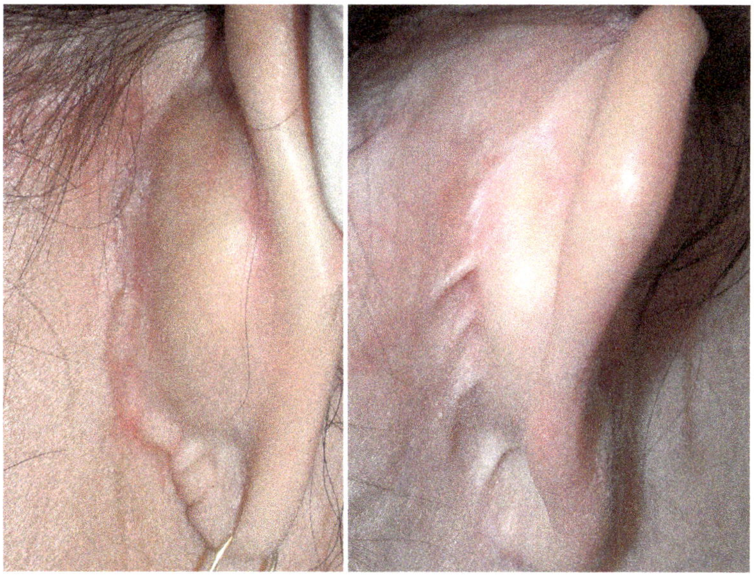

Fig. 12.95. This image shows common areas of contour irregularities on the posterior auricular region including the posterior lobe (*left* image) and the sulcus (*right* image). Concave regions are frequently problematic for wound closure.

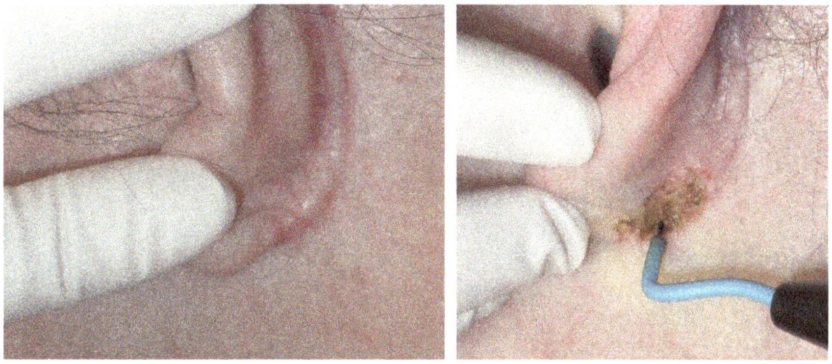

Fig. 12.96. These images show hypertrophic tissue in the posterior auricular region being recontoured with radio wave tissue ablation. Laser tissue reduction can also be used.

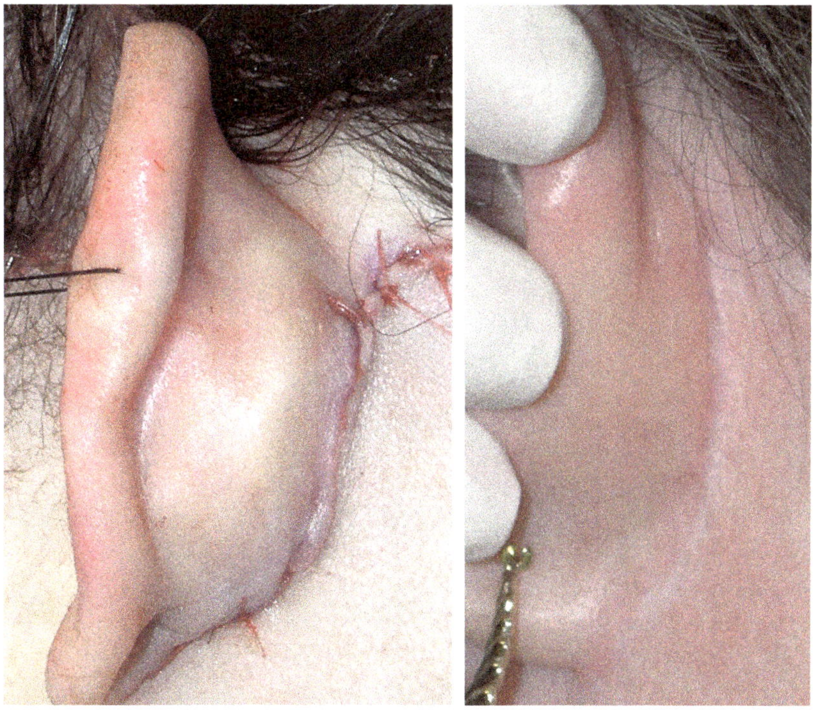

Fig. 12.97. The *left* image shows the posterior auricular intrasulcular incision closed with a running 4-0 gut running subcuticular suture and wound eversion and the *right* image shows the excellent healing that can be produced by this type of suturing.

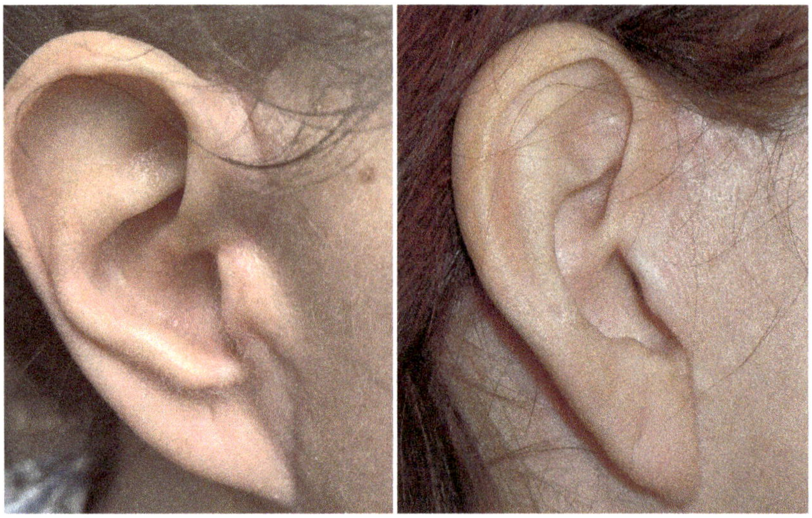

Fig. 12.98. These two images from other surgeons show extended and stretched earlobes known as pixie lobes. This is a very unpleasant stigma of facelift surgery and is usually a result of improper skin cutback and lobe placement of the earlobe during surgery.

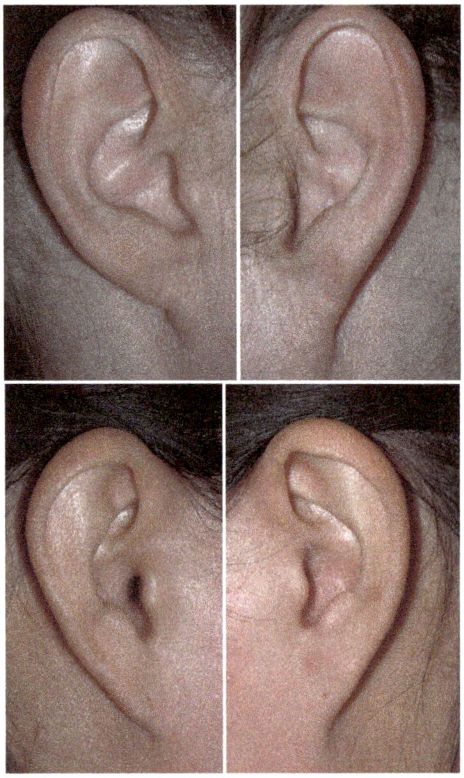

Fig. 12.99. These images show patients who have congenitally attached earlobes.

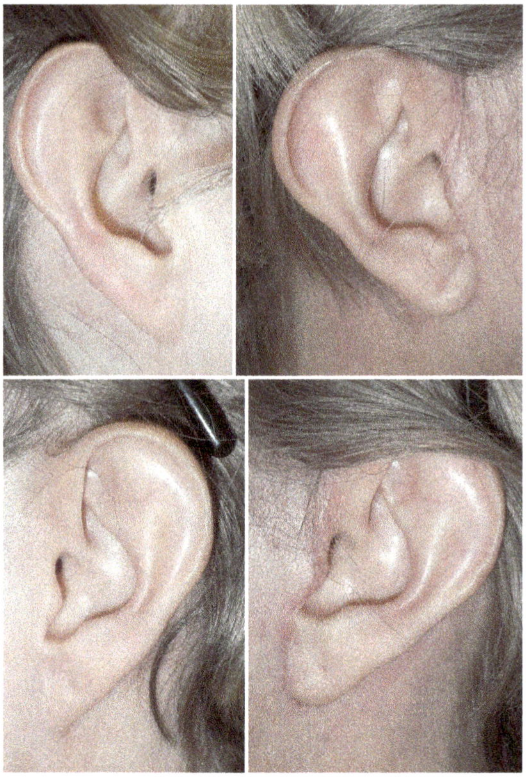

Fig. 12.100. These images show a patient with congenitally attached earlobes who desired to have unattached lobes after surgery. The *left* images are preoperative, and the *right* images are postoperative, showing the conversion from attached to unattached lobes by the author.

"elfin" earlobe is one of the most dreaded complications for patients (Fig. 12.98).

Some patients have congenitally attached and pointed earlobes before surgery (Fig. 12.99). Preoperative discussion with these patients is important as their earlobe architecture can be changed by the surgeon, where pointed and attached lobes can be converted to a rounded normal-appearing earlobe (Fig. 12.100). Personally, I favor changing the patient's earlobe during the procedure because a postoperative facelift patient with a pointed and attached lobe (even knowing this was a presurgical condition) may appear as a complication and reflect negatively on the competence of the surgeon. Some patients may wish to retain their preoperative lobes, as in Chinese culture it is believed that long ears signify nobility and predict a long life and thick earlobes predict greater wealth. Fig. 12.97 shows a case where a congenitally attached lobes were converted to rounded lobes by the author.

A significant amount of ink and paper in this book have been devoted to the discussion of natural and unnatural earlobes in the

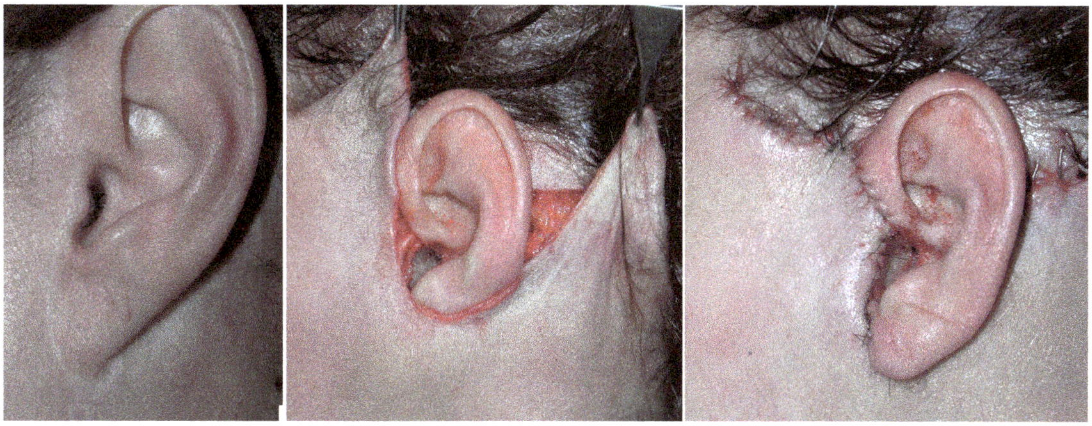

Fig. 12.101. The left image shows a pixie earlobe where the surgery was performed by another surgeon. The patient presented to my office for correction and the previous incisions were opened and the flaps dissected and the skin retracted (*middle* image). The *right* image shows the completed surgery with the flap and lobe repositioned superiorly to a normal position and shape.

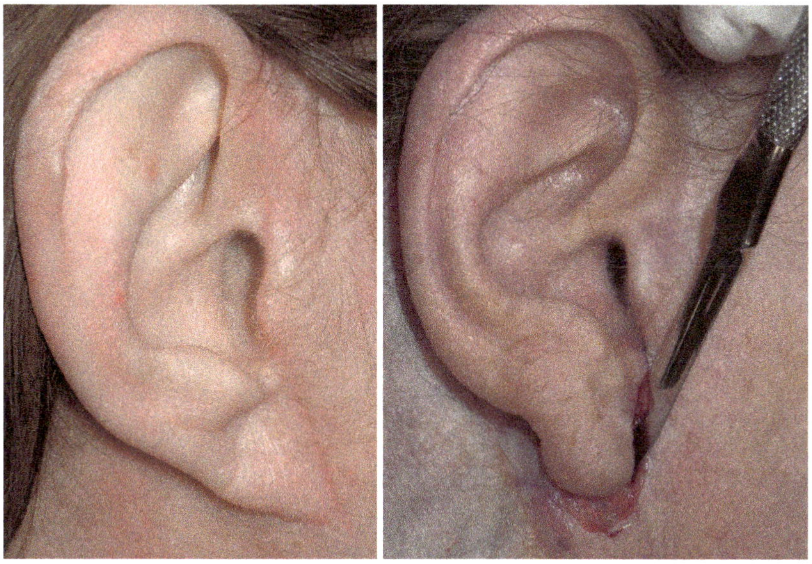

Fig. 12.102. This patient from another surgeon presented with a pixie earlobe. Pixie earlobe is repaired by incising around the base of the lobe and releasing the scar to retract the lobe superiorly.

performance of facelift surgery. By this point I would assume that the reader understands the significant impact earlobes have on the surgeon and patient. Severe earlobe distortion or "pixie" earlobes are the mortal sin of facelift surgery. Surgeons who routinely experience pixie-type earlobe deformities probably need continuing education. Having said this, a distorted or pixie lobe can occasionally occur in the best of hands. Although I most often repair pixie earlobes that were caused by other surgeons, I have had to revise my own work several times over the years. Although unusual, wound contracture can induce tension on a well-positioned lobe. There are numerous ways to repair a pixie earlobe described in the literature. The most accurate means of repair is to redirect the entire facelift incision, remove some excess skin, and reposition the entire flap and lobe. This can sometimes be done with relatively conservative flap dissection and skin excision (Fig. 12.101). This is usually not possible immediately after facelift surgery because there is not enough excess skin to be redirected to accommodate the lengthened lobe. In my opinion, to do this properly, the patient has to wait until enough excess skin is present so the flaps can be opened, and the skin retracted to properly position the earlobe.

The most comprehensive way to repair a pixie lobe is to redissect the facelift flap to reposition the flap superiorly and release and reattach the lobe in the normal position (Fig. 12.101). The problem with this method is there needs to be enough skin excess to redrape and when pixie lobes occur immediately after surgery, this in many cases is not possible and the patient would have to wait several years for more skin laxity.

A more conservative way to repair a pixie ear deformity is to incise and release the earlobe, which will retract superiorly (Figs. 12.102–12.106). This will leave a "V"-shaped trough at the base of the ear, which is brought together by primary closure. The "V" is undermined with lateral dissection and the edges sutured, which creates a straight line. The lobe is then placed superiorly and sutured. In effect, the patient is achieving normal lobe position at the expense of a small vertical scar under the lobe. At 4–6 weeks the scar is treated with CO_2 laser resurfacing and in most cases blends imperceptibly (Fig. 12.105).

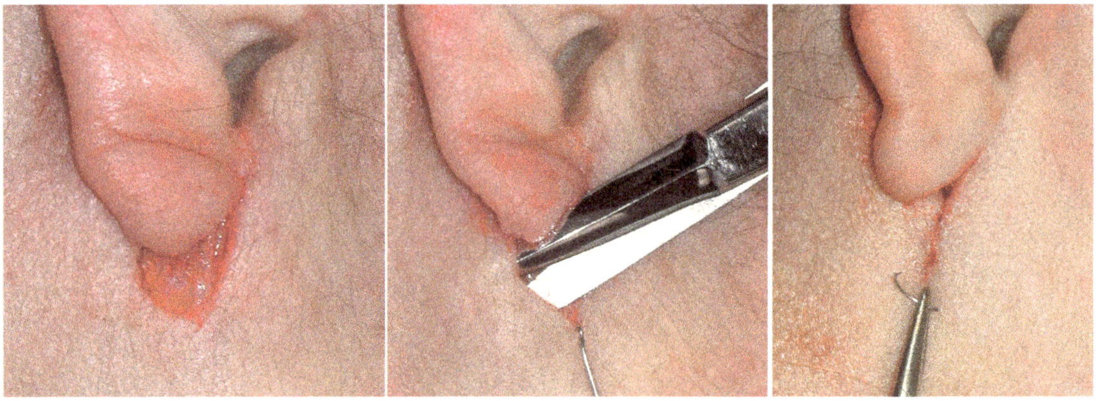

Fig. 12.103. The vertical lobe incision is then undermined and closed, and the ear is repositioned superiorly and sutured to the cheek at the top of the incision.

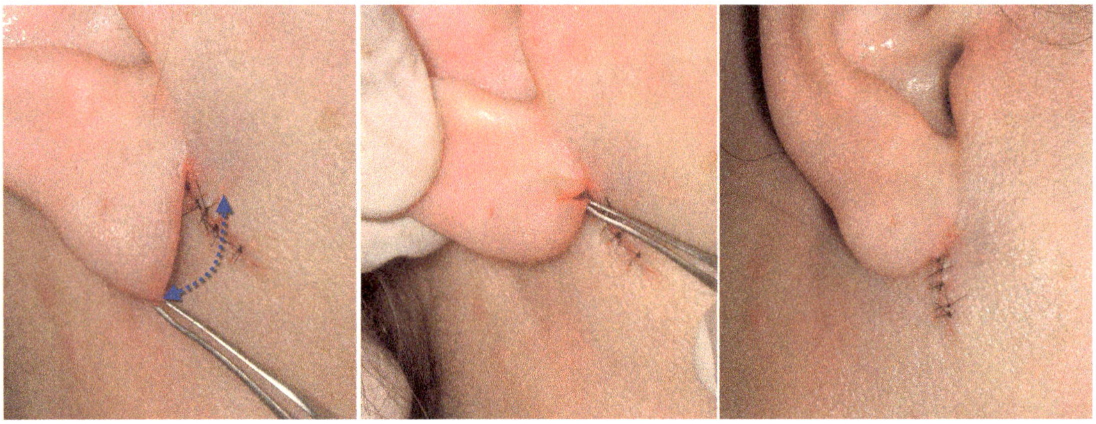

Fig. 12.104. After the vertical incision is closed, the lobe is rotated superiorly to its normal position (*left* and *center* images), and the final skin closure is performed (*right* image).

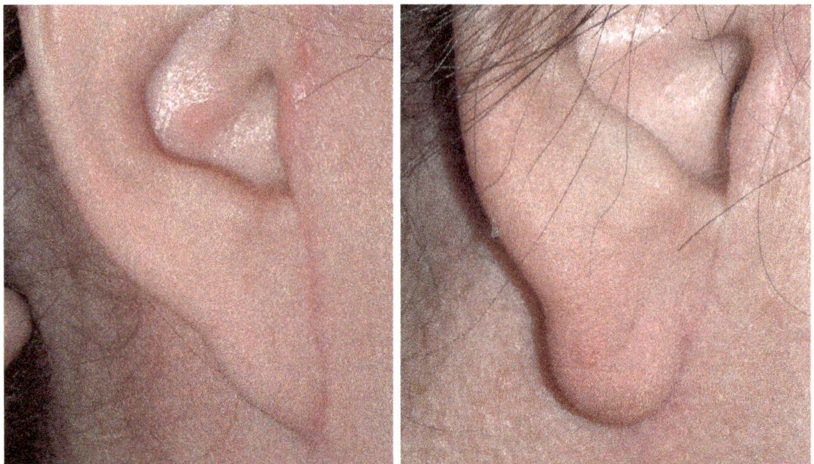

Fig. 12.105. This image shows a pixie lobe repair treated by the author that has been treated with the CO_2 laser at final healing. Lasering the vertical release scar generally produces an acceptable aesthetic result.

Some patients can experience significant earlobe swelling immediately after surgery and have a very large and deformed earlobe. This mega lobe situation is a temporary phenomenon, and the patient must be reassured that with further healing their lobes will return to normal size (Fig. 12.107).

Tragal blunting was discussed in the operative part of this chapter. It is important to gently handle cartilage and allow some subcutaneous fat to overlay the tragus to provide a cushion (Fig. 12.108). Blunted tragi can be difficult if not impossible to correct on a revision procedure. If the patient already presents with a blunted tragus, the surgeon must decide whether to try to improve the situation with another retrotragal incision tragal, which could also worsen it. If the blunting is moderate, I always use a pretragal incision. When attempting to improve a

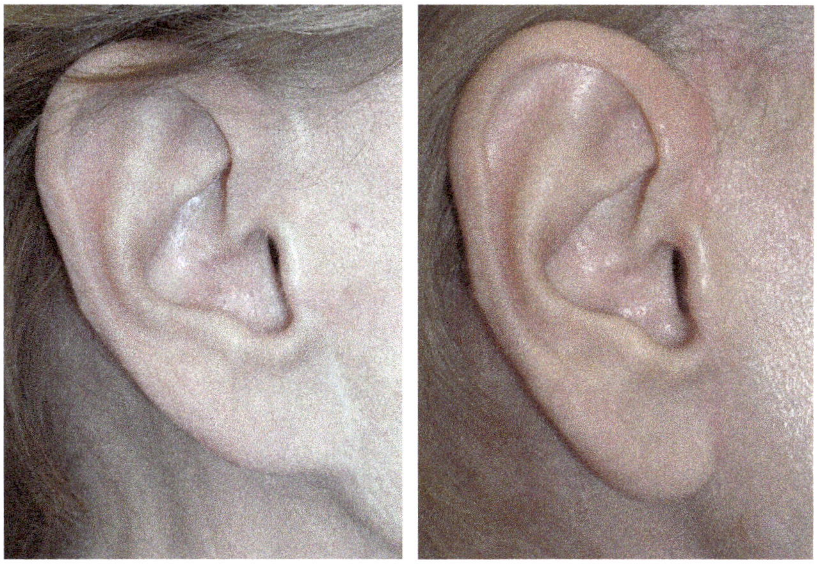

Fig. 12.106. This figure shows another before-and-after image of a pixie earlobe performed by the author.

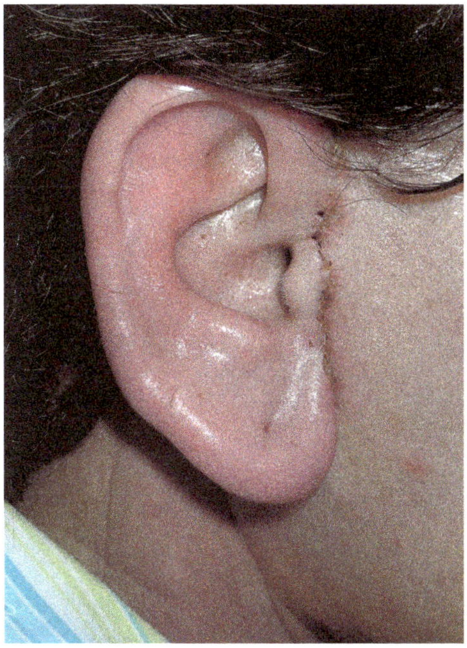

Fig. 12.107. Some patients can have significant swelling of the earlobe in the early postoperative period. This can be very worrisome to the patient, and they need reassured that their lobes will return to normal size after further healing.

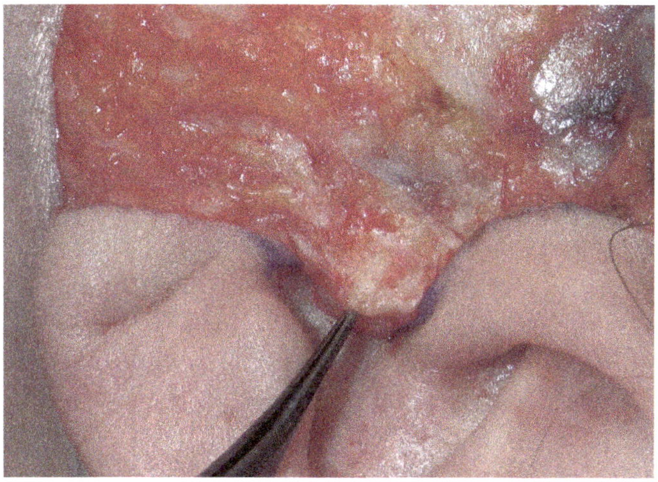

Fig. 12.108. Leaving a cushion of fat over the tragal cartilage helps prevent camouflage contour irregularities and prevents skeletonization visible through the skin, enabling a more naturally appearing tragus.

blunted tragus with a retrotragal incision, the skin of the underside of the tragus is freed from the cartilage to allow mobility. Frequently the tragal cartilage is warped in a curved fashion from anterior contraction and can be relaxed by scoring the superior cartilaginous surface with a #15 scalpel blade (Fig. 12.109). It is also important to leave generous skin over the tragus as wound contracture will ensue, possibly making the situation worse.

I personally have had mixed results when trying to improve a blunted tragus. I have had moderate success using permanent fillers such as injectable silicone in this area to plump up postoperatively and add some contour to a blunted tragus.

I have been experimenting with a tragal implant, which is a silicone analogue of a normal tragus that is placed and sutured over the cartilage with the skin redraped and trimmed over the implant (Figs. 12.110 and 12.111).

The best way to end up with an anesthetic tragus is to use careful techniques in handling the tragus when using a pretragal incision. As stated earlier, I frequently prefer the pretragal incision. It normally heals very well and can be touched up with CO_2 laser if a minor scar is present. This is desirable over the possibility of a blunted tragus when using a retrotragal incision, which is a situation that is much more difficult to repair. My decision to do pre- or posttragal incision is based upon patient preference and the size and shape of the preoperative tragus. A petite or ill-defined tragus may recontour after surgery, and in those cases I always use a pretragal incision. I also use a pretragal incision for patients whose tragus angles outward anteriorly. In these patients one can already see "inside" the external

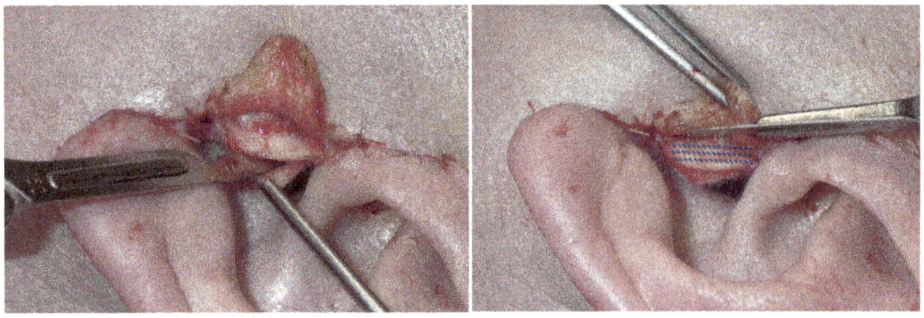

Fig. 12.109. When reoperating on a blunted tragus, the underside of the tragal skin can be undermined and the anterior surface of the tragal cartilage can be scored to help flatten the cartilage, which tends to curve upward with wound contracture. Leaving a generous amount of skin over the tragus when trimming this area will also discourage further wound contraction.

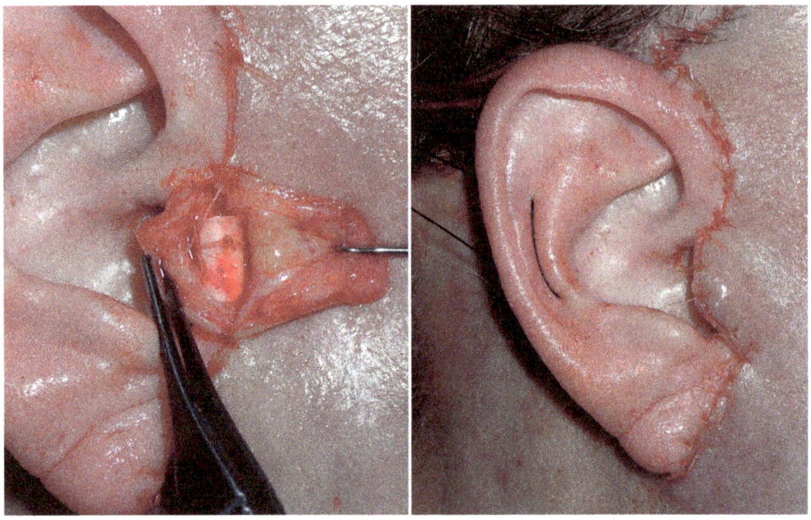

Fig. 12.110. The author has experimented with silicone tragal implants to restore normal tragal anatomy in the case of reoperation with tragal blunting. The *left* image shows the silicone implant zone in place, and the *right* image shows the immediate wound closure.

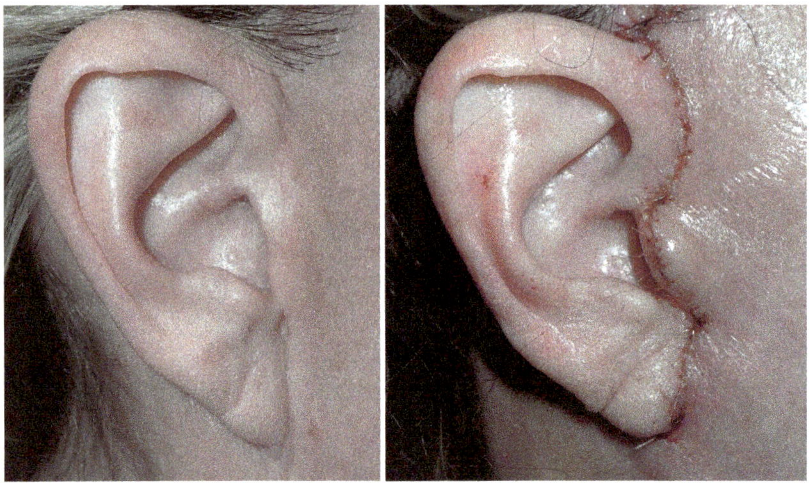

Fig. 12.111. The same patient shown in Fig. 12.110 is shown with her blunted tragus before surgery (*left*) and a well-formed tragus over the implant at 2 weeks postsurgery (*right*).

auditory canal, and by altering this already compromised situation, it could worsen. Normally the tragus hides most of the external auditory canal. Exposing the canal so one can "see inside the canal" is not a desirable postoperative result.

Surgical Scars

As surgeons we do a lot of work in multiple tissue planes on the inside of somebody's face during a facelift, but the only thing that the patient and those around them will ever see are their scars. The surgeon's scars are their signature, and they are extremely important in terms of quality of facelift surgery. A great facelift with poor scars is not a great facelift. One of the biggest compliments a facelift surgeon can receive is when a patient states that their hairdresser said that the scars are excellent. Hairdressers get to see everybody's scars, good and bad.

All surgical incisions will produce scars, and some patients simply heal more gracefully than others regardless of the competence of the surgeon. Like all recovery factors, the patient's care or lack thereof can also affect the outcome of scars and healing. Ethnicity and skin type can predispose patients to healing problems Is a well-known fact that darker skin types may have thicker scars, hypertrophic scars, or keloid scars, but unfavorable

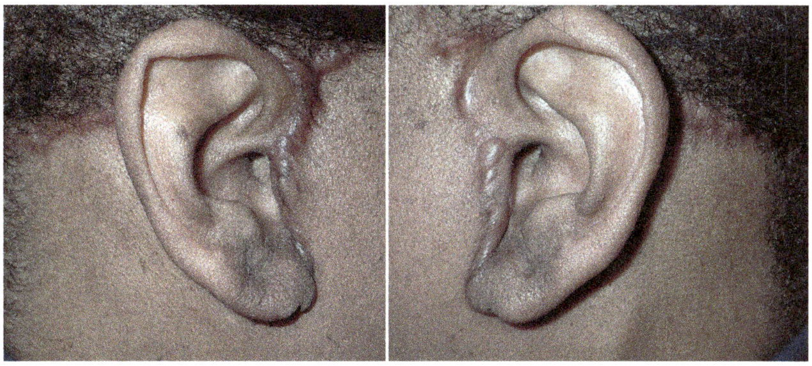

Fig. 12.112. This image shows an African American patient with hypertrophic scarring following facelift surgery. Discussion of the possibility of scarring and its related treatment postoperatively is imperative in the consent process. These scars usually improve greatly with steroid and/or 5-fluorouracil injection and the passage of time.

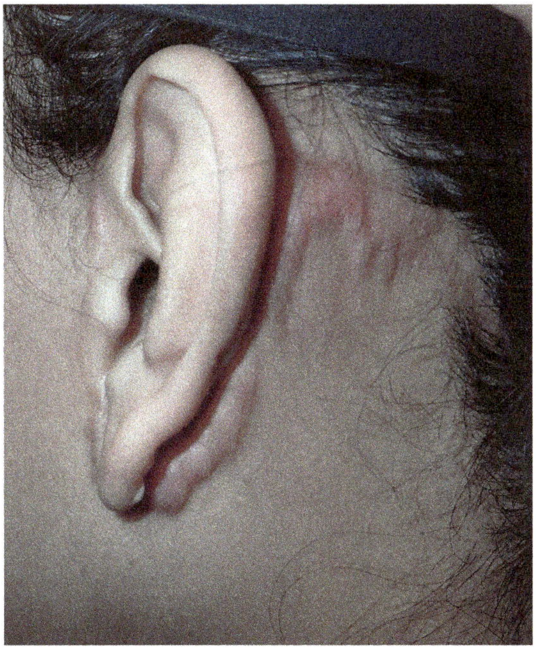

Fig. 12.113. Hypertrophic or keloid scarring is not 100% limited to darker skin types and may occur in other skin types as well. Besides steroid and 5-fluorouracil injections, CO_2 laser resurfacing can be used to improve scars on lighter-skinned patients.

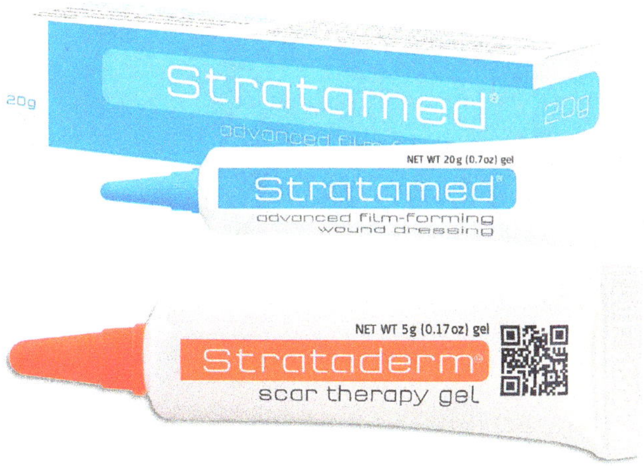

Fig. 12.114. Stratamed and Strataderm are useful wound-healing adjuncts. Stratamed is used until the wound is complete (not raw anymore), and Strataderm is used on the healing wound.

scarring in not limited to any single situation (Figs. 12.112 and 12.113). As stated earlier, scarring has a potential to be worse over concavities or anatomic contour transitions.

It is important to discuss this preoperatively with patients that may have predispositions for problematic facelift scars. In this type of patient, I explained that they may or may not scar gracefully, and if they do not, we will need to perform intensive scar management. Obviously for all patients it is important not to close wounds under tension and that is a given. In lighter-skinned patients I always use resorbable sutures, but I do not use this type of suture in darker skin types as I believe it initiates more of an inflammatory response. Instead, I use the smallest-gauge nylon sutures I can and remove them approximately a week after surgery. I also recommend that all patients use Stratamed (a silicone-based scar gel; Stratamed.com) for the first 8–12 weeks of their healing. Stratamed is a silicone gel approved by the Food and Drug Administration that can be placed on open, raw, or healing tissue. The patient purchases this from my office in advance and begins treatment immediately after surgery with the Stratamed product until the wounds are healed. At that point they use another preparation by the same company known as Strataderm, which is designed to improve scarring in healed wounds (Fig. 12.114). There are obviously scores of various scar preparations, and I am not saying that this product is miraculous, but I do feel that this product or others that are similar assist in aesthetic scar formation. I do recommend these preparations to all facelift patients, not just those who are predisposed to ungraceful scarring.

At the first sign of scar hypertrophy, I begin using topical clobetasol, which is a potent topical steroid as well as performing intralesional injections every three weeks with triamcinolone 10 mg/mL or 5-fluorouracil. The 5-fluorouracil can be injected directly from the vial or mixed with Kenalog in equal parts as some practitioners prefer. Kenalog 40 mg/mL can be injected in the extremely hypertrophic scars but at that concentration it is imperative to stay away from any underlying subcutaneous fat as severe and permanent fat atrophy and/or hypopigmentation can occur with high concentrations. When injecting Kenalog 10 or 5-fluorouracil, a 32 gauge needle can be used. A 25 gauge

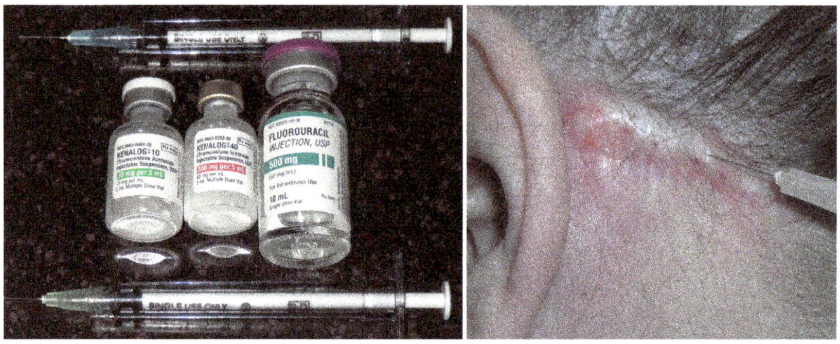

Fig. 12.115. The *left* image shows the common scar treatment preparations used to treat hypertrophic scarring (from *left* to *right*: Kenalog 10 mg/mL, Kenalog 40 mg/mL, 5-Flurouracil). The *right* image shows an intralesional injection into a hypertrophic scar. Note the blanching and the containment of the medication intralesionally.

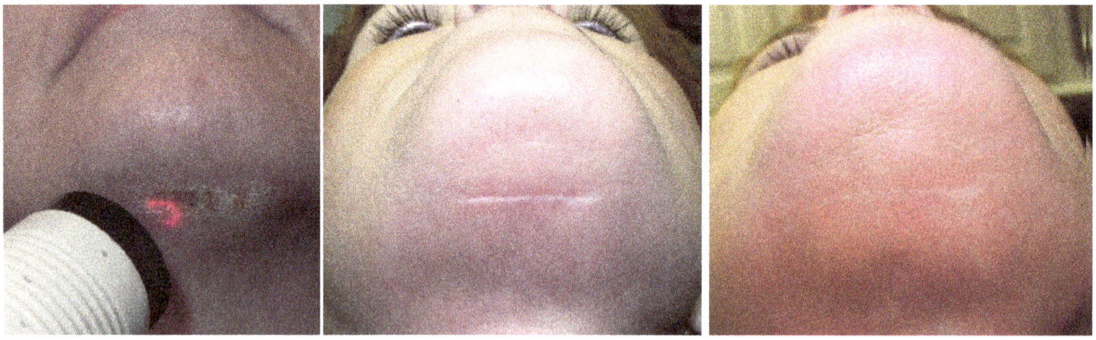

Fig. 12.116. The *left* image shows a noticeable submental incision scar. The *middle* image show CO_2 laser resurfacing to the scar and the *right* image shows the improved scar 8 weeks later.

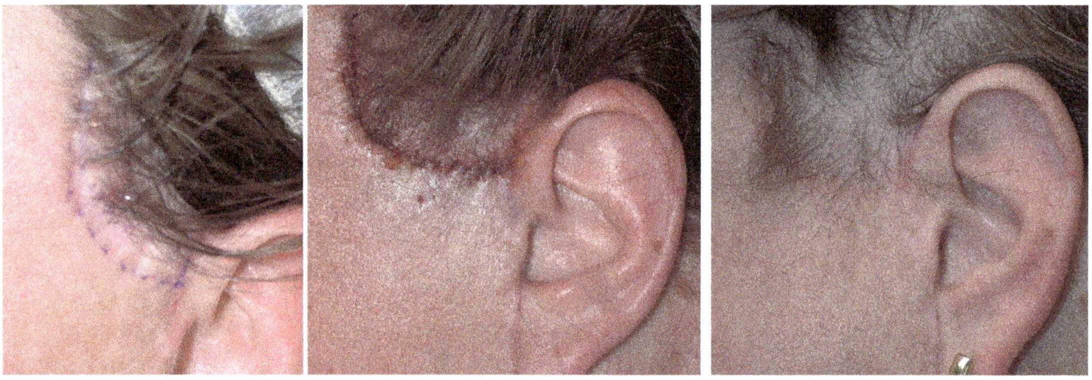

Fig. 12.117. The *left* image shows a visible depressed and hypopigmented scar at the sideburn incision. The *middle* image shows this scar excised and the wound resutured. The *right* image shows the same patient 6 weeks after scar revision.

needle is recommended when using Kenalog 40 mg/mL due to its particulate nature. When injecting Kenalog or 5-fluorouracil, it is important that the injections remain intralesional as that is where the fibroblastic scarring is occurring. Generally, enough medication is injected to blanch the scar as shown in Fig. 12.115

I also have the patient wear adhesive silicone sheeting at night or when possible at home. In my experience most hypertrophic surgical scars will become much better overtime with conservative treatment but they can be challenging for the patient, the surgeon, and the staff. Again, discussing this with patients that may be prone to scar problems is imperative.

CO_2 laser resurfacing and fractional laser resurfacing can also be used to treat scars as well as various wavelengths including intense pulse light or vascular lasers (Figs. 12.116 and 12.117).

Surgical scars can be hypertrophic, depressed hyperpigmented, and hypopigmented, and some scars require surgical excision as the preferred treatment (Fig. 12.117).

Pigmentation problems can occur after incision and dissection or wound breakdown. Hyperpigmentation is more easily treated with bleaching agents and light chemical peel or laser treatment. Hypopigmentation is more problematic and frequently permanent. Fractional laser treatments may stimulate melanocytes (Fig. 12.118). *There is some evidence that Latisse (bimatoprost) applied immediately to the lasered skin can assist repigmentation.* Cosmetic tattooing can also be used to add color to hypopigmented skin. In this day and age of tattoo popularity, many businesses will perform cosmetic camouflaging tattoo services.

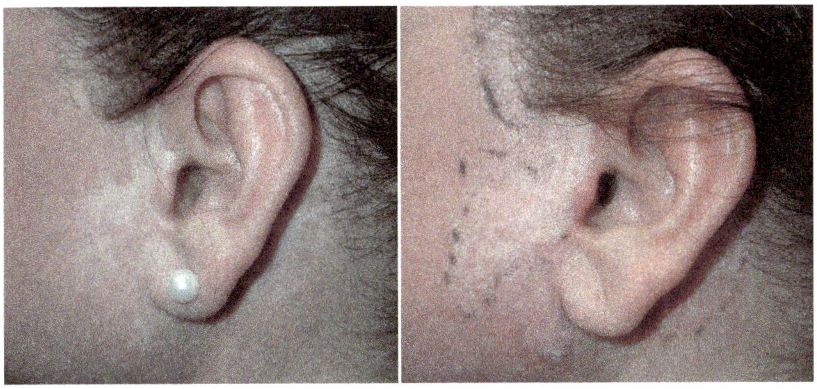

Fig. 12.118. The *left* image shows hypopigmentation after wound breakdown. Fractional or light laser resurfacing can be used to blend the color and texture. Some surgeons feel that Latisse (bimatoprost) applied immediately to the lasered skin can assist repigmentation. Cosmetic tattoo can also be an option to blend the color. The *right* image shows the patient after immediate light laser resurfacing of the hypopigmented regions.

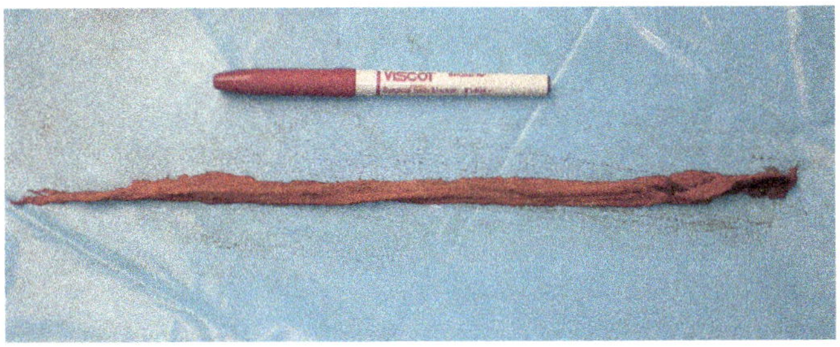

Fig. 12.119. This previously placed gauze was undetectable when our gauze count was off. It took significant exploration to locate it in the most inferior portion of the anterior neck. This can happen; always use gauze with radiographic markers.

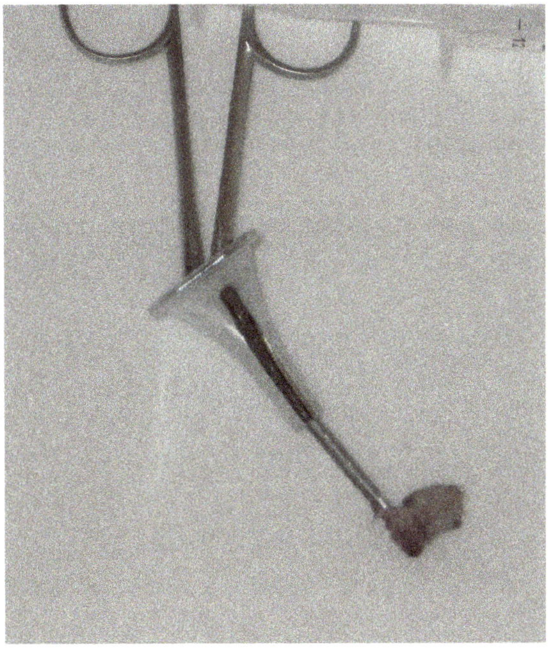

Fig. 12.120. This cotton ball packing was inadvertently left in place after facelift, and the patient complained of an earache a week later. It was successfully retrieved and a lesson learned. What goes in must be accounted for, and what comes out must match.

Retained Foreign Bodies

All surgeons and staff must be vigilant about leaving foreign bodies in any surgical site. Although it would be rare to leave an instrument in the small confines of a facelift, needles, scalpel blades, broken instrument tips, and retained gauze can be inadvertently left in the wound. Although some surgeons do not use gauze with radiopaque markers, I personally feel it is a big mistake as retained sponges have been left in facelift wounds and an unmarked gauze can be impossible to document on simple radiographs. Gauze counts should be routinely performed, and radiopaque marked sponges should be the standard of care. It is difficult to identify retained unmarked gauze in the face or neck. I have retrieved a missing gauze at the end of a case that was unraveled and smaller than the size of a pencil (Fig. 12.119). It was originally packed in the anterior inferior neck for hemostasis and was so small we missed it until the gauze count prompted further exploration. Always use gauze with radiographic markers!

Other retained foreign bodies can include sutures, ear plugs, and staples. I have personally seen several cases where a cotton earplug was inadvertently left in the external auditory canal after surgery causing significant pain a week later (Fig. 12.120). It is important to document what you put in at surgery and what you take out at surgery.

Corneal Abrasion

A prime objective of the surgeon is to protect the patient throughout all phases of the surgical experience. The corneas are subject to damage during the entire operative experience including anesthesia, surgical prep, laser and light devices and incidental abrasion, anesthesia emergence, and recovery room activity (Fig. 12.121). If blepharoplasty or browlift procedures are planned, then corneal shields should be used. Plastic shields are used with electrical devices such as cautery or radio wave incision, and metal shields are used with laser procedures. It is important to remove shields as soon as the procedure is completed to avoid abrasion or compromised corneal oxygenation. I personally experienced more corneal abrasions when using a lubricant with the shields than when using plain saline. It is also imperative to visually inspect the shields before as well as feel the surfaces for any palpable burrs or defects that could scratch the cornea. Any of smallest scratches or irregularities can cause corneal damage. It is also imperative to keep corneal shields separate in their own protective container and not dump them in a sink with other heavy or rough instruments.

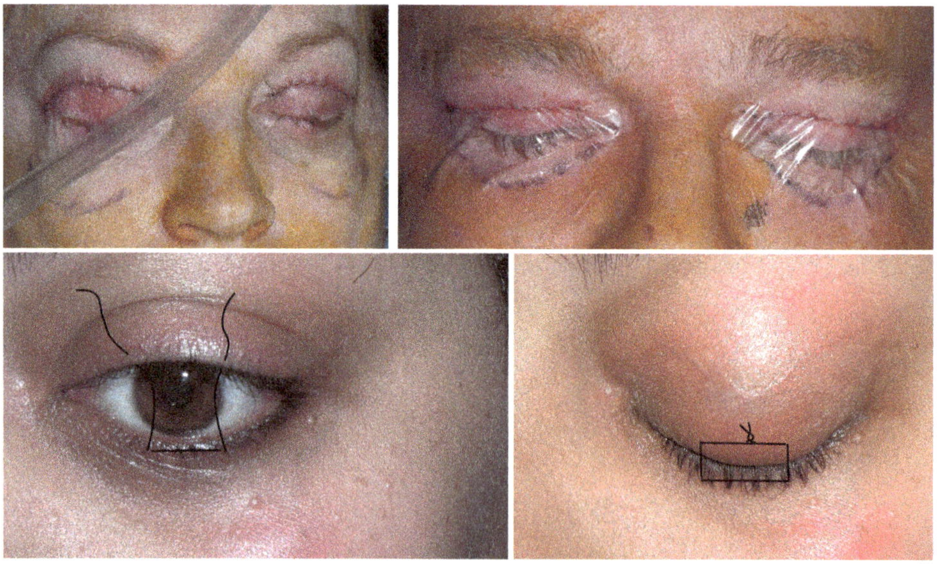

Fig. 12.121. The *left upper* image is closed with a tarsorrhaphy suture to protect from abrasion from hoses, sleeves, and so on. The *upper right* image shows the eyes protected with a surgical membrane such as Tagaderm (3M.com). The *lower* images show how a tarsorrhaphy suture is placed. I usually use 6-0 gut suture for this procedure.

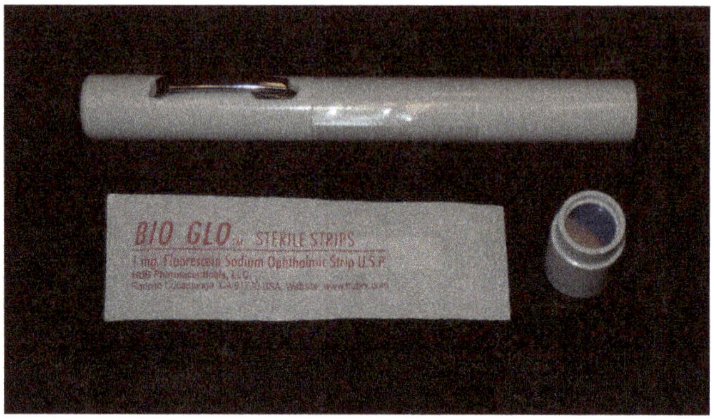

Fig. 12.122. This image shows a simple exam light with a cobalt lens and a pack of fluorescein eye strips.

If no blepharoplasty procedures are being performed, the lids are closed with tape, adhesive breathable membrane (Fig. 12.121, *upper* images), or tarsorrhaphy (Fig. 12.121, *lower* images). Acute abrasions can be identified by symptoms of pain and the feeling of "sand in the eye" and verified with fluorescein dye strips that show the abraded cornea under blue light. Initial treatment is antibiotic ophthalmic ointment and double patching the eye. The abrasions usually heal in 24 hours. The reason for the double patch is to exert light pressure on the lid so the patient does not open and reabrade the corneal on a single loose patch.

A beautifully performed facelift can be make a miserable postoperative experience with corneal abrasion. It is an acutely painful situation and requires treatment. It is generally recognized immediately after surgery or in the postanesthesia care unit. Patients complain of severe pain and a foreign body sensation like sand in the eye.

Every surgical office should have a corneal abrasion kit, which consists of a flashlight with a cobalt lens and fluorescein eye strips (Fig. 12.122).

The first step is to gently touch the fluorescein eye strip on the wet part of the cornea or tuck under the lower eyelid until the dye is dispersed (Fig. 12.123, *top left*). Fig. 12.123 (*middle*) shows the green stain of the abrasion showing up under the cobalt lens filter. The *right* image in Fig. 12.123 shows the place of erythromycin (or other suitable) ophthalmic ointment. Fig. 12.124 shows the special patching procedure to protect the cornea.

The eye patch is usually left in place 24–48 hours as corneal abrasions heal very fast when properly treated.

A new phenomenon has emerged in facelift complications from the continual wearing of surgical masks in the COVID-19 crisis. Several patients wore surgical masks after surgery, and the elastic loops eroded the posterior auricular incisions (Fig. 12.125).

Revision Facelift Surgery

"Revision facelift" is a broad term that includes numerous variables, and common reasons will be discussed. By definition a revision facelift is an additional procedure to address insufficiencies from a previous procedure. When I have a patient that needs a touch-up in the first year postoperatively, I refer to it as a revision procedure. If I did a facelift 10 years ago and the patient presents for another facelift, I do not refer to this as a revision but as "second facelift."

Any given surgeon who performs a high volume of facelifts and has consistently natural and long-lasting results can develop a good reputation for the procedure. In this day and age of the Internet and social media, an excellent reputation can be local, national, and international. I have seen this happen in my own practice. In the first decade of my practice, my patients were local; toward the end of the second decade, I was seeing out-of-state patients, and at the beginning of my third decade, 60% of my facelifts fly in from out of town and sometimes internationally. Talented surgeons will see numerous requests to improve a

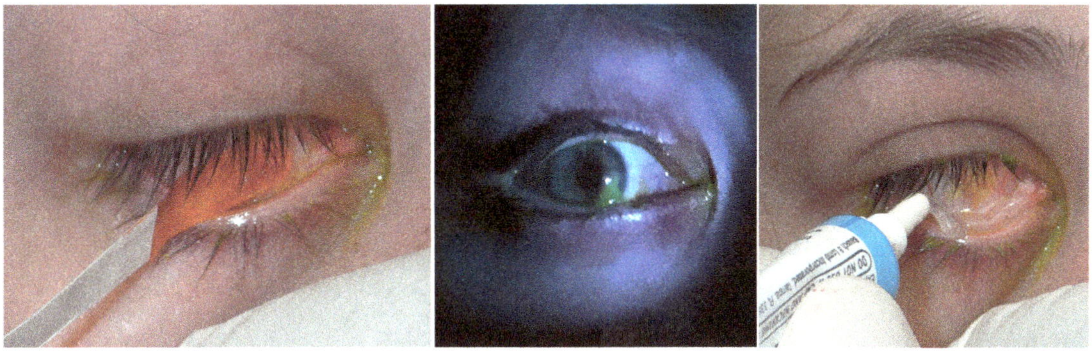

Fig. 12.123. The *left* image shows the fluorescein application, the *middle* images shows the abrasion under cobalt light, and the *right* image shows the application of ophthalmic ointment prior to patching.

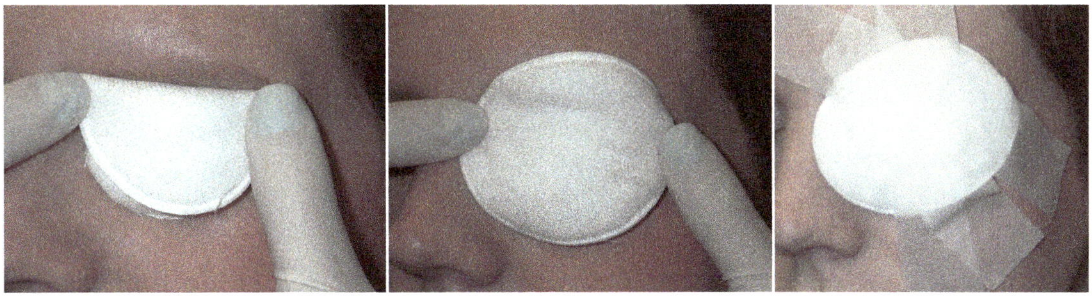

Fig. 12.124. A double patch is required to properly protect they eye. If using a single patch, there is a danger of the patient opening and closing their eye and making the abrasion worse. To prevent this, the first patch is folded in half a (*left* image) and then a second eye patch is placed with light pressure (*middle* picture) and both patches are taped in place with paper tape (*right* image).

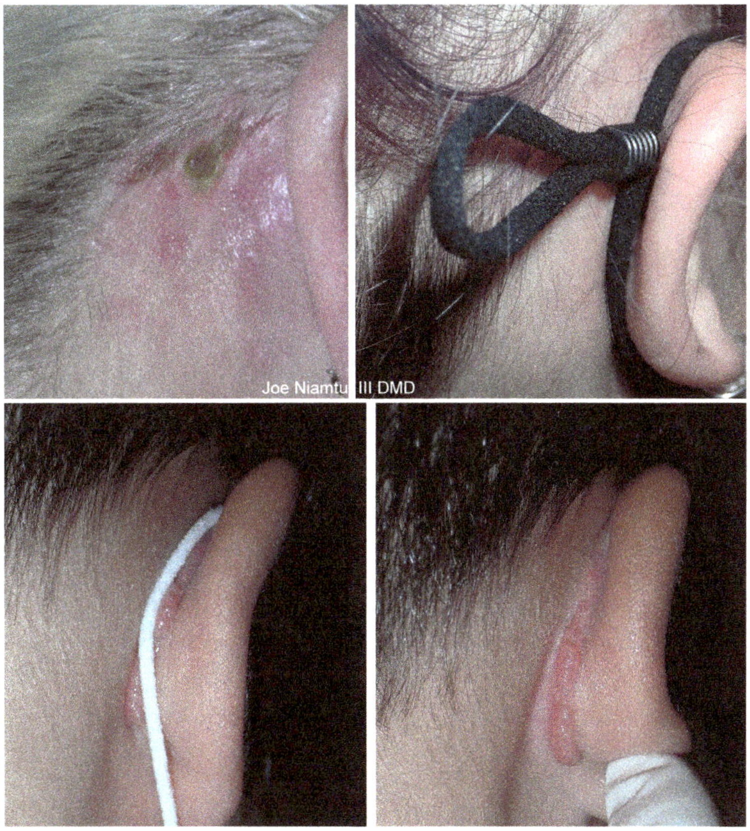

Fig. 12.125. These patients disrupted their posterior auricular facelift suture lines by wearing surgical masks with elastic ear bands during the COVID-19 crisis. In cases where a patient must wear a mask, the "four-string" type mask that ties around the back of the head and around the neck should be used.

poor outcome from another surgeon. These requests may be shortly after the patient's surgery or years later. Having the reputation and ability to improve a substandard result is an honor; however, it can also have drawbacks. I have had numerous patients with poor facelift results from elsewhere come to my office for consultation for improvement. These patients may present on a busy day with a full waiting room, and some other new facelift consultation patients have commented to my staff that "they did not want to look unnatural, like the lady sitting in the reception room." My patients thought these patients represented my work when in reality they were here for repair. This is something a surgeon and staff can keep in mind and discreetly handle. It is a great feeling for a surgeon and staff to take a poor result and convert it to good one and make a happy patient. One problem is that many times, the patient may present with problems that, although can be improved, will never look natural. In cases like this, that last surgeon to operate on such a patient (you or me) will now become "the surgeon." This can be a problem as although the patient was improved, the result will never be great and the last surgeon to touch the patient may come under criticism that can affect their brand. This can be more of a problem with local patients that mingle with other local patients. I once had a local patient who had a poor facelift from a local surgeon. The patient had severe temporal balding, severe pixie earlobes, and residual neck skin and jowls. I retreated this patient, and she and I were both extremely pleased with the improvement. Unfortunately, despite my improvement, the patient still had stigmata of poor facelift surgery from her previous procedure. If someone sees her result, they may feel that I caused the hairline problems, even though I know I actually improved them. Surgeons that perform significant revision surgery need to find ways to explain this to future and current prospective patients.

When I started seeing patients requesting revision, I was honored and felt that I had made an impact in the field of facelift surgery. At first it was challenging and exciting to be "the hero." After a while, however, I realized that I was seeing a lot of "problem patients." They were already unhappy with a result and were frequently at odds with their previous surgeon. Anyone reading this page understands the stress of having a schedule full of problem patients. As my facelift practice grew and I was doing over 100 lifts a year, I (like all high-volume practices) had my own revision patients. By and large these were small revisions of my own surgery, but nonetheless, they were problem patients. So, while dealing with my own revisions, I began to have less interest in seeing outside patients with problems and now try not to become involved in revisions from other surgeons.

A certain number of facelift surgeries (or any surgery for that matter) will have areas that did not heal as expected. These are frequently manifested as skin or jowl excess and can be minor or major. This is an unexpected phenomenon and causes anxiety for the patient and the surgeon. I tell every patient that this experience is about their face and my reputation. Sometimes it is the patient who points out the problem and other times they are actually happy but it is me that tells them that the outcome is not as good as it should be. We, as surgeons, have to remember that if our patients don't look good, then we don't look good. If I purchase a wide-screen TV from a major big box store and I get it home and it does not work, I am 100% confident they will replace it. Although surgery is far different from electronics, reputable surgeons back up their work. The devil can be in the details. A patient that has just paid $20,000–$40,000 for a facelift (or combined procedures) will not be excited about paying again for the same thing. Every surgeon will have to deal with revisions, and this must be addressed in the preoperative period. My consent defines the possibility of revision surgery and that there will be a surgical and anesthetic fee for the retreatment. I have to say that even though patients have signed off on this, they have short memories and many refuse to pay anything for "making it right." They can become downright belligerent with the thought of paying more money. I personally approach this in two ways. In a perfect situation, the patient will pay a reasonable fee for surgery plus the anesthesia. Although some patients are willing to pay $5,500 for revision plus $1,200 for the anesthesia, many are not. When a patient refuses to pay for a revision, a turning point may have been reached. If the surgeon stands fast on charging, the patient may seek assistance at another office while simultaneously punishing the original surgeon on social media. In my mind it is simply not worth losing the ability to correct one's work and losing my reputation with patients and competitors. I personally will do whatever it takes to retain the patient. Sometimes they will agree to pay the anesthesia fee only and I drop my fee. Again, I am maintaining my reputation. There have been rare times where a patient refused any payment for revision and I simply stood down and fixed my work. There are also cases where patients are being unreasonable or have traits that make me not want to keep them in the practice. For those patients, I will offer a revision for reduced fee or a refund or partial refund. Some patients simply cannot be made happy. All surgeons are going to have wins and losses, just like sports. We need to relish our wins and learn from our defeats.

Renowned plastic surgeon Val Lambros authored an article on "serial facelifts." His thought process explains that revision surgery is part of any surgery and general surgeons may not punish themselves for a failed hernia repair or an orthopod does not chastise themselves for a fracture nonunion; nature happens. We, as cosmetic surgeons, however, live in a world of elective surgery and ultimate pride and precision. For these reasons, we may perceive revisions as an embarrassing loss. In reality, some patients will simply need a second lift for reasons of skin excess or elasticity. One procedure is just not enough to treat the patient. In effect, they need a "serial facelift." As this is more of a situation with patients with higher body mass index or those with extreme excess skin, I discuss this concept both in my written and verbal consents. So, what is the bottom line? Some patients need touch-ups, some will agree to pay, and others will not. I have pretty much started a situation where I tell the patient that if they will need a revision in the first year after surgery, I will do it with "no surgical fee." They will pay the anesthesia and the operating room materials fee. This has worked well, but again, sometimes I get paid and sometimes I do not. What does happen is that I maintain my reputation and make unhappy patients happy. We have to back up our work!

I once had a younger visiting plastic surgeon who was observing in my office, and we saw a 3-month follow-up after facelift surgery. The patient was very happy with her result, but I brought up several small problems I wanted to correct at no charge to the patient. This doctor was a bit taken back with my comments and asked, "If a patient thinks their result is good and they are happy, then why did you bring up a deficiency?" The answer is simple: a great result is positive marketing and a result that does not meet my personal standards may be negative marketing and brand damage. If it can be better, then make it better! It will pay off many times over in the long run.

The other side of this coin is the patient that truly does have an acceptable result and is not happy. This multifactorial situation is addressed in previous chapters. This type of patient may be unhappy because they had unrealistic expectations, or a jealous friend spoke negatively of their result, or they did not get a job promotion or meet a new dating partner. Some of this type of reasoning is unfixable and is a quick reminder that the surgeon may have operated on the wrong patient. If a patient is unhappy, it does not help me or my brand, so I want to try to make them happy within reason. Sometimes it is as simple as reviewing their before-and-after pictures and explaining that they have very positive changes and pointing them out. Also, sometimes the patient must understand that the result is the best I can do with their anatomic situation. Sometimes the old joke "this is a scalpel, not a magic wand" applies. We weigh all of our postoperative patients at each follow-up appointment as part of our vital sign workup. I have had patients present unhappy at 4 months only to find out they have gained 25 lbs. This now gives me a leg to stand on, which can shift responsibility to the patient. Another pitfall is to see a postoperative patient that is several months out of surgery without first immediately reviewing their before pictures before entering the consult room. I have made this mistake several times where I walked in a room to see a patient that was 3 months out of surgery and did not feel the result was up to my standards. Perhaps I brought up some deficiencies. Then when I looked at the before pictures, I realized that the patient had extreme aging with skin and fat excess, and the result is actually pretty darn good. There is a lesson here. When my staff informs me that there is a postoperative facelift patient for follow-up, the first thing we do is review the before pictures before going into the appointment. This is especially important for busy practices and patients that present months after a procedure. It is hard to remember what they looked like at the beginning of the journey. It is also important for the patient to see the results, and I make before-and-after pictures on all my patients. Most of the results are excellent, but in some pictures, I see things that could be improved. It is the surgeon's quality control!

Despite my accuracy and diagnosis, a small percentage of patients will heal with skin excess in the submental region. On some patients, it seems that regardless of the vectors of pull on the pre- and postauricular flaps, a small area in the submental region is resistant to improvement. This can be a result of the shape of the mandible and simple physics of the flap vectors. As stated earlier, removing a small ellipse of skin with the submental incision may assist in addressing this area. When patients undergo a large facelift and heal with minor submental skin redundancy, conservative local submental skin excision may be all that is necessary. Trying to "piecemeal" a revision is a prescription for further failure. The only thing that makes a patient more unhappy than a revision is another revision. In the past I have attempted to open only the preauricular flaps or the postauricular flaps, but the result was rarely adequate. At this point in my career, I now open all incisions and flaps and basically redo the lift. This also usually means more liposuction, more SMAS treatment, and more jowl treatment. What it does mean is a successful revision. Although no surgeon welcomes revision surgery, every time I have performed a comprehensive revision, I have an improved result and a happy patient. Trying shortcuts may sound good but is not a good plan. I have never performed a revision where the result was not improved. In addition I look at it this way: I get to do another facelift (which I love) and I have restored confidence in my patient. The best thing to do is always the "right thing."

Revisions are usually much easier for patients in terms of recovery for several reasons. One, they have undergone the procedure previously and know what to expect, and two, a revision is usually much less invasive. I have actually had revision facelift patients drive to the office the next day for their 24-hour follow-up.

Some minor revision cases may only require minor liposuction or buccal fat reduction to improve the result such as with jowl or submental fat excess (Figs. 12.126 and 12.127).

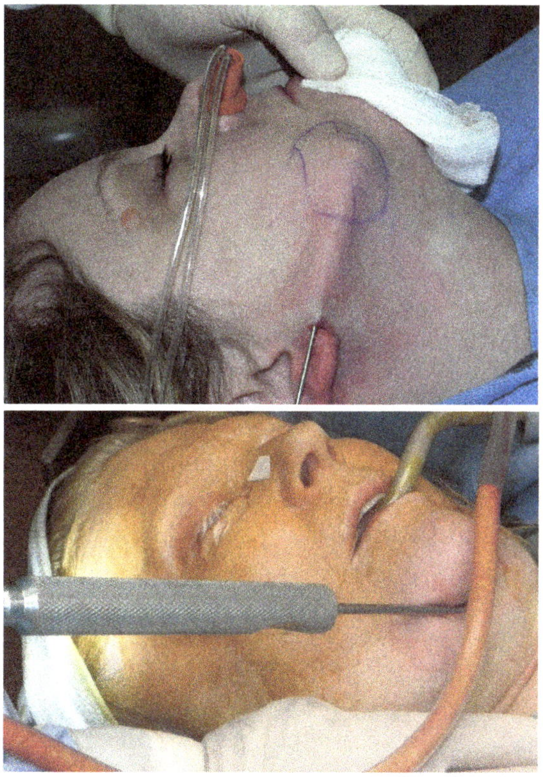

Fig. 12.126. Redundant adipose tissue can produce a suboptimal result or asymmetry from one side to another. Revision liposuction of the jowls and submental region or neck is an additional simple and minimally invasive method to improve the results of selected cases. Buccal fat reduction can also improve jowl excess in some patients.

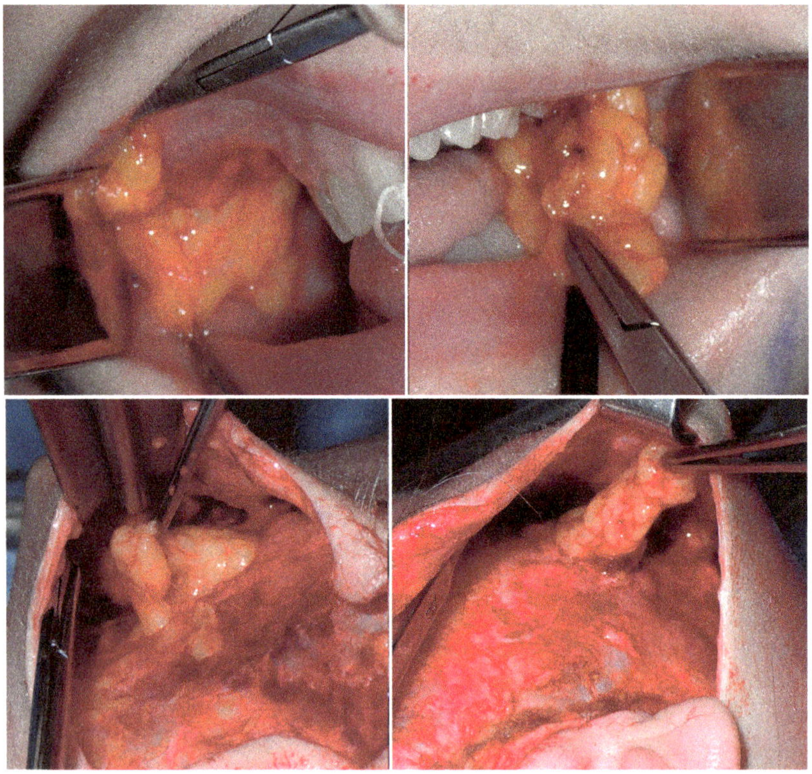

Fig. 12.127. The more facelifts I perform, the more times I am treating the buccal fat pads, especially on patients with heavy jowling. The buccal fat can be accessed through the oral cavity (*upper* images) or through facelift flap (*bottom* images).

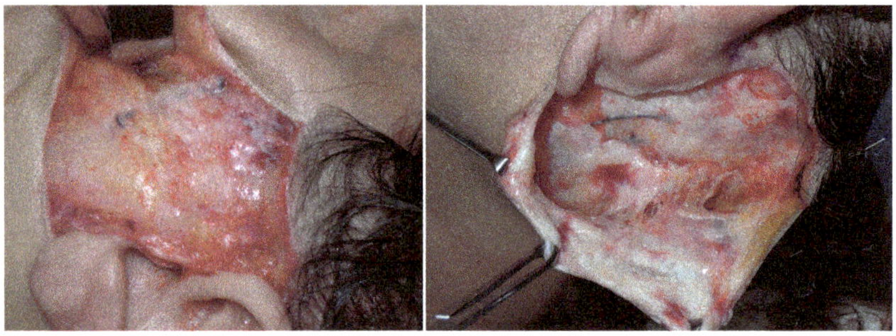

Fig. 12.128. The *left* image shows scar tissue and previous sutures on a secondary facelift 20 years after the initial lift. This type of tissue usually dissects with relative ease. Note that there is very little SMAS to manipulate. The *right* image shows significant scar tissue in another patient, and this type of fibrosis can be very difficult to dissect.

Revising a facelift is similar to the previous surgery but may be easier or harder in numerous ways. Reopening previous incisions can produce tragal, hairline, and lobe changes, and this should be discussed with patients. This does not mean that these areas will be changed, but multiple surgeries can induce changes to these areas. Secondary surgery can be easier or harder due to scar tissue from previous surgery. In some circumstances, the scar tissue forms a "glide plane" and the dissection is very simple with little tissue resistance (Fig. 12.128, *left*). In other cases, the scar tissue can be extreme and make dissection complicated and offer significant resistance (Fig. 12.128, *right*). Older female patients' scarcity of adipose tissue may exist in the subcutaneous plane. Due to this, any contour irregularities or uneven tissue below the skin may be more visible after surgery.

Scarring and friability of the SMAS is common in the previously operated patient. Due to the fragility of the previously operated SMAS, open SMAS-ectomy procedures may not be possible, and thus plication may be the only option. In rare cases, the scar tissue is so plentiful that it is impossible to manipulate the SMAS at all.

Let's talk revisions

> As stated, revision surgery can be a result of undertreatment by the surgeon or simply the inability to address all excess tissues intraoperatively. The latter refers to patients with unusually large skin or fat excess or exceedingly elastic skin. This is seen when the surgeon did the procedure correctly but a single procedure was not adequate to correct all of the excess. A second procedure or serial facelift may be required (Fig. 12.129).

Figs. 12.130–12.136 illustrate revision surgery cases performed by the author.

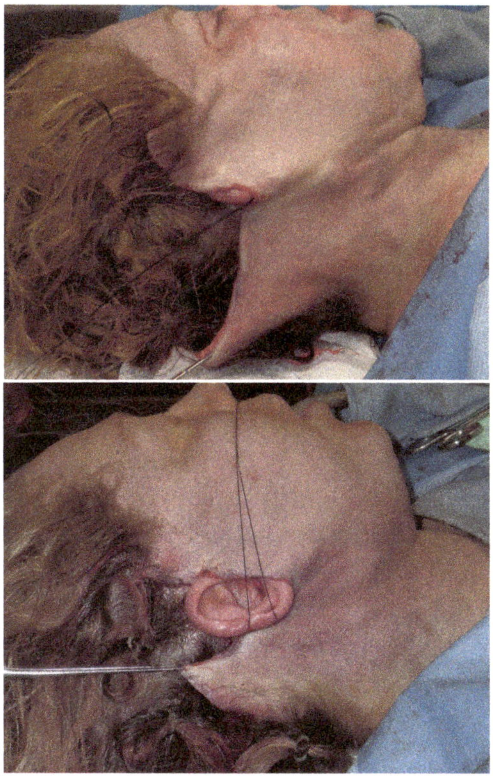

Fig. 12.129. Patients with remarkable skin excess should understand preoperatively that a revision procedure may be necessary. This patient's skin excess is shown at her primary facelift (*top* image). The *bottom* image shows the much smaller amount of skin excess at her revision 6 months after her primary surgery. Such cases most commonly require anterior and posterior auricular incisions and significant undermining. They may or may not require readdressing this superficial musculoaponeurotic system or platysma. In essence a revision surgery is sometimes a replication of the original procedure, hence the concept of "serial facelift."

Readdressing a Good Result That Has Changed Over the Years From the Natural Aging Process

Of the types of revisions mentioned, redoing a lift on a happy patient 12 years later is much less complicated situation. Reasonable patients realize they will continue to age after their facelift and in time require another procedure. They are generally quite happy and probably had a good surgical experience with the initial surgery. They are educated on the procedure and recovery from the first surgery and understand that it is simply time for another lift. Although facelift surgery is a predictable long-lasting procedure, it is not permanent. The longevity of a surgical procedure is influenced by many variables, including the patient's age, surgical procedure and technique, patient genetics, skin quality, and how the result is maintained or protected after surgery. A well-done cervicofacial rhytidectomy with medial and lateral platysmaplasty and SMAS-ectomy or deep plane SMAS can last 10–12 years and in some cases beyond. Most patients understand and prepare for this. This longevity is so variable, and although one patient may get 15 years out of a facelift, another patient could experience postsurgical change several years after the procedure. Although the surgeon has some component of control over longevity, no one can control nature. All consultations, consents, and perioperative discussions should address the variability of facelift "shelf life." One way to communicate this to a patient is as follows: "If a facelift lasts 10 years, this means that the patient loses 10% of the result each year. So, at year 5 there would be

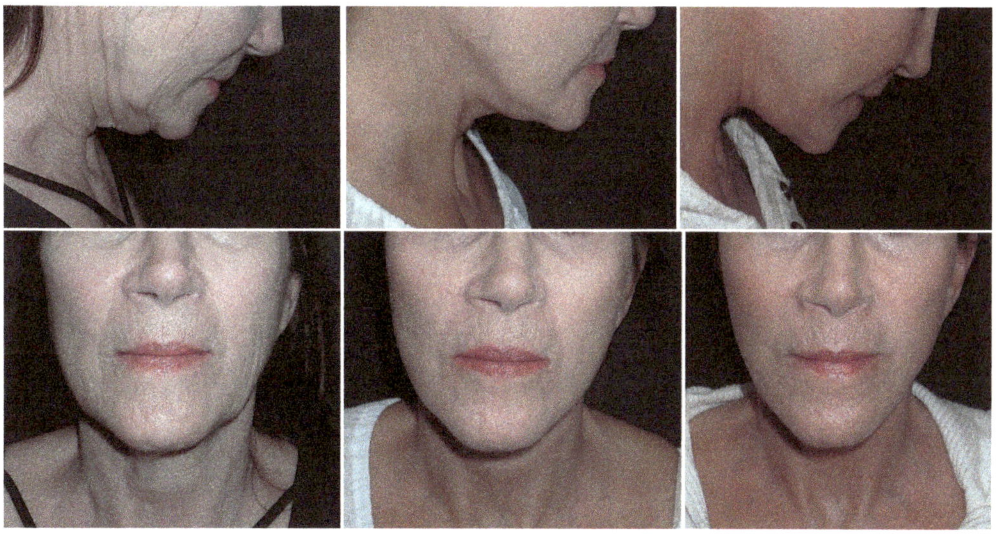

Fig. 12.130. This 70-year-old female is shown before deep plane facelift and neck lift (*left* images), 3 months after the procedure (*center* images), and 4 months after deep plane revision surgery (*right* images).

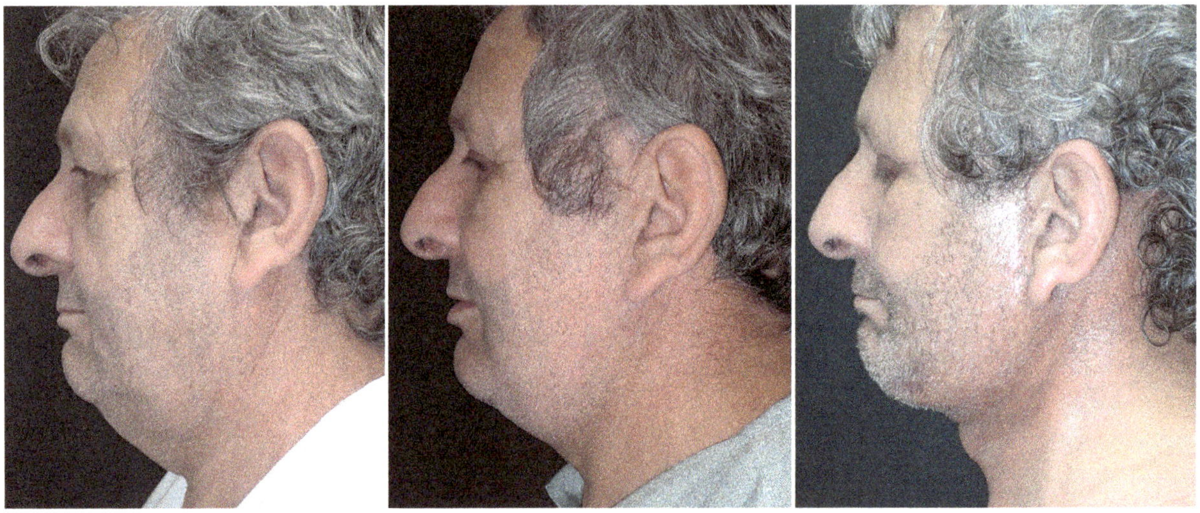

Fig. 12.131. This 65-year-old male is a very large man with large and thick anatomy. The *left* image shows the before pictures, the *center* image is after deep plane facelift and neck lift, and the *right* image is 2 weeks after deep plane revision.

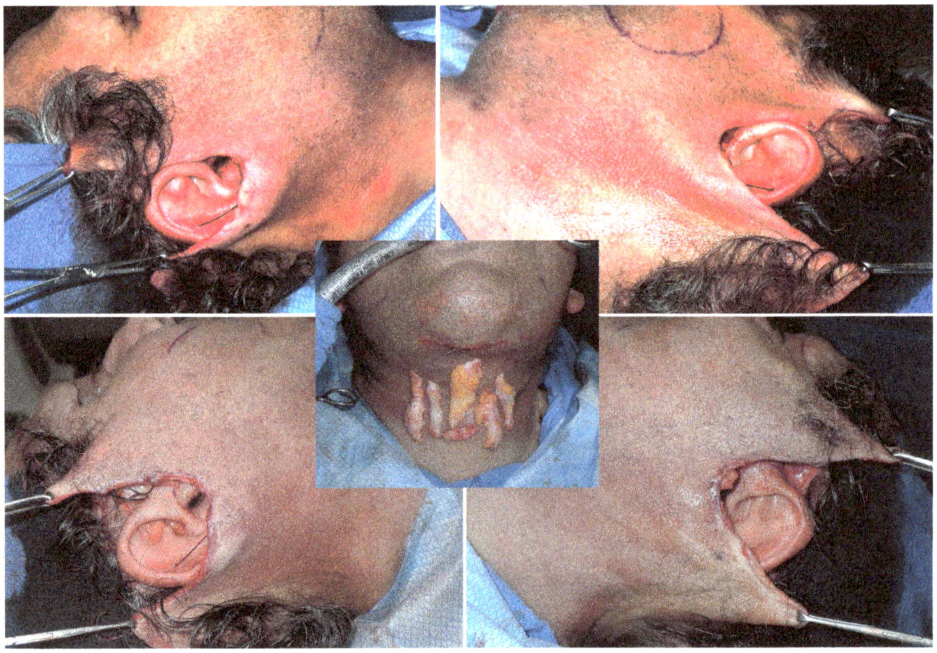

Fig. 12.132. The skin excess from original surgery and revision of the same patient shown in Fig. 12.131 is shown. The *upper* images show the skin excess on the original surgery. The *lower* images show the skin excess from the revision surgery, and the *inset* shows fibro/muscular/fatty tissues removed to slim his neck at the revision surgery.

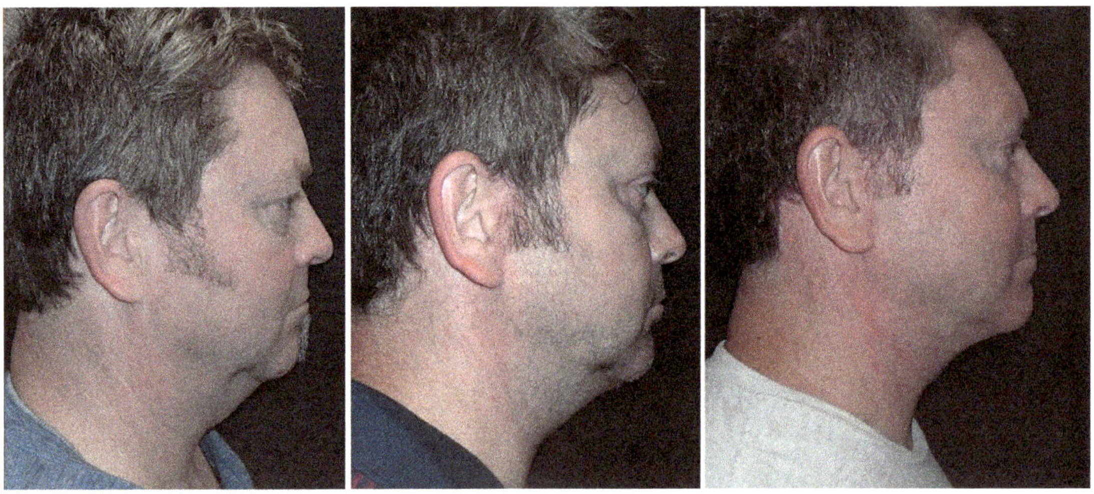

Fig. 12.133. This 58-year-old male patient is shown before any surgery (*left*), after facelift and neck lift (*middle*), and after revision of improved result (*right* image).

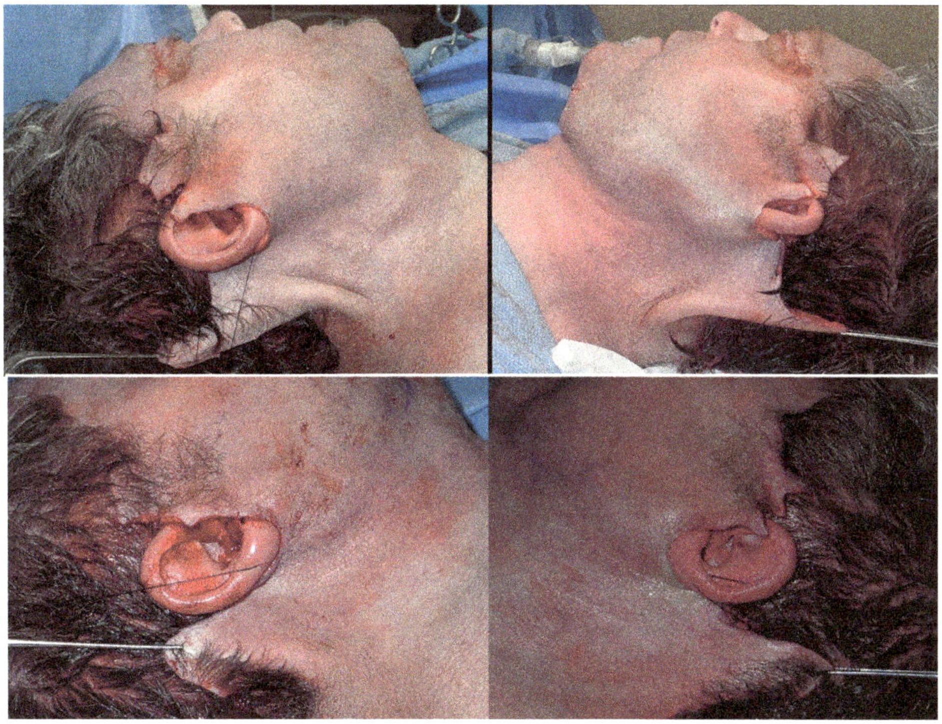

Fig. 12.134. This is the same patient shown in Fig. 12.133. The *upper* pictures are the skin excess at his original surgery, and the *bottom* images are the skin excess at his revision some 6 months later. Some patients simply have a lot of skin and a lot of skin elasticity.

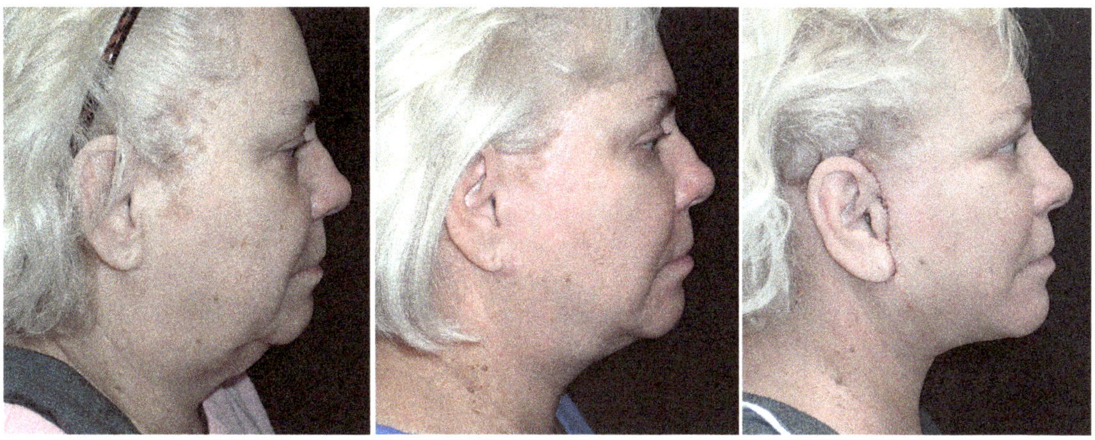

Fig. 12.135. This 65-year-old female is shown before facelift surgery (*left*), after her procedure (*middle*), and after revision to correct deficiencies (*right*). Although the *middle* picture was better, it was not good enough for me as a surgeon.

a 50% change in the original postoperative result." This helps patients understand the aging experience and develop realistic expectations. Figs. 12.137–12.139 show patients spanning a decade of aging.

Conclusion

Mastering facelift and neck lift surgery is a lifetime journey. Nothing replaces experience, and there are no shortcuts to gaining experience. Astute surgeons will study the entire realm of facelift surgery from the understanding of aging, anatomy, surgical technique, anesthesia, postoperative care, and patient management. I feel that surgeons with high-volume facelift practices have a special dedication to this procedure, and although they perform other procedures, this is their "happy place." I personally feel it takes at least 1000 facelift procedures for a surgeon to truly master the art. And after this, we all should celebrate our victories and learn from our defeats. It is said that excellence is a journey, not a destination, which means you never really arrive there. It makes sense, you just keep getting better. Always strive for patient safety with predictable outcomes and do the right thing.

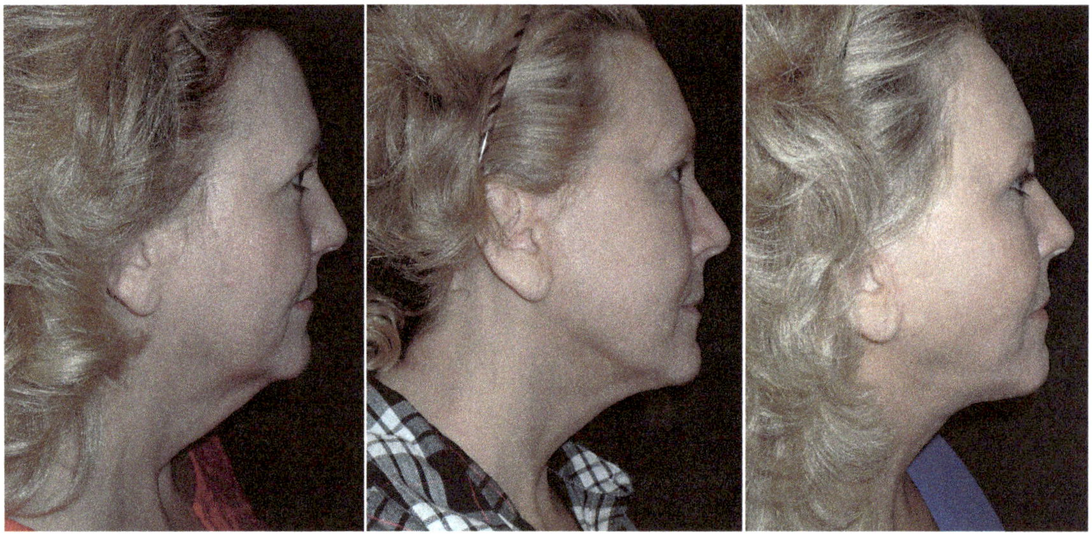

Fig. 12.136. This 51-year-old female is shown before surgery (*left*), after her facelift (*middle*), and after her revision (*right*) to improve deficiencies. Although no surgeon relishes performing revision surgery, it is imperative to deliver the best result to the patient and maintain a reputation for excellence.

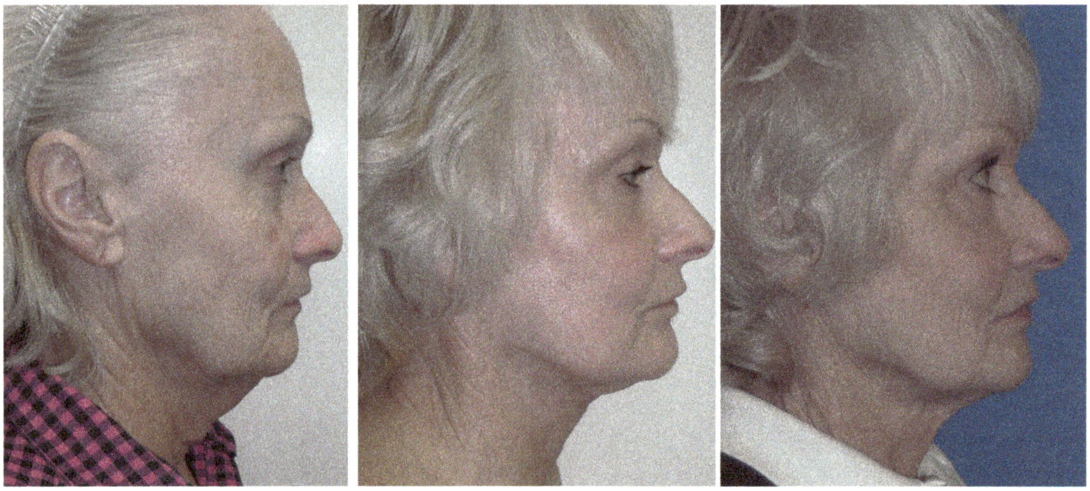

Fig. 12.137. This patient is shown before (*left* image), 3 months after facelift and CO_2 laser (*center* image), and 10 years after her original surgery (*right*) showing the natural aging progression. This is a typical postsurgical change over a decade.

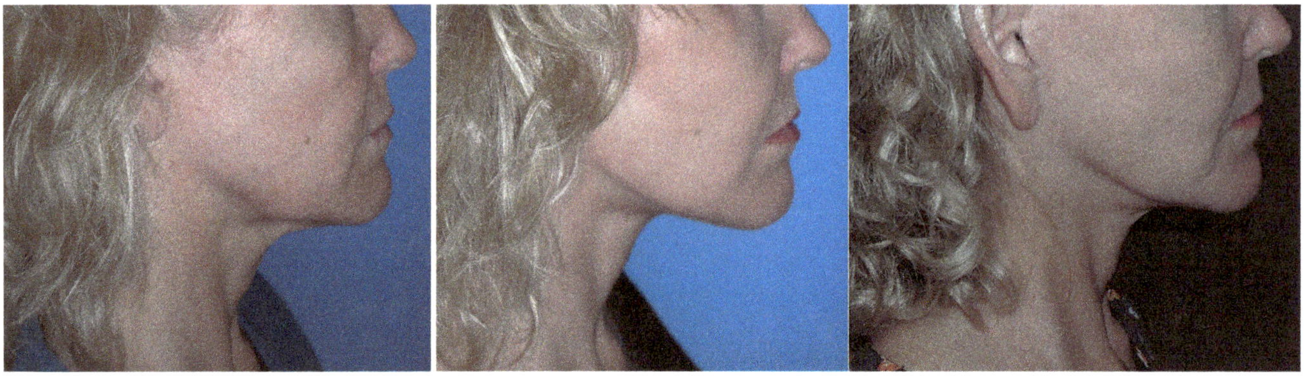

Fig. 12.138. This patient is shown before facelift surgery in the *left* image, 3 months after I performed facelift surgery on her in the *center* image, and 10 years after my facelift procedure on the *right* image. Cases like this illustrate the predictability and longevity of a properly done lift with platysmaplasty and proper superficial musculoaponeurotic system treatment.

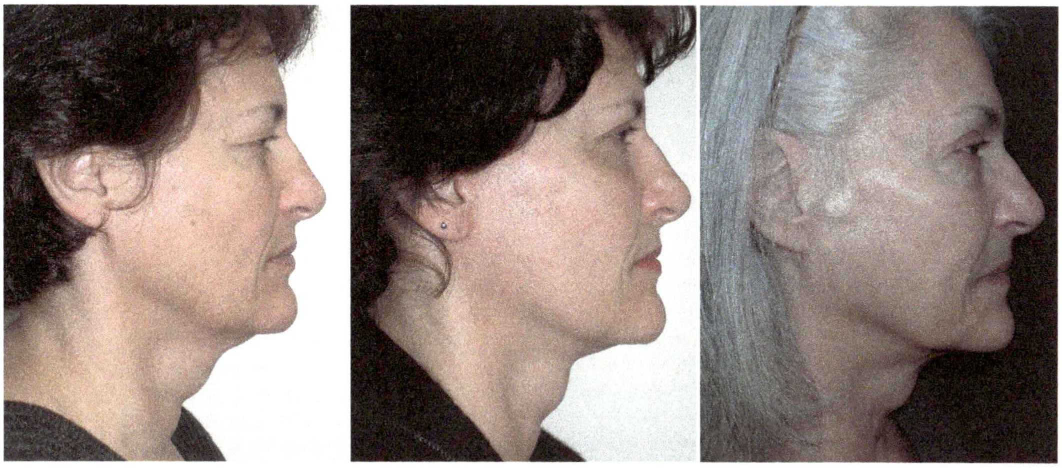

Fig. 12.139. This patient is shown before facelilft (*left* image), 3 months after facelift (*middle* image), and 15 years after facelift (*right* image). This progression shows normal aging but much of her result has persisted.

Index

Page numbers followed by "*f*" indicate figures, and "*b*" indicate boxes.

T

U

V

W

Y

Z